THE KIDNEY AND HYPERTENSION IN DIABETES MELLITUS

FOURTH EDITION

THE KIDNEY AND HYPERTENSION IN DIABETES MELLITUS

Fourth Edition

EDITED BY

CARL ERIK MOGENSEN
Medical Department M
(Diabetes & Endocrinology)
Aarhus Kommunehospital
Aarhus University Hospital
Aarhus C, Denmark

Editorial Assistant

ANNA HONORÉ

SPRINGER-SCIENCE+BUSINESS MEDIA, B.V.

Library of Congress Cataloging-in-Publication Data

The kidney and hypertension in diabetes mellitus / edited by Carl Erik Mogensen; editorial assistant, Anna Honore. -- 4th ed.
P. Cm.
Includes bibliographical references and index.

ISBN 978-1-4757-6754-4 ISBN 978-1-4757-6752-0 (eBook)
DOI 10.1007/978-1-4757-6752-0

1. Diabetic nephropathies. 2. Renal hypertension. 3. Diabetes--Complications. I. Mogensen, Carl Erik.
[DNLM: 1. Diabetic Nephropathies. 2. Hypertension, Renal. 3. Diabetes Mellitus--complications. 4. Kidney Diseases--etiology. WK 835K458 1998]
RC918.D53.K53 1998
616.4 ' 62--dc21
DNLM/DLC
For Library of Congress 98-8769
CIP

Originally published by Kluwer Academic Publishers in 1998
Softcover reprint of the hardcover 4th edition 1998

Printed on acid-free paper.

This book is dedicated to the memory of Knud Lundbæk (born 1912 - †1995), distinguished diabetologist, my friend and mentor, and a great inspiration for all of us. He also became strongly engaged in exciting and penetrating new studies in the field of sinology, his second science.

CEM

TABLE OF CONTENTS

SOME KEYS TO THE LITERATURE

S.-E. Bachman, ed. *Le Rein des Diabétiques* (Thesis). Paris: Librairie J.-B. Baillière et Fils, 1936.

H. Rifkin, L. Leiter, J. Berkman, eds. *Diabetic Glomerulosclerosis. The specific renal disease of diabetes mellitus.* Springfield, Illinois, USA: Charles C. Thomas Publisher, 1952.

L. Scapellato, ed. *La Nefropatia Diabetica.* Roma: Luigi Pozzi, 1953

K. Lundbæk, ed. Long-Term Diabetes. The clinical picture in diabetes mellitus of 15-25 years' duration with a follow-up of a regional series of cases. Copenhagen: Ejnar Munksgaard, 1953.

Å.Chr. Thomsen, ed. *The Kidney in Diabetes Mellitus. A clinical and histological investigation base on renal biopsy material* (Thesis). Copenhagen: Munksgaard, 1965.

G. Ditscherlein, ed. *Nierenveränderungen bei Diabetikern.* Jena: VEB Gustav Fischer Verlag, 1969

D.E. McMillan, J. Ditzel, eds. Proceedings of a Conference on Diabetic Microangiopathy. April 6-10, 1976. Santa Ynez Valley, California. Diabetes 1976; 25: Suppl. 2.

C.E. Mogensen, ed. Diabetes Mellitus and the Kidney. Kidney Int 1982; 21: 673-791.

H. Keen, M. Legrain, eds. *Prevention and treatment of Diabetic Nephropathy.* Boston, The Hague, Dordrecht, Lancaster: MTP Press Limited, 1983.

D.E. McMillan, J. Ditzel, ed.. Proceedings of a Conference on Diabetic Microangiopathy. Diabetes 1983; 32: Suppl. 2: 1-104.

P. Weidmann, C.E. Mogensen, E. Ritz, eds. Diabetes and Hypertension. Proceedings of the First International Symposium on Hypertension Associated with Diabetes Mellitus. June 22-23, 1984. Hypertension 1985; 7: Part II: S1-S174.

P. Passa, C.E. Mogensen, eds. Microalbuminuria in Diabetes Mellitus. Proceedings of an international workshop. Chantilly, France, May 8-9, 1987. Diabete Metab 1988; 14: Suppl.: 175-236.

H.U. Janka, E. Standl, eds. Hypertension in Diabetes Mellitus: Pathogenesis and clinical impact. Proceedings of an International Symposium. Munich, Germany, May 3, 1989. Diabete Metab 1989; 15: Suppl.: 273-366.

R.A. DeFronzo, ed. Diabetic Nephropathy. Semin Nephrol 1990; 10: 183-304.

W.J. Howard, G.C. Viberti, eds. When to treat? A workshop to address the threshold of treatment of hypertension in diabetes. Diabetes Care 1991; 14: Suppl. 4: 1-47.

R.A. DeFronzo, E. Ferrannini, eds. Diabetes Care 1991; 14: 173-269.
Proceedings of the International Symposium on Diabetic Nephropathy, July 24-25 1990, Otsu, Japan. J Diabetic Complications 1991; 5: 49-203.

B. Charbonnel, J.M. Mallion, A. Mimran, Ph. Passa, P.F. Plouin, G. Tchobroutsky, eds. Hypertension, diabète et systèmes rénine-angiotensine tissulaires. Aspects fondamentaux et conséquences thérapeutiques. Diabete Metab 1992; 18: 127-186.

A.S. Krolewski, ed. Third International Symposium on Hypertension Associated with Diabetes Mellitus. J Am Soc Nephrol 1992; 3: Suppl.: S1-S139.

G.C. Viberti, W.B. White, eds. What to treat? The structural basis for renal and vascular complications and hypertension, and the role of angiotensin converting enzyme inhibition. J Hypertens 1992; 10: Suppl. 1: S1-S51.

S. M. Mauer, C.E. Mogensen, G.C. Viberti, eds. Symposium on the Progress in Diabetic Nephropathy. Kidney Int 1992: 41: 717-929

R.A. DeFronzo, ed. Diabetes Care 1992; 15: 1125-1238.

G. Crepaldi, R. Nosadini, R. Mangili, eds. Proceedings of the International Meeting »State of the art and new perspective sin Diabetic Nephropathy« University of Padua, 6-7 March, 1992. Acta Diabetol 1992; 29: 115-279.

C.E. Mogensen, C. Berne, E. Ritz, G.-C. Viberti, eds. Proceedings of the Symposium Diabetic Renal Disease in Type 2 Diabetic Patients. A major worldwide health problem. Prague, 7 September, 1992. Diabetologia 1993; 36: 977-1117.

F. Belfiore, R.N. Bergman, G.M. Molinatti, eds. *Current Topics in Diabetes Research. 4th International Diabetes Conference, Florence, March 18-20, 1992. Frontiers in Diabetes, Vol. 12.* Basel, Freiburg, Paris, London, New York, New Delhi, Bangkok, Singapore, Tokyo, Sydney: Karger, 1993.

M.M. Avram, S. Klahr, eds. Proceedings from the Long Island College Hospital. Symposium on Lipids and Vasoactive Agents in Renal Disease. Am J Kidney Dis 1993; 22: 64-239.

E. Ferrannini, ed. Insulin Resistance Syndrome. Cardiovasc Risk Factors 1993; 3: 1-81.

D. Batlle, ed. The Diabetes/Hypertension Connection. Cardiovasc Risk Factors 1993; 3: 145-187.

C. Hasslacher, C.G. Brilla, eds. Renin-angiotensin-system and collagen metabolism in diabetes mellitus and arterial hypertension. Clin Investig 1993; 71: Suppl.: S1-S50.

E. Ferrannini, ed. *Insulin Resistance and Disease. Baillière's Clinical Endocrinology and Metabolism. International Practice and Research. Vol. 7.* London, Philadelphia. Sydney, Tokyo, Toronto: Baillière Tindall, 1993.

C.E. Mogensen, E. Standl, eds. *Research Methodologies in Human Diabetes. Part 1*, Berlin, New York: Walter de Gruyter, 1994.

P.T. Sawicki, ed. *Hemmung der Progression diabetischer Nephropathie.* Mainz: Verlag Kirchheim, 1994.

W.F. Keane, B.M. Brenner, H.H. Parving, eds. Progression of Renal Disease. Kidney Int 1994; Suppl. 45: S1-S180.

Journal of Diabetes and Its Complications. Special Issue: Selected presentations from Epidemiology of Microalbuminuria, Mortefontaine, France, 13 November 1993. July-September 1994; 8: No. 3.

H.J.G. Bilo, G.C. Viberti, eds. *Diabetic Nephropathy. de Weezenlanden Series, No. 2. Zwolle 1994.* Den Haag: CIP-Gegevens Koninklijke Bibliotheek, 1994.

Ch. Hasslacher, ed. *Der Hypertensive Typ-II-Diabetiker. Pathophysiologie, Diagnostik, Komplikationen und Differentialtherapie.* Berlin/New York: Walter de Gruyter, 1994.

L.M. Ruilope et al. Microalbuminuria in clinical practice. Kidney: A current survey of world literature 1995; 4: 211-216.

C.E. Mogensen, E. Standl, eds. *Research Methodologies in Human Diabetes. Part 2*, Berlin, New York: Walter de Gruyter, 1995.

Journal of Diabetes and Its Complications. Special Section: Proteinuria and Progressive Renal disease. Second International Symposium, Vienna, Austria, 2 July 1994. January-March 1995; 9: No. 1.

Journal of Diabetes and Its Complications. Special Issue: Proceedings of the Fourth International Symposium on Hypertension Associated with Diabetes Mellitus, A Satellite Symposium of the 15th International Diabetes Fedration Congress, Otsu, Japan, 4-5 November 1994. October-December 1995; 9: No. 4.

R. Nosadini, ed. Symposium on diabetic nephropathy. Diab Nutr Metab 1995; 8: 129-185.

H.B. Lee, ed. Pathogenesis of Diabetic Nephropathy: Experimental approaches. Kidney Int 1995; Suppl. 51.

E. Ritz, P.U. Weidmann, eds. Hypertension and the Kidney. 29th Deidesheimer Gespräch, April 29, 1995. Nephrol Dial Transplant 1995; 10: Suppl. 9.

H.-H. Parving, R. Østerby, P.W. Anderson, W.A. Hsueh. »Diabetic nephropathy.« In *The Kidney.* Brenner BM, Rector F, eds. W.B. Saunders Co., 1995; pp 1864-1892.

R.A. DeFronzo. Diabetic nephropathy: etiologic and therapeutic considerations. Diabetes Rev 1995; 3: 510-564.

H. Koide, I. Ichikawa, eds. *Progression of Chronic Renal Diseases. International Symposium, Shizuoka, May 20-23, 1995.* Contributions to Nephrology, vol. 118. Basel, Freiburg, Paris, London, New York, New Delhi, Bangkok, Singapore, Tokyo, Sydney: Karger, 1996.

C.E. Mogensen, R. Turner, eds. Proceedings of the Symposium: Improving Prognosis in NIDDM. Stockholm, 11-12 September, 1995. Diabetologia Diabetologia 1996; 39: 1539-1678.

Grossman E, Messerli FH. Diabetic and hypertensive heart disease. Ann Intern Med 1996; 125: 304-310.

R. Østerby. Lessons from Kidney Biopsies. Diabetes/Metabolism Reviews 1996; 12: 151-174.

Chronic Complications of Diabetes. Endocrinology and Metabolism Clinics of North America 1996; 25: 217-438.

B. Bauduceau, G. Chatellier, D. Cordonnier, M. Marre, A. Mimran, L. Monnier, J.-P. Sauvanet, P. Valensi, N. Balarac. Hypertension artérielle et diabète. Diabetes & Metabolism (Paris) 1996; 22: 64-76.

Journal of Diabetes and Its Complications. Special Section: Diabetic Complications and Early Treatment using ACE Inhibitors. May-June 1996; 10: No. 3: 124-153

G.M. Reaven, Y-D.I. Chen. Insulin resistance, its consequences, and coronary heart disease. Must we choose one culprit? Circulation 1996; 93: 1780-1783.

H. Taegtmeyer. Insulin resistance and atherosclerosis. Common roots for two common diseases? Circulation 1996; 93: 1777-1779.
G.M. Reaven, H. Lithell, L. Landsberg. Hypertension and associated metabolic abnormalities - the role of insulin resistance and the sympathoadrenal system. N Engl J Med 1996; 334: 374-381.

C.E. Mogensen, ed. *Microalbuminuria. A Marker for Organ Damage.* 2nd ed. London: Science Press, 1996.
A.H. Barnett, P.M. Dodson, eds. *Hypertension and Diabetes.* 2nd ed. London: Science Press, 1996.

M. Mauer, C.E. Mogensen. »Diabetic nephropathy.« In *Diseases of the Kidney*, vo. III, R.W. Schrier, C.W. Gottschalk. eds. Boston: Little, Brown and Company, 1996; Chapter 73: p. 2019-2062.

R. Pedrinelli. Microalbuminuria in hypertension (Editorial). Nephron 1996; 73: 499-505.

R. Pontremoli. Microalbuminuria in essential hypertension - its relation to cardiovascular risk factors (Editorial Comment). Nephrol Dial Transplant 1996; 11: 2113-2115.

C.E. Mogensen, ed. Over-Mortality in NIDDM. Journal of Diabetes and Its Complications 1997; 11: 59-143.

C.E. Mogensen, P. Weidmann, eds. Hypertension and Diabetes: a risky alliance. How can drug therapy improve clinical outcome? Am J Hypertens 1997; 10: no. 9, pt. 2, suppl.: 171S-217S.

P.E. de Jong, Dick de Zeeuw, C.E. Mogensen, eds. Proteinuria and Progressive Renal Disease. June 1996. Amsterdam, The Netherlands. Nephrol Dial Transplant 1997; 12: suppl. 2: 1-85.

F.A. Gries, T. Koschinsky, D. Tschöpe, D. Ziegler, eds. Current State and Perspectives of Diabetes Research: Chronic Complications. Diabetes 1997; 46: suppl. 2: S1-S134.

R.W. Bilous, P. Fioretto, P. Czernichow, K. Drummond. Growth factors and diabetic nephropathy: kidney structure and therapeutic interventions. Diabetologia 1997; 40: B68-B73.

T. Baba, S. Neugebauer, T. Watanabe. Diabetic Nephropathy. Its relationship to hypertension and means of pharmacological intervention. Durgs 1997; 54: 197-234.

E.J. Lewis, ed. Prevention of Diabetic Nephropathy. Sem Nephrol 1997; 17: 77-147.

H.B. Lee, H. Ha, eds. Experimental Approaches to Diabetic Nephropathy. The Third Hyonam Kidney Laboratory International Symposium. Seoul, South Korea, January 24-25, 1997. Kidney Int 1997; 51: suppl. 60: 1-103.

W.F. Keane, B.M. Brenner, K. Kurokawa, eds. Progression of Renal Disease: Clinical Patterns, Therapeutic Options, and Lessons from Clinical Trials, Coolum, Australia, May 31-June 3, 1997. Kidney Int 1997; 52: suppl. 63: 1-243.

J.C. Pickup, G. Williams, eds. Textbook of Diabetes, 2nd ed. Section 13, Chapters 52-54. Blackwell Science 1997.

D.J. Barnes, J.R. Pinto, G.-C. Viberti. The Kidney in systemic disease. The patient with diabetes mellitus. In A.M. Davision, J.S. Cameron, J.-P. Grünfeld, D.N.S. Kerr, E. Ritz, C.G. Winearls, eds. Oxford Textbook of Clinical Nephrology, 2nd ed. Oxford, New York, Tokyo; Oxford University Press 1998; 723-776.

American Diabetes Association. Diabetic Nephropathy. Diabetes Care 1998; 21: suppl. 1: S50-S53.

L.P. Aiello, T.W. Gardner, G.L. King, G. Blankenship, J.D. Cavallerano, F.L. Ferris III, R. Klein. Diabetic Retinopathy. Diabetes Care 1998; 21: 143-156.

C.E. Mogensen, ed. Proceedings from 4th Symposium on Proteinuria and Progressive Renal Disease. September 1997. Montreux, Switzerland. Nephrol Dial Transplant 1998; April.

C.E. Mogensen. Microalbuminuria and diabetic renal disease. Original and development of ideas. Diabetologia, 1998. In press (including newest literature).

Relevant review articles in DIABETES ANNUAL

E.N. Ellis, S.M. Mauer. »Diabetic nephropathy.« In *The Diabetes Annual/1*. Alberti KGMM, Krall LP, eds. Amsterdam, New York, Oxford: Elsevier Science Publishers B.V., 1985; pp 309-322.

C.E. Mogensen. »Early diabetic renal involvement and nephropathy. Can treatment modalities be predicted from identification of risk factors?« In *The Diabetes Annual/3*. Alberti KGMM, Krall LP, eds. Amsterdam, New York, Oxford: Elsevier Science Publishers B.V., 1987; pp 306-324.

A.R. Christlieb, A.S. Krolewski, J.H. Warram. »An update on hypertension in patients with diabetes mellitus.« In *The Diabetes Annual/4*. Alberti KGMM, Krall LP, eds. Amsterdam, New York, Oxford: Elsevier Science Publishers B.V., 1988; pp 384-393.

C.E. Mogensen. »Diabetic renal involvement and disease in patients with insulin-dependent diabetes.« In *The Diabetes Annual/4*. Alberti KGMM, Krall LP, eds. Amsterdam, New York, Oxford: Elsevier Science Publishers B.V., 1988; pp 411-448.

G.C. Viberti. »New insights into the genesis of diabetic kidney disease in insulin-dependent diabetic patients.« In *The Diabetes Annual/5*. Alberti KGMM, Krall LP, eds. Amsterdam, New York, Oxford: Elsevier Science Publishers B.V., 1990; pp 301-311.

P.L. Drury. »Hypertension in diabetes.« In *The Diabetes Annual/5*. Alberti KGMM, Krall LP, eds. Amsterdam, New York, Oxford: Elsevier Science Publishers B.V., 1990; pp 362-372.

S.M. Marshall. »Diabetic nephropathy.« In *The Diabetes Annual/6*. Alberti KGMM, Krall LP, eds. Amsterdam, London, New York, Tokyo: Elsevier Science Publishers B.V., 1991; pp 302-325.

H.-H. Parving. »Hypertension and diabetes.« In *The Diabetes Annual/7*. Marshall SM, Home PD, Alberti KGMM, Krall LP, eds. Amsterdam, New York, Oxford: Elsevier Science Publishers B.V., 1993; pp 301-311.

G. Jerums, R. Gilbert. »Renal tubular dysfunction in diabetes mellitus.« In *The Diabetes Annual/7*. Marshall SM, Home PD, Alberti KGMM, Krall LP, eds. Amsterdam, New York, Oxford: Elsevier Science Publishers B.V., 1993; pp 146-165.

A.R.G. Humphrey, P.Z. Zimmet, R.F. Hamman. »The epidemiology of diabetes mellitus.« In *The Diabetes Annual/9*. Marshall SM, Home PD, Rizza RA, eds. Amsterdam, Lausanne New York, Oxford, Shannon, Tokyo: Elsevier Science Publishers B.V., 1995; pp 1-31.

H. Vlassara, R. Bucala. »Advanced glycation and diabetes complications: an update.« In *The Diabetes Annual/9*. Marshall SM, Home PD, Rizza RA, eds. Amsterdam, Lausanne, New York, Oxford, Shannon, Tokyo: Elsevier Science B.V., 1995; pp 227-244.

A.S. Reddi. »The basement membrane in diabetes.« In *The Diabetes Annual/9*. Marshall SM, Home PD, Rizza RA, eds. Amsterdam, Lausanne, New York, Oxford, Shannon, Tokyo: Elsevier Science B.V., 1995; pp 245-263.

P. Ruggenenti, G. Remuzzi. »Anti-hypertensive agents and incipient diabetic nephropathy.« In *The Diabetes Annual/9*. Marshall SM, Home PD, Rizza RA, eds. Amsterdam, Lausanne New York, Oxford, Shannon, Tokyo: Elsevier Science Publishers B.V., 1995; pp 295-317.

CONTRIBUTING AUTHORS

Sharon Anderson, M.D.
Division of Nephrology and Hypertension
PP262
Oregon Health Sciences University
3314 SW US Veterans Hospital
Portland, OR 97201
USA
Tel: +1-503-494-8490
Fax: +1-503-721-7810
e-mail: anderssh@aol.com

George L. Bakris, MD, F.A.C.P
Rush University Hypertension Center
Rush-Presbyterian-St. Luke's Medical Center
1725 West Harrison Street
Suite #119
Chicago, IL 60612-3833
USA
Tel: +1 312 563 2195
Fax: +1 312 942 4464

Hans-Jacob Bangstad, M.D.
Department of Pediatric
Aker sykehus
0514 Oslo 5
Norge
Tel: +47 2289 4585
Fax: +47 2289 4204

Staffan Björck, M.D.
Njurmottagningen
Sahlgrenska sjukhuset
S-413 45 Göteborg
Sverige
Tel: +46 31 60 26 11
Fax: +46 31 41 23 32

Rudy W. Bilous, MD, FRCP
Consultant Physician
Diabetes Care Centre
Middlesbrough General Hospital
Ayresome Green Lane
Middlesbrough
Cleveland TS5 5AZ
United Kingdom
Tel: +44 1 642 854146
Fax: +44 1 642 854148

Knut Borch-Johnsen, M.D.
Steno Diabetes Center
Niels Steensens Vej 2
2820 Gentofte
Tel: +45 44439415
Fax: +45 44438233
e-mail: KBJO@Novo.DK

Nishi Chaturvedi, M.D.
University College London
Department of Epidemiology & Public Health
1-19 Torrington Place
London WC1E 6BT
United Kingdom
Tel: +44 171 391 1724/1725/1726 (direct line)
Eurodiab fax: +44 171 813 0288
e-mail: eurodiab@public-health.ucl.ac.uk

Vito M. Campese, M.D.
Assoc Chief Div Nephrol
LAC/USC Medical Center
1200 North State St.
Los Angeles, CA 90033
USA
Tel: +1 213 226 7307
Fax: +1 213 226 5390
e-mail: campese@hsc.usc.edu

Mark Cooper, M.D.
The University of Melbourne
Department of Medicine
Austin and Repatriation Medical Centre -
Repatriation Campus
West Heidelberg 3081
Australia
Tel: +61 3 9496 2347
Fax: +61 3 9497 4554
e-mail cooper@austin.unimelb.edu.au

Pedro Cortes, M.D.
Department of Internal Medicine
Henry Ford Hospital & Medical Centers
Nephrology and Hypertension
2799 West Grand Boulevard
Detroit, Michigan 48202
USA
Tel: +1 313 876 2711
Fax: +1 313 876 2554

Torsten Deckert, M.D.
Steno Diabetes Center
Niels Steensensvej 2
2820 Gentofte
Tel: +45 3168 0800
Fax: +45 3168 2322

Bo Feldt-Rasmussen, M.D.
Medical Department P 2132
Rigshospitalet
Blegdamsvej 9
DK-2100 København Ø
Denmark
Tel: +45 3545 2135
Fax: +45 3545 2240

Ele Ferrannini, M.D.
Istituto di Fisiologia Clinica del CNR
CNR Institute of Clinical Physiology
Consiglio Nazionale delle Ricerche - C.N.R.
c/o Università di Pisa
Via Savi, 8
I-56100 Pisa
Italy
Tel: +39 50 500087
Fax: +39 50 553235

Paola Fioretto, M.D.
Istituto di Medicina Interna
Università di Padova
Via Giustiniani, 2
I-35128 Padova
Italy
Tel: +39 49 821 2150
Fax: +39 49 821 2151

Allan Flyvbjerg, M.D.
Medical Department M
Diabetes & Endocrinology
Aarhus Kommunehospital
Aarhus University Hospital
DK-8000 Aarhus C
Denmark
Tel: +45 8949 2019
Fax: +458949 2010
e-mail: AKH.GRP02S.AFG@AAA.DK

Eli A. Friedman, M.D.
Division of Renal Disease
Department of Medicine
State University of New York Health Science
Center at Brooklyn
450 Clarkson Avenue, Box 52
Brooklyn, NY 11203
USA
Tel: +1 718 270 1584
Fax: +1 718 270 3327
e-mail: elifriedmn@aol.com

Norman K. Hollenberg, M.D., Ph.D.
Brigham and Women's Hospital
75 Francis Street
Boston, MA 02115
USA
Tel: +1 617 732 6682
Fax: +1 617 232 2869

Per-Henrik Groop, M.D., Ph.D.
Department of Medicine
Division of Nephrology
Helsinki University Central Hospital
Kasarminkatu 11-13
Fin-00130 Helsinki
Finland
Tel: +358 9 471 8203
Fax: +358 9 471 8400
e-mail: ph.groop@pp.fimnet.fi

Klavs Würgler Hansen, M.D.
Medical Department M
Diabetes & Endocrinology
Aarhus Kommunehospital
Aarhus University Hospital
DK-8000 Aarhus C
Denmark
Tel: +45 8949 2023
Fax: +45 8949 2010
e-mail: AKH.GRP02S.KWH@AAA.DK

John L. Kitzmiller, M.D.
Chief, Maternal Fetal Medicine
Good Samaritan Health System
Perinatal Associates of Santa Clara Valley
2425 Samaritan Drive
San Jose, California 95124
USA
Tel: +1 408 559 2258
Fax: +1 408 559 2658

Allan Kofoed-Enevoldsen, M.D.
Department of Endocrinology
Amtssygehuset i Herlev
Herlev Ringvej 75
DK-2730 Herlev
Denmark
Tel: +45 4453 5300
Fax: +45 4453 5332

William C. Knowler, M.D., Dr.P.H.
Diabetes and Arthritis Epidemiology Section
Department of Healthy & Human Services
National Institutes of Health
National Institute of Diabetes and Digestive
and Kidney Diseases
1550 East Indian School Road
Phoenix, Arizona 85014
USA
Tel: +1 602 200 5206
Fax: +1 602 200 5225
e-mail: kcw@cu.nih.gov

Daisuke Koya, M.D.
Third Department of Medicine
Shiga University of Medical Science
Seta
Otsu
Shiga 520-21
JAPAN
Tel: +81 775 48 2222
Fax: +81 775 43 3858
e-mail: koya@belle.shiga-med.ac.jp

Michel Marre, M.D.
Service de Médecine B
Centre Hospitalier Universitaire
49033 Angers Cedex 01
France
Tel: +33 241 35 44 99
Fax: +33 24(1) 73 82 30
e-mail: M.MARRE@unimedia.fr

Carl Erik Mogensen, M.D.
Medical Department M
Diabetes & Endocrinology
Aarhus Kommunehospital
Aarhus University Hospital
DK-8000 Aarhus C
Denmark
Tel: +45 8949 2011
Fax: +45 8613 7825/8949 2010
e-mail: AKH.GRP02S.CAM@AAA.DK

Henrik Bindesbøl Mortensen, M.D.
Pediatric Department L
Amtssygehuset i Glostrup
Ndr. Ringvej
DK-2600 Glostrup
Denmark
Tel: +45 4363 2466 ext. 6010
Fax: +45 4323 2967

Gerjan J. Navis, M.D.
Department of Medicine
Division of Nephrology
University Hospital
Hanzeplein 1
9700 RB Groningen
The Netherlands
Fax: +31 50 3169310
e-mail: g.j.navis@int.azg.nl

Søren Nielsen, M.D.
Medical Department M
Diabetes & Endocrinology
Aarhus Kommunehospital
Aarhus University Hospital
DK-8000 Aarhus C
Denmark
Tel: +45 8949 2019
Fax: +45 8949 2010

Jens Randel Nyengaard, M.D.
Stereological Research Laboratory
Bartholinbygningen
Aarhus University
DK-8000 Aarhus C
Denmark
Tel: +45 8949 3654
Fax: +45 8949 3650
e-mail: stereo@svfcd.aau.dk

James A. O'Hare, M.D., FRCPI, MRCP
Mid-Western Health Board
Regional General Hospital
Dooradoyle
Limerick
Ireland
Tel: +353 61 301111
Fax: +353 61 301165

Steen Olsen, M.D.
Department of Pathology-Anatomy
Aarhus Kommunehospital
Aarhus University Hospital
DK-8000 Aarhus C
Denmark
Tel: +45 8949 3701
Fax: +45 8949 3700

D.G. Oreopoulos, M.D.
Director - Peritoneal Dialysis Unit
University of Toronto
The Toronto Hospital (Western Division)
Division of Nephrology
399 Bathurst Street
Toronto, Ontario
Canada M5T 2S8
Tel: +1 416 364 9974
Fax: +1 416 360 8127

Margrethe Mau Pedersen, M.D.
Medical Department M
Diabetes & Endocrinology
Aarhus Kommunehospital
Aarhus University Hospital
DK-8000 Aarhus C
Denmark
Tel: +45 8949 2019
Fax: +45 8949 2010

David J. Pettitt, M.D.
Sansum Medical Research Foundation
2219 Bath Street
Santa Barbara, CA 93105
USA
Tel: +1 805 682 7640
Fax: +1 805 682 3332
e-mail: dpettitt@workmail.com

Per Løgstrup Poulsen, M.D.
Medical Department M
Diabetes & Endocrinology
Aarhus Kommunehospital
Aarhus University Hospital
DK-8000 Aarhus C
Denmark
Tel: +45 8949 2019
Fax: +45 8949 2010

Eberhard Ritz, M.D.
Sektion Nephrologie
Klinikum der Universität Heidelberg
Medizinische Klinik
Bergheimer Strasse 56a
D-69115 Heidelberg
Germany
Tel: +49 6221 91120
Fax: +49 6221 162476

Peter Rossing, M.D.
Steno Diabetes Center
Niels Steensensvej 2
DK-2820 Gentofte
Denmark
Tel: +45 3968 0800
Fax: +45 4443 8232
e-mail: prossing@inet.uni2.dk

D.J.F. Rowe, M.D.
Department of Chemical Pathology
Southampton University Hospital
Tremona Road
Southampton SO166YD
United Kingdom
Tel: +44 1 703 796437/8
Fax: +44 1 703 796339

Peter T. Sawicki, M.D.
Medizinische Einrichtungen
der Heinrich-Heine Universität
Abteilung für Ernährung und Stoffwechsel
Moorenstr. 5
40225 Düsseldorf
Germany
Tel: +49 211 81 17836
Fax: +49-211-81 18772

Erwing Schleicher, M.D.
Institute of Internal Medicine
Dep. Of Endocrinology, Metabolism and
Pathobiochemistry
University of Tübingen
Otfried-Müller-Str. 10
D-72076 Tübingen
Germany
Tel: +49 7071 29 87599
Fax: +49 7071 29 5646

Anita Schmitz, M.D.
Medical Department M
Diabetes & Endocrinology
Aarhus Kommunehospital
Aarhus University Hospital
DK-8000 Aarhus C
Denmark
Tel: +45 8949 2019
Fax: +45 8949 2010

Coen D.A. Stehouwer, M.D.
Department of Internal Medicine
Free University Hospital
De Boelelaan 1117
1081 HV Amsterdam
The Netherlands
Tel: +31 20 444 0531
Fax: +31 20 444 0502

Roberto Trevisan, M.D.
Cattedra Malattie del Ricambio
Università di Padova
U.L.S.S. 21
Divisione Malattie del Ricambio
Via Giustiniani, 2
I-35128 Padova
Italy
Tel: +39 49 821 2335/8762121
Fax: +39 49 821 2151

GianCarlo Viberti, M.D.
Division of Medicine
Guy's and St Thomas's Medical and Dental School
Unit for Metabolic Medicine
Diabetes, Endocrinology, Metabolism
Floor 4 Hunt's House, Guy's Hospital
London Bridge, London SE1 9RT
United Kingdom
Tel: +44 1 71 955 4826
Fax: +44 1 71 955 2985
e-mail: g.viberti@umds.ac.uk

James Walker, M.D.
Department of Diabetes
The Royal Infirmary of Edinburgh
Lauriston Place
Edinburgh EH3 9YW
Scotland
Tel: +44 1 31 536 1000
Fax: +44 1 31 536 1001

James H. Warram, M.D.
Joslin Diabetes Center
One Joslin Place
Boston
Massachusetts 02215
USA
Tel: +1 617 732 2668
Fax: +1 617 732 2593

Giulio Zuanetti, M.D.
Department of Cardiovascular Research
Istituto Mario Negri
via Eritrea 62
I-20157 Milan
Italy
Tel: +39 2 3901 4454
Fax: +39 2 3320 0049
e-mail: zuanetti@irfmn.mnegri.it

Fuad N. Ziyadeh, M.D.
Renal-Electrolyte and Hypertension Division
700 Clinical Research Building
University of Pennsylvania Medical Center
415 Curie Boulevard
Philadelphia, PA 19104-6144
USA
Tel: +1 215 662 7900
Fax: +1 215 898 0189
e-mail: ziyadeh@mail.med.upenn.edu

PREFACE, first edition

The first sporadic observations describing renal abnormalities in diabetes were published late in the 19th century, but systematic studies of the kidney in diabetes started only half a century ago after the paper by Cambier in 1934 and the much more famous study by Kimmelstiel and Wilson in 1936. These authors described two distinct features of renal involvement in diabetes: early hyperfiltration and late nephropathy. Diabetic nephropathy is, despite half a century of studies, still a very pertinent problem, renal disease in diabetes now being a very common cause of end-stage renal failure in Europe and North America and probably throughout the world. It is a very important part of the generalized vascular disease found in long-term diabetes as described by Knud Lundbæk in his monograph *Long-term Diabetes* in 1953, published by Munksgaard, Copenhagen.

Surprisingly, there has not been a comprehensive volume describing all aspects of renal involvement in diabetes, and the time is now ripe for such a volume summarizing the very considerable research activity within this field during the last decade and especially during the last few years.

This book attempts to cover practically all aspects of renal involvement in diabetes. It is written by colleagues who are themselves active in the many fields of medical research covered in this volume: epidemiology, physiology and pathophysiology, laboratory methodology, and renal pathology. New studies deal with the diagnosis and treatment of both incipient and overt nephropathy by metabolic, antihypertensive, and dietary invention. Considerable progress has been made in the management of end-stage renal failure and also in the management and treatment of nephropathy in the pregnant diabetic woman. Diabetic nephropathy is a world-wide problem, but it is more clearly defined in Europe and North America where facilities for the diagnosis and treatment of diabetes and its complications are readily available. Much more work needs to be done in other parts of the world, as it appears from this book.

It is hoped that we now have a handbook for the kidney and hypertension in diabetes and that further progress can be made in clinical work in diagnosing and treating diabetic patients. Much more work still needs to be done regarding patient education with respect to complications. Many diabetics have now been trained to take part in the management of their metabolic control; they should also be trained to take part in the follow-up and treatment of complications.

This volume also underlines the considerable need for future research. So far, research in this field has been carried out in relatively few countries and centres in the world. The editor is sure that this volume will also stimulate further advancement in clinical science within the field of diabetic renal disease.

In 1952, the book *Diabetic Glomerulosclerosis, The Specific Renal Disease in Diabetes Mellitus,* by Harold Rifkin and co-workers, published by Charles C. Thomas, Springfield, Illinois, USA, summarized all current knowledge on the diabetic kidney in about 100 short pages, including many case histories. Much more space is needed now and the many disciplines involved will undoubtedly attract many readers.

Carl Erik Mogensen

PREFACE, second edition

The sum of clinical problems caused by diabetic renal disease has been steadily increasing since the first edition of this book was published in 1988. Indeed, it is now estimated that throughout the world about 100,000 diabetic individuals are receiving treatment for end-stage renal failure. Obviously, this means a burden with respect to human suffering, disease and premature mortality, but additionally these treatment programmes are extremely costly, so costly that in many areas resources are not available for this kind of care. It is therefore clear, that every efforts should be made to prevent or postpone the development of end-stage disease.

The years since the first edition appeared we have seen a tremendous progress in research activities. Importantly, this also includes improvement in the treatment programmes to prevent end-stage renal failure. Thus it has become clear that the diabetic kidney is extremely pressure-sensitive, responding to effective antihypertensive treatment by retarded progression of disease. Some agents may be more beneficial in this respect than other, although the effective blood pressure reduction per se is crucial throughout the stages of diabetic renal disease. However, the prime cause of diabetic renal disease is related to poor metabolic control and it is now documented beyond doubt that good metabolic control is able to postpone or perhaps even prevent the development of renal disease. However, in many individuals we are not able to provide such a quality of control that will prevent complications, and therefore non-glycaemic intervention remains important. Maybe in the future non-glycaemic intervention will become the most important research area in diabetic nephropathy.

With respect to the exact mechanisms behind poor metabolic control and development of renal disease, much information is now being gained. It is likely that a combination of genetic predisposition and metabolic and haemodynamic abnormalities explain the progression to renal disease, seen in about 30% of the diabetic individuals. Much of this development probably relates to modifiable genetic factors, such as blood pressure elevation or haemodynamic aberrations. However, mechanisms related to the response to hyperglycaemia are also of clear importance as is the possibility that these metabolic or haemodynamic pathway may be inhibited.

This volume review older data as well as the progress seen within the research of diabetic nephropathy over the last five years and provides a state of the art of the development. However, we are still far from the main goal, which is the abolition of end-stage renal disease in diabetic individuals. Obviously, much work still needs to be done and one of the intentions of this book is to stimulate further research in this area where so many sub-disciplines of medical science are involved from the extremes of genetic and molecular biology to clinical and pharmacological research trials.

January 1994

Carl Erik Mogensen

PREFACE, third edition

Many new dimensions have been added to the concepts regarding diabetic renal disease in the past few years. In addition some considerably amounts of new studies have been published since the second edition of this book. Therefore, there is a clear need to update the issue on diabetic renal disease. Ever more focus is placed on pressure-induced and metabolic related aberration, in relation to genetic abnormalities and also changes developing in fetal life. New chapters also include exercise, lipidemia and retinopathy in diabetic renal disease. New data are also included regarding structural changes in NIDDM-patients. Much of the development in diabetic renal disease is also relevant to non-diabetic renal disease, and therefore chapters comparing diabetic and non-diabetic renal disease have been included.

As a result of the studies on pathogenesis of treatment of diabetic renal disease, new guidelines have been published as recently reviewed in the Lancet 1995. These guidelines are also included in this new edition, where the editor has tried to focus on all major issues relevant to diabetic renal disease.

Many groups are working within this field, but the most cited authors are the following as recently reviewed by JDF (for the years 1981-95).

Measure Diabetes Research 1981-95
Hypertension, Nephropathy (T-10)

		Cites	Papers	C/P
USA	Brenner B	2499	33	76
DK	*Christiansen JS*	2659	115	23
DK	*Deckert T*	4229	157	27
USA	Knowler WC	2975	127	23
USA	Krolewski AS	2220	74	30
USA	Mauer SM	2307	101	23
DK	*Mogensen CE*	3456	146	24
DK	*Parving HH*	4702	216	22
F	*Passa P*	1570	196	8
UK	*Viberti GC*	2820	119	24

August 1996

Carl Erik Mogensen

PREFACE, fourth edition

We have witnessed a rapid development within the field of the kidney and hypertension in diabetes mellitus. A lot of work within the traditional areas has been published, and several new dimensions are now being developed, mostly in the experimental setting as discussed in several chapters. Therefore, there is now a need for an updated edition of this volume. A clear policy has been to have completely updated versions of the book, at disposal for the clinicians and the scientists in the area.

New guidelines are being developed within the field of hypertension and also in the field of diabetes mellitus, where new definitions are being introduced, mainly relevant for type 2 diabetes. The number of patients entering end-stage renal failure programmes are still increasing, underscoring the need for better management of these patients. The number of patients with diabetes is predicted to increased over the next decade, mainly due to changing patterns of life-style and an older population. Therefore, we need to be even more prepared to look after these patients, also with respect to renal, hypertensive and cardiovascular complications.

Since diabetic nephropathy is in most cases associated with heart disease and with retinopathy, new chapters on this aspect have been added. Very importantly, there is now more and more scientific support for early treatment in normotensive patients with microalbuminuria with ACE-inhibitors. This treatment seems beneficial also for diabetic heart disease and diabetic retinopathy according to new studies, also discussed in the book. The maxim is that diabetic nephropathy, retinopathy and heart disease often go together. The same seems to be the case regarding treatment and prevention, with focus on good glycemic control.

January 1998

Carl Erik Mogensen

1. HISTORICAL ASPECTS OF DIABETES AND DIABETIC RENAL DISEASE

Torsten Deckert
Steno Diabetes Center, Copenhagen, Denmark.

The eldest description of the diabetic syndrome is seen in Papyrus Ebers from Luxor in Egypt about 1550 BC. The term diabetes, however, was coined by the roman physician Aretæus of Cappadokia 200 AD.[1]. He wrote: "Diabetes is a wonderful affection, not very frequent among men, being a melting down of the flesh and limbs into urine, the patients never stop making water, but the flow in incessant, as if opening of aqueducts, life is short, disgusting and painful".

Naturally polyuria attracted the attention of physicians, but old Indians discovered why also flies were interested in the urine of diabetic patients. However not before 1775 Matthew Dobson [2] from Britain proofed that the sweetness of the urine was due to sugar. Also blood of diabetic patients sometimes had a sweet taste. Therefore, in order to distinguish diabetes with sweet urine from diabetes with insipid urine, his contemporary John Rollo [3] proposed the suffix "mellitus" to diabetes, honey-like. When the famous French physician Appollinaires Bouchardat in 1839 found that the sweetness of serum was due to glucose and that even normal men seemed to have glucose in the blood, it was not believed by the scientific society including Claude Bernard. Under the chairmanship of professor Dumas the French Academy appointed a committee to investigate the question. The result was negative: only in patients with diabetes glucose was present in the blood the committee decided [4]. However already around 1855 the understanding of carbohydrate metabolism was pushed forward by two observations. The French doctor C.Chauveau proofed that fasting healthy men do have glucose in the blood, about 0.10 % and Claude Bernard demonstrated that the liver was able to secrete glucose from glycogen [4]. Now more specific speculations regarding the cause of blood glucose elevation in diabetes started. But where was the seat of the trouble?

Galenus (130 - 201 AD), imperial physician of Marcus Aurelius, believed diabetes to be a kidney disease. This believe was unanimously accepted until John Rollo seventeen hundred years later hypothesized that diabetes was a digestive disease which could be relieved by dieting, blood pudding, for example. Dieting continued, but the hypothesis changed when Claude Bernard suggested diabetes to be the result of hepatic dysfunction [5]. Thereafter young men took over. At Strassburg in 1889 at the department of Bernhard Naunyn a young Russian doctor Oscar Minkowsky (30 years) had a bet with his elder colleague Joseph van Mering [6] on whether a dog could survive without pancreas. Minkowsky won but found that the dog developed diabetes. The two physicians, therefore, continued their experiments. They found that diabetes could be prevented when only a very small part of the removed pancreas together with its blood supply was implanted in the subcutaneous tissue of the dog. This observation drew the attention to the islets of pancreas tissue described by Paul Langerhans (22 years) at Virchows laboratory in Berlin 1869 [7]. In a series of beautiful experiments another Russian research fellow, Leonid Szobolev (25 years), was able to proof in 1901, that the islets of Langerhans and not the exocrine tissue were involved in the pathogenesis of diabetes [8].

Since then several attempts were made to isolate the antidiabetic principle [9]. As well the German practitioner G.L.Zuelzer (1906), the young Rockefeller scientist I.Kleiner (1919) as professor Nicolas Paulesco from Bucharest(1921) extracted insulin and demonstrated its capacity to reduce glucosuria and hyperglycaemia in a reproducible way. However their extracts induced fever due to impurities and therefore were inapplicable for the treatment of diabetes. Not before the young biochemist J.B.Collip(29 years) from Atlanta University on his sabbatical at Toronto became involved in Banting(30 years) and Bests(22 years) experiments by professor Macleod(45 years) the problems were solved. Collip found that the impurities could be removed by precipitating the extracts containing insulin with concentrated alcohol. Since he was unwilling to tell his observation to Mr. Banting he was knocked down. Banting was jealous. In fact Banting and Best did not contribute with anything in the development of insulin preparations but energy and endurance. It is tempting to believe that Banting was proposed to the Nobel Prize because the press and the public liked him. His father was poor, he served as a soldier during the first world war, had trouble with his sweet-heart, sold every thing he had to get money for the experiments in Toronto, believed strongly in his success and shed a flattering light on an absolute unknown university in the New World, certainly a good American fellow. In my opinion the Nobel Prize should have been given to Paulesco and Collip, but neither of them was recommended.

The discovery of applicable insulin preparations had an enormous impact on the life of diabetic patients. The amount of carbohydrates and calories in the diet could now be increased without impairment of diabetes regulation. Before the discovery of insulin, Joslin [10] wrote in his famous textbook of 1917: "It is desirable in peace but a duty in war, for every diabetic patient to keep sugar free. The food which the untreated diabetic patient wastes in a week would feed a soldier for a day." After the discovery of insulin, starvation was not longer necessary and most patients were happy to inject insulin, though many of them hated the large needles and the local side effects after injection. Also the doctors were happy. Voltaire's slogan:" The art of medicine is to amuse the patient until nature has healed him" could now be rejected. Much could be done and the life of diabetic patients was prolonged. But the prolongation of life resulted in an increasing incidence of diabetic complications.

Until 1930 diabetic complications were not very well known in spite of the fact that Avicenna already about 1000 AD. had described gangrene and the "collapse of sexual function" in diabetic patients. Rollo added cataract [11]. Albuminuria was so frequently seen that it was not regarded as a serious prognostic token. It was regarded as an unimportant consequence of metabolic poisoning of the tubuli, reversible by improvement of metabolic control [12]. Still in 1941 the famous Danish nephrologist Iversen who invented the needle for kidney biopsy, maintained, that proteinuria in diabetics was so common, that no particular significance should be attached to it [13]. Brights disease with severe albuminuria and hypertension was rare (about 2 - 3 % in Joslins material) and mostly seen in elderly patients. Among 497 fatal cases of diabetes followed by Joslin until 1916 only 3 % died from renal diseases. Also von Noorden, the most famous European diabetologist in 1927 did not describe the clinical syndrome of diabetic nephropathy [12]. If albuminuria, edema, hypertension and retinopathy were present in diabetic patients, it was regarded as complicating malignant nephrosclerosis or glomerulonephritis. The term diabetic nephropathy was for the first time used by Aschoff in 1911 [12], but only to characterize the frequent minor albuminuria which was believed to be due to the glycogen deposits within the tubuli described by Armanni in 1877 [14].

The situation changed totally after 1936 when Kimmelstiel and Wilson described nodular glomerulosclerosis in patients characterized by long duration of diabetes, heavy albuminuria, hypertension, edema and renal insufficiency [15]. Similar lesions had been mentioned by Inglessis (1885) and Waku (1928) from Japan [16], but Kimmelstiel&Wilson were the first to relate the clinical symptoms of nephropathy to a specific histopathology. In 1953 Lundbæk [17] demonstrated, that diabetic nephropathy was part of a generalized specific diabetic vascular disease, characterized by basement membrane thickening. Now a more systematic study of diabetic complications started. These studies resulted in a precise description of epidemiology [18], clinic [16] and morphology [19] of diabetic nephropathy. It was demonstrated that diabetic histopathology is present even in long-term diabetics without clinical signs of nephropathy, but more pronounced in patients with albuminuria. It was found that mesangial expansion correlated best with GFR [20] and that only patients with albuminuria demonstrated a decline of GFR, which in patients not treated with anti-hypertensive therapy was found to be about 10 ml/min./year [21]. Finally the Steno group demonstrated clearly that over-mortality and over-morbidity among IDDM patients was almost exclusively confined to patients with albuminuria [18].

These observation resulted in an increased interest for the pathogenesis of diabetic nephropathy. The old observation by Fichtner in 1888 of renal hypertrophy in diabetes [22] was rediscovered and supplemented by the finding of glomerular hypertrophy and renal hyperfiltration in patients without albuminuria [23]. These observations contributed to the ongoing debate on the role of glomerular hyperperfusion and hypertension in the pathogenesis of diabetic nephropathy. Also the old observation by Hitzenberger from 1921 [24] of the high prevalence of hypertension in diabetes was confirmed and it was demonstrated, that in IDDM patients this was due to the frequent occurrence of diabetic nephropathy [25] whereas in NIDDM the association was more complicated. Keen found that diabetes and hypertension were bad companions [26] and the appearance of new antihypertensive drugs stimulated Mogensen and Parving to conduct controlled trials with antihypertensive therapy in patients with albuminuria [27]. The effect was very convincing, showing a dramatic reduction of the fall rate of GFR. Besides the progress within the treatment of ESRD these studies represented the first progress in the treatment of diabetic nephropathy. Shortly after several European centres demonstrated that besides antihypertensive therapy strict metabolic control significantly reduced the progression of early nephropathy [28], and the DCCT study finally proofed that strict metabolic control could prevent the development of nephropathy in patients with IDDM [29]. Together these discoveries resulted in an enormous increase of life expectancy in IDDM patients.

A further progress was the development of sensitive methods for the quantitation of small amounts of protein in the urine and the resulting concept of microalbuminuria in 1984 [30]. This enabled the clinician to identify patients at risk for nephropathy and cardiovascular complications rather early and to start preventive efforts. But identification of patients with persistent and increasing microalbuminuria also helped to study the initial steps in the development of diabetic nephropathy. The application of molecular biologic technology recently in the study of the pathogenesis [31] and genetic disposition [32] of diabetic vasculopathy will hopefully result in the development of new more specific preventive drugs and bring the patients nearer to the goal: The normalization of life expectancy and quality of life.

REFERENCES

1. Poulsen J E. Features of the history of diabetology. Munksgaard, Copenhagen 1982
2. Dobson M. Experiments and observations on the urine in diabetes. Med Obs Inq 1776, 5:298 - 316
3. Rollo J. An account of two cases of the diabetes mellitus. London 1797
4. Bang I. Der Blutzucker. Bergmann, Wiesbaden 1913
5. Bernard C. Lecon de physiologie experimentales. Balliere, Paris 1855
6. Mering J von, Minkowski O. Diabetes mellitus nach Pancreasextirpation. Arch Exper Path Pharm 1890, 26: 371 - 387
7. Langerhans P. Beitrage zur mikroskopischen Anatomi der Bauchspeicheldruse. Inaugural-Dissertation zur Erlangung der Doctorwurde. Lange, Berlin 1869
8. Szobolew L W. Zur normalen und pathologischen Morphologie der inneren Sekretion der Bauchspeicheldruse. Virchows Arch 1902, 48: 168 - 180
9. Bliss M. The discovery of insulin. Harris, Edinburgh 1982
10. Joslin E.P. The treatment of diabetes insulin. Lea&Febiger, Philadelphia & New York, 1917
11. Macfarlane I A. The millenia before insulin. In: Textbook of diabetes. Blackwell Scientific Publications. Oxford 1991
12. Noorden C von, Isaach S. Die Zuckerkrankheit und ihre Behandlung. Springer, Berlin 1927
13. Iversen P, Bjerrin T, Bing J. De medicinske nyrelidelser. Munksgaard, København 1941
14. Armanni . In: Cantani A. Der Diabetes Mellitus. Berlin 1877
15. Kimmelstiel P, Wilson C. Intercapillary lesions in the glomeruli of the kidney. Am J Path 1936, 12: 83 – 95
16. Thomsen Å Chr. The kidney in diabetes mellitus. Thesis. Munksgaard, København 1965
17. Lundbæk K. Long-term diabetes. Munksgaard, København 1953.
18. Borch-Johnsen K. The prognosis of insulin-dependent diabetes mellitus. Thesis Lægeforeningens forlag. København 1989
19. Østerby R, Gundersen HJG, Nyberg G, Aurell M. Advanced diabetic glomerulopathy. Quantitative

structural characterisation of non-occluded glomeruli. Diabetes 1987, 36: 612 - 619
20. Mauer SM, Barbosa J, Sutherland DER, Brown DM, Goetz FC. Structural-functional relationships in diabetic nephropathy. J Clin Invest 1984,74: 1143 - 1155
21. Mogensen CE. Progression of nephropathy in long-term diabetics with proteinuria and initial anti-hypertensive treatment. Scand J Clin Lab Invest 1976, 36: 383 - 388
22. Fichtner R. Zur pathologischen Anatomie der Niere beim Diabetes mellitus. Virchows Arch. 1888, 114: 400 - 420
23. Hirose K, Tsuschida H, Østerby R, Gundersen HJG. A strong correlation between glomerulat filtration rate and filtration surface in diabeteic kidney hyperfunction. J Lab Invest 1980, 43: 434 - 437
24. Hitzenberger K. Uber den Blutdruck bei Diabetes mellitus. Wien Arch Inn Med 1921, 2: 461 - 466
25. Nørgaard K, Feldt-Rasmussen B, Borch-Johnsen K, Sælan H, Deckert T. Prevalence of hypertension in type I(insulin dependent) diabetes mellitus. Diabetologia 1990, 33: 407 - 410
26. Keen H, Track IVS, Sowry GSC. Arterial pressure in clinically apparent diabetics. Diab Metab 1975, 1: 159 - 178
27. Mogensen CE. Diabetic renal disease. The quest for normotension - and beyond. Diab Med 1995, 12: 756 - 769
28. Wang PH, Lau J, Chalmers TC. Metanalysis of the effect of insulin therapy of nephropathy in type I diabetes mellitus. Lancet
29. DCCT Reasearch group. The effect of intensive treatment of diabetes on the development and progression of long-term complications in insulin-dependent diabetes mellitus. N Engl J Med 1993, 329: 977 - 986
30. Mathiesen ER, Oxenbøl B, Johansen K, Svendsen PA, Deckert T. Incipient nephropathy in type I(insulin-dependent) diabetes. Diabetologia 1984, 26: 406 - 410
31. Yokoyama H, Deckert T. Central role of TGF-beta in the pathogenesis of diabetic nephropathy and macrovascularcomplications:Ahypothesis.DiabMed, 1996; 13:313-3232.
32. Hansen PM, Chowdhury T, Deckert T, Hellgren A, Bain SC, Pociot F. Genetic variation of the heparan sulphate proteoglycan gene(perlecan gene)- association to urinary albumin excretion in IDDM patients. Diabetes, 1997; 46: 1658-59

2. THE NATURE OF THE DIABETIC GLOMERULUS: PRESSURE-INDUCED AND METABOLIC ABERRATIONS

Pedro Cortes and Bruce L. Riser
Henry Ford Hospital, Detroit, Michigan USA

Early clinical and experimental studies on the pathogenesis of diabetic glomerulosclerosis identified specific mechanisms believed to be unique and crucial in the development and progression of the glomerular lesion. The relative importance of these mechanisms, broadly classified as hemodynamic or metabolic, has been long debated. The hemodynamic factors included systemic arterial hypertension [1-3], glomerular hyperfunction and increased glomerular capillary hydrostatic pressure [4-6]. The metabolic factors related to changes associated with glomerular hypertrophy [7-9], hyperlipidemia [10, 11] and the effects of hyperglycemia exerted either directly [12-14] or through the formation of advanced glycosylation end products [15-17] and increased polyol pathway activity [18]. More recent studies have demonstrated that stimulated cytokine expression is also an important pathogenetic component [19-21]. These cytokines, specially transforming growth factor-β (TGF-β) and platelet-derived growth factor (PDGF) have been shown to induce extracellular matrix (ECM) deposition in glomeruli and to stimulate the mesangial cell synthesis of ECM components [22-25].

As a better understanding of the pathogenesis of diabetic renal disease has been achieved, it is now recognized that diverse alterations in glomerular hemodynamics, metabolic activity and in the action of growth factors are intimately intertwined. Increased plasma glucose concentration, for example, directly stimulates mesangial cell ECM synthesis by activating transcription factors modulated by diacylglycerol-protein kinase C (PKC) [26]. However, PKC may also stimulate TGF-β secretion [27] and TGF-β action, in turn, may contribute to the development of glomerular hypertrophy [28, 29]. Further, this glomerular hypertrophy, will intensify the hemodynamic stress of diabetes [4] leading to further TGF-β stimulation and enhanced ECM synthesis [30]. Not surprisingly, it is the concerted effect of multiple factors that conspire to the glomerular ECM accumulation and mesangial expansion of diabetes, although the relative importance of these may vary depending on the specific clinical or experimental

Mogensen, C.E. (ed.), THE KIDNEY AND HYPERTENSION IN DIABETES MELLITUS.

conditions.

HYPERFUNCTION, INTRAGLOMERULAR PRESSURE AND THE ELASTIC PROPERTIES OF THE GLOMERULUS

Although increased glomerular capillary pressure is a long recognized alteration closely associated with the local deposition of ECM, it has been only recently that information has emerged on the mechanisms involved. A number of distinct sequential steps are part of the process by which the mechanical stimulus of altered hemodynamics is translated into metabolic events. These steps include the application of specific mechanical stimuli, a sensing mechanism and the translation of the signal to evoke changes in protein expression and enzymatic activity. In terms of the causative stimuli, initial studies suggesting increased trafficking and impaired clearance of macromolecules by the mesangium as an important pathogenetic event have been conflictive [31, 32]. More recently, it has been suggested that activation or injury by shear stress of the endothelium lining dilated capillaries near the glomerular vascular pole may be the initial triggering event [33]. Studies in endothelial cells in culture have shown that laminar shear stress results in generation of active TGF-β1, PDGF and altered ECM deposition [34-36].

Additional mechanisms for the coupling of hemodynamic strain and metabolic events have emerged following the demonstration of the unique elastic properties of the glomerular structure and the response of mesangial cells when subjected to mechanical stretch in tissue culture. The elasticity of glomeruli was implied, although not so recognized, from the early histological observations on glomerular size. Mean glomerular volume and mean peripheral capillary wall surface area are 62% and 41%, respectively, greater in histological specimens from kidneys perfused and fixed in situ as compared to values in specimens fixed by immersion, i. e. fixed in the presence (perfusion-fixation) or absence (immersion-fixation) of intraglomerular pressure [37]. Conclusive evidence of glomerular elasticity has been provided by studies in isolated microperfused glomeruli *ex vivo* [38]. As the intraglomerular pressure is increased from zero to levels approximating those observed in the diabetic and in the remnant kidney, glomerular volume increases by about 30% [39]. In addition, due to the high elasticity of the glomerular structure, volume changes reach their maximum within 3-4 seconds following alteration in intraglomerular pressure [40]. This elasticity, therefore, implies the occurrence of significant volume changes even with the most transient variations in intraglomerular pressure.

Glomerular expansion is, obviously, associated with the stretching of its structural components, including the ECM and the cellular constituents. Because both capillary lumina and mesangial regions equally participate in the overall increase in glomerular volume [40], endothelial, mesangial and epithelial cells will all be subjected to stretch as intraglomerular pressure increases. While distentional strain of the epithelial cells may be important as an injurious stimulus in the pathogenesis of some forms of focal glomerulosclerosis [41], it is likely that the mechanical stimulation of the mesangial cell is most important in the development of diabetic mesangial expansion. Due to the central location of the mesangial regions within the glomerular lobule, mesangial cells, in particular, experience substantial mechanical strain. Detailed morphological studies have demonstrated how numerous cytoplasmic projections emerging from the mesangial cell body extend between adjacent capillaries and firmly attach to the perimesangeal regions of the glomerular basement membrane [42]. Therefore, the centrifugal displacement of these regions during glomerular expansion is expected to result in marked tridimensional mesangial cell stretch.

MESANGIAL CELL MECHANICAL STRETCH AND METABOLIC RESPONSE

A vast body of information has been accumulated in recent years demonstrating remarkable morphologic and metabolic alterations resulting from the application of mechanical stimuli in various cell types.

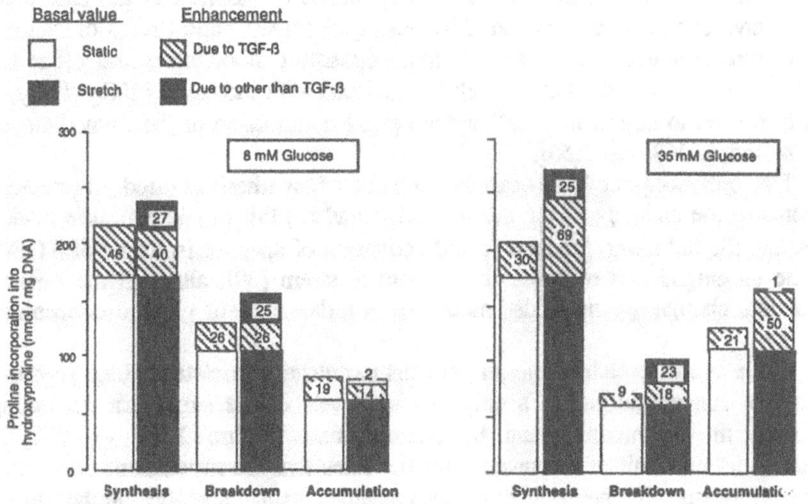

Figure 2-1. Contribution of TGF-β activity to the stretch-altered metabolism of collagen in mesangial cells in tissue culture. A summarv is presented of experiments in which mesangial cells were subjected to cyclic stretch under conditions of different medium glucose concentration. The contribution of the activation of TGF-β and that resulting from other factors on the collagen metabolic response stimulated by stretch was calculated after the addition of specific TGF-β neutralizing antibodies to the culture medium. Mesangial cell stretch in an environment of high glucose concentration markedly increased collagen synthesis without a corresponding increase in breakdown. This resulted in significant net collagen accumulation in the incubation medium which was attributable to TGF-β action. (Modified from ref. 57. Reproduced with permission)

These studies have targeted cells which are under some form of obvious mechanical strain *in vivo*, such as urinary tract, vascular smooth muscle cells, vascular endothelial cells, osteocytes and myocytes. In these cells, cyclic mechanical stretch has been frequently linked to the overproduction of ECM [43, 44]. It has been proposed that both, integrin-related cellular transmembrane molecules and their association with specific extracellular components and the cytoskeleton [45-47] or the opening of stretch-activated ion channels [48] act as the mechanisms sensing the mechanical force. The transmission of the mechanical signal is presumably via the cytoskeleton, specially the actin-myosin stress fibers and the associated signaling molecules [49]. Signaling molecules, including protein kinase C and the inositol phospholipid-specific phospholipase C are rapidly activated during mechanical stretch [50, 51]. Interestingly, mesangial cells in culture demonstrate a PKC-dependent disassembly of the actin cytoskeleton when exposed to high glucose concentrations [52]. Finally, induction of c-*fos* protooncogenes and other immediate, early genes also has been described in mesangial cells subjected to cyclic stretch [53].

Because of the recognition of glomerular distensibility, now mesangial cells can be included among those cells which may alter their metabolism when subjected to mechanical stretch. In fact, many of the stretch-induced metabolic changes described in other cells have been also demonstrated in mesangial cells. Cyclic stretch of mesangial cells in culture stimulates the synthesis and deposition of collagen and other ECM constituents [38, 54]. In addition, it is also associated with increased PKC activity, and temporally related to augmented Ca^{2+} uptake and the induction of the immediate early genes c-*fos* and *zif*268/*erg*-1 [55].

The enhancement of mesangial cell ECM synthesis caused by stretch is proportional to the intensity of the mechanical stimulus [38]. In addition, new evidence indicates that the autocrine production and activation of specific isoforms of TGF-β is part of the mesangial cell response to mechanical strain [30], although the metabolic effects of this change are markedly modulated by the ambient glucose concentration [56].

While cyclic stretch of mesangial cells in culture stimulates collagen synthesis at all glucose concentrations, it is only at high levels of the sugar that net collagen accumulation in the medium can be demonstrated (Figure 2-1) [56, 57]. This accumulation is the result of enhanced catabolic rates that are insufficient to match the increased synthesis. In neutralization experiments using specific antibodies, the potentiating effect of glucose on collagen accumulation has been demonstrated to be mediated via increased TGF-β action [57]. TGF-β neutralization in cells cultured in low glucose reduces collagen synthesis, breakdown and accumulation to a similar extent in static and stretched cultures. However, this neutralization does not modify a portion of the enhanced collagen turnover in stretched cells which is, therefore, attributable to other effects, independently of TGF-β action. In contrast, after using the same antibodies in cells stretched in high glucose concentration, it is evident that an increased TGF-β activity is responsible for the significantly additional increment in the stretch-induced synthesis of collagen which results in net medium accumulation (Figure 2-1). It may be therefore concluded, that the additive overexpression of this growth factor is responsible for the accentuated metabolic effects of mechanical stretch in a milieu of high glucose concentration.

DETERMINANTS OF GLOMERULAR EXPANSION

Because cellular mechanical strain is the consequence of cyclic variations in glomerular volume, it is important to understand which factors control glomerular expansion. These factors have been recently outlined, and their relative importance assessed [40]. As depicted in Table 2-1, the magnitude of glomerular distention will depend on the balance between elements opposing (overall stiffness) and the forces promoting (capillary wall tension) deformation. The degree of glomerular stiffness is primarily determined by the rigidity of the glomerular scaffold, i. e., peripheral basement membrane and mesangial matrix, with a probable small contribution of the non contractile cellular cytoskeletal component [40, 58]. The composition and distribution of the ECM is probably the most important determinant of the glomerular mechanical properties [40]. Mesangial cells are known to maintain cell tone in tissue culture and to be responsible for the contractile activity of isolated, suspended (non perfused) glomeruli [59]. However, under conditions of physiological intraglomerular pressure levels, their maximal contraction only reduces glomerular volume by 3.8%. This, therefore, suggests that mesangial cell tone is only a small contributor to overall glomerular rigidity and volume control.

Table 2-1. Factors determining glomerular expansion

Limiting Glomerular Distention	Favoring Glomerular Distention
Glomerular Stiffness a) Passive component: Intrinsic elasticity of the capillary wall and mesangial matrix b) Active component: Mesangial cell tone	Capillary Wall Tension a) Glomerular size Capillary diameter b) Increased intraglomerular hydrostatic pressure

Increased capillary wall tension is, obviously, the force causing distention of the elastic glomerulus. This wall tension depends on the level of intraluminal hydrostatic pressure and the diameter of the vessel, as defined by the LaPlace's principle [60]. Thus, for any given pressure, glomerular expansion will be greater in large glomeruli containing capillaries with increased vessel radius than in smaller glomeruli formed by capillaries of smaller radius. However, independently of the prevalent stiffness and capillary diameter, it is the wide oscillation in intraglomerular pressure the force which ultimately may cause the repeating glomerular expansion/contraction that causes mesangial mechanical injury. Under normal conditions these oscillations are not expected to occur. Due to the precise adjustment of afferent arteriole contractility, intraglomerular pressure is finely regulated, varying little with alterations in renal perfusion pressure [61]. It is only after this autoregulation is compromised when systemic perfusion pressure may be freely transmitted into the glomerular capillary network.

Glomerular autoregulation of pressure is impaired early in disease processes that eventually lead to glomerulosclerosis, such as in the kidney remnant [61] and in experimental insulin-deficient diabetes [62, 63]. If systemic hypertension is present, this deficient autoregulation will permit the transmission into the glomerulus of, not only a higher mean pressure, but also the wide moment-to-moment variations in arterial pressure which are commonly observed in conditions with hypertension [1, 2, 64]. These variations, and their potential injurious properties, have been only recognized after the availability of continuous blood pressure monitoring. The large oscillations in intraglomerular pressure are particularly significant during the early stages of glomerulosclerosis following subtotal nephrectomy. Contrary to what might have been predicted, the rigidity of the passive component of glomerular stiffness is diminished in these sclerosing glomeruli. Thus, it may be anticipated that the oscillations in intraglomerular pressure will cause periods of glomerular distention/contraction with levels of expansion approximating 18-fold greater than that in normal conditions [40]. This large difference is likely to be of biological significance, imposing an vastly exaggerated mechanical strain on glomerular cells and thus, triggering cytokine activation and metabolic alterations.

In diabetes, glomerular compliance could be expected to be decreased, because non enzymatic glycation and the formation of advanced glycosylation end products increase the maximal stiffness of structures rich in collagen [65, 66]. This change would protect the glomerulus from excessive distention, even when afferent arteriolar autoregulation is impaired. However, direct measurement of compliance in diabetic animals has demonstrated that diabetic glomeruli are as prone to distention as normal glomeruli because both the passive and active components of glomerular stiffness are unaltered [56].

CONCLUSION

The hemodynamic glomerular injury of diabetes is closely related to the loss of afferent arteriole autoregulation of pressure, the presence of increased mean arterial pressure and the occurrence of large moment-to-moment oscillations in systemic arterial pressure. This mechanical injury is possible due to the preservation of a high elasticity of the glomerular structure permitting the repeated stretch/relaxation of the cellular component. The cellular response to this mechanical stimulus is one leading to the enhanced action of growth factors and the increased synthesis of ECM. These processes are further aggravated by an environment of high glucose concentration inducing increased TGF-β activity and collagen accumulation.

REFERENCES

1. Bidani AK, Mitchel KD, Schwatz MM, Navar LG, Lewis EJ. Absence of glomerular injury or nephron loss in a normotensive rat remnant kidney model. Kidney Int 1990; 38: 28-38.
2. Bidani AK, Griffin KA, Picken M, Lansky DM. Continuous telemetric blood pressure monitoring and glomerular injury in the rat remnant kidney model. Am. J Physiol 1993; 265 (Renal Fluid Electrolyte Physiol 34): F391-F398.
3. Gaber L, Walton C, Brown S, Bakris G. Effects of different antihypertensive treatments on morphologic progression of diabetic nephropathy in uninephrectomized dogs. Kidney Int 1994; 46: 161-169.
4. Hostetter TH, Olson JL, Rennke HG, Venkatachalam MA, Brenner BM. Hyperfiltration of remnant nephrons: a potentially adverse response to renal ablation. Am J Physiol 1981; 241(Renal Fluid Electrolyte Physiol 10): F85-F93.
5. Miller PL, Rennke HG, Meyer TW. Hypertension and glomerular injury caused by focal glomerular ischemia. Am J Physiol 1990; 259 (Renal Fluid Electrolyte Physiol 28): F239-F245.
6. Zatz R, Dunn BR, Meyer TW, Anderson S, Rennke HG, Brenner BM. Prevention of diabetic glomerulopathy by pharmacological amelioration of glomerular capillary hypertension. J Clin Invest 1986; 77: 1925-1930.
7. Miller PL, Rennke HG, Meyer TW. Glomerular hypertrophy accelerates hypertensive glomerular injury in rats. Am J Physiol 1991; 262 (Renal Fluid Electrolyte Physiol 30): F459-F465.
8. Yoshida H, Mitarai T, Kitamura M, Suzuki T, Ishikawa H, Fogo A, Sakai O. The effect of selective growth hormone defect in the progression of glomerulosclerosis. Am J Kidney Dis 1994; 23: 302-312.
9. Østerby R, Gundersen HJG. Fast accumulation of basement membrane material and the rate of morphological changes in acute experimental diabetic glomerular hypertrophy. Diabetologia 1980; 18: 493-500.
10. Joles JA, van Goor H, Braam B, Willekes-Koolschijn N, Jansen EHJM, van Tol A, Koomas HA. Proteinuria, lipoproteins and renal apolipoprotein deposits in uninephrectomized female analbuminemic rats. Kidney Int 1995; 47: 442-453.
11. Kasiske BL, O'Donnell MP, Cleary MP, Keane WF. Effects of reduced renal mass on tissue lipids and renal injury in hyperlipidemic rats. Kidney Int 1989; 35: 40-47.
12. Fumo P, Kuncio GS, Ziyadeh FN. PKC and high glucose stimulate collagen a1(IV) transcriptional activity in a reporter mesangial cell line. Am J Physiol 1994; 267 (Renal Fluid Electrolyte Physiol 36): F632-F638.
13. Danne T, Spiro MJ, Spiro RG. Effect of high glucose on type IV collagen production by cultured glomerular epithelial, endothelial and mesangial cells. Diabetes 1993; 42: 170-177.
14. Kreisberg JI, Garoni JA, Radnik R, Ayo SH. High glucose and $TGF\beta_1$ stimulate fibronectin gene expression through a cAMP response element. Kidney Int 1994; 46: 1019-1020.
15. Soulis-Liaparota T, Cooper M, Papazoglou D, Clarke B, Jerums G. Retardation by aminoguanidine of development of albuminuria, mesangial expansion, and tissue fluorescence in streptozotocin-induced diabetic rat. Diabetes 1991; 40: 1328-1334.
16. Yang C-W, Vlassara H, Striker GE, Striker LJ. Administration of AGEs *in vivo* induces genes implicated in diabetic glomerulosclerosis. Kidney Int 1995; 47 (Suppl 49): S55-S58.
17. Cohen MP, Sharma K, Jin Y, Hud E, Wu V-Y, Tomaszewski J, Ziyadeh FN. J Clin Invest 1995; 95: 2338-2345.
18. Goldfarb S, Ziyadeh FN, Kern EFO, Simmons DA. Effects of polyol pathway inhibition and dietary *myo*-inositol on glomerular hemodynamic function in experimental diabetes mellitus in rats. Diabetes 1991; 40: 465-471.
19. Nakamura T, Fukui M, Ebihara I, Osada S. Nagakoa I, Tomino Y, Koide H. mRNA expression of growth factors in glomeruli from diabetic rats. Diabetes 1993; 42: 450-456.
20. Sharma K, Ziyadeh FN. Hyperglycemia and diabetic kidney disease. The case for transforming growth factor-β as a key mediator. Diabetes 1995; 44: 1139-1146.

21. Young BA, Johnson RJ, Alpers CE, Eng E, Gordon C, Floege J, Couser WG. Cellular events in the evolution of experimental diabetic nephropathy. Kidney Int 1995; 47: 935-944.
22. Isaka Y, Fujiwara Y, Ueda N, Kaneda Y, Kamada T, Imai E. Glomerulosclerosis induced by in vivo transfection of transforming growth factor-β or platelet-derived growth factor gene into the rat kidney. J Clin Invest 1993; 92: 2597-2601.
23. Yamamoto T, Nakamura T, Noble NA, Ruoslahti E, Border WA. Expression of transforming growth factor β is elevated in human and experimental diabetic nephropathy. Proc Natl Acad Sci USA 1993; 90: 1814-1818.
24. Floege J, Eng E, Young BA, Alpers CE, Barret TB, Bowen-Pope DF, Johnson RJ. Infusion of platelet-derived growth factor or basic fibroblast growth factor induces selective glomerular mesangial cell proliferation and matrix accumulation in rats. J Clin Invest 1993; 92: 2952-2962.
25. Ziyadeh FN, Sharma K, Ericksen M, Wolf G. Stimulation of collagen gene expression and protein synthesis in murine mesangial cells by high glucose is mediated by autocrine activation of transforming growth factor-?. J Clin Invest 1994; 93: 536-542.
26. Kreisberg JI, Kreisberg SH. High glucose activates protein kinase C and stimulates fibronectin gene expression by enhancing a cAMP response element. Kidney Int 1995; 48 (Suppl. 51): S3-S11.
27. Koya D, Jirousek MR, Lin Y-W, Ishii H, Kuboki K, King GLUT1. Characterization of protein kinase C β isoform activation on gene expression of transforming growth factor β, extracellular matrix components, and prostanoids in the glomeruli of diabetic rats. J Clin Invest 1997; 100: 115-126.
28. Sharma K, Jin Y, Guo J, Ziyadeh FN. Neutralization of TGF-β by anti-TGF-β antibody attenuates kidney hypertrophy and the enhanced extracellular matrix gene expression in STZ-induced diabetic mice. Diabetes 1996; 45: 522-530.
29. Wolf G, Schroeder R, Ziyadeh FN, Thaiss F, Zahner G, Stahl RAK. High glucose stimulates expression of $p27^{Kip1}$ in cultured mouse mesangial cells: relationship to hypertrophy. Am J Physiol 1997; 273 (Renal Physiol 42): 348-356.
30. Riser BL, Cortes P, Heiligh C, Grondin J, Ladson-Wofford S, Patterson D, Narins RG. Cyclic stretching force selectively up-regulates transforming growth factor-β isoforms in cultured rat mesangial cells. Am J Pathol 1996; 148: 1915-1923.
31. Grond J, Koudstaal J, Elema JD. Mesangial function and glomerular sclerosis in rats with aminonucleoside nephrosis. Kidney Int 1985; 27: 405-410.
32. Schwartz MM, Bidani AK. Mesangial structure and function in the remnant kidney. Kidney Int 1991; 40: 226-237.
33. Lee LK, Meyer TW, Pollock AS, Lovett DH. Endothelial cell injury initiates glomerular sclerosis in the rat remnant kidney. J Clin Invest 1995; 96: 953-964.
34. Ohno M, Cooke JP, Dzau VJ, Gibbons GH. Fluid shear stress induces endothelial transforming growth factor beta-1 transcription and production. J Clin Invest 1995; 95: 1363-1369.
35. Mitsumata M, Fishel RS, Nerem RM, Alexander RW, Berk BC. Fluid shear stress stimulates platelet-derived growth factor expression in endothelial cells. Am J Physiol 1993; 265 (Heart Circ Physiol 34): H3-H8.
36. Thoumine O, Nerem RM, Girard PR. Changes in organization and composition of the extracellular matrix underlying cultured endothelial cells exposed to laminar steady shear stress. Lab Invest 1995; 73: 565-576.
37. Miller P, Meyer TW. Methods in laboratory investigation. Effects of tissue preparation on glomerular volume and capillary structure in the rat. Lab Invest 1990; 63: 862-866.
38. Riser BL, Cortes P, Zhao X, Bernstein J, Dumler F, Narins RG. Intraglomerular pressure and mesangial stretching stimulate extracellular matrix formation in the rat. J Clin Invest 1992; 90: 1932-1943.
39. Cortes P, Riser BL, Zhao X, Narins RG. Glomerular volume expansion and mesangial cell mechanical strain: mediators of glomerular pressure injury. Kidney Int 1994; 45 (Suppl 45): S11-S16.
40. Cortes P, Zhao X, Riser BR, Narins RG. Regulation of glomerular volume in normal and partially nephrectomized rats. Am J Physiol 1996; 270 (Renal Fluid Electrolyte Physiol 39): F356-F370.

41. Kriz W, Elger M, Nagata M, Kretzler M, Uiker S, Koeppen-Hagemann I, Tenschert S, Lemley KV. Kidney Int 1994; 45 (Suppl 42): S64-S72.
42. Kriz W, Elger M, Lemley K, Sakai T. Structure of the glomerular mesangium: A biomechanical interpretation. Kidney Int 1990; 38 (Suppl 30): S2-S9.
43. Baskin L, Howard PS, Macarak E. Effect of mechanical forces on extracellular matrix synthesis by bovine urethral fibroblasts in vitro. J Urol 1993; 150: 637-641.
44. Kollros PR, Bates SR, Mathews MB, Horwitz AL, Glagov S. Cyclic AMP inhibits increased collagen production by cyclically stretched smooth muscle cells. Lab Invest 1987; 56: 410-417.
45. Ingber D. Integrins as mechanochemical transducers. Curr Opinion Cell Biol 1991; 3: 841-848.
46. Duncan RL, Turner CH. Mechanotransduction and the functional response of bone to mechanical strain. Calcif Tissue Int 1995; 57: 344-358.
47. Wilson E, Sudhir K, Ives HE. Mechanical strain of rat vascular smooth muscle cells is sensed by specific extracellular matrix/integrin interactions. J Clin Invest 1995; 96: 2364-2372.
48. Naruse K, Sokabe M. Involvement of stretch-activated ion channels in Ca^{2+} mobilization to mechanical stretch in endothelial cells. Am J Physiol 1993; 264 (Cell Physiol 33): C1037-C1044.
49. Burridge K, Chrzanowska-Wodnicka M. Focal adhesions, contractility and signaling. Ann Rev Cell Dev Biol 1996; 12:463-519.
50. Persson K, Sando JJ, Tuttle JB, Steers WD. Protein kinase C in cyclic stretch-induced nerve growth factor production by urinary tract smooth muscle cells. Am J Physiol 1995; 269 (Cell Physiol 38): C1018-C1024.
51. Matsumoto H, Baron CB, Coburn RF. Smooth muscle stretch-activated phospholipase C activity. Am J Physiol 1995; 268 (Cell Physiol 37): C458-C465.
52. Zhou X, Li C, Kapor-Drezgic J, Munk S, Whiteside C. Mesangial cell actin disassembly in high glucose mediated by protein kinase C and the polyol pathway. Kidney Int 1997; 51: 1797-1808.
53. Komuro I, Jayazaki T, Tobe K, Maemura K, Kadowski T, Nagai R. Role of protein kinase system in the signal transduction of stretch-mediated protooncogene expression and hypertrophy of cardiac myocytes. Mol Cell Biochem 1993; 119: 11-16.
54. Harris RC, Haralson MA, Badr KF. Continuous stretch-relaxation in culture alters rat mesangial cell morphology, growth characteristics, and metabolic activity. Lab Invest 1992; 66: 548-554.
55. Akai Y, Homma T, Burns KD, Yasuda T, Badr KF, Harris RC. Mechanical stretch/relaxation of cultured rat mesangial cells induces protooncogenes and cyclooxygenase. Am J Physiol 1994; 267 (Cell Physiol 36): C482-C490.
56. Cortes P, Zhao X, Riser BL, Narins RG. Role of glomerular mechanical strain in the pathogenesis of diabetic nephropathy. Kidney Int 1997; 51: 57-68.
57. Riser B, Cortes P, Yee J, Sharba AK, Asano K, Rodriguez-Barbero A, Narins RG. Mechanical strain- and high glucose-induced alterations in mesangial cell collagen metabolism: role of TGF-β. J Am Soc Nephrol (in press).
58. Welling LW, Grantham JJ. Physical properties of isolated perfused renal tubules and tubular basement membranes. J Clin Invest 1972; 51: 1063-1075.
59. Iversen BM., Kvam FI, Matre K, M¿rkrid L, Horvei G, Bagchus W, Grond J, Ofstad J. Effect of mesangiolysis on autoregulation of renal blood flow and glomerular filtration rate in rats. Am J Physiol 1992; 262 (Renal Fluid Electrolyte Physiol 31): F361-F366.
60. Nave CR, Nave BC. Physics for the Health Sciences. Philadelphia, London and Toronto, WB Saunders Company; 1980, p. 111.
61. Pelayo JC, Westcott JY. Impaired autoregulation of glomerular capillary hydrostatic pressure in the rat remnant nephron. J Clin Invest 1991; 88: 101-105.
62. Ohishi K, Okwueze MI, Vari RC, Carmines PK. Juxtamedullary microvascular dysfunction during the hyperfiltration stage of diabetes mellitus. Am J Physiol 1994; 267 (Renal Fluid Electrolyte Physiol 36): F99-F105.
63. Hayashi K, Epstein M, Loutzenhiser, Forster H. J Am Soc Nephrol 1992; 2: 1578-1586.
64. Parati, G, Omboni S, Di Rienzo M, Frattola A, Albini F, Mancia G. twenty-four hour blood pressure variability: Clinical implications. Kidney Int 1992; 41 (Suppl 37): S24-S28.

65. Menzel EJ, Reihsner R. Alterations of biochemical and biomechanical properties of rat tail tendons caused by non-enzymatic glycation and their inhibition by dibasic amino acids arginine and lysine. Diabetologia 1991; 34:12-16.
66. Huijberts MSP, Wolffenbuttel BHR, Struijker-Boudier HAJ, Crijns FRL, Nieuwenhuijzen-Kruseman AC, Poitevin P, L vy BI. Aminoguanidine treatment increases elasticity and decreases fluid filtration of large arteries from diabetic rats. J Clin Invest 1993; 92:1407-1411.

3. DEFINITION OF DIABETIC RENAL DISEASE IN INSULIN-DEPENDENT DIABETES MELLITUS BASED ON RENAL FUNCTION TESTS

Carl Erik Mogensen
Medical Department M, Aarhus Kommunehospital, Aarhus, Denmark

Defining renal disease and renal involvement in diabetes appeared not to be an easy task, mainly because of the wide range of changes seen. The different degree of abnormalities, often with the same duration of disease, seemingly same quality of long-term metabolic control, and the same type of diabetes, may according to older literature indeed be striking [1-2]. However, with better techniques and more well-defined patients [3] much more consistency is found, although the situation in very long-term diabetes with normoalbuminuria still needs further clarification [4].

The main criteria for a suitable system of definition are outlined in table 3-1: (a) the parameters should have strong prognostic or predictive power with respect to progression of disease, (b) clear pathophysiologic relevance, (c) relation to structural or ultrastructural abnormalities, and (d), because of the generalized disease process of complications, the system should be related to other microvascular and also macrovascular lesions of diabetes. (e) It should also be clinically relevant and treatment-orientated.

Table 3-1. Definition of diabetic renal disease

	Hyperfiltration	Micro-albuminuria	Clinical proteinuria	Structural lesions
Predictive power	Yes/No	Strong	Strong	Likely
Relationship to patho-physiology	Likely	Yes	Yes	Not yet defined
Relationship to structural damage	Not clearly	Yes	Yes	
Associated with other vascular lesions	?	Yes	Yes	Likely

During the last ten years, a diagnostic system has been elaborated [5] that seems to fulfil the criteria indicated above. This system was mainly worked out on the basis of the predictive power of urinary albumin excretion (UAE) as well as knowledge of the pathophysiology of renal changes in diabetes. Structural changes appear still to be secondary elements in the system, but importantly microalbuminuria clearly correlate to structural lesions [6,7]. The »subclinical« level of increased albumin excretion is termed microalbuminuria [8]. So far this system is mainly relevant to insulin-dependent patients, but can also to some extent be used in non-insulin-dependent diabetes.

1. LONGITUDINAL AND FOLLOW-UP STUDIES IN INSULIN-DEPENDENT DIABETICS

Three centres documented the predictive power of raised UAE [8-11]. If UAE is above a certain limit, excretion rate tends to increase with time and spontaneous reversal occurs only in relatively few patients. The exact level above which albumin excretion rate tends to rise with time is not clearly defined [5], but even patients with upper-normal level tends to progress [12]. The level is likely to vary with methods of urine collection, e.g. the critical level of albumin excretion rate was 30 μg/min in a study using overnight urine collection procedure, 70 μg/min in a study using 24-h urine collection, and as low as 15 μg/min in another study using short-term collection during the daytime in hospital. Usually albuminuria is lower during night (lower BP, lower GFR and recumbency), than during the day. The procedure of urine collection seems to be more important than the method used for measuring albumin, but duration of follow-up is also likely to be of significance in these studies.

The risk for future clinical nephropathy over the next decade is markedly higher (≈80%) in the presence of microalbuminuria, compared with patients with a completely normal excretion rate (≈5%). Thus it is now possible to identify, early in the course of diabetes, patients prone to the development of overt renal disease. Longitudinal studies in patients with microalbuminuria have revealed a rather slow rate of progression, as measured by yearly increase in UAE. In recent longitudinal studies, the yearly percentage increase in albumin excretion on conventional insulin treatment was around 15%-20% [13,14]. the yearly increase rate in albumin excretion rate was related to BP elevation [13,14] as well as metabolic control during the observation period [14,15].

The recognition of the ability of microalbuminuria to predict future diabetic nephropathy (DN) leads to the definition of a new stage in the development of renal disease in diabetics, namely, incipient DN [5]. Obvious, effective antihypertensive treatment as well as intensified diabetes treatment reduces microalbuminuria or risk of development of microalbuminuria [6,14,15]. This is likely to change also long-term prognosis.

2. URINARY ALBUMIN EXCRETION IN YOUNG NORMAL SUBJECTS AND PROCEDURE OF URINE COLLECTION

In one study, the UAE measured in 24-h samples in 23 normal men and 20 normal women (aged 22-40 years) averaged 4.7±4.7 µg/min (SD) (range, 2.6-12.6) and 4.3±4.8 (range, 1.1-21.9), respectively [16]. The day-to-day variation in UAE of 24 normal subjects, estimated as the coefficient of variance of 24-h samples, was 31.3%. The mean UAE at rest (short-term collections over several hours, or overnight n=180) was similar (5.8±1.4 µg/min). Similar values have been obtained by other authors, but usually overnight excretion rates are somewhat lower than day-time values, even at complete rest: median daytime UAE: 6.2 µg/min; overnight 3.7 µg/min for men, and similar values for women. There is not very precise correlation between UAE and urinary albumin creatinine ratio or albumin concentration as seen in figure 3-1 [E. Vestbo et al., personal communication].

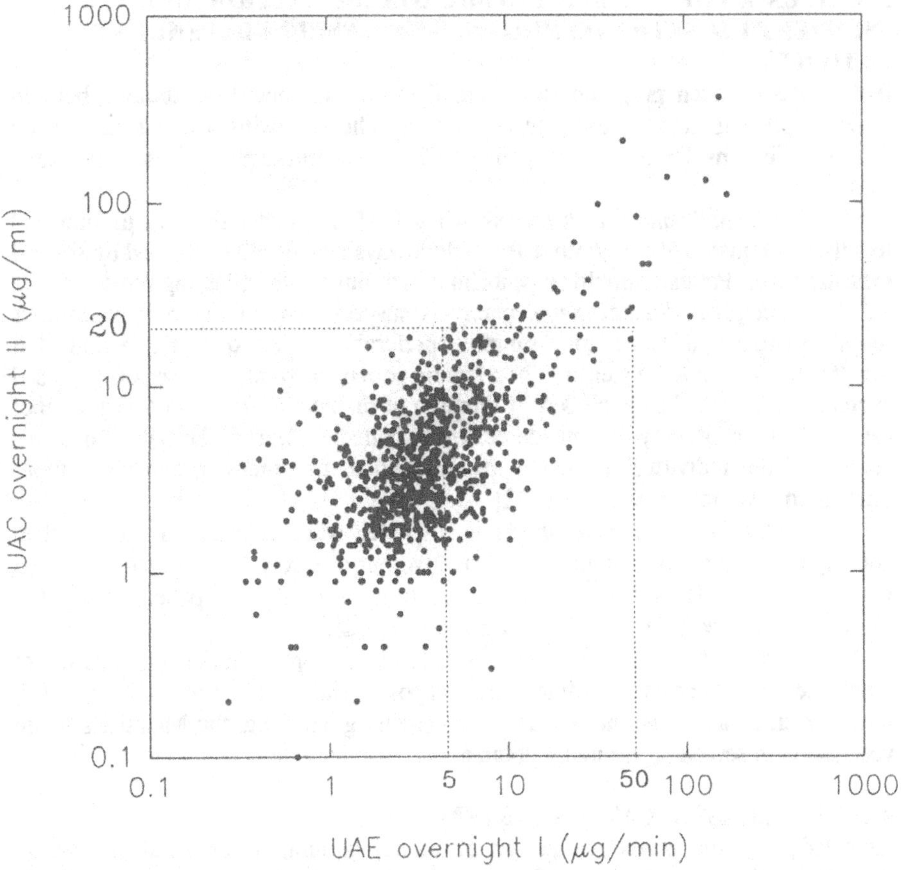

Figure 3-1. Relationship between UAE overnight I and UAC overnight II. Spearmans R = 0.53). (E. Vestbo with permission).

Higher values for UAE are recorded in some elderly non-diabetic individuals in population studies, as related to BP and other risk factors [17]. Because the UAE varies with posture [18] and with exercise [19] and after heavy water drinking [20], evaluation should be carried out only on urine collected under very standardized conditions.

Each of the following procedures is considered acceptable: (a) overnight (approximately 8-h) urine collection, (b) short-term collections over one or several hours in the laboratory or clinic, (c) a 24-h collection, and (d) an early morning urine sample using albumin concentration or possibly corrected for urine flow by creatinine measurements, using albumin creatinine ratio. The latter procedure is gaining more and more acceptance.Because the coefficient of variance in UAE is between 30%-45%, at least three urine collections are recommended [21]. Studies among diabetics should always include measurements in comparable healthy controls, with exactly the same procedures.

3. CRITERIA FOR DIAGNOSING MICROALBUMINURIA AND INCIPIENT DIABETIC NEPHROPATHY IN INSULIN-DEPENDENT PATIENTS

It has recently been proposed that more firm criteria should be applied, both in research projects and in the clinical setting. The following criteria have been proposed for insulin-dependent patients [21], and subsequently used in many studies.

Microalbuminuria is present when UAE is greater than 20 μg/min and less than or equal to 200 μg/min. BP should always be carefully recorded by several measurements. Patients should be peaceful conditions while collecting urine.

Incipient diabetic nephropathy is suspected when microalbuminuria is found in two out of three urine samples, preferably collected over a period of 6 months. Urine should be sterile in non-ketotic patients and other causes of increased excretion rate should be excluded. If duration of diabetes is less than 6 years, other causes should especially be considered. Urine collection during the typical diabetes control of the individual patient is recommended. Long-term prognosis without intensified treatment may be poor [22].

Overt diabetic nephropathy is suspected when UAE rate is greater than 200 μg/min (macroalbuminuria) in at least two out of three urine samples collected within 6 months. Urine samples should be sterile in non-ketotic patients and other causes of increased UAE rate should again be excluded.

Dipsticks for urinary protein should not be applied in the classification of renal disease in diabetes according to this proposal. The dipstick procedure is useful, however, in clinical laboratories, and new screening tests, e.g. the Micral-test® are very useful in screening for microalbuminuria.

4. A NEW CLASSIFICATION SYSTEM

Knowledge of the predictive power of microalbuminuria for renal disease in diabetes, and the description of glomerular hyperfiltration and hypertrophy in diabetes present already at diagnosis, have underlined the need for redefinition of renal involvement in diabetes and DN. A redefinition is most easily achieved by defining new stages in the development of renal changes. These stages, as well as their main characteristics, and outlined in table 3-2. The following stages can be defined:

1. *Glomerular hyperfunction and hypertrophy stage* present at diagnosis. It should be mentioned that certain features in this stage will also accompany diabetes of longer duration when metabolic control is not completely perfect.
2. *The silent stage with normal albumin excretion*, but with structural lesions being present. This stage may last many years; in fact, most patients will continue in this stage throughout their lifetime. Occasionally, in stress situations, e.g. during episodes of very poor metabolic control or during moderate exercise, albumin excretion rate may increase, but this is a readily reversible phenomenon. Transition to stage 3 is seen in 2-4% of cases per year, associated with poor metabolic control, and high level of normoalbuminuria [12,23].
3. *Incipient diabetic nephropathy* is characterized by persistent and, with long observation period, usually increasing microalbuminuria, Patients with microalbuminuria have a very high risk of subsequent development of overt DN.

   However, intervention (e.g. optimized metabolic control as well as antihypertensive treatment) may certainly change the so-called natural history, reversing functional and maybe even stabilizing structural changes. In patients with long-standing diabetes progression may be slower.
4. *Overt diabetic nephropathy* is characterized by proteinuria, hypertension and subsequent fall in glomerular filtration rate (GFR) [24-27]. A decrease in incidence has been reported [28].

   Beta-2-microglobulin excretion starts to increase in the stage of overt DN, at UAE of around 1000 μg/min [13]. Dextran clearance is according to older as well as most recent study only abnormal with advanced proteinuria [5,29].
5. *End-stage-renal-failure* (ESRF). This entity is now the most common cause of uraemia in the US, and very common also elsewhere. Treatment options are also discussed in the final chapters of the book. Recently scepticisms has been expressed about combined pancreas-kidney transplantation, which with the exception of selected patients, may be regarded as experimental medicine [30].

   Systematic screening for early renal involvement is clearly advisable in the diabetes clinic, e.g. by annual measurement of albuminuria in all ranges, or possibly at each visit; more frequent monitoring should be done if UAE is elevated.

4.1 The traditional clinical definition of diabetic nephropathy

The clinical definition can also, as by tradition, be based on measurement of total protein excretion over three 24-h periods. If mean excretion rate is more than 0.5 g over 24 h, DN is likely in a patient with more than 8-10 years' of diabetes, especially with the presence of retinopathy. This level corresponds approximately to >200

Table 3 –2 Microalbuminuria and diabetic nephropathy stages in diabetic renal involvement and nephropathy (DN)

Stage	Designation	Main characteristics	Main structural changes	GFR (ml/min)	UAE	Blood pressure	Suggested main pathophyiologic change
Stage I	Hyperfunction/ hypertrophy[a]	Glomerular hyperfiltration	Glomerular hypertrophy	≈150	May be increased	N	Glomerular volume and pressure increase
Stage II	Normo-albuminuria	Normal UAE	Increasing basal membrane (bm) thickness	Hyperfiltration[a]	N (high in stress situations)	N	changes as indicated above but quite variable
Transition from I→II	Transition phase	High normal UAE	Not known	Hyperfiltration	Increasing	Increasing	Somewhat poor metabolic control
Stage III	Incipient DN, microalbuminuria	Elevated UAE	UAE correlated to structural damage	Still high GFR	20→200μg/min	Elevated compared to stage II	Advancing glomerular lesions. Permeability defect not located.
Stage IV	Overt DN	Clinical proteinuria or UAE > 200 μg/min	Advanced structural damage	"Normal" to advanced reduction	>200 μg/min	Often frank hypertension increase by ≈ 5% yearly	High rate of glomerular closure advancing and severe mesangial expansion.

[a]Changes present probably in all states when control imperfect and in stage II marker of future nephropathy (if GFR > 150 ml/min). The scheme is valid in the "untreated situation" without antihypertensive treatment. BP reduction often reduces albuminuria (Proteinuria →Microalbuminuria→Normoalbuminuria). Stage V is ESRD. Progression associated to HbA_{1c} in all stages (incl. IV).

μg/min in UAE or 300 mg/24h.

With a non-typical course, e.g. short duration of diabetes in patients without retinopathy or rapid progression of disease (e.g. great fall in GFR, very rapid increase in proteinuria, or sudden onset of proteinuria) - renal biopsy would be appropriate in order to diagnose non-diabetic renal disorders. Measurement of total proteinuria is now usually being replaced by measurement specific for albuminuria.

4.2. Abnormalities associated with microalbuminuria

Several abnormalities have been documented in patients with incipient DN.

1. During the stages of incipient DN, the GFR is most often elevated above normal [4]. As microalbuminuria progresses to proteinuria, GFR returns to the »normal« range, which is in fact usually abnormally low IDDM-patients. Patients who enter the stage of clinical proteinuria exhibit gradual decreases in both GFR and renal plasma flow (RPF).
2. Several groups have recognized that elevated BP is an early accompaniment of incipient DN; the magnitude of the elevation is in the range of 10%-15% above values in control subjects and normoalbuminuric diabetics [12,31-33]. Disturbed salt sensitivity may exist [34,35].
3. Diabetic retinopathy is more advanced in patients with microalbuminuria than in patients with silent stage II disease. Importantly, patients at risk for proliferative diabetic retinopathy can be identified on the basis of microalbuminuria [36].
4. Transcapillary escape rate of albumin is increased in incipient DN [37], and plasma lipid abnormalities may be found. Atherosclerotic vascular disease may be predicted [38].
5. A multitude of other features of vascular, cardiac and neurological damage is seen in these patients [39]. Plasma prorenin may also be associated to microalbuminuria [40] but its significance is still not clearly defined [41].

At the time of diagnosis of microalbuminuria or incipient DN, HbA_{1c} is often elevated by in mean by 10%-20% compared to normoalbuminuric diabetics [4]. Patients with microalbuminuria are obviously likely to have been in poorer control, also during many years earlier in the course of diabetes [12,23,33,42,43]. A decreasing incidence has been suggested [28] but recently disputed [44].

5. PROBLEMS RELATED TO DIAGNOSING DIABETIC NEPHROPATHY ON THE BASIS OF URINARY ALBUMIN EXCRETION

There are a number of other causes of raised UAE rate in diabetic patients [23]. UAE may increase during very poor metabolic control [21], and it may also be slightly increased at the time of clinical diagnosis [18]. Such elevations are usually readily reversible. Urinary tract infection may also be present and may cause some elevation of UAE. Other vascular diseases such as essential hypertension and cardiac failure should also be considered [45]. Moderate exercise causes increases in UAE more readily in diabetics than in non-diabetics and is thus a confounding factor [19]. It has also been shown that UAE increases temporarily (less than one hour) after drinking large amounts of water, e.g. 1 litre [20]. Therefore, urine flow and UAE should be stable sometime after the start of water drinking (2 h are advisable) when evaluating patients during, e.g. renal clearance procedures [4].

A special problem regarding interpretation of data is borderline increase of UAE. Some patients do show an excretion rate of around 15-30 μg/min and classification may be difficult during a short observation period. The risk of progression is, however, high [12,46].

6. PROGRESSION OF CHANGES

It is important to note that progression of nephropathy in the incipient phase is rather slow: yearly mean increase rate in UAE is around 15%-20%. GFR probably starts to decline late in this stage. Progression is more rapid in overt nephropathy without treatment and GFR declines at a mean value of 12 ml/min/year [47,48]. To have clinical relevance, studies of the spontaneous course as well as studies on the effect of intervention should be sufficiently long, e.g. at least 2-3 years or even longer. A given treatment modality may also be difficult to sustain for a prolonged period without any other intervention: e.g. can optimized insulin treatment be given without considering BP elevation? Of course the final end point would be prevention of development of ESRF. In any patients under study, however, development of renal failure would last one or more decades. Therefore ESRF is not really a feasible test parameter. Increasing albuminuria and especially fall in GFR are satisfactory intermediate end-points

7. GLOMERULAR FILTRATION RATE IN THE DEFINITION OF DIABETIC NEPHROPATHY

An isolated GFR is not a very appropriate parameter to use in the definition of DN. Both metabolic control and structural lesions have a profound effect on GFR. A low GFR (e.g. 110 ml/min), accompanied by totally normal UAE (≈4 μg/min), usually indicates an excellent prognosis. A similar low GFR may be found in patients with even marked proteinuria. Such a patient is likely to have experienced a decline in GFR, e.g. from 170 to 110 ml/min. The situation may be more complex in patients with normoalbuminuria and long-term diabetes.

When optimizing metabolic control, GFR usually falls, as does an even borderline elevated UAE, whereas a completely normal UAE does not change. Progression of structural lesions also results in reduction of GFR, but in this case UAE increases considerably. Antihypertensive treatment reduces GFR acutely.

Importantly, hyperfiltration in well-defined patients with and without microalbuminuria usually carries poorer prognosis [10,49]. In the follow-up of patients, it is extremely important to *monitor* GFR along with UAE, but the definition of DN should be based upon UAE (in patients without antihypertensive treatment and in their usual glycaemic control).

The coefficient of variance in GFR measurements using a constant infusion technique with 3-6 periods may vary according to the degree of renal involvement or vascular and neuropathic damage in general. In normoalbuminuric and microalbuminuric patients, the coefficient is low, on the order of 5%-8% [4]. In some situations it is not possible to use a constant infusion technique in patients with advanced nephropathy because of voiding problems. Six or more collection periods are usually advisable in such patients and, if the coefficient of variance is high (>15%), this procedure for measuring GFR simply cannot be used. Single-shot measurement of GFR, e.g. using [Cr]EDTA clearance, is then clearly advisable [50,51].

Several more detailed reviews on different aspects of microalbuminuria and diabetic renal disease is available elsewhere [5,23,52-71].

New avenues of prevention and treatment of diabetic renal disease (and other vascular complication) are now in the horizon. Protein kinase C may be involved in genesis of renal complication and inhibitors are now developed [72]. Interestingly agents that cleave glucose-derived protein crosslinks in vitro and in vivo may offer a new potential therapeutic approach [73,74]. This is a somewhat different principle than the inhibitor aminoguanidine, earlier used in experimental diabetes, but recently explored in non-diabetic rats, preventing cardiovascular and renal pathology of ageing [75]. It is also being examined in patients on dialysis [76].

8. NEW DEFINITIONS

New definitions of diabetes has recently been developed [77], as outlined in Fig 3-2. Fasting plasma glucose is now a key parameter. Individuals with repeated values over 7.0 are now by definition diabetes and values between 6.1 and 6.9 are designated impaired fasting plasma glucose [77]. Obviously fasting plasma glucose, not related to age-unlike values during glucose tolerance tests is a continuum. Borderline-values and especially values higher than 6.1 are often related to syndrome X or the metabolic syndrome.

Figure 3-2 New Criteria for diagnosis according to fasting plasma glucose types, definitions, and specificities in diabetes.

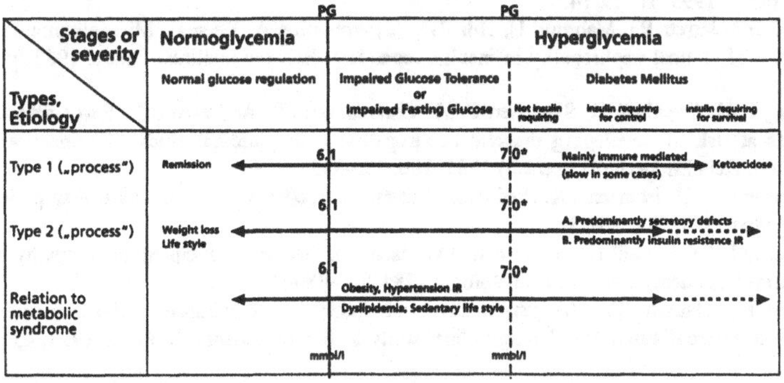

* or casual plasma glucose (PG) ≥11.1 (+symptoms) or 2h PG≥11.1 mmol/l (varies with age)
Blood glucose show lower values.

Blood pressure abnormalities are being redefined, also for diabetics, according to the new Joint National Committee [78-79], with the sixth report. Regarding treatment the following is stated: Antihypertensive drug therapy should be initiated along with life-style modifications, especially weight loss, to reduce arterial blood pressure to below 130/85 mmHg. Angiotensin-converting enzyme inhibitors, α-blockers, calcium antagonists, and diuretics in low doses are preferred because of fewer adverse effects on glucose homeostasis, lipid profiles, and renal function.. Although β-blockers may have adverse effects on peripheral blood flow, prolong hypoglycemia, and mask hypoglycemic symptoms, patients with diabetes who are treated with diuretics and β-blockers experience a similar or greater reduction of CHD and total cardiovascular events compared with persons without diabetes. In patients with diabetic nephropathy, ACE inhibitors are preferred. If ACE inhibitors are contraindicated or are not well tolerated, angiotensin II receptor blockers may be considered. Renoprotection also has been shown by the use of a calcium antagonists.

REFERENCES

1. Thomsen OF, Andersen AR, Christiansen JS, Deckert T. Renal changes in long-term type 1 (insulin-dependent) diabetic patients with and without clinical nephropathy: a light microscopic, morphometric study of autopsy material. Diabetologia 1984; 26: 361-365.
2. Mauer SM, Steffes MW, Ellis EN, Sutherland DER, Brown DM, Goetz FC. Structural-functional relationships in diabetic nephropathy. J Clin Invest 1984; 74: 1143-1155.
3. Hansen KW, Mau Pedersen M, Christensen CK, Schmitz A, Christiansen JS, Mogensen CE. Normoalbuminuria ensures no reduction of renal function in type 1 (insulin-dependent) diabetic patients. J Intern Med 1992; 232: 161-167.
4. Poulsen PL, Ebbehøj E, Mogensen CE. Elevated blood pressure in microalbuminuric IDDM patients is associated with low renal plasma flow (Abstract). Diabetologia 1996; 39: Suppl. 1: A301.
5. Mogensen CE, Christensen CK, Vittinghus E. The stages in diabetic renal disease. With emphasis on the stage of incipient diabetic nephropathy. Diabetes 1983; 32: Suppl. 2: 64-78.
6. Bangstad H-J, Østerby R, Dahl-Jørgensen K, Berg KJ, Hartmann A, Hanssen KF. Improvement of blood glucose control retards the progression of morphological changes in early diabetic nephropathy. Diabetologia 1994; 37: 483-490.
7. Østerby R. Microalbuminuria in diabetes mellitus: Is there a structural basis? (editorial). Nephrol Dial Transpl 1995; 10: 12-14.
8. Viberti GC, Jarrett RJ, Mahmud U, Hill RD, Argyropoulos A, Keen H. Microalbuminuria as a predictor of clinical nephropathy in insulin-dependent diabetes mellitus. Lancet 1982; i: 1430-1432.
9. Parving H-H, Oxenbøll B, Svendsen PAA, Christiansen JS, Andersen AR. Early detection of patients at risk of developing diabetic nephropathy: a longitudinal study of urinary albumin excretion. Acta Endocrinol (Copenh) 1982; 100: 550-555.
10. Mogensen CE, Christensen CK. Predicting diabetic nephropathy in insulin-dependent patients. N Engl J Med 1984; 311: 89-93.
11. Mathiesen ER, Oxenbøll B, Johansen K, Svendsen PA, Deckert T. Incipient nephropathy in type I (insulin-dependent) diabetes. Diabetologia 1984; 26: 406-410.
12. Poulsen PL, Hansen KW, Mogensen CE. Ambulatory blood pressure in the transition from normo- to microalbuminuria. A longitudinal study in IDDM patients. Diabetes 1994; 43: 1248-1253.
13. Christensen CK, Mogensen CE. The course of incipient diabetic nephropathy: Studies of albumin excretion and blood pressure. Diabetic Med 1985; 2: 97-102.
14. Feldt-Rasmussen B, Mathiesen E, Deckert T. Effect of two years of strict metabolic control on the progression of incipient nephropathy in insulin-dependent diabetes. Lancet 1986; ii: 1300-1304.
15. The Diabetes Control and Complications Trial Research Group. The effect of intensive treatment of diabetes on the development and progression of long-term complications in insulin-dependent diabetes mellitus. New Engl J Med 1993; 329: 977-986.

16. Mogensen CE. »Microalbuminuria and kidney function in diabetes: Notes on methods, interpretation and classification.« In *Methods in Diabetes Research, volume II: Clinical Methods*, W.L. Clarke, J. Larner, S.L. Pohl, eds. New York, Chichester, Brisbane, Toronto, Singapore: John Wiley & Sons, 1986; pp 611-631.
17. Vestbo E, Damsgaard EM, Frøland A, Mogensen CE. Urinary albumin excretion in a population based cohort. Diabetic Med 1995; 12: 488-493.
18. Mogensen CE. Urinary albumin excretion in early and long-term juvenile diabetes. Scand J Clin Lab Invest 1971; 28: 183-193.
19. Christensen CK, Mogensen CE. Acute and long-term effect of antihypertensive treatment on exercise-induced albuminuria in incipient diabetic nephropathy. Scand J Clin Lab Invest 1986; 46: 553-559.
20. Viberti GC, Mogensen CE, Keen H, Jacobsen FK, Jarrett RJ, Christensen CK. Urinary excretion of albumin in normal man. The effect of water loading. Scand J Clin Lab Invest 1982; 42: 147-152.
21. Mogensen CE, Chachati A, Christensen CK, Close CF, Deckert T, Hommel E, Kastrup J, Lefebvre P, Mathiesen ER, Feldt-Rasmussen B, Schmitz A, Viberti GC. Microalbuminuria: an early marker of renal involvement in diabetes. Uremia Invest 1985-86; 9: 85-95.
22. Messent JWC, Elliott TG, Hill RD, Jarrett RJ, Keen H, Viberti GC. Prognostic significance of microalbuminuria in insulin-dependent diabetes mellitus: A twenty-three year follow-up study. Kidney Int 1992; 41: 836-839.
23. Mogensen CE, Vestbo E, Poulsen PL, Christiansen C, Damsgaard EM, Eiskjær H, Frøland A, Hansen KW, Nielsen S, Mau Pedersen M. Microalbuminuria and potential confounders. A review and some observations on variability of urinary albumin excretion. Diabetes Care 1995; 18: 572-581.
24. Rossing P, Hommel E, Smidt UM, Parving H-H. Impact of arterial blood pressure and albuminuria on the progression of diabetic nephropathy in IDDM Patients. Diabetes 1993; 42: 715-719.
25. Rossing P, Hommel E, Smidt UM, Parving H-H. Reduction in albuminuria predicts a beneficial effect on diminishing the progression of human diabetic nephropathy during antihypertensive treatment. Diabetologia 1994; 37: 511-516.
26. Rossing P, Hommel E, Smidt UM, Parving H-H. Reduction in albuminuria predicts diminished progression in diabetic nephropathy. Kidney Int 1994; Suppl. 45: S145-149.
27. Parving H-H, Rossing P, Hommel E, Smidt UM. Angiotensin-converting enzyme-inhibition in diabetic nephropathy - 10 years experience. Am J Kidney Dis 1995; 26: 99-107.
28. Bojestig M, Arnqvist HJ, Hermansson G, Karlberg BE, Ludvigsson J. Declining incidence of nephropathy in insulin-dependent diabetes mellitus. N Engl J Med 1994; 330: 15-18.
29. Deckert T, Kofoed-Enevoldsen A, Vidal P, Nørgaard K, Andreasen HB, Feldt-Rasmussen B. Size- and charge selectivity of glomerular filtration in IDDM patients with and without albuminuria. Diabetologia 1993; 36: 244-251.
30. Remuzzi G, Ruggenenti P, Mauer SM. Pancreas and kidney/pancreas transplants: experimental medicine or real improvement? Lancet 1994; 343: 27-31.
31. Mogensen CE, Christensen CK. Blood pressure changes and renal function changes in incipient and overt diabetic nephropathy. Hypertension 1985; 7: II-64-II-73.
32. Mogensen CE. Diabetic Renal Disease: The quest for normotension - and beyond. Diabetic Med 1995; 12: 756-769.
33. Molitch ME, Steffes MW, Cleary PA, Nathan DM. Baseline analysis of renal function in the diabetes control and complications trial. Kidney Int 1993; 43: 668-674.
34. Strojek K, Grzeszczak W, Lacka B, Gorska J, Keller CK, Ritz E. Increased prevalence of salt sensitivity of blood pressure in IDDM with and without microalbuminuria. Diabetologia 1995; 38: 1443-1448.
35. Gerdts E, Svarstad E, Myking OL. Lund-Johansen P, Omvik P. Salt sensitivity in hypertensive type-1 diabetes mellitus. Blood Pressure 1996; 5: 78-85.
36. Vigstrup J, Mogensen CE. Proliferative diabetic retinopathy: at risk patients identified by early detection of microalbuminuria. Acta Ophthalmol 1985; 63: 530-534.
37. Feldt-Rasmussen B. Increased transcapillary escape rate of albumin in type 1 (insulin-dependent) diabetic patients with microalbuminuria. Diabetologia 1986; 29: 282-286.

38. Deckert T, Yokoyama H, Mathiesen E, Rønn B, Jensen T, Feldt-Rasmussen B, Borch-Johnsen K, Jensen JS. Cohort study of predictive value of urinary albumin excretion for atherosclerotic vascular disease in patients with insulin dependent diabetes. BMJ 1996; 312: 871-874.
39. Mogensen CE, Christensen CK, Christensen PD, Hansen KW, Mølgaard H, Mau Pedersen M, Poulsen PL, Schmitz A, Thuesen L, Østerby R. »The abnormal albuminuria syndrome in diabetes.« In *Current Topics in Diabetes Research. Front Diabetes*, F. Belfiore, R.N. Bergman, G.M. Molinatti, eds. Basel: Karger, 1993; pp 86-121.
40. Franken AAM, Derkx FHM, Man in't Veld AJ, et al. High plasma prorenin in diabetes mellitus and its correlation with some complications. J Clin Endocrinol Metab 1990; 71: 1008-1015.
41. Matinlauri IH, Rönnemaa T, Koskinen PJ, Aalto MA, Viikari JSA, Irjala KMA. Elevated serum total renin is insensitive in detecting incipient diabetic nephropathy. Diabetes Care 1995; 18: 1357-1361.
42. Mathiesen ER, Rønn B, Storm B, Foght H, Deckert T. The natural course of microalbuminuria in insulin-dependent diabetes: a 10-year prospective study. Diabetic Med 1995; 12: 482-487.
43. Krolewski AS, Laffel LMB, Krolewski M, Quinn M, Warram JH. Glycosylated hemoglobin and the risk of microalbuminuria in patients with insulin-dependent diabetes mellitus. N Engl J Med 1995; 332: 1251-1255.
44. Rossing P, Rossing K, Jacobsen P, Parving H-H. Unchanged incidence of diabetic nephropathy in IDDM patients. Diabetes 1995; 44: 739-743.
45. Christensen CK, Krusell LR, Mogensen CE. Increased blood pressure in diabetes: essential hypertension or diabetic nephropathy? Scand J Clin Lab Invest 1987; 47: 363-370.
46. Microalbuminuria Collaborative Study Group UK. Risk factors for development of microalbuminuria in insulin dependent diabetic patients: a cohort study. BMJ 1993; 306: 1235-1239.
47. Mogensen CE. Angiotensin converting enzyme inhibitors and diabetic nephropathy (editorial). BMJ 1992; 304: 227-228.
48. Mogensen CE. Long-term antihypertensive treatment inhibiting progression of diabetic nephropathy. BMJ 1982; 285: 685-688.
49. Rudberg S, Persson B, Dahlquist G. Increased glomerular filtration rate as a predictor of diabetic nephropathy - An 8-year prospective study. Kidney Int 1992; 41: 822-828.
50. Brøchner-Mortensen J. Current status on assessment and measurement of glomerular filtration rate. Clin Physiol 1985; 5: 1-17.
51. Jones SL, Viberti GC. »Methodologies to assess renal function in diabetes mellitus.« In *Research Methodologies in Human Diabetes. Diabetes Forum Series, Volume V*, C.E. Mogensen, E. Standl, eds. Berlin: Walter de Gruyter, 1994; pp 359-385.
52. Mogensen CE, Hansen KW, Sommer, S, Klebe J, Christensen CK, Marshall S, Schmitz A, Mau Pedersen M, Christiansen JS, Pedersen EB. »Microalbuminuria: Studies in diabetes, essential hypertension, and renal diseases as compared with the background population.« In *Advances in Nephrology, Vol. 20*, J.P. Grünfeld, J.F. Bach, J.-L. Funck-Brentano, M.H. Maxwell, eds. St. Louis, Baltimore, Boston, Chicago, London, Philadelphia, Sydney, Toronto: Mosby Year Book, 1991; pp 191-228.
53. Mogensen CE. Management of renal disease and hypertension in insulin-dependent diabetes, with an emphasis on early nephropathy. Curr Opin Nephrol Hypertens 1992; 1: 106-115.
54. Mauer SM, Mogensen CE, Viberti GC. Introduction. Symposium on the Progression Diabetic Nephropathy. Kidney Int 1992; 41: 717-718.
55. Mogensen CE, Hansen KW, Østerby R, Damsgaard EM. Blood pressure elevation versus abnormal albuminuria in the genesis and prediction of renal disease in diabetes. Diabetes Care 1992; 15: 1192-1204
56. Mogensen CE, Damsgaard EM, Frøland A, Hansen KW, Nielsen S, Mau Pedersen M, Schmitz A, Thuesen L, Østerby R. Reduced glomerular filtration rate and cardiovascular damage in diabetes: a key role for abnormal albuminuria. Acta Diabetol 1992; 29: 201-213.
57. Mogensen CE, Poulsen PL, Heinsvig EM. «Abnormal albuminuria in the monitoring of early renal changes in diabetes.» In *Concepts for the Ideal Diabetes Clinic. Diabetes Forum Series, Volume 4*, C.E. Mogensen, E. Standl, eds. Berlin, New York: Walter de Gruyter, 1993; pp 289-313.

58. Mogensen CE, Hansen KW, Nielsen S, Mau Pedersen M, Rehling M, Schmitz A. Monitoring diabetic nephropathy: Glomerular filtration rate and abnormal albuminuria in diabetic renal disease - reproducibility, progression, and efficacy of antihypertensive intervention. Am J Kidney Dis 1993; 22: 174-187.
59. Mogensen CE, Berne C, Ritz E, Viberti G-C. Preface. The kidney in Type 2 (non-insulin-dependent) diabetes mellitus. Diabetologia 1993; 36: 977.
60. Mogensen CE. Microalbuminuria, early blood pressure elevation and diabetic renal disease. Curr Opin Endocrinol 1994; 4: 239-247.
61. Mogensen CE. Systemic blood pressure and glomerular leakage with particular reference to diabetes and hypertension. J Intern Med 1994; 235: 297-316.
62. Mogensen CE. Microalbuminuria in prediction and prevention of diabetic nephropathy in insulin-dependent diabetes mellitus patiens. J Diabetes and Its Complications 1995; 9: 337-349.
63. Alzaid AA. Microalbuminuria in patients with NIDDM: An overview. Diabetes Care 1996; 19: 79-89.
64. Gilbert RE, Cooper ME, McNally PG, O'Brien RC, Taft J, Jerums G. Microalbuminuria: Prognostic and therapeutic implications in diabetes mellitus. Diabetic Med 1994; 11: 636-645.
65. DeFronzo RA. Diabetic nephropathy: etiologic and therapeutic considerations. Diabetes Rev 1995; 3: 510-564.
66. Breyer JA. Medical management of nephropathy in type I diabetes mellitus: Current recommendations. J Am Soc Nephrol 1995; 6: 1523-1529.
67. Gosling P. Microalbuminuria: a marker of systemic disease. Br J Hosp Med 1995; 54: 285-290.
68. Raskin GS, Tamborlane WV. Molecular and physiological aspects of nephropathy in type I (insulin-dependent) diabetes mellitus. J Diabetes and Its Complications 1996; 10: 31-37.
69. Clark CM, Lee DA. Prevention and treatment of the complications of diabetes mellitus. N Engl J Med 1995; 332: 1210-1217.
70. Mogensen CE. »Management of the diabetic patient with elevated blood pressure or renal disease. Early screening and treatment programs: albuminuria and blood pressure.« In *Hypertension: Pathology, Diagnosis & Management. 2nd ed*, J.H. Laragh, B.M. Brenner, eds. New York: Raven Press Ltd., 1995; pp 2335-2365.
71. Leese GP, Vora JP. The management of hypertension in diabetes: with special reference to diabetic kidney disease. Diabetic Med 1996; 13: 401-410.
72. Ishii H, Jirousek MR, Koya D, Takagi C, Xia P, Clermont A, Bursell S-E, Kern TS, Ballas LM, Heath WF, Stramm LE, Feener EP, King GL. Amelioration of vascular dysfunctions in diabetic rats by an oral PKC β inhibitor. Science 1996; 272: 728-731.
73. Drickamer K. Breaking the curse of the AGEs. Nature 1996; 382: 211-212.
74. Vasan S, Zhang X, Zhang X, Kapurniotu A, Bernhagen J, Teichberg S, Basgen J, Wagle D, Shih D, Terlecky I, Bucala R, Cerami A, Egan J, Ulrich P. An agent cleaving glucose-derived protein crosslinks in vitro and in vivo. Nature 1996; 382: 275-278.
75. Li YM, Steffes M, Donnelly T, Liu C, Fuh H, Basgen J, Bucala R, Vlassara H. Prevention of cardiovascular and renal pathology of aging by the advanced glycation inhibitor aminoguanidine. Proc Natl Acad Sci USA 1996; 93: 3902-3907.
76. Friedman EA. Will pimagidine improve survival of diabetics on dialysis? Nephrol Dial Transplant 1996; 11: 1524-1527.
77. The Expert Committee on the Diagnosis and Classification of Diabetes Mellitus. Report of the Expert Committee on the Diagnosis and Classification of Diabetes Mellitus. Diabetes Care 1997; 20: 1183-1197.
78. The sixth report of the Joint National Committee on Prevention, Detection, Evaluation and Treatment of High Blood Pressure. Arch Intern Med 1997; 157: 2413-2446.
79. Fagan TC. Evolution of the Joint National Committee Reports, 1988-1997. Evolution of the Science of Treating Hypertension. Arch Intern Med 1997; 157: 2401-2402

4. RETINOPATHY IN RELATION TO ALBUMINURIA AND BLOOD PRESSURE IN IDDM

Nish Chaturvedi, John H Fuller
EURODIAB, Department of Epidemiology and Public Health, University College London, UK

The microvascular complications of diabetes, retinopathy and nephropathy, are often considered as a single entity, with the implicit assumption of a close correlation between these complications, both in terms of occurrence, and in terms of putative risk factors 1-3. It is certainly true that patients with one complication will generally demonstrate signs of the other, and that glycaemic control and duration of diabetes are clear risk factors for each of these complications4-10. But in contrast, current evidence indicates that while the majority of patients with IDDM will develop retinopathy (estimates vary from 70% to 100%) [11-13], only about a third of patients will develop detectable nephropathy [2,14], even when glycaemic control is poor, and the duration of diabetes is long [2,15].

Raised blood pressure is an important associated factor with even relatively early stages of diabetic renal disease [16,17]. But while blood pressure and albuminuria are unquestionably closely related [18], there is still controversy about whether increases in blood pressure result in renal damage, or whether albuminuria precedes the rise in blood pressure, or whether in fact each of these variables could be risk factors for the other [19]. Several studies have demonstrated a relationship between retinopathy and blood pressure [6,9,20-23], but whether this relationship is confounded by renal disease or is truly independent remains unclear [23-25]

This chapter will describe the relationship between retinopathy and nephropathy, and examine the role of blood pressure in this association, both in terms of aetiology and intervention. One major difficulty in assessing these relationships is the near ubiquity of retinopathy in people with diabetes. However, the EURODIAB and Diabetes Control and Complications Trial studies have shown that this need not necessarily be so [26,27]. The EURODIAB study, a cross-sectional survey of 3250 people with IDDM, drawn from 31 centres across Europe, had substantial numbers of people without retinopathy. This is probably due to several design features of that study. The first is that the sampling of IDDM patients in all clinics was stratified by age, sex, and most importantly duration of diabetes, thus about a third of patients had a very short duration of diabetes (less than 8 years). This is in contrast with other study populations, which are generally biased towards those with a relatively long duration of diabetes. Secondly, glycaemic control in this study was relatively good. This is probably a reflection of the current clinical acceptance of the importance of tight glycaemic control in the avoidance of diabetes related complications.

Thus in the EURODIAB study, the prevalence of any retinopathy was 82%, even after 20 years duration of diabetes [26]. In contrast, only 30% of these participants had either micro- or macroalbuminuria. In those with macroalbuminuria, 89% had some degree of retinopathy, compared with 30% in the normoalbuminuric group. However, in those with proliferative retinopathy, only 63% had albuminuria, compared to 20% in those without retinopathy. This confirms that albuminuria without retinopathy is rare, while retinopathy without albuminuria is common [2].

There is now evidence that the key to understanding the association between retinopathy and nephropathy is blood pressure [2,9,15,18,23]. The EURODIAB study showed that the prevalence of retinopathy was positively correlated with blood pressure, in those with and without nephropathy, but the increase in prevalence of retinopathy with blood pressure was more marked in those with nephropathy than those without[15]. Others have claimed that this relationship is confined to those with nephropathy [23,24], but on closer inspection, this may not necessarily be true. In the study by Norgaard et al [23], in those without nephropathy, the prevalence of advanced retinopathy was 17% in the hypertensive group, and 9% in the normotensive group; a clinically important effect even if not statistically significant. Similarly, Krolewski et al claimed that there was no relationship between isolated retinopathy and blood pressure [24], but blood pressure on average was 6mmHg higher than those without complications.

More strikingly, Stephenson et al, demonstrated an important new feature in the relationship between blood pressure and albumin excretion rate (AER). In people with retinopathy, AER increased exponentially with increasing blood pressure, and the curve describing this relationship is very similar to that describing the relationship for the whole EURODIAB population (figure 4-1) [15]. However, in those without retinopathy, there was no rise in AER with increasing blood pressure. From these data, it would appear that the relationship between blood pressure and nephropathy is dependent upon retinopathy. Differences in diabetes duration or glycaemic control could not account for this observation, as these were adjusted for in the analysis. Furthermore, when retinopathy status was stratified by good or poor glycaemic control, any effect of glycaemic control was confined to those with retinopathy. The effect of blood pressure on nephropathy was most marked in those with poor glycaemic control, and attenuated (although still present) in those with good control. In people without retinopathy, the relationship between blood pressure and AER was identical in those with good and poor glycaemic control.

How can we account for this difference in relationship between blood pressure and AER by retinopathy status? and what does it mean for further research and clinical practice?

This relationship has not been demonstrated in other studies for two reasons, firstly, others have not stratified by retinopathy status when examining the blood pressure/AER relationship, and secondly, there have not been sufficient numbers of people without retinopathy to examine the relationship in this subgroup separately. But it is unlikely that this is a chance finding, due to the large numbers of patients both with and without retinopathy in the EURODIAB study, and the clear clinical and statistical significance of these findings.

Studies of clinic based populations are often criticised because they are often prone to bias. This is an unlikely explanation for the observed findings in this case however, as one would have to postulate a rather complicated patient selection bias, i.e. patients with retinopathy were somehow selected for their propensity to show a relationship between blood pressure and nephropathy, whilst those without retinopathy were selected on the basis that they had no relationship between blood pressure and nephropathy. This seems highly unlikely, particularly as this relationship was observed in all centres which took part in the EURODIAB study, indicating that such a selection bias would have had to have taken place in each centres.

A further explanation is that this relationship could be due to confounding. People with retinopathy tend to have poorer glycaemic control, and have had diabetes for longer. Thus the relationship of blood pressure and AER could simply be a reflection of the poor control and long duration of diabetes in people with diabetes. Whilst these factors were adjusted for in the above analysis, there remains the possibility of residual confounding. It is well known that duration of diabetes is poorly estimated in studies of people with diabetes, and there is no easy way of assessing the duration of the pre-diagnostic phase. Glycaemic control was measured by a central assessment of

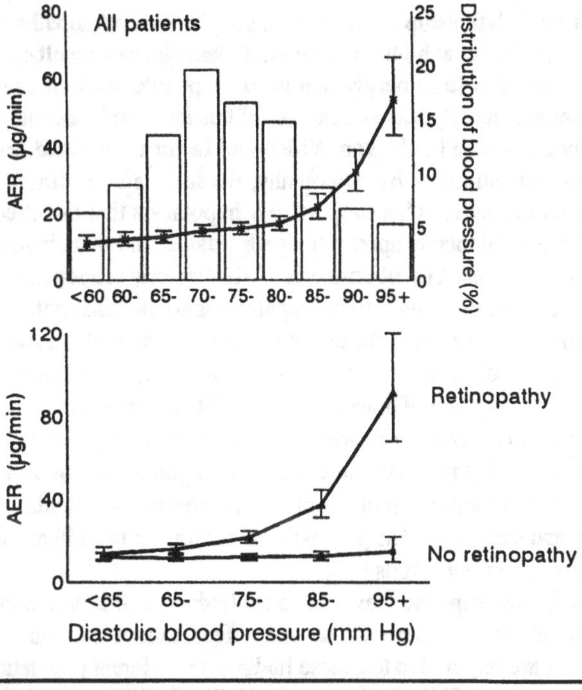

Figure 4-1. Geometric mean AER by diastolic blood pressure in all patients (top, n=3046) and in those with (n=1098) and without (n=1280) retinopathy (bottom). Geometric means with 95% confidence intervals are adjusted for duration of diabetes and HbA_{1c}. With permission from Diabetologia.

glycated haemoglobin, which is a good measure of glycaemic control in the previous three months, and is likely to be correlated with previous glycaemic control, but is obviously not as good as repeated measures of glycaemic control throughout the history of disease. Thus adjustment for these measured variables does not fully adjust for duration and glycaemic control, and a degree of confounding remains. An indication of the likely effect of residual confounding can be obtained from comparing the unadjusted and adjusted effects. In this case, the unadjusted levels of AER by blood pressure and retinopathy status were similar to those of the adjusted effects, and residual confounding is an unlikely explanation for this observation. There may however be other confounders, such as smoking, which were not controlled for in this analysis. Again, it is unlikely that these factors can account for this relationship, as they are less strongly related to complications than duration of diabetes and glycaemic control, and would therefore have a minimal effect in any adjustment.

It is therefore possible that this may be a true and independent association. There is clear evidence that hyperglycaemia is associated with an unfavourable lipid profile and increased blood pressure, as part of a syndrome of insulin resistance[28]. Even in people with diabetes, those with glucose levels at the higher end of the spectrum were more likely to have an unfavourable lipoprotein pattern than those with relatively good control [29,30] These disturbances contribute to vascular damage, as evidenced by raised von Willebrand factor and other indicators of endothelial damage[30,32]. This vascular damage is reflected in the kidney, with resulting protein excretion in the urine [10,31,33,34]. But we hypothesise that this relationship is stronger in people with retinopathy, in other words people with retinopathy are at higher risk of renal damage, as a result of disturbances in vascular risk factors due to hyperglycaemia, than people without retinopathy. The presence of retinopathy merely acts as a marker of this increased susceptibility. When we plot the association between lipids, von Willebrand factor or glycated haemoglobin and albumin excretion rate stratified by retinopathy, we show a very similar picture to that observed for blood pressure. This supports our hypothesis that the effect of these risk factors on renal disease depends upon retinopathy status, and that changes in these risk factors occur before the onset of albuminuria. What exactly retinopathy is a marker for is unclear. A genetic predisposition to retinopathy cannot be ruled out. Those who have this predisposition will have some degree of retinopathy, even if duration of diabetes is short and glycaemic control good. Others will only develop retinopathy if glycaemic control is poor, or the duration of diabetes is long. This observation might explain why the risk of retinopathy cannot fully be accounted for by glycaemic control and duration of diabetes, and indicates that no matter how well blood glucose is controlled, retinopathy will always be found in a subgroup of people with diabetes. A candidate for this gene is not yet available, and studies of ACE gene polymorphism, the most likely candidate so far, have produced disappointing results [35].

The final, most important caveat of these findings is that they were demonstrated in a cross-sectional study, where cause and effect cannot be concluded. Further longitudinal studies are required to test these findings on different populations, with better measures of confounders. If these findings are replicated in other studies, we need to search for the pathogenetic mechanism, and consider what this means for clinical practice.

With increasing recognition of the importance of tight glycaemic control in reducing the risk of retinopathy, it is likely that the proportion of people without retinopathy will increase [27]. The identification of those who develop or who are at risk of developing retinopathy, despite good control, would be of importance in ensuring that interventions are instituted early, at relatively low levels of blood pressure, and which would reduce the progression of renal disease, and thus the risk of nephropathy and perhaps even macrovascular disease.

One such important intervention which currently has clear evidence of benefit for at least nephropathy is the use of ACE inhibitors[36]. Given the relationships between blood pressure, nephropathy and retinopathy, it is reasonable to suggest that this class of agent may be of value in retinopathy as well. Trials in IDDM [37,39] as well as NIDDM patients [40] all demonstrate a clinically important effect in terms of progression of retinopathy. A combined analysis of these trials suggests that a halving in the risk of progression of retinopathy can be observed over a period as short as two years (figure 4-2). The largest trial by far in this group of studies is the EUCLID study, which together with a halving in progression of retinopathy associated with ACE inhibitor treatment also demonstrated a reduction in the incidence of retinopathy by 30% [39].

These are extremely important findings, both in terms of understanding the pathogenesis of microvascular complications, and in terms of clinical practice. It is clear that for nephropathy in IDDM, ACE inhibitors are superior to other classes of antihypertensive agent, despite similar achieved reductions in systemic blood pressure. This would indicate that other mechanisms are involved. No direct comparisons between ACE

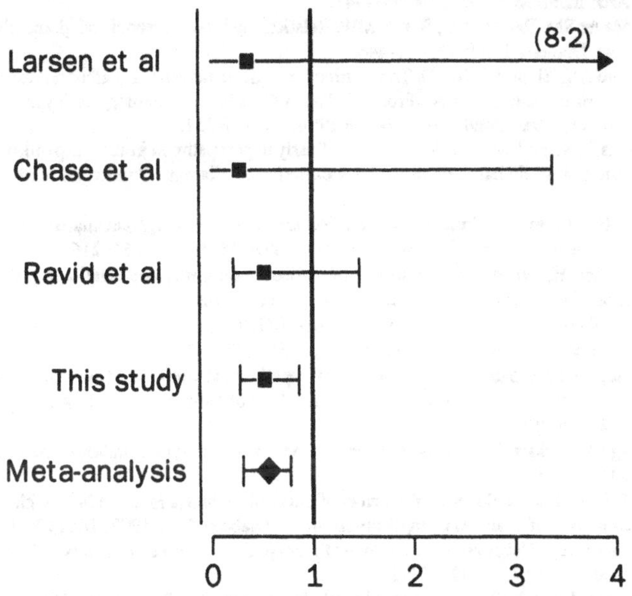

Figure 4-2. Odds ratios (95% CI) for progression of retinopathy for both groups in EUCLID and previous studies. (With permission, the Lancet)

inhibitors and other classes of agent have been made in terms of retinopathy, but in the EUCLID study, adjustment for changes in systemic blood pressure had little impact on the observed beneficial treatment effect. This should not be the case if the reduction in risk of retinopathy progression in the treatment arm is solely due to changes in systemic blood pressure. A likely explanation for these findings is the existence of local renin-angiotensin systems in the eye and the kidney[41].

Thus it is hypothesised that the usually efficient blood-retina barrier is breached in the presence of diabetes[42], and that the leakage of angiotensin II has a direct effect on the genesis of diabetic retinopathy. Direct administration of ACE inhibitors reduce this leakage[42].

Both EUCLID and earlier studies on retinopathy have limitations which would not support immediate changes in current prescribing. However, the implications of these findings for clinical practice are enormous. If the EUCLID findings were to be replicated in further, adequately powered clinical trials, it would not be unreasonable to suggest that all IDDM patients should receive ACE inhibitors, regardless of their complication status. The beneficial effects of ACE inhibitors on retinopathy were not restricted to patients with microalbuminuria at baseline; equivalent beneficial effects were observed in both normoalbuminuric and microalbuminuric patients. So to restrict ACE inhibitors to those patients at risk of nephropathy would exclude many patients who may stand to benefit in terms of retinopathy. The outcome of such trials is keenly awaited.

REFERENCES

1. Root HF, Pote WH, Frehner H. Triopathy of diabetes: a sequence of neuropathy, retinopathy and nephropathy. Arch Intern Med 1954; 94: 931-941.
2. Chavers BM, Mauer SM, Ramsay RC, Steffes MW. Relationship between retinal and glomerular lesions in IDDM patients. Diabetes 1994; 43: 441-446.
3. Johansen J, Sjolie AK, Elbol P, Eshoj O. The relation between retinopathy and albumin excretion rate in insulin-dependent diabetes mellitus. From the Funen County Epidemiology of Type 1 Diabetes Complications Survey. Acta Ophthalmol Copenh 1994; 72: 347-351.
4. Watts GF, Harris R, Shaw KM. The determinants of early nephropathy in insulin- dependent diabetes mellitus: a prospective study based on the urinary excretion of albumin. Quarterly J Med 1991; 79: 365-378.
5. Klein R, Klein BE, Moss SE, Cruickshanks KJ. Relationship of hyperglycaemia to the long-term incidence and progression of diabetic retinopathy. Arch Intern Med 1994; 154: 2169-2178.
6. Teuscher A, Scnhell H, Wilson PW. Incidence of diabetic retinopathy and relationship to baseline plasma glucose and blood pressure. Diabetes Care 1988; 11: 246-251.
7. Knuiman MW, Welborn TA, McCann VJ, Stanton KG, Constable IJ. Prevalence of diabetic complications in relation to risk factors. Diabetes 1986; 35: 1332-1339.
8. Nielsen NV. Diabetic retinopathy I. The course of retinopathy in insulin-treated diabetics. A one year epidemiological cohort study of diabetes mellitus. The Island of Falster, Denmark. Acta Ophthalmol Copenh 1984; 62: 256-265.
9. Chase HP, Garg SK, Jackson WE. Blood pressure and retinopathy in type 1 diabetes. Ophthalmology 1990; 97: 155-159. P8`4
10. Coonrod BA, Ellis D, Becker DJ, et al. Predictors of microalbuminuria in individuals with IDDM. P ittsburgh Epidemiology of Diabetes Complications Study. Diabetes Care 1993; 16: 1376-1383.
11. Danielsen R, Jonasson F, Helgason T. Prevalence of retinopathy and proteinuria in type 1 diabetics in Iceland. Acta Med Scand 1982; 212: 277-280.
12. Dwyer MS, Melton LJ3d, Ballard DJ, Palumbo PJ, Trautmann JC, Chu CP. Incidence of diabetic retinopathy and blindness: a population-based study in Rochester, Minnesota. Diabetes Care 1985; 8: 316-322.

13. Klein R, Klein BE, Moss SE, Davis MD, DeMets DL. The Wisconsin epidemiologic study of diabetic retinopathy. II. Prevalence and risk of diabetic retinopathy when age at diagnosis is less than 30 years. Arch Ophthalmol 1984; 102: 520-526.
14. Andersen AR, Christiansen JS, Andersen JK, Kreiner S, Deckert T. Diabetic nephropathy in type I (insulin-dependent) diabetes: an epidemiologic study. Diabetologia 1983; 25: 496-501.
15. Stephenson JM, Fuller JH, Viberti GC, Sjolie AK, Navalesi R, EURODIAB IDDM Complications Study Group . Blood pressure, retinopathy and urinary albumin excretion in IDDM: the EURODIAB IDDM Complications Study. Diabetologia 1995; 38: 599-603.
16. Parving HH, Smidt UM, Frisberg B, Bonnevie-Nielsen V, Andersen AR. A prospective study of glomerular filtration rate and arterial blood pressure in insulin- dependent diabetes with diabetic nephropathy. Diabetologia 1981; 20: 457-461.
17. Mogensen CE, Christensen CK. Predicting diabetic nephropathy in insulin-dependent patients. N Engl J Med 1984; 311: 89-93.
18. Krolewski AS, Canessa M, Warram JH. Predisposition to hypertension and susceptibility to renal disease in insulin-dependent diabetes mellitus. N Engl J Med 1988; 318: 140-145.
19. Mogensen CE, Osterby R, Hansen KW, Damsgaard EM. Blood pressure elevation versus abnormal albuminuria in the genesis and prediction of renal disease in diabetes. Diabetes Care 1992; 15: 1181-1204.
20. West KM, Erdreich LJ, Stober A. A detailed study of risk factors for retinopathy and nephropathy in diabetes. Diabetes 1980; 29: 501-508.
21. Janka HU, Warram JH, Rand LI, Krolewski AS. Risk factors for progression of background retinopathy in long-standing IDDM. Diabetes 1989; 38: 460-464.
22. Klein BE, Klein R, Moss SE, Palta M. A cohort study of the relationship of diabetic retinopathy to blood pressure. Arch Ophthalmol 1995; 113: 601-606.
23. Norgaard K, Feldt-Rasmussen B, Deckert T. Is hypertension a major risk factor for retinopathy in type 1 diabetes? Diabetic Med 1991; 8: 334-337.
24. Krolewski AS, Warram JH, Cupples A, Gorman CK, Szabo AJ, Christlieb AR. Hypertension, orthostatic hypotension and the microvascular complications of diabetes. J Chronic Dis 1985; 38: 319-326.
25. Vigstrup J, Mogensen CE. Proliferative diabetic retinopathy: at risk patients identified by early detection of microalbuminuria. Acta Opthalmol 1985; 63: 530-534. P8`4
26. The EURODIAB IDDM Complications Study Group . Microvascular and acute complications in IDDM patients: the EURODIAB IDDM Complications Study. Diabetologia 1994; 37: 278-285.
27. The Diabetes Control and Complications Trial Research Group . The effect of intensive treatment of diabetes on the development and progression of long-term complications in insulin-dependent diabetes mellitus. N Engl J Med 1993; 329: 977-986.
28. Reaven GM. Role of insulin resistance in human disease. Diabetes 1988; 37: 1595- 1607.
29. Sosenko JM, Breslow JL, Miettinen OS, Gabbay KH. Hyperglycaemia and plasma lipid levels: a prospective study of young insulin-dependent diabetic patients. N Engl J Med 1980; 302: 650-654.
30. Jensen T, Stender S, Deckert T. Abnormalities in plamsa concentrations of lipoproteins and fibrinogen in type 1 (insulin-dependent) diabetic patients with increased urinary albumin excretion. Diabetologia 1988; 31: 142-145.
31. Jones SL, Close CF, Mattock MB, Jarrett RJ, Keen H, Viberti GC. Plasma lipid and coagulation factor concentrations in insulin dependent diabetics with microalbuminuria. Br Med J 1989; 298: 487-490.
32. Stehouwer CD, Stroes ES, Hackeng WH, Mulder PG, Den-Ottolander GJ. von Willebrand factor and development of diabetic nephropathy in IDDM. Diabetes 1991; 40: 971-976.
33. Stehouwer CD, Fischer HR, van-Kuijk AW, Polak BC, Donker AJ. Endothelial dysfunction precedes development of microalbuminuria in IDDM. Diabetes 1995; 44: 561- 564.
34. Winocour PH, Durrington PN, Ishola M, Anderson DC, Cohen H. Influence of proteinuria on vascular disease, blood pressure, and lipoproteins in insulin dependent diabetes mellitus. Br Med J 1987; 294: 1648-1651.
35. Tarnow L, Cambien F, Rossing P, et al. Lack of relationship between an insertion/deletion polymorphism in the angiotensin I-converting enzyme gene and diabetic nephropathy and proliferative retinopathy in IDDM patients. Diabetes 1995; 44: 489-393.
36. Kasiske BL, Kalil RS, Ma JZ, Liao M, Keane BF. Effect of antihypertensive therapy on the kidney in patients with diabetes: a meta-regression analysis. Ann Intern Med 1993; 118: 129-138.

37. Chase HP, Garg SK, Harris S, Hoops S, Jackson WE, Holmes DL. Angiotensin- Converting Enzyme Inhibitor Treatment for Young Normotensive Diabetic Subjects: A Two-Year Trial. Ann Opthalmol 1993; 25: 284-289.
38. Larsen M, Hommel E, Parving HH, Lund-Andersen H. Protective effect of captopril on the blood-retina barrier in normotensive insulin-dependent diabetic patients with nephropathy and background retinopathy. Graefes Arch Clin Exp Ophthalmol 1990; 228: 505-509.
39. Chaturvedi N, Sjolie A-K, Stephenson JM, et al. Effect of lisinopril on progression of retinopathy in normotensive people with type 1 diabetes. Lancet 1998; 351: 28-31.
40. Ravid M, Savin H, Jutrin I, Bental T, Katz B, Lishner M. long-term stabalising effect of angiotensin-converting enzyme inhibition on plasma creatinine and on proteinuria in normotensive type II diabetic patients. Ann Intern Med 1993; 118: 577-581.
41. Wagner J, Danser AHJ, Derkx FHM, et al. Demonstration of renin mRNA, angiotensin mRNA, and angiotensin converting enzyme mRNA expression in the human eye: evidence for an intraocular renin-angiotensin system. Br J Ophthalmol 1996; 80: 159-163.
42. Danser AHJ, Derkx FHM, Admiraal PJJ, Deinum J, De Jong PTVM, Schalekamp MADH. Angiotensin levels in the eye. Invest Ophthalmol Vis Sci 1994; 35: 1008-1018.

5. MICROALBUMINURIA AND CARDIOVASCULAR DISEASE

S.M. Thomas, G.C. Viberti.
Department for Endocrinology, Diabetes and Metabolic Medicine, Guy's Hospital, London, UK

INTRODUCTION

Classical risk factors for cardiovascular disease (CVD) mortality, such as cholesterol, blood pressure and smoking operate both in diabetic and non -diabetic subjects. However the absolute risk of cardiovascular death for men with diabetes, principally Type 2 diabetes, is up to three times higher and is progressively greater with each additional risk factor than in non-diabetic men [81]. Similarly the CVD mortality in a cohort of subjects with type 1 diabetes mellitus rises significantly in both men and women after the age of 30 reaching a two-fold excess, compared with non - diabetic subjects from the Framingham study [46].

The development of persistent proteinuria in Type 1 diabetes patients increases early mortality from CVD approximately 9-fold and the risk of developing coronary artery disease is 15 times higher compared to those patients without proteinuria [17]. In Type 2 diabetes although CVD is frequently present at diagnosis, this relationship with proteinuria persists.

This relationship between the renal and cardiovascular complications of diabetes is also present at lower levels of urinary albumin excretion. Microalbuminuria, defined as a urinary albumin excretion rate of 20-200μg/min or 30 - 300 mg/day, is associated with a substantially increased risk of CVD in both diabetic and non- diabetic populations.

In this chapter, we will discuss the associations between microalbuminuria and CVD in diabetes, hypertension and the general population. We shall examine some of the reasons for the strong relationship between the two and review some of the treatment strategies available.

MICROALBUMINURIA AND CARDIOVASCULAR DISEASE IN TYPE 2 DIABETES

Several cross - sectional [30,3,54], retrospective [57,38,78] and prospective studies [52,60,55,20] have shown the predictive value of microalbuminuria for mortality, an association that may be independent of other conventional risk factors. In all of these studies, the predominant cause of death was vascular disease.

This relationship is true in both European and Non -European subjects. In European Type 2 diabetes, the presence of an elevated UAE increases the relative risk of all cause mortality to between 1.6 and 2.7-fold (Table 5-1). In a recent 7 year prospective study of a hospital-based cohort, coronary heart disease (CHD) was the cause of death in 72% of patients with microalbuminuria as compared with 39% of patients with normoalbuminuria. Microalbuminuria, in this study, was an independent predictor of early mortality if cholesterol and HBA1c were entered as categorical variables but not when these same parameters were analysed as continuous variables [53]. Whether under all circumstances microalbuminuria is an independent predictor of CHD has also been questioned by other investigators [84]. A combined analysis of total mortality using all available studies in 1995 yielded a pooled odds ratio of 2.5 (95% Confidence Interval 1.8 - 3.60) [23]. In non - European Type 2 Diabetes, where the diabetes often develops at a younger age, this relationship persists although as the prevalence of large vessel disease in these studies has been lower, microalbuminuria is a predictor predominantly of renal disease [45].

Table 5-1. Microalbuminuria as a predictor of mortality in Type 2 Diabetes.

Study Design	Follow-up /years)	Outcome Relative risk of death (95% Confidence Interval)
Retrospective		
Jarret et al 1984	14	2.72* (1.3 B 5.74)
Mogensen 1984	9	1.57* (1.2 B 2.03)
Schmitz et Vaeth	10	2.28** (unavailable)
Prospective		
Mattock et al	7	2.73** (1.3 B 5.73)
Damsgaard et al	8 B 9	1.57* (1.17 – 2.11)
Macleod et al	8 B 9	1.7* (1.34 - 2.16)
Neil et al	6	2.15** (1.27 B 3.65)

* Relative risk calculated after Mattock et al (Excerpta Medica 2/93)
** Survival Analysis

MICROALBUMINURIA AND CARDIOVASCULAR DISEASE IN TYPE 1 DIABETES.

Microalbuminuria is strongly predictive of the development of overt diabetic nephropathy and its associated excess of coronary, cerebrovascular and peripheral arterial disease [85]. In prospective studies those with microalbuminuria have a significantly higher risk of dying from a cardiovascular cause (Relative Risk 2.94 95% Confidence Interval 1.18 - 7.34) [71,56]. Myocardial involvement may even be present at the stage of microalbuminuria, aerobic work capacity can be reduced in patients with microalbuminuria [40] and significant coronary lesions may be present [27].

MICROALBUMINURIA IN THE NON DIABETIC POPULATION.

General Population

In non - diabetic individuals the prevalence of microalbuminuria is around 3 - 5%, 2.2% in those aged 20 - 65 years to 13 - 20% in those rising from aged 60 - 74 years [87, 21]. In the Islington heart study an elevated albumin excretion increased rate (AER) was found in 9% of non - diabetic patients over 40 years of age. Those with an elevated AER had more coronary disease (73% versus 32% odds ratio 5.7), more peripheral vascular disease (PVD) (44 versus 9% odds ratio 7.45) and an increased mortality after 3.6 years (33% versus 2% odds ratio 24.3) [90].

Table 5-2.. The relationship between microalbumiuria in the non-diabetic population and cardiovascular risk factors

Study Design	Follow-up Years	Cardiovascular Outcome	Relative Risk (95% Confidence Interval)
Cross sectional			
Winocour et al 1987	N/A	Blood pressure/ECG abnormalities	
Haffner et al 1990	N/A	Myocardial infarction/ blood pressure	
Gould et al 1993	N/A	blood pressure	2.13 in men 1.85 in women
Retrospective			
Yudkin et al 1988	3-4	coronary heart disease/ peripheral vascular disease/mortality	2.43(5.4-109.7)
Prospective			
Damsgaard et al, 1992	5-7	Mortality	2.87

This relationship between microalbuminuria and cardiovascular end-points such as blood pressure and ischaemic heart disease has also been confirmed in other population-based studies [87, 36] (Table5-2).

Essential Hypertension

In essential hypertension, the prevalence of microalbuminuria varies between 5 and 25% in treated hypertension and up to 40% in untreated hypertension [64,50,31,12]. Hypertensive patients with microalbuminuria show more evidence of target organ damage such as increased carotid wall thickness and retinopathy [75,14,29]. Several studies have shown a marked correlation between both clinic and ambulatory blood pressure levels and AER. Salt sensitive hypertensive patients, in particular, have higher albumin excretion rates than salt - resistant patients [13,15]. Effective blood pressure treatment can lower the AER suggesting a causal relationship [74,73,8,9].

In the few histological studies performed involving patients with essential hypertension and microalbuminuria, no special renal lesions were seen as compared with normoalbuminuric controls [83].

Elderly

Microalbuminuria is a marker of increased mortality in the elderly [91] and of the subsequent development of coronary heart disease (CHD) especially in those with high circulating insulin levels [47].

FACTORS THAT MAY CONTRIBUTE TO CARDIOVASCULAR DISEASE IN DIABETIC AND NON– DIABETIC SUBJECTS WITH MICROALBUMINURIA.

The reason for the interaction between microalbuminuria and cardiac disease is uncertain. The observed aggregation of conventional cardiovascular risk factors does not explain all of the excess risk [55].

Familial Dispositions

Positive family histories of hypertension or CVD in the non-diabetic parents are related to the development of albuminuria in the diabetic proband emphasising the shared predisposition to these two conditions. These associations hold true for both Type 1 and Type 2 diabetes after adjustment for age, sex and duration of diabetes [25,24]. There is also some evidence for a familial predisposition to develop microalbuminuria in association with essential hypertension. Children with one hypertensive parent have a higher AER than children of a normotensive parent while normotensive adults with at least one hypertensive parent have an elevated AER compared to normotensive adults with a negative family history [35,29].

Smoking

There is a higher prevalence of heavy cigarette smokers amongst non – diabetic individuals with microalbuminuria. In addition in both Type 1 and Type 2 diabetes, smoking is an independent risk factor for the development of microalbuminuria. Calculations indicate however that excess smoking is only partly responsible for the excess cardiovascular risk.

Blood Pressure

In some studies non –diabetic subjects with microalbuminuria have higher DBP [68] while in others both systolic blood pressure (SBP) and DBP were higher [36]. Several studies have shown the correlation to be best with 24 hour ambulatory blood pressure monitoring with higher 24 hour mean levels, lower day: night ratios and greater variability of pressure readings [14,9]. Studies in both Type 1 and Type 2 diabetes indicate that elevations in blood pressure occur early as the AER rises within the normal range in those patients who develop microalbuminuria [37].

Left Ventricular Hypertrophy

Left ventricular hypertrophy (LVH) is a predictor of morbidity and mortality in diabetic and non- diabetic individuals. Microalbuminuria is associated with LVH in non – diabetic subjects and those with both Type 1 and Type 2 diabetes

[70,66,18,76] and in the latter group this effect seems independent of clinic measured SBP or DBP [80].

Lipid Abnormalities

In both Type 1 and Type 2 diabetes, an unfavourable lipid profile is present at a very early stage of albuminuria. The concentrations of total cholesterol, VLDL cholesterol LDL cholesterol, triglycerides and fibrinogen rise with increasing UAE in patients with Type 1 diabetes (11 - 14 % higher in microalbuminuria 26 - 87% higher in macroalbuminuria) [41]. In addition, there is an increase in LDL mass and atherogenic small dense LDL particles, which correlates with the plasma triglyceride concentrations. HDL levels also tend to be reduced with a disadvantageous alteration in their composition [84,43,63,83,48]. Lipoprotein (a) is reported to be elevated by some though not all authors [34,44,32,27]

Similarly in the non -diabetic population, those with elevated UAE have increased Lipoprotein (a), LDL: HDL cholesterol ratios and lower Apolipoprotein A-1 and HDL cholesterol levels [28,14].

Insulin Resistance

In both non - diabetic subjects and in those with Type 1 and Type 2 diabetes, persistent microalbuminuria is associated with insulin resistance [89,11,10,2]. Thus, microalbuminuria may form part of a metabolic syndrome that predisposes to accelerated atherogenesis. Interestingly insulin resistance, essential hypertension and microalbuminuria have all been associated with elevations in cation membrane transport systems [79,72,61,62,519] which may be important in cell growth and pH regulation.

Endothelial dysfunction and Haemostatic abnormalities

Levels of Von Willebrand factor (vWF), PAI1, Factor VII and fibrinogen are higher in patients with microalbuminuria as compared with controls suggesting associated endothelial activation and a hypofibrinolytic, hypercoagulable state [42,33,22,43,67]. Recent evidence suggests that the increase in vWF may precede the onset of microalbuminuria in type 1 diabetes [82]. In addition, there is a generalised increase in vascular permeability in both the non – diabetic and diabetic population indicated by an increased transcapillary escape of albumin.

Autonomic Neuropathy

Autonomic neuropathy is associated with an alteration in the perception of cardiac symptoms [27] and abnormalities in the Q-T interval possibly predisposing to ventricular arrhythmias [77] although this remains uncertain. In addition, studies in diabetes show autonomic neuropathy to be an independent predictor of CVD [88,27].

INTERVENTION

Microalbuminuria fulfils many of the Bradford Hill criteria for causality for cardiovascular complications [86] with strong consistent evidence of the association, an appropriate temporal relationship, and a biological gradient. There is however, a relative lack of intervention studies looking at risk factor reduction in microalbuminuria in relation to CVD outcome. Many of the studies performed to date have been small, have centred on renal outcome and the results have been conflicting.

Glycaemic Control

The question of whether improved glycaemic control is of benefit in preventing CVD in either Type 1 Diabetes or Type 2 diabetes remains unresolved. In the Diabetes Control and Complications Trial intensive insulin therapy lowered the risk of microalbuminuria and concomitantly reduced development of hypercholesterolaemia with a 41% reduction in the risk of macrovascular disease (combined cardiovascular and peripheral vascular). The number of outcome events was small however as the trial was carried out in relatively young subjects with Type 1 Diabetes and the difference was not statistically significant. In Type 2 diabetes there is some evidence that improved glycaemic control may protect against renal progression but not against CVD although these have not focussed on those with microalbuminuria [1].

The UK Prospective Diabetes Study (UKPDS), a multi-centre prospective randomised intervention trial of newly-diagnosed patients with Type 2 Diabetes randomised to either diet or "active" treatment with insulin or an oral hypoglycaemic agent may also provide information on this area.

Lipid lowering therapy.

A sub-analysis of 202 subjects with mainly Type 2 diabetes in the Scandinavian Simvastatin Survival study (4S) revealed a reduction of 24% in total cholesterol, 37% in LDL cholesterol, 11 % in triglyceride and a 7% increase in HDL cholesterol. There was a reduction in both total and CHD mortality, with a risk reduction for "major" CHD over the course of the study of 36-54% [69]. This study did not however addres the issue of lipid lowering therapy in diabetic patients with microalbuminuria or albuminuria.

Blood Pressure Reduction

Many of the studies of blood pressure focus on renal end points where ACE inhibition has been shown to reduce AER and prevent progression to overt proteinuria.

In diabetes effective blood pressure treatment is able to lower urinary albumin excretion and reduce the risk of progression to macroalbuminuria. There is also evidence for a specific benefit AER lowering effect of ACE inhibitors [58,49] and in the Euclid study the rise in AER was delayed by ACE inhibition [6]. To date however no study has had a CVD mortality end-point.

Studies in non – diabetic people have also shown a benefit of anti – hypertensive treatment in reducing microalbuminuria and suggested that inhibition of the renin – angiotensin system may have specific benefits in renal protection [73,14,7]. However, again there are no specific studies with CVD mortality end points available.

Finally, in patients with diabetes and proteinuria, cohort studies show a reduction in cumulative mortality, from over 50 per cent to 18 per cent at 10 years in patients receiving anti-hypertensive treatment [65].

SUMMARY

Microalbuminuria is associated with an excess all cause and cardiovascular mortality in both diabetic and non-diabetic people. An intensive strategy of risk factor reduction may be necessary to tackle this problem and specific studies that address the issue of risk reversibility are required.

REFERENCES

1. Abraira, C., J. Colwell, F. Nuttall, C.T. Sawin, W. Henderson, J.P. Comstock, N.V. Emanuele, S.R. Levin, I. Pacold, and H.S. Lee. "Cardiovascular events and correlates in the Veterans Affairs Diabetes Feasibility Trial. Veterans Affairs Cooperative Study on Glycemic Control and Complications in Type II Diabetes." Archives of Internal Medicine 157(1997):181-188.
2. Agewall, S., B. Persson, O. Samuelsson, S. Ljungman, H. Herlitz, Fagerberg, and B. "Microalbuminuria in treated hypertensive men at high risk of coronary disease. The Risk Factor Intervention Study Group." Journal of Hypertension 11(1993):461-469.
3. Allawi, J. and R.J. Jarrett. "Microalbuminuria and cardiovascular risk factors in type 2 diabetes mellitus." Diabetic Medicine 7(1990):115-118.
4. Microalbuminuria Collaborative Study Group United Kingdom. "Risk factors for development of microalbuminuria in insulin dependent diabetic patients: a cohort study." *BMJ* 306(1993a):1235-1239.
5. The Diabetes Control and Complications Trial Research Group. "The effect of intensive treatment of diabetes on the development and progression of long-term complications in insulin-dependent diabetes mellitus." New England Journal of Medicine 329(1993b):977-986.
6. The EUCLID Study Group. "Randomised placebo-controlled trial of lisinopril in normotensive patients with insulin-dependent diabetes and normoalbuminuria or microalbuminuria." Lancet 349(1997):1787-1792.
7. Bianchi, S., R. Bigazzi, G. Baldari, and V.M. Campese. "Microalbuminuria in patients with essential hypertension. Effects of an angiotensin converting enzyme inhibitor and of a calcium channel blocker." American Journal of Hypertension 4(1991):291-296.
8. Bianchi, S., R. Bigazzi, G. Baldari, and V.M. Campese. "Microalbuminuria in patients with essential hypertension: effects of several antihypertensive drugs." American Journal of Medicine 93(1992):525-528.
9. Bianchi, S., R. Bigazzi, G. Baldari, G. Sgherri, and V.M. Campese. "Diurnal variations of blood pressure and microalbuminuria in essential hypertension." American Journal of Hypertension 7(1994a):23-29.
10. Bianchi, S., R. Bigazzi, C. Valtriani, I. Chiapponi, G. Sgherri, G. Baldari, A. Natali, E. Ferrannini, and V.M. Campese. "Elevated serum insulin levels in patients with essential hypertension and microalbuminuria." Hypertension 23(1994b):681-687.
11. Bianchi, S., R. Bigazzi, A. Quinones Galvan, E. Muscelli, G. Baldari, N. Pecori, D. Ciociaro, E. Ferrannini, and A. Natali. "Insulin resistance in microalbuminuric hypertension. Sites and mechanisms." Hypertension 26(1995):789-795.

12. Bigazzi, R., S. Bianchi, V.M. Campese, and G. Baldari. "Prevalence of microalbuminuria in a large population of patients with mild to moderate essential hypertension." *Nephron* 61(1992):94-97.
13. Bigazzi, R., S. Bianchi, D. Baldari, G. Sgherri, G. Baldari, and V.M. Campese. "Microalbuminuria in salt-sensitive patients. A marker for renal and cardiovascular risk factors." Hypertension 23(1994):195-199.
14. Bigazzi, R., S. Bianchi, R. Nenci, D. Baldari, G. Baldari, and V.M. Campese. "Increased thickness of the carotid artery in patients with essential hypertension and microalbuminuria." Journal of Human *Hypertension* 9(1995):827-833.
15. Bigazzi, R., S. Bianchi, G. Baldari, and V.M. Campese. "Clustering of cardiovascular risk factors in salt-sensitive patients with essential hypertension: role of insulin." American Journal of Hypertension 9(1996):24-32.
16. Bigazzi, R. and S. Bianchi. "Microalbuminuria as a marker of cardiovascular and renal disease in essential hypertension." Nephrology, Dialysis, Transplantation 10 Suppl 6(1995):10-14.
17. Borch-Johnsen, K. and S. Kreiner. "Proteinuria: value as predictor of cardiovascular mortality in insulin dependent diabetes mellitus." British Medical Journal Clinical Research Ed 294(1987):1651-1654.
18. Cerasola, G., S. Cottone, G. Mule, E. Nardi, M.T. Mangano, G. Andronico, A. Contorno, M. Li Vecchi, P. Galione, F. Renda, G. Piazza, V. Volpe, Lisi, A, L. Ferrara, N. Panepinto, and R. Riccobene. "Microalbuminuria, renal dysfunction and cardiovascular complication in essential hypertension." Journal of Hypertension 14(1996):915-920.
19. Chaturvedi, N., J.M. Stephenson, and J.H. Fuller. "The relationship between smoking and microvascular complications in the EURODIAB IDDM Complications Study." *Diabeteland, O.D. Jorgensen, and C.E. Mogensen. "Microalbuminuria as predictor of increased mortality in elderly people."* BMJ 300(1990):297-300.
20. Damsgaard, E.M., A. Froland, O.D. Jorgensen, and C.E. Mogensen. "Eight to nine year mortality in known non-insulin dependent diabetics and controls." Kidney International 41(1992):731-735.
21. Damsgaard, E.M. and C.E. Mogensen. "Microalbuminuria in elderly hyperglycaemic patients and controls." Diabetic Medicine 3(1986):430-435.
22. Deckert, T., B. Feldt-Rasmussen, K. Borch-Johnsen, T. Jensen, and A. Kofoed-Enevoldsen. "Albuminuria reflects widespread vascular damage. The Steno hypothesis." Diabetologia 32(1989):219-226.
23. Dineen, S. and H. Gerstein. "Microalbuminuria and mortality in NIDDM: a systematic overview of the literature." Diabetes 44(1995):458(Abstract)
24. Earle, K. and Viberti G.C. "Familial, hemodynamic and metabolic factors in the predisposition to diabetic kidney disease." Kidney International 45(1994):434-437.
25. Earle, K.A., J. Walker, C. Hill, and Viberti G.C. "Familial clustering of cardiovascular disease in patients with insulin-dependent diabetes and nephropathy." *New England Journal of Medicine* 326(1992):673-677.
26. Earle, K.A., M. Mattock, A. Morocutti, D. Aravanitis, and G.C. Viberti. "Lipoprotein(a) and atherosclerotic disease in insulin-dependent diabetic patients with declining glomerular filtration rate [letter]." Diabetic Medicine 13(1996a):1071-1072.
27. Earle, K.A., M. Mishra, A. Morocutti, D. Barnes, E. Stephens, J. Chambers, and G.C. Viberti. "Microalbuminuria as a marker of silent myocardial ischaemia in IDDM patients." Diabetologia 39(1996b):854-856.
28. Erley, C.M. and T. Risler. "Microalbuminuria in primary hypertension: is it a marker of glomerular damage?" Nephrology, Dialysis, Transplantation 9(1994):1713-1715.
29. Fauvel, J.P., A. Hadj-Aissa, M. Laville, G. Fadat, M. Labeeuw, P. Zech, and N. Pozet. "Microalbuminuria in normotensives with genetic risk of hypertension [letter]." Nepanscapillary Escape of albumin in Type 1 (insulin-dependent) diabetic patients with microalbuminuria." Diabetologia 29(1986):282-286.

30. Gatling, W., S. Tufail, M.A. Mullee, T.A. Westacott, and R.D. Hill. "Mortality rates in diabetic patients from a community-based population compared to local age/sex matched controls." Diabetic Medicine 14(1997):316-320.

31. Gerber, L.M., C. Shmukler, and M.H. Alderman. "Differences in urinary albumin excretion rate between normotensive and hypertensive, white and nonwhite subjects." Archives of Internal Medicine 152(1992):373-377.

32. Groop, P.H., Viberti G.C., T.G. Elliott, R. Friedman, A. Mackie, C. Ehnholm, M. Jauhiainen, and M.R. Taskinen. "Lipoprotein(a) in type 1 diabetic patients with renal disease." Diabetic Medicine 11(1994):961-967.

33. Gruden, G., P. Cavallo-Perin, M. Bazzan, S. Stella, V. Vuolo, and G. Pagano. "PAI-1 and Factor VII activity are higher in IDDM patients with microalbuminuria." *Diabetes* 43(1994a):426-429.(Abstract)

34. Gruden, G., M. Veglio, P. Cavallo-Perin, C. Olivetti, A. Mormile, Cassader, M, and G. Pagano. "Lipoprotein(a) in non-insulin-dependent diabetic patients with normo- and microalbuminuria." Hormone & Metabolic Research 26(1994b):489-490.

35. Grunfeld, B., E. Perelstein, R. Simsolo, M. Gimenez, and J.C. Romero. "Renal functional reserve and microalbuminuria in offspring of hypertensive parents." Hypertension 15(1990):257-261.

36. Haffner, S.M., M.P. Stern, M.K. Gruber, H.P. Hazuda, B.D. Mitchell, Patterson, and JK. "Microalbuminuria. Potential marker for increased cardiovascular risk factors in nondiabetic subjects?" Arteriosclerosis 10(1990):727-731.

37. Haneda, M., R. Kikkawa, M. Togawa, D. Koya, N. Kajiwara, T. Uzu, and Y. Shigeta. "High blood pressure is a risk factor for the development of microalbuminuria in Japanese subjects with non-insulin-dependent diabetes mellitus." Journal of Diabetes & its Complications 6(1992):181-185.

38. Jarrett, R.J., Viberti G.C., A. Argyropoulos, R.D. Hill, U. mortality in non-insulin-dependent diabetics." Diabetic Medicine 1(1984):17-19.

39. Jensen, J.S., K. Borch-Johnsen, G. Jensen, and B. Feldt-Rasmussen. "Microalbuminuria reflects a generalized transvascular albumin leakiness in clinically healthy subjects." Clinical Science 88(1995):629-633.

40. Jensen, T., E.A. Richter, B. Feldt-Rasmussen, H. Kelbaek, and T. Deckert. "Impaired aerobic work capacity in insulin dependent diabetics with increased urinary albumin excretion." British Medical Journal Clinical Research Ed . 296(1988a):1352-1354.

41. Jensen, T., S. Stender, and T. Deckert. "Abnormalities in plasmas concentrations of lipoproteins and fibrinogen in type 1 (insulin-dependent) diabetic patients with increased urinary albumin excretion." *Diabetologia* 31(1988b):142-145.

42. Jensen, T., J. Bjerre-Knudsen, B. Feldt-Rasmussen, and T. Deckert. "Features of endothelial dysfunction in early diabetic nephropathy." *Lancet* 1(1989):461-463.

43. Jones, S.L., C.F. Close, M.B. Mattock, R.J. Jarrett, H. Keen, and Viberti G.C. "Plasma lipid and coagulation factor concentrations in insulin dependent diabetics with microalbuminuria." *BMJ* 298(1989):487-490.

44. Kapelrud, H., H.J. Bangstad, K. Dahl-Jorgensen, K. Berg, and K.F. Hanssen. "Serum Lp(a) lipoprotein concentrations in insulin dependent diabetic patients with microalbuminuria." *BMJ* 303(1991):675-678.

45. Knowler, W.C., R.G. Nelson, and D.J. Pettitt. Diabetes, hypertension and kidney disease in the Pima Indians. In: *The Kidney and Hypertension in Diabetes Mellitus.* Edited by Mogensen, C. Boston, Dordrecht, London: Kluwer Academic, 1997, p.53.

46. Krolewski, A.S., E.J. Kosinski, J.H. Warram, O.S. Leland, E.J. Busick, A.C. Asmal, L.I. Rand, A.R. Christlieb, R.F. Bradley, and C.R. Kahn. "Magnitude and determinants of coronary artery disease in juvenile-onset, insulin-dependent diabetes mellitus." American Journal of Cardiology 59(1987):750-755.

47. Kuusisto, J., L. *Mykkanen*, K. Pyorala, and M. Laakso. "Hyperinsulinemic microalbuminuria. A new risk indicator for coronary heart disease." Circulation 91(1995):831-837.

48. Lahdenpera, S., P.H. Groop, M. Tilly-Kiesi, T. Kuusi, T.G. Elliott, Viberti G.C., GC, and M.R. Taskinen. "LDL subclasses in IDDM patients: relation to diabetic nephropathy." Diabetologia 37(1994):681-688.
49. Lewis, E.J., L.G. Hunsicker, R.P. Bain, and R.D. Rohde. On behalf of The Collaborative Study Group. "The effect of angiotensin-converting-enzyme inhibition on diabetic nephropathy." New England Journal *of Medicine* 329(1993):1456-1462.
50. Ljungman, S. "Microalbuminuria in essential hypertension." American Journal of Hypertension 3(1990):956-960.
51. Lopes de Faria, J.B., S.L. Jones, F. Macdonald, J. Chambers, and M.B. Mattock. "Sodium-lithium countertransport activity and insulin resistance in normotensive IDDM patients." Diabetes 41(1992):610-615.
52. Macleod, J.M., J. Lutale, and S.M. Marshall. "Albumin excretion and vascular deaths in NIDDM." Diabetologia 38(1995):610-616.
53. Mattock, M., D.J. Barnes, Viberti G.C., H. Keen, D. Burt, J. Hughes, A.P. Fitzgerald, B. Sandhu, and P.G. Jackson. "Microalbuminuria and coronary heart disease in non - insulin dependent diabetes mellitus: an incidence study." Submited for Publication (1998)(Abstract)
54. Mattock, M.B., H. Keen, Viberti G.C., M.R. el-Gohari, T.J. Murrells, G.S. Scott, J.R. Wing, and P.G. Jackson. "Coronary heart disease and urinary albumin excretion rate in type 2 (non-insulin-dependent) diabetic patients." Diabetologia 31(1988):82-87.
55. Mattock, M.B., N.J. Morrish, Viberti G.C., H. Keen, A.P. Fitzgerald, and G. Jackson. "Prospective study of microalbuminuria as predictor of mortality in NIDDM." Diabetes 41(1992):736-741.
56. Messent, J.W., T.G. Elliott, R.D. Hill, R.J. Jarrett, H. Keen, and Viberti G.C. "Prognostic significance of microalbuminuria in insulin-dependent diabetes mellitus: a twenty-three year follow-up study." Kidney International 41(1992):836-839.
57. Mogensen, C.E. "Microalbuminuria predicts clinical proteinuria and early mortality in maturity-onset diabetes." New England Journal of Medicine 310(1984):356-360.
58. Mogensen, C.E., W.F. Keane, P.H. Bennett, G. Jerums, H.H. Parving, P. Passa, M.W. Steffes, G.E. Striker, and Viberti G.C. "Prevention of diabetic renal disease with special reference to microalbuminuria." *Lancet* 346(1995):1080-1084.
59. Nannipieri, M., L. Rizzo, A. Rapuano, A. Pilo, G. Penno, and R. Navalesi. "Increased transcapillary escape rate of albumin in microalbuminuric type II diabetic patients." Diabetes Care 18(1995):1-9.
60. Neil, A., M. Hawkins, M. Potok, M. Thorogood, D. Cohen, and J. Mann. "A prospective population-based study of microalbuminuria as a predictor of mortality in NIDDM." Diabetes Care 16(1993):996-1003.
61. Ng, L.L., C. Dudley, J. Bomford, and D. Hawley. "Leucocyte intracellular pH and Na+/H+ antiport activity in human hypertension." Journal of Hypertension 7(1989):471-475.
62. Ng, L.L., J.E. Davies, M. Siczkowski, F.P. Sweeney, P.A. Quinn, B. Krolewski, and A.S. Krolewski. "Abnormal Na+/H+ antiporter phenotype and turnover of immortalized lymphoblasts from type 1 diabetic patients with nephropathy." Journal of Clinical Investigation 93(1994):2750-2757.
63. Nielsen, F.S., A.I. Voldsgaard, M.A. Gall, P. Rossing, E. Hommel, P. Andersen, and H.H. Parving. "Apolipoprotein(a) and cardiovascular disease in type 2 (non-insulin-dependent) diabetic patients with and without diabetic nephropathy." Diabetologia 36(1993):438-444.
64. Parving, H.H., C.E. Mogensen, H.A. Jensen, and P.E. Evrin. "Increased urinary albumin-excretion rate in benign essential hypertension." Lancet 1(1974):1190-1192.
65. Parving, H.H., P. Jacobsen, K. Rossing, U.M. Smidt, E. Hommel, and P. Rossing. "Benefits of long-term antihypertensive treatment on prognosis in diabetic nephropathy." Kidney International 49(1996):1778-1782.

66. Pedrinelli, R., V.D. Bello, G. Catapano, L. Talarico, F. Materazzi, Santoro, G, C. Giusti, F. Mosca, E. Melillo, and M. Ferrari. "Microalbuminuria is a marker of left ventricular hypertrophy but not hyperinsulinemia in nondiabetic atherosclerotic patients." Arteriosclerosis & Thrombosis 13(1993):900-906.

67. Pedrinelli, R., O. Giampietro, F. Carmassi, E. Melillo, G. Dell'Omo, G. Catapano, E. Matteucci, L. Talarico, M. Morale, F. De Negri, and et al. "Microalbuminuria and endothelial dysfunction in essential hypertension." Lancet 344(1994):14-18.

68. Pontremoli, R., V. Cheli, A. Sofia, A. Tirotta, M. Ravera, C. Nicolella, N. Ruello, C. Tomolillo, G.C. Antonucci, D. Bessarione, and et al. "Prevalence of micro- and macroalbuminuria and their relationship with other cardiovascular risk factors in essential hypertension." Nephrology, Dialysis, Transplantation 10 Suppl 6(1995):6-9.

69. Pyorala, K., T.R. Pedersen, J. Kjekshus, O. Faergeman, A.G. Olsson, and G. Thorgeirsson. "Cholesterol lowering with simvastatin improves prognosis of diabetic patients with coronary heart disease. A subgroup analysis of the Scandinavian Simvastatin Survival Study (4S)." Diabetes Care 20(1997):614-620.

70. Redon, J., M.A. Gomez-Sanchez, E. Baldo, M.C. Casal, M.L. Fernandez, Miralles, A, C. Gomez-Pajuelo, J.L. Rodicio, and L.M. Ruilope. "Micro-albuminuria is correlated with left ventricular hypertrophy in male hypertensive patients." Journal of Hypertension - Supplement 9(1991):S148-9.

71. Rossing, P., P. Hougaard, K. Borch-Johnsen, and H.H. Parving. "Predictors of mortality in insulin dependent diabetes: 10 year observational follow up study." BMJ 313(1996):779-784.

72. Rosskopf, D., R. Dusing, and W. Siffert. "Membrane sodium-proton exchange and primary hypertension." Hypertension 21(1993):607-617.

73. Ruilope, L.M., J.M. Alcazar, E. Hernandez, M. Praga, V. Lahera, and J.L. Rodicio. "Long-term influences of antihypertensive therapy on microalbuminuria in essential hypertension." Kidney International *Supplement* 45(1994):S171-3.

74. Ruilope, L.M. and J.L. Rodicio. "Clinical relevance of proteinuria and microalbuminuria." Current Opinion in Nephrology & Hypertension 2(1993):962-967.

75. Ruilope, L.M. and J.L. Rodicio. "Hypertension, atherosclerosis and microalbuminuria in ELSA. European Lacidipine Study of Atherosclerosis." Blood Pressure Supplement. 4(1996):48-52.

76. Sampson, M.J., J.B. Chambers, D.C. Sprigings, and P.L. Drury. "Regression of left ventricular hypertrophy with 1 year of treatment in type 1 diabetic patients with early." Diabetic Medicine 8(1991):106-110.

77. Sawicki, P.T. "Mortality in diabetic nephropathy: the importance of the QT interval." Nephrology, Dialysis, Transplantation 11(1996):1514-1515.

78. Schmitz, A. and M. Vaeth. "Microalbuminuria: a major risk factor in non insulin dependent diabetes. A 10 year follow up study of 503 patients." Diabetic Medicine 5(1988):126-134.

79. Semplicini, A., M. Canessa, M.G. Mozzato, G. Ceolotto, M. Marzola, F. Buzzaccarini, P. Casolino, and A.C. Pessina. "Red blood cell Na+/H+ and Li+/Na+ exchange in patients with essential hypertension." American Journal of Hypertension 2(1989):903-908.

80. Spring, M.W., A. Raptis, J. Chambers, and Viberti G.C. "Left ventricular structure and function are associated with microalbuminuria independently of blood pressure in Type II diabetes." Diabetes 46(1997):109A-A0426.(Abstract)

81 Stamler, J., O. Vaccaro, J.D. Neaton, and D. Wentworth. "Diabetes, other risk factors, and 12-yr cardiovascular mortality for men screened in the Multiple Risk Factor Intervention Trial." Diabetes Care 16(1993):434-444.

82. Stehouwer, C.D., H.R. Fischer, A.W. van Kuijk, B.C. Polak, and A.J. Donker. "Endothelial dysfunction precedes development of microalbuminuria in IDDM." Diabetes 44(1995):561-564.

83. Steiner, G. "The dyslipoproteinemias of diabetes." Atherosclerosis 110 Suppl(1994):S27-33.

Titov, V.N., A.V. Tarasov, R.I. Sokolova, E.I. Volkova, and G.G. Arabidze. "A comparison of selective microproteinuria with histomorphology of the kidneys in patients with arterial hypertension." Laboratornoe Delo (1989):43-48.

84. Uusitupa, M.I., L.K. Niskanen, O. Siitonen, E. Voutilainen, and K. Pyorala. "Ten-year cardiovascular mortality in relation to risk factors and abnormalities in lipoprotein composition in type 2 (non-insulin-dependent) diabetic and non-diabetic subjects." Diabetologia 36(1993):1175-1184.
85. Viberti G.C., R.D. Hill, R.J. Jarrett, A. Argyropoulos, U. Mahmud, and H. Keen. "Microalbuminuria as a predictor of clinical nephropathy in insulin-dependent diabetes mellitus." Lancet 1(1982):1430-1432.
86. Viberti G.C. "Outcome variables in the assessment of progression of diabetic kidney disease." Kidney International - Supplement 45(1994):S121-4.
87. Winocour, P.H., J.O. Harland, J.P. Millar, M.F. Laker, and K.G. Alberti. "Microalbuminuria and associated cardiovascular risk factors in the community." Atherosclerosis 93(1992):71-81.
88. Wirta, O., A. Pasternack, J. Mustonen, and P. Laippala. "Renal and cardiovascular predictors of 9-year total and sudden cardiac mortality in non -insulin dependent diabetic subjects." Nephrology, Dialysis, Transplantation 12(1997):2612-2617.(Abstract)
89. Yip, J., M.B. Mattock, A. Morocutti, M. Sethi, R. Trevisan, and Viberti G.C. "Insulin resistance in insulin-dependent diabetic patients with microalbuminuria." Lancet 342(kson. "Microalbuminuria as predictor of vascular disease in non-diabetic subjects. Islington Diabetes Survey." Lancet 2(1988):530-533.
90. Yudkin JS, Forrest RD, Jackson CA. 1988. Microalbuminuria as a predictor of vascular disease in non-diabetic subjects. Islington Diabetes Survey. Lancet ii: 530-533.
91. Damsgaard EM, Frøland A, Jørgensen OD, Mogensen CE, 1990. Microalbuminuria as a predictor of increased mortality in elderly people. BMJ 300: 297-300.

6. THE HEART IN DIABETES: RESULTS OF TRIALS

Giulio Zuanetti, Roberto Latini
Istituto Mario Negri, Milano

Aldo P Maggioni
Centro Studi ANMCO, Firenze, Italy

It has been known for many years that diabetes has profound consequences on the cardiovascular system leading to increased morbidity and mortality in diabetic patients [1]. In the last years, the completion of several large trials allowed to gather critical information on the efficacy and safety of different drugs in patients with a variety of cardiovascular diseases. In most of these trials diabetic patients, generally identified on the basis of clinical history and with no distinction between type 1 and type 2 diabetes, represented an important proportion of the randomized population, ranging between 10 and 25 % in most cases. In this brief review, we will summarize how these trials helped in widening our knowledge of the pathophysiology, prognosis and pharmacological treatment of diabetic patients with cardiovascular disease. Table 6-1 shows the meaning of the acronyms of the trials quoted in this review, where three specific settings will be discussed: acute myocardial infarction (MI); congestive heart failure (CHF) and treatment of myocardial ischemia with coronary angioplasty (PTCA).

1. ACUTE MYOCARDIAL INFARCTION IN DIABETICS IN THE FIBRINOLYTIC ERA

The widespread use of fibrinolytic agents and aspirin led to a marked improvement in the prognosis of acute MI patients. This notwithstanding, the difference in post-MI survival between diabetic and non-diabetic patients, documented by several studies performed before the introduction of fibhnolysis [2,3] remains mostly unaffected. Data from the GISSI-2 [4], GUSTO-1 [5] and TIMI2 [6] trials, in which all patients received fibrinolytic agents, show a 30 to 100% higher in-hospital mortality in diabetic patients of both genders compared to non-diabetics.

Although concomitant risk factors such as hypertension, hyperlipidemia and increased body mass index may all contribute to a decreased survival post-MI, diabetes *per se* exerts an independent negative role, as consistently documented in all studies.

Efficacy of pharmacological treatment

So far, only one prospective study, the DIGAMI trial [7,8], evaluated specifically the effect of pharmacological treatment on prognosis of diabetic patients after acute MI. In this study, diabetic patients were randomized to receive either standard treatment or an intensive treatment with insulin-glucose infusion targeted to achieve a tight control of glycemic levels. The insulin treatment was then continued long-term. Data showed that this "intensive" hypoglycemic treatment was associated with a lower 1 year morbidity and mortality and that the beneficial effect was even more evident during long-term follow-up.

Most of the information on the effect of commonly used cardiovascular drugs in diabetics with MI has been obtained only from retrospective subgroup analyses of some large trials or as non-randomized comparisons between control and drug-treated patients. The evidence for several classes of drugs, summarized in Table 6-2, will be discussed below.

Table 6-1. Significance of acronyms of trials quoted

AIRE=	The Acute Infarction Ramipril Efficacy
CARE=	Cholesterol and Recurrent Events
CCS-1=	Chinese Cardiac Study Collaborative Groups I
CONSENSUS2=	Co-operative New Scandinavian Enalapril Survival Study II
DIGAMI=	Diabetes Mellitus Insulin-Glucose Infusion in Acute Myocardial Infarction
GISSI-2=	Gruppo Italiano per lo Studio delta Sopravvivenza nell'infarto miocardico 2
GISSI-3=	Gruppo Italiano per lo Studio delia Sopravvivenza nell'infarto miocardico 3
GUSTO-1=	Global Utilization of Streptokinase and Tissue Plasminogen Activator for Occluded Coronary Arteries 1
ISIS-2=	International Study of Infarct Survival 2
MOCHA=	Multicentric Oral Carvedilol Heart Failure Assessment
PURSUIT=	Platelet IIb/IIIa in Unstable angina: Receptor Suppression Using Integrilin Therapy
SAVE=	Survival and Ventricular Enlargement
SOLVD=	Studies of Left Ventricular Dysfunction
TAMI=	Thrombolysis and Angioplasty in Myocardial Infarction
TIMI-2=	Thrombolysis in Myocardial Infarction 2
TRACE=	Trandolapril Cardiac Evaluation
4S=	Scandinavian Simvastatin Survival Study

Fibrinolytic agents

Based on their tendency toward a more thrombogenic, less profibrinolytic state [9], it may be expected that thrombolytic treatment would be less effective in diabetic patients. However, the relative decrease in mortality of diabetics with fibrinolytic treatment has been at least similar to that observed in non diabetics: the overview of fibrinolytic trials in acute MI [10] found that fibrinolytic treatment was associated with a 35 days mortality of 13.6% vs 17.3% in diabetics (-21.7%, or 37 lives saved per 1 000 treated patients) and 8.7% vs 10.2% in non diabetics (-14.3% or 15 lives saved per 1 000 treated patients). One of the major concerns in administering thrombolytic treatment to diabetic patients was the possibility of a higher incidence of adverse effects, particularly stroke and retinal hemorrage. The incidence of stroke in diabetics (1.9% in fibrinolytic treated patients vs 1.3% in control) is higher than in non-diabetics (1.0% vs 0.6% respectively); however, this increased risk is by far outweighed by the beneficial effect on mortality. Also, no retinal hemorrages in diabetics treated with fibrinolysis were observed in the TAMI trial [11], despite presence of documented retinopathy in several patients, thus diabetes can not be considered a contraindication to fibrinolytic treatment, as suggested when thrombolysis was introduced in clinical practice.

The relative efficacy of newer fibrinolytic treatment regimens in this population remains to be determined.

Aspirin and other antiplatelet agents

The role of aspirin as first-line therapy in the treatment of patients with acute MI has been firmly established [12]. However, the optimal dosage in the diabetic population remains unclear, since these patients have a higher platelet aggregability. Interestingly, in ISIS-2 [12] there was no reduction in mortality among diabetic patients receiving aspirin 160 mg daily compared with a 20% reduction in non-diabetic patients. On the other hand aspirin 325 mg in GISSI-3 trial (a non-randomized treatment) was associated to an independent beneficial effect on 6-week mortality [unpublished data]. Finally, the antiplatelet trialists collaboration overview [13] on patients with unstable angina, acute MI, prior MI, stroke or transient ischemic attack indicate a similar benefit (38 vs 36 vascular events saved /1 000 treated patients) in diabetics vs non-diabetics. Taken together, these data would suggest that the beneficial effect of aspirin is maintained in diabetics, but the optimal dosage remains undefined.

Attention has recently shifted toward selective antiplatelet agents, such as the glycoprotein IIb/IIIa antagonists. Preliminary data from subgroup analysis of the several trials in acute coronary syndromes recently completed, such as PURSUIT [unpublished data], appear to suggest that these agents are as effective in diabetic as in non diabetic patients.

Beta-blockers

Beta-blockers are able to reduce mortality post-MI in diabetic patients, with an absolute and relative beneficial effect in most cases larger than that observed in non-diabetics. However, current evidence is based on subgroup analysis of several trials performed during the eighties and on non-randomized studies [14]. Further, in these trials the population of patients with diabetes was scarcely represented. However, the pooled data indicate a 37% mortality reduction during the acute phase (13% in non diabetics) and a 48% mortality reduction post-discharge (33% in non-diabetics). Since all these studies have been performed before the advent of fibrinolytic therapy, the question remains whether this marked beneficial effect is still present in more "updated" populations. Data from a subgroup analysis of DIGAMI study [15], where beta-blockers were not randomized, suggest that this is the case.

ACE-inhibitors

Several recent trials used ACE-inhibitors as a new therapeutic strategy in the attempt to reduce mortality and morbidity after acute MI. The studies in which ACE--inhibitors have been started within 24 to 36 hrs after the onset of symptoms showed an overall reduction of about 5 deaths for 1,000 treated patients. In the GISSI 3 study [16] information on diabetic status was available for 18,294 patients (97% of total population); 2.7% of patients had an IDD (n=496) and 12.5 % had a NIDD (n=2294). In this study, treatment with lisinopril was associated with a decreased 6-week mortality in both IDD (1 1.8% vs 21.1 %, p<0.05) and NIDD (8.0% vs 10.6%, p<0.05) patients corresponding to a 44.1 and 24.5% reduction respectively [17]. The treatment was associated with an increased incidence of persistent hypotension and renal dysfunction, an effect similar to that observed in the general population. The meta-analysis by the "ACE-inhibitor in MI Collaborative Group" [unpublished data], including data from GISSI-3, CCS-1 and CONSENSUS 2, confirmed that the subgroup of diabetic patients experienced a 30 days lower mortality (10.3 vs 12.0 %, or 17.3 lives saved per 1 000 patients) when treated early with an ACE-inhibitor.

Statins

Two recent studies, the 4S [18] and the CARE [19] trials, evaluated the effect of statins in reducing morbidity and mortality in patients with an history of ischemic heart disease (mainly previous MI). The main difference between these two trials lies in the cut-off of cholesterol level for enrolment, that were much tighter for 4S than for CARE. A total of 202 diabetics (4.5% of the total population) were enrolled in 4S and of 586 (14% of the total population) in CARE. In both trials diabetics had a worsened outcome compared to non-diabetics; also, in both trials, the reduction in mortality was proportionally at least similar to that observed in non-diabetics. In the 4S study a 42% reduction in the incidence of death was observed in diabetic patients compared to 27% in non-diabetics; in the CARE study mortality reductions were -25% for non-diabetics, -23% for diabetics. Despite of the obvious limitations of this post-hoc analyses, these data suggest that statins confer long-term protection from cardiovascular events in diabetic patients recovering from MI at least to the same extent as in non-diabetics.

2. CONGESTIVE HEART FAILURE

The interest toward this clinical condition has grown recently mainly due to the increasing prevalence of this disease as a consequence of chronic ischemic heart disease, to the better understanding of pathophysiological mechanisms responsible for its evolution and to the availability of drugs that appear to improve prognosis markedly.

Again, data obtained in diabetic patients with CHF have been gathered mainly through the post-hoc analysis of clinical trials in patients with overt or silent heart failure. There is strong evidence indicating that ischemic heart disease in diabetics, particularly the post-MI setting, is associated with an increased incidence of CHF. This has been documented even in the fibrinolytic era by data from the GISSI -2 [4] as well as other studies.

Also, analysis of crude mortality and morbidity rates in diabetics vs non--diabetics with CHF again indicates that diabetics have a worse outcome. For example, the meta-analysis of the major trials in this setting, including about 13,000 patients from SAVE [25], AIRE [26], TRACE [27] and a subpopulation of SOLVD [22,23] trials showed mortality of 36.4% in diabetics and 24.7% in non diabetics [unpublished data]. The relative role of concomitant risk factors in this setting remains undefined.

Efficacy of pharmacological treatment

Beside the use of diuretics, which remain the mainstay of pharmacological treatment, and of digitalis, which remains a recommended treatment particularly in patients with atrial fibrillation, two classes of drugs appear as critical in the management of patients with heart failure: ACE-inhibitors, which are now indicated in all classes of CHF patients, and beta-blockers, whose efficacy in reducing morbidity and mortality has rapidly emerged from the latest trials [20].

Table 6-2. Efficacy of pharmacological agents in diabetic patients with acute MI

	In-hospital	Post-discharge
Fibrinolytics	++	NA
Aspirin	+	++
ACE-inhibitors	+++	++*
Beta-blockers	+++	+++
Statins	NA	++
Nitrates	+?	NA
Calcium antagonists	?	?

* efficacy evaluated only in patients with left ventricular dysfunction
+++ efficacy higher than that in non-diabetics
++ efficacy similar to that in non-diabetics
\+ efficacy lower than that in non-diabetics
NA not applicable
? data for diabetics not available from clinical trials performed

ACE-inhibitors

The landmark studies in the evaluation of the efficacy of ACE-inhibitors have been performed in the eighties and early nineties, when the CONSENSUS [21], SOLVD treatment [22] and SOLVD prevention [23] trials were completed. A sub-analysis of the SOLVD trial showed that ACE-inhibitors are as effective in diabetics as in non - diabetics in reducing mortality and hospitalization rates [24]. More recently, the attention of researchers shifted toward patients with overt CHF and/or with left ventricular dysfunction resulting from acute MI. All the "long-term" studies enrolling patients with left ventricular dysfunction some time after MI have shown a significant benefit of ACE-inhibitor therapy, with a risk reduction in mortality of 19 to 27% over a 2.5-4 years follow-up. The meta-analysis of the major trials in this setting mentioned earlier indicate that the beneficial effect of ACE inhibitors documented in the overall population is present also when limiting the analysis to patients with a history of diabetes. More in detail, the benefit per 1,000 patients was

36 in the 10,501 non diabetics and 48 in the 2,282 diabetics [unpublished data].

Beta-blockers

For many years beta-blockers have been contraindicated in CHF patients, and even more so in diabetic patients, where the accentuation of altered lipid levels induced by these drugs and the fear of masking hypoglycemic episodes have been considered strong contraindications to their use; however, the pioneering work performed in the seventies and the eighties particularly by Scandinavian groups [28] led the way to their targeted use in patients with asymptomatic or overt CHF. A retrospective analysis performed by Kjeskhus et al [29] showed that diabetic patients with CHF post-MI benefited even more than those with preserved left ventricular function. Recently, the investigators of the MOCHA trial [30] reported that the effect of treatment with carvedilol was associated to a dramatic decrease in mortality, that was most evident in diabetic patients, with a 6.1 % mortality after a median of 6 months, compared to a 30% mortality in the control group. Although the small sample size and short follow-up of the study or perhaps the ancillary properties of carvedilol, including a vasodilating and antioxidant activity, may have contributed to this outstanding result, these data would suggest that diabetic patients with CHF are among the ones who benefit most from treatment with betablockers.

3. CORONARY ANGIOPLASTY (PTCA)

A history of diabetes is associated with a higher incidence of complications during PTCA and to increased morbidity and mortality during follow-up. The mechanisms responsible for an increased incidence of restenosis are several, as well reviewed by Aronson et al [31]. Interestingly, in the BARI trial [32] comparing PTCA and coronary bypass surgery (CABG) in patients with multivessel disease, diabetic patients treated with PTCA had a higher mortality (35 vs 19%, $p<0.02$) as compared with CABG, whereas no difference was observed in non diabetic patients using the two different approaches. Also, older data derived from the TIMI-2 trial showed that primary angioplasty in patients with acute MI (a rapidly emerging new treatment of acute MI patients) was associated with a higher mortality than in patients treated with a more conservative strategy [6]. A prospective reassessment of the use of PTCA in diabetic patients with newer techniques is therefore warranted. Specifically the role of stenting implantation after direct PTCA is not yet completely defined either in non-diabetic or in diabetic patients, despite the extended use in clinical practice.

Efficacy of pharmacological treatment

So far, no conclusive data are available to indicate the best pharmacological treatment to prevent restenosis in this setting. Patients are usually treated with aspirin as a standard treatment with or without ticlopidine. Studies with ACE-inhibitors, calcium antagonists or statins usually failed to show any consistent effect of these agents in reducing the incidence of restenosis or morbidity during long-term follow-up. On the other hand data obtained with antithrombotic agents suggest that drugs such as abciximab [33] are effective in the general population. Due to the rapid evolution in the technique used for this intervention, including the use of stents and other devices, targeted to achieve a more stable vessel lumen after angioplasty, it is extremely difficult to quantitate the value of results obtained and published even very recently. Overall, there has been a lack of focus of the researchers on diabetic patients as a relevant subgroup to study in this setting and thus data on diabetic patients are scanty. Available unpublished data do suggest that the efficacy (or lack of efficacy) of different agents is similar irrespective of the diabetic status of the patients. Thus, currently the treatment of diabetic patients undergoing PTCA mirrors that of non-diabetic patients. In particular, no data are available to indicate whether a careful control of blood glucose during the peri-intervention period would decrease morbidity and mortality after PTCA.

4. IMPLICATIONS FOR CLINICAL PRACTICE

The continuous progress in the management of patients with cardiovascular diseases have radically changed their prognosis. This is particularly true for diabetic patients, whose rate of morbidity and mortality has now been shown to be beneficially affected by a variety of interventions, as summarized in this review. Several issues however should be underlined. First, most of these data have been obtained as post-hoc subgroup analysis of trials performed in a general population of patients with cardiovascular disease. This would imply the need to confirm these findings in appropriate prospective studies; although some ongoing studies with ACE-inhibitors target diabetic patients as a predefined subgroup where drug efficacy will be assessed [34], no further studies are ongoing or planned with most of the agents reviewed in this article, indicating that the evidence so far gathered will be the one to rely upon. Second, the application of these research findings in clinical practice remains a major challenge, since drugs consistently documented to be effective in specific patients population are often under-used in clinical practice. Finally, the burden of morbidity and mortality of diabetic patients with cardiovascular disease remains high and deserves testing novel therapeutic approaches targeting several pathophysiological alterations present in diabetic patients with cardiovascular diseases.

5. CALCIUM CHANNEL BLOCKERS

The role of calcium channel blockers in patients with acute MI is controversial. In the last decade several clinical trials have been performed to evaluate the role of these drugs in affecting prognosis post MI, with mixed results; short-acting nifedipine tended to increase mortality; diltiazem had a dicotomic effect of mortality, depending upon absence or presence of congestive heart failure and verapamil had a positive effect in patients without heart failure and a neutral effect in patients with heart failure were observed. Unfortunately, although diabetic patients represented between 5 and 23% of the enrolled population in the above trials, data on this subgroup of patients in these trials are lacking.

Some intriguing findings on a possible detrimental effect of calcium channel blockers have been recently published in NIDD patients with hypertension enrolled in the Appropriate Blood Pressure Control in Diabetes (ABCD) trial [35] where patients were treated with nisoldipine or enalapril. After 5 years of follow-up hypertensive patients randomized to nisoldipine had a fivefold higher incidence of fatal and non-fatal myocardial infarction, compared to patients allocated enalapril. The evidence from this trial is in agreement with preliminary data from the Fosinopril vs. Amlodipine Cardiovascular Event Trial (FACET) and other epidemiological evidence [36] suggesting that diabetic patients treated with dihydropiridine calcium antagonists experience cardiovascular events more frequently than patients treated with other antihypertensive agents (not placebo). Clearly, this intriguing finding need confirmation from the large studies currently ongoing.

REFERENCES

1. Jacoby RM, Nesto RW. Acute myocardial infarction in the diabetic patient: pathophysiology, clinical course and prognosis. J Am Coll Cardiol 1992; 20:736-44.
2. Smith JW, Marcus FI, Serokman R, Multicenter Postinfarction Research Group. Prognosis of patients with diabetes mellitus after acute myocardial infarction. Am J Cardiol 1984; 54:718-21.
3. Stone PH, Muller JE, Hartwell T, et al. The effect of diabetes mellitus on prognosis and serial left ventricular function after acute myocardial infarction: contribution of both coronary disease and diastolic left ventricular dysfunction to the adverse prognosis. J Am Coll Cardiol 1989; 14:49-57.
4. Zuanetti G, Latini R, Maggioni AP, Santoro L, Franzosi MG, GISSI-2 Investigators. Influence of diabetes on mortality in acute myocardial infarction: data from the GISSI-2 study. J Am Coll Cardiol 1993; 22:1788-94.
5. Lee KL, Woodlief LH, Topol EJ, Weaver D, Betriu A, Col J, Simoons M, Aylward P, Van de Werf F, Califf RM, for the GUSTO-1 Investigators. Predictors of 30-day mortality in the era of reperfusion for acute myocardial infarction. Results from an international trial of 41 021 patients. Circulation 1995; 91:1659-68.
6. Mueller HS, Cohen LS, Braunwald E, Forman S, Feit F, Ross A, Schweiger M, Cabin H, Davison R, Miller D, Solomon R, Knatterud GL, for the TIMI Investigators. Predictors of early morbidity and mortality after thrombolytic therapy of acute myocardial infarction. Analyses of patient subgroups in the thrombolysis in myocardial infarction (TIMI) trial, phase 11. Circulation 1992; 85:1254-64.
7. Malmberg K, Rydén L, Efendic S, Herlitz J, Nicol P, Waldenström A, Wedel H, Welin L, on behalf of the DIGAMI Study Group. Randomized trial of insulin glucose infusion followed by subcutaneous insulin treatment in diabetic patients with acute myocardial infarction (DIGAMI Study): effects on mortality at 1 year. J Am Coll Cardiol 1995; 26:57-65.
8. Malmberg K for the DIGAMI (Diabetes Mellitus Insulin Glucose Infusion in Acute Myocardial Infarction) Study Group. Prospective randomised study of intensive insulin treatment on long term survival after acute myocardial infarction in patients with diabetes mellitus. BMJ 1997; 314:1512-5.
9. Aoki 1, Shimoyama K, Aoki N, Homori M, Yanagisawa A, Nakahara K, Kawai Y, Kitamura S, Ishikawa K. Platelet-dependent thrombin generation in patients with diabetes mellitus: effects of glycemic control on coagulability in diabetes. J Am Coll Cardiol 1996; 27:560-6.
10. Fibrinolytic Therapy Trialists' (FTT) Collaborative Group. Indications for fibrinolytic therapy in suspected acute myocardial infarction: collaborative overview of early mortality and major morbidity results from all randomised trials of more than 1000 patients. Lancet 1994; 343:311-22.
11. Granger CB, Califf RM, Young S, Candela R, Samaha J, Worley S, Kereiakes DJ, Topol EJ, and the Thrombolysis and Angioplasty in Myocardial Infarction (TAMI) Study Group. Outcome of patients with diabetes mellitus and acute myocardial infarction treated with thrombolytic agents. J Am Coll Cardiol 1993; 21:920-5.
12. ISIS-2 Collaborative Group. Randomized trial of intravenous streptokinase, oral aspirin, both or neither among 17187 cases of suspected acute myocardial infarction: ISIS 2 Lancet 1988; ii:349-60.
13. Antiplatelet Trialists' Collaboration. Collaborative overview of randomised trials of antiplatelet therapy-I: prevention of death, myocardial infarction, and stroke by prolonged antiplatelet therapy in various categories of patients. Br Med J 1994; 308:81-106.

14. Kendall MJ, Lynch KP, Hjaimarson A, Kjekshus J. B-Blockers' and sudden cardiac death. Ann Intern Med 1995; 123:358-67.
15. Malmberg K, Ryden L. Intense metabolic control decreases long-term mortality in diabetics with acute myocardial infarction: predictors of one year mortality. J Am Coll Cardiol 1996; 27 Suppl. A, 82A.
16. Gruppo Italiano per lo Studio della Sopravvivenza nell'infarto Miocardico. GISSI-3: effects of lisinopril and transdermal glyceryl trinitrate singly and together on 6-week mortality and ventricular function after acute myocardial infarction. Lancet 1994; 343:1115-22.
17. Zuanetti G, Latini R, Maggioni AP, Franzosi MG, Santoro L, Tognoni G, on behalf of GISSI-3 Investigators. Effect of the ACE-inhibitor lisinopril on mortality in diabetic patients with acute myocardial infarction: the data from the GISSI-3 study. Circulation 1997; 96:4239-45.
18. Pyorala K, Pedersen TR, Kjekshus J, Faergeman 0, Oisson AG, Thorgeirsson G, The Scandinavian Simvastatin Survival Study (4S) Group. Cholesterol lowering with simvastatin improves prognosis of diabetic patients with coronary heart disease. A subgroup analysis of the Scandinavian Simvastatin Survival Study (4S). Diabetes Care 1997; 20:614-20.
19. Sacks FM, Pfeffer MA, Moye LA, Rouleau JL, Rutherford JD, Cole TG, Brown L, Wamica JW, Arnold JMO, Wun C-C, Davis BR, Braunwald E, for the Cholesterol and Recurrent Events Trial Investigators. The effect of pravastatin on coronary events after myocardial infarction in patients with average cholesterol levels. N Engl J Med 1996; 335:1001-9.
20. Packer M, Bristow MR, Cohn JN. The effect of carvedilol on morbidity and mortality in patients with chronic heart failure. N Engl J Med 1987; 316:1429-35.
21. The CONSENSUS Trial Group. Effects of enalapril on mortality in severe congestive heart failure. Results of the Cooperative North Scandinavian Enalapril Survival Study (CONSENSUS). N Engl J Med 1987; 316:1429-35.
22. The SOLVD Investigators. Effect of enalapril on survival in patients with reduced left ventricular ejection fractions and congestive heart failure. N Engl J Med 1991; 325:293-302.
23. The SOLVD Investigators. Effect of enalapril on mortality and the development of heart failure in asymptomatic patients with reduced left ventricular ejection fractions. N Engl J Med 1992; 327:685-91.
24. Shindier DM, Kostis JB, Yusuf S, Quinones MA, Pitt B, Stewart D, Pinkett T, Ghali JK, Wilson AC, for the SOLVD Investigators. Diabetes mellitus, a predictor of morbidity and mortality in the studies of left ventricular dysfunction (SOLVD) trials and registry. Am J Cardiol 1996; 77:1017-20.
25. Moyé LA, Pfeffer MA, Wun CC, Davis BR, Geltman E, Hayes D, Farnham DJ, Randall OS Dinh H, Arnold JMO, Kupersmith J, Hager D, Glasser SP, Biddle T, Hawkins CM, Braunwald E, for the SAVE Investigators. Uniformity of captopril benefit in the SAVE study: subgroup analysis. Eur Heart J 1994; 15:2-8
26. The Acute Infarction Ramipril Efficacy (AIRE) Study Investigators. Effect of ramipril on mortality and morbidity of survivors of acute myocardial infarction with clinical evidence of heart failure. Lancet 1993; 342:821-28.
27. Torp-Pedersen C, Kober L, Carisen J, on behalf of the TRACE Study Group. Angiotensin-converting enzyme inhibition after myocardial infarction: the Trandolapril Cardiac Evaluation Study. Am Heart J 1996; 132:235-43.
28. Waagstein F, Hjalmarson A, Varnauskas E, Wallentin J. Effect of chronic betaadrenergic receptor blockade in congestive cardiomyopathy. Br Heart J 1975; 37:1022-36.
29. Kjeskhus J, Gilpin E, Cali G, Blackey AR, Henning H, Ross J Jr. Diabetic patients and betablockers after acute myocardial infarction. Eur Heart J 1990; 11:43-50.
30. Bristow MR, Gilbert EM, Abraham WT, Adams KF, Fowler MB, Hershberger R, Kybo SH, Narahara KA, Robertson AD, Krueger S, for the MOCHA Investigators. Effect of carvedilol on left ventricular function and mortality in diabetic versus non-diabetic patients with ischaemic or non-ischaemic dilated cardiomyopathy. Eur Heart J 1996; 17(Suppl.):78.
31. Aronson D, Bloomgarden Z, Rayfield EJ. Potential mechanisms promoting restenosis in diabetic patients. J Am Coll Cardiol 1996; 27:528-35.
32. The Bypass Angioplasty Revascularization Investigation (BARI) Investigators. Comparison of coronary bypass surgery with angioplasty in patients with multivessel disease. N Engl J Med 1996; 335:217-25.

33. Topol EJ, et al. Long-term protection from myocardial ischemic events in a randomized trial of brief integrin β3 blockade with percutaneous coronary intervention. JAMA 1997; 278:479-84.
34. The HOPE Study Investigators. The HOPE (Heart Outcomes Prevention Evaluation) Study: The design of a large, simple randomized trial of an angiotensin-converting enzyme inhibitor (ramipril) and vitamin E in patients at high risk of cardiovascular events. Can J Cardiol 1996; 12:127-37.
35. Estacio RO, Jeffers BW, Hiatt WR, Biggerstaff SL, Gifford N, Schrier RW. The effect of nisoldipine as compared with enalapril on cardiovascular outcomes in patients with non-insulin-dependent diabetes and hypertension. N Engl J Med 1998; 338:645-52.
36. Pahor M, Psaty BM, Furberg C. Treatment of hypertensive patients with diabetes. Lancet 1998; 351:689-690.

7. ALBUMINURIA IN NON-INSULIN-DEPENDENT DIABETES - RENAL OR EXTRARENAL DISEASE ?

Anita Schmitz
Medical Department, Horsens Sygehus, Horsens, Denmark

Microalbuminuria and overt proteinuria in IDDM have been decisively established as indicators of various stages in diabetic renal disease. Persistent microalbuminuria defines the stage of 'incipient nephropathy', that is the stage that heralds progression to overt nephropathy in more than 80 percent of cases within a decade, with proteinuria and relentless decline in kidney function, unless intervention is undertaken. Subsequent research concerning patients with NIDDM has clearly demonstrated, that the course of complications and the implication of albuminuria differ in several respects between the two types of diabetes [1-3].

Microalbuminuria and proteinuria are frequent in NIDDM amounting to 20-40% and 5-15% [4-8] respectively. This pertain also to newly or recently diagnosed patients [4,8-13], though at that point elevated albuminuria is reversible to some degree [12,14,15]. As an apparent paradox the incidence of renal impairment is of a low order of magnitude, 3-8% (in Caucasian NIDDM patients) [3,4,16]. Because of the large and increasing number of patients with NIDDM, however, renal failure constitutes an important health care problem [17-19], yet the poorer prognosis in NIDDM is due mainly to cardiovascular disease. As an additional ambiguity microalbuminuria has been brought into focus as a marker of cardiovascular disease and probably also increased mortality among non-diabetic subjects. Furthermore microalbuminuria may precede or even predict the onset of NIDDM [20].

The first reports that microalbuminuria is associated with an increased mortality in NIDDM appeared in 1984 [21,22].

1. MICROALBUMINURIA - A MAJOR RISK MARKER.

We investigated the prognostic influence of microalbuminuria, also in relation to other potential risk factors in a 10-year follow-up study [5] of 416 Caucasian non-insulin-dependent patients with urinary albumin concentration (UAC) ≤ 200µg/ml [23]. UAC was measured in first morning urine samples at each outpatient attendance during one year. Inclusion criteria were: age 50-75 years, age at diagnosis ≥ 45 years, and treatment managed without insulin for a period of at least 2 years. Clinical data are presented in table 7-1; 15 µg/ml was chosen as the upper limit of a normal UAC, and the patients were divided into three categories accordingly. Weight recorded during all visits, was related to "ideal" and treatment modality was recorded as the most "severe" (insulin > tablets > diet) during the 10-year period, since treatment modality often changes over time.

It appears that the only significant differences between the groups were higher level of plasma glucose ($r = 0.17$, $p < 0.001$) and serum creatinine ($r = 0.26$, $p < 0.001$) in patients with elevated UAC. Blood pressures (BP) were comparable and hypertensive (BP > 160 mmHg systolic or > 95 mmHg diastolic, n= 255) and normotensive (n=161) patients had mean UAC values of 11.0 µg/ml x/÷ 2.8 and 9.3 µg/ml x/÷ 2.8 respectively. Frequency of retinopathy tended to be higher in the groups with microalbuminuria.

After 10 years 219 patients had died. The prognostic influence of the variables listed in table 7-1 was first evaluated separately using a log rank test, and subsequently by Cox regression analyses. The significant independent prognostic variables and hazard ratios are given in Table 7-2. By these analyses, the remaining variables had no significant influence on survival.

	Urinary albumin concentration (µg/ml)			
	≤15 n = 290	>15-≤40 n = 72	>40-≤200 n = 54	
Age (years)	65.6±6.5 50-75	66.9±5.7 50-75	67.2±5.0 54-75	NS[e]
Age at diagnosis (years)	59.4±7.2 45-75	59.8±6.6 47-74	59.8±6.9 46-71	NS
Known diabetes duration (years)	6.2±4.9 0-23	7.1±5.4 0-22	7.5±5.2 1-21	NS
Systolic blood pressure (mmHg)	159±23 113-250	162±23 108-210	166±26 110-231	NS
Diastolic blood pressure (mmHg)	91±12 60-130	92±14 60-134	94±12 70-128	NS
Fasting plasma glucose (mmol/liter)	8.8±2.1 4.6-15.8	9.5±2.6 4.4-15.8	9.6±2.5 6.1-17.6	p=0.005
Fasting plasma glucose (all visits) (mmol/liter)	8.7±1.6 5.3-14.1	9.3±1.9 6.4-13.6	9.3±1.8 5.8-16.3	p=0.002
Relative weight (all visits) (%)	111±18 73-207	114±22 76-231	111±16 82-163	NS
Serum creatinine (mg%)[a]	0.9×/÷1.2 0.6-2.8	1.0×/÷1.3 0.6-3.1	1.1×/÷1.4 0.7-3.3	p=0.000
Sex (M/F)[b]	126/164	35/37	23/31	NS
Retinopathy (N/B/P)[c]	238/42/0	51/16/0	43/10/0	NS
Treatment (D/T/I)[d]	33/201/56	8/44/20	5/34/15	NS

[a]Geometric mean ×/÷ tolerance factor.
[b]M/F, male/female.
[c]N/B/P, normal/background/proliferative.
[d]D/T/I, diet/tablet/insulin.
[e]NS, not significant.

Table 7-1. Clinical data.

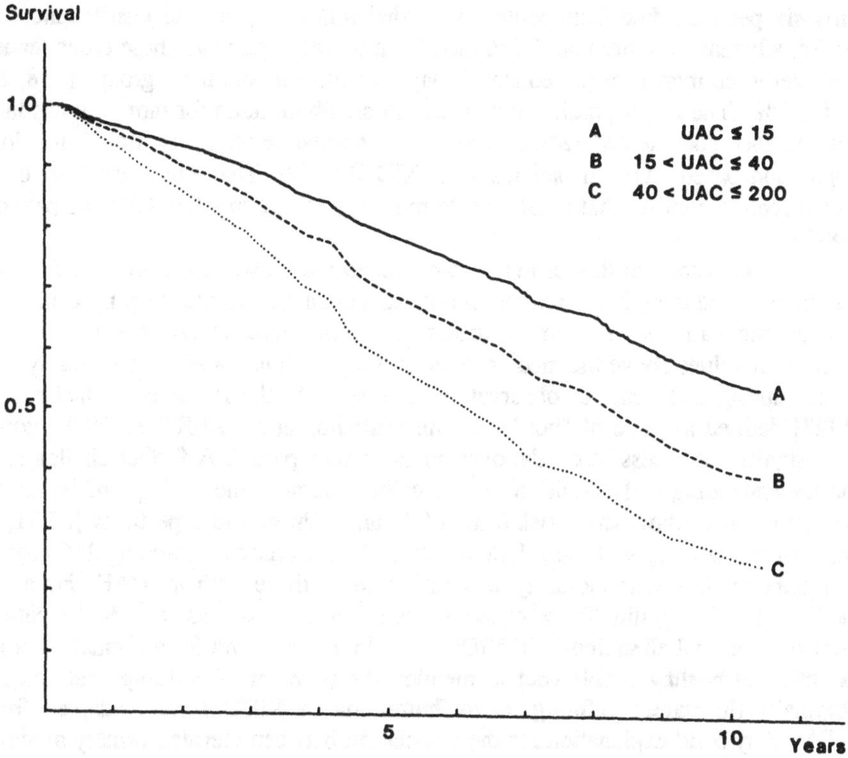

Figure 7-1. Survival curves for the three UAC groups, after correction for the other independent significant prognostic variables;age, known diabetes duration and serum creatinine. N=407,(subjects with missing value(s) excluded).

Table 7-2 Significant prognostic variables and the way they were presented in the Cox regression analyses.

Risk factor		Regression coefficient	p-value	Relative risk
Age	in years	0.070	0.0000	1.07
Diabetes duration	>10	0.385	0.015	1.47
Serum creatinine	>1.3	0.463	0.043	1.59
UAC	>15	0.503	0.003	1.65
UAC	>40	0.382	0.078	1.46
			(0.000002)	(2.41)

The haxard ratios in the groups with elevated UAC relative to those with UAC≤15μg/ml were 1.65 (p=0.003) and 2.41 (p=0.000002) respectively.

Figure 7-1 presents the survival curves for the three UAC categories after correction for the influence of the other independent prognostic variables. From this it is clear, that even a minor increase in albuminuria , i.e. UAC 16-40 μg/ml, predicts a significantly reduced survival probability. A further increase in albuminuria i.e. 41-

200μg/ml, is associated with a worse prognosis. No additional increase in mortality was detected in patients with UAC > 200 μg/ml [5], but the latter were few (n = 25). Fifty-six per cent died from acute myocardial infarction, cardiac insufficiency, or stroke, whereas no more than 2.3% died from or with uraemia. These cases tended however to be increasingly frequent through the three albuminuria groups (0.8, 2.1 and 7.5 %).The major predictive power of microalbuminuria for mortality has later been further documented [24-26] and a very similar relative risk was found in a population based study in patients with NIDDM [27]. That study and also more recent reports confirm that renal disease mortality is rare in white NIDDM patients [28-29].

Considering the results in two prospective outpatient cohort studies, attention is called to high *normo*albuminuria carrying a risk. In the study by Gall et al. [29] among patients with normal urinary albumin excretion (AER <30 mg/24h), those with values above the median AER of 8 mg/24 h had a relative mortality risk of 2.7 during five years of observation, compared to the remainder. MacLeod et al.[28] defined a group of "borderline microalbuminuria": AER 10.6-29.9 μg/min with significant excess of deaths over an eight year period. A further challenge to the understanding and definition of microalbuminuria is the findings of increased prevalence of cardiovascular risk factors [30] and reduced life expectancy [25,31] in non-diabetic persons with raised albuminuria. In one study [25] among 216 elderly non-diabetics 8-9 year mortality was increased in those with an UAE above the median of 7.52 μg/min. These observations raises questions as regards the cut-off level of abnormal albuminuria in NIDDM, including the limit for a normal albumin excretion in healthy people (not to mention the problem of defining healthiness). Originally the values defining microalbuminuria in NIDDM were adapted from IDDM. Any solid explanation for the association between elevated urinary albumin excretion and cardiovascular disease and death has so far not emerged. Albuminuria in non-insulin-dependent patients is predominantly of glomerular origin [32], but the exact mechanism behind the increased escape of albumin is not known in either type of diabetes [33-35]. Elevated albumin excretion is associated with both coronary heart disease, cardiac failure (even minor degrees of left ventricular dysfunction), as well as peripheral vascular disease [3,10,36-39]. A number of cardiovascular risk factors have been linked also with albuminuria, such as lipoprotein abnormalities, hyperinsulinemia and markers of endothelial dysfunction as well as hypertension. It is predominantly systolic BP (also isolated systolic hypertension), that carries the risk [3,35,40-46]. None of these factors, however either alone or in combination have been able to "explain" the increased cardiovascular mortality in diabetic patients with microalbuminuria [3,35,40]. Consequently new risk factors are suggested [47].

2. ALBUMINURIA AND GLOMERULAR STRUCTURE

Diabetic glomerulopathy definitely does develop in non-insulin-dependent diabetes leading in some cases to renal impairment [48,49]. Information concerning the relationship between quantitative glomerular morphology and clinical renal parameters is however scarce in NIDDM.

In order to study the possible relation between urinary albumin excretion and glomerular structure [50] autopsy kidney tissue was sampled from 19 NIDDM patients, without other known renal disease, who had died within 18 months, mean 9 months, after UAC had been measured. They were aged 76 years (59-89),(mean, (range)), with known diabetes duration of 11 years (2-24), and UAC 29.7 μg/ml x/÷ 5.5 (1.4-710). Autopsy kidney tissue from 19 consecutive comparable non-diabetics was sampled for control.

A quantitative light-microscopic examination was performed on periodic-acid-Schiff- (P.A.S.) stained sections. The classic diabetic glomerulopathy is characterized by increased amounts of basement membrane and mesangial matrix (P.A.S.-positive) in the glomerular tuft (Chapter 23). The volume of P.A.S.-positive material as percent of tuft volume (defined as the minimal convex circumscribed polygon), estimated by point counting, was significantly increased in the group of diabetics. In this series there was no correlation between the quantitative structural parameters obtained and UAC, figure 7-2. Notably, a high UAC was not necessarily associated with more advanced glomerulopathy. In a later light- and electron microscopic study of biopsies from 20 NIDDM patients with proteinuria [51],

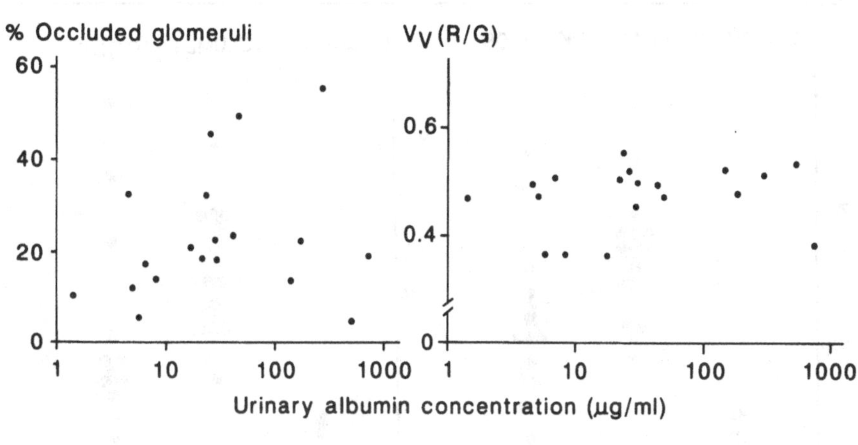

Figure 7-2. Relationship between urinary albumin concentration (μg/ml) and frequency of glomerular occlusion (left panel) and volume fraction of P.A.S. positive material in the glomerular tuft (Vv(R/G)) in 19 NIDDM patients.Data obtained from light-microscopic studies on autopsy kidneys. Reproduced with permission from the American Diabetes Association, Inc.

the degree of glomerulopathy was estimated by measurement of basement membrane thickness, mesangial and matrix volume fractions (i.e volume per glomerular volume), and frequency of glomerular occlusion. Patients were aged 55 years (37-67), known diabetes duration was 8 years (1-19), urinary albumin excretion (UAE) 1.5 g/24h (0.3-8.7) and glomerular filtration rate (GFR) 90 ml/min/1.73 m^2 (24-146). Data were compared with previous data on 22 IDDM patients aged 35 years (24-47), diabetes duration 20 years (12-31), UAE 1.4 g/24h (0.3-7.9) and GFR 57 ml/min/-1.73m^2 (16-104). Also, reference was made to 13 (age 51 years (21-68)) non-diabetic living renal transplant donors. There was a striking variation in the severity of glomerulopathy among NIDDM patients, and some proteinuric patients presented structural parameters within the normal range, figures 7-3 and 7-4. When retinopathy was taken into account, patients with this complication all showed a glomerulopathy index (index is a calculated expression of the sum of changes in peripheral basement membrane and mesangium) above normal. In those without retinopathy approximately half had a normal glomerular structure. Notably, GFR was rather well preserved in NIDDM compared with the younger IDDM patients, with the same degree of proteinuria.

In accordance with our findings Fioretto in a biopsy study on NIDDM patients with microalbuminuria found approximately 30% with a normal or near normal structure (see chapter 25). In our study kidney function was certainly associated with the structure, as an inverse correlation obtained between severity of glomerulopathy (index) and current glomerular filtration rate. Also the structural index correlated with the ensuing rate of decline in GFR (r = 0.84). No clear association between the structural quantities and albuminuria was however seen. Interestingly in three different studies around 60 percent of NIDDM patients with proteinuria had no retinopathy [5-7].

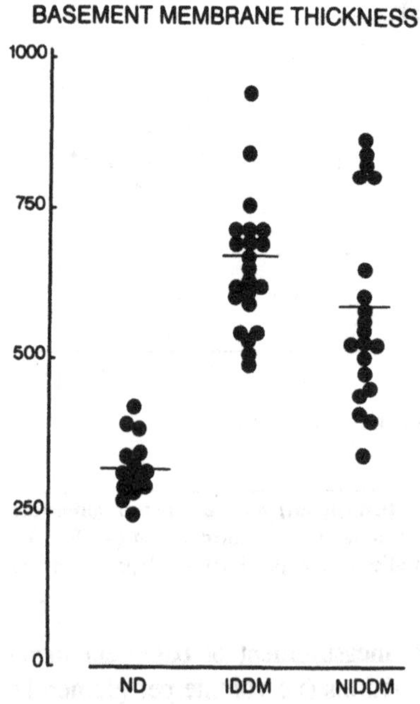

Figure 7-3 Basement membrane thickness in non-diabetic kidney transplant donors (ND) and IDDM and NIDDM patients with proteinuria. Data obtained from electron microscopic studies on kidney biopsies.

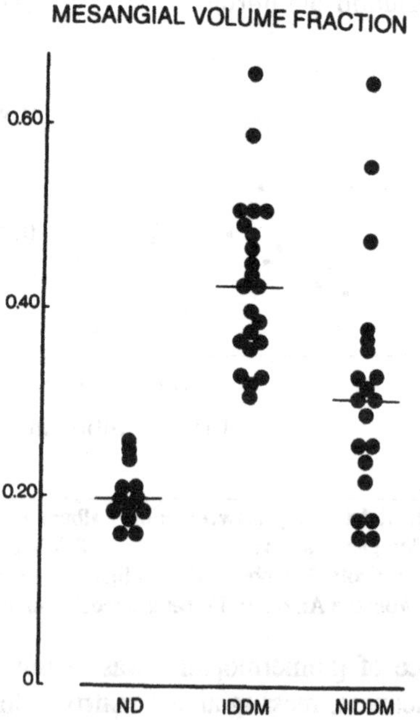

Figure 7-4 Mesangial volume perglomerulus (defined as the minimal convex polygon). See legend to figure 7-3.

These observations underline the rather poor relation between albuminuria and microvascular complications compared to conditions in IDDM, and thus imply, that albuminuria has also causes other than diabetic glomerulopathy. Renal diseases unrelated to diabetic nephropathy may contribute, and has been reported to be present in as much as 30% [52,53], though others did not confirm this high frequency [54-55] but rather around 12%. As commented above, abnormalities in albumin excretion may reflect cardiovascular disorders and essential hypertension.
Noticeable in this context, is the relation between systolic blood pressure and albumin excretion, which is demonstrated in several studies [3,5,6,9,27,43,56], whereas the relation to diastolic pressure is modest. Systolic hypertension expresses reduced vascular compliance, rather than "real" hypertension. Both systolic BP and albuminuria are related to coronary heart disease [3,57] in NIDDM as well as in non-diabetic subjects.

Albuminuria may thus express widespread vascular disease [3,35]. To elucidate why an increased urinary albumin excretion reflects non-renal complications, several hypotheses have been suggested. One recent remarkable clue for explaining this relation between albuminuria and atherosclerosis, was the finding of an increased transcapillary escape rate of albumin in otherwise clinically healthy subjects with elevated albuminuria [58]. Thus, NIDDM patients and non-diabetic persons share a relation between abnormal albuminuria and cardiovascular risk factors and disease. Transcapillary escape rate of albumin was increased in one study in NIDDM [59] but we were not able to confirm this [60]. Further research are needed to explain these matters.

3. ALBUMINURIA AND FUTURE RENAL FUNCTIONAL DETERIORATION

As in IDDM, microalbuminuria in NIDDM obviously also progresses to overt proteinuria, but overall does so to a less extent, around 20 % over a decade [61]. Also, the cumulative risk for renal failure 10 years after the appearance of proteinuria, was reported to be 11% in a population based study, [62] far more rare than in IDDM. Elevated UAE is associated both with nephropathy and large-vessel disease, and it is possible that even less severe renal changes may aggravate the latter. Either the rate of progression to renal failure is misjudged as many patients are selected out by death from other causes, or the development of diabetic glomerulopathy is indeed a slower process perhaps with a better potential for compensation [51]. The implication of microalbuminuria in a single individual is thus difficult to decide disabling the notion "incipient nephropathy" [63] in NIDDM.
(For further on the clinical course of renal function see Chapter 8).

4. PROGRESSION OF ALBUMINURIA

Although important for the evaluation of intervention measures, the knowledge of the rate of progression of albuminuria and factors with influence on this progression is modest. We followed of cohort of 278 NIDDM patients [64] during 6 years and estimated the average relative rate of increase to 17% per year, but with considerable interindividual variation. Systolic blood pressure and level of albuminuria were with significant influence on the rate of progression, but only a modest fraction of the variation between subjects could be explained by these factors. Progressors were then defined as those who both changed category of albuminuria (e.g. normo → micro) and increased more than 20%. These patients were characterised by elevated systolic blood pressure (165 vs 156 mmHg) a higher level of albuminuria as well as a more poor glycemic control (HbA_{1C} 8.2 vs 7.7%) as compared to their non-progressing counterparts. It should be noted though that a few progressors had a very low initial level of albuminuria (1μg/ml) stressing that serial measurements are imperative. In a more recent study [65] rather analogous differences were seen at baseline, only blood pressure did not appear as an independent predictor of progression of albuminuria.

Overall however, it is plausible from these and few other data [66], that progression of albuminuria is on average associated with a higher level of albumin excretion, more poor glycemic control and a higher blood pressure, especially the systolic. These factors are items for intervention.

5. PERSPECTIVES FOR INTERVENTION

There are no longer any doubts that microalbuminuria is a major independent marker of a poor prognosis. The predominant problem in intervention is though, that the cause(s) of albuminuria and the mechanism behind the relations to cardiovascular diseases and its risk factors still remain largely unknown, and the benefits from early intervention have yet to be proven. Obviously, reducing albuminuria would be a goal for the distressed physician, and numerous studies documented this to be rather easily obtainable by antihypertensive treatment and optimised glycemic control [3,56,63,67-68]. Most studies so far were however short-term without demonstrating any improvement in health or survival. Yet Ravid, in a now 7-year prospective study [69] demonstrates, that antihypertensive treatment with an ACE-inhibitor probably retards the decline in kidney function, at least in younger NIDDM patients. As expected, but finally shown in the DCCT [70] study, improving glycemic control was of benefit as regards microvascular complications, only this trial did not include NIDDM's.

During 14 years mortality was reduced in NIDDM's receiving intensive insulin therapy [71]. In this study aggressive cardiac screening was also introduced; the authors conclude that intensive insulin therapy does not increase cardiac mortality, a concern which has been put forward, but they could not prove a beneficial effect of the blood glucose reduction per se. The relation between poor glycaemic control and the development of macrovascular complications has indeed been disputed. Follow-up studies do indicate a relation as the incidence of cardiac events and mortality were higher in those with the most poor control [72-73]. But the concern whether insulin treatment accelerates atheroscleroses is still not solved [74] and this effect and the plausible beneficial effect of normalizing glycaemic control may neutralize each other. Further prospective intervention studies are needed and awaited [75-77]. The best possible control should though be aimed for in the individual patient and intervention against other plausible risk factors also seem prudent especially in regard to atherosclerosis, such as including lipid-lowering agents and aspirin [78]. The results from the 4S study [79] in the subgroup of diabetics showed a beneficial effect in those with CHD, but whether primary prevention should be undertaken is unknown, studies in progress [80]. Overall an intensive multifactorial intervention seems warranted [81].

REFERENCES

1 Mogensen CE, Schmitz O. The diabetic kidney: From hyperfiltration and microalbuminuria to endstage renal failure. Med Clin North Am 1988; 72:1465-1492.

2 Mogensen CE, Damsgaard EM, Frøland A, Nielsen S, de Fine Olivarius N, Schmitz A. Microalbuminuria in non-insulin-dependent diabetes. Clin. Nephrol 1992; 38: s28-s39.

3 Schmitz A. The kidney in non-insulin-dependent diabetes. Studies in glomerular structure and function and the relationship between microalbuminuria and mortality. Acta Diabetol 1992; 29: 47-69.

4 Fabre J, Balant LP, Dayer PG, Fox HM, Vernet AT. The kindney in maturity onset diabetes mellitus: A clinical study of 510 patients. Kidney Int. 1982; 21:730-738.

5 Schmitz A, Væth M. Microalbuminuria: A major risk factor in non-insulin-dependent diabetes. A 10-year follow-up study of 503 patients. Diabetic Med 1988; 5:126-134.

6 Gall M-A, Rossing P, Skøtt P, Damsbo P, Vaag A, Bech K, Dejgaard A, Lauritzen M, Lauritzen E, Hougaard P, Beck-Nielsen H, Parving H-H. Prevalence of micro- and macroalbuminiuria, arterial hypertension, retinopathy and large vessel disease in European Type 2 (non-insulin-dependent) diabetic patients. Diabetologia 1991; 34: 655-661.

7 Marshall SM, Alberti KGMM. Comparison of the prevalence and associated features of abnormal albumin excretion in insulin-dependent and non-insulin-dependent diabetes. Q J Med 1989; 70: 61-71.

8 Damsgaard EM. »Prevalence and incidence of microalbuminuria in non-insulin-dependent diabetes: Relations to other vascular lesions.« In *The Kidney and Hypertension in Diabetes Mellitus, 1. ed..*, C.E. Mogensen, ed. Boston: Martinus Nijhoff Publishing, 1988; pp 59-63.

9 Olivarius N de F, Andreasen AH, Keiding N, Mogensen CE. Epidemiology of renal involvement in newly-diagnosed middle-aged and elderly diabetic patients. Cross-sectional data from the population-based study " Diabetes care in Generel Practice", Denmark. Diabetologia 1993; 36: 1007-1016.

10 Standl E, Stiegler H. Microalbuminuria in a random cohort of recently diagnosed Type 2 (non-insulin-dependent) diabetic patients living in the Greater Munich area. Diabetologia 1993; 36: 1017-1020.

11 Ballard DJ, Humphrey LL, Melton LJ III, Frohnert PP, Chu C-P, O'Fallon WM, Palumbo PJ. Epidemiology of persistent proteinuria in type II diabetes mellitus. Population-based study in Rochester, Minnesota. Diabetes 1988; 37: 405-412.

12 Schmitz A, Hvid Hansen H, Christensen T. Kidney function in newly diagnosed Type 2 (non-insulin-dependent) diabetic patients, before and during treatment. Diabetologia 1989; 32: 434-439.

13 Uusitupa M, Siitonen O, Penttilä I, Aro A, Pyörälä K. Proteinuria in newly diagnosed type II diabetic patients. Diabetes Care 1987; 10: 191-194.

14 Martin P, Hampton KK, Walton C, Tindall H, Daview JA. Microproteinuria in Type 2 diabetes mellitus from diagnosis. Diabetic Med 1990; 7:315-318.

15 Patrick AW, Leslie PJ, Clarke BF, Frier BM. The natural history and associations of microalbuminuria in type 2 diabetes during the first year after diagnosis. Diabetic Med 1990; 7: 902-908.

16 Tung P, Levin SR. Nephropathy in non-insulin-dependent diabetes mellitus. Am J Med 1988; 85: Suppl 5A: 131-136.

17 Mauer SM, Chavers BM. »A Comparison of kidney disease in Type 1 and Type II diabetes.« In *Comparison of Type 1 and Type II Diabetes. Similarities and dissimilarities in etiology, pathogenesis, and complications*, M. Vranic, C.H. Hollenberg, G. Steiner, eds. New York, London: Plenum Press, 1985; pp 299-303.

18 Rosansky SJ, Eggers PW. Trends in the US end-stage renal disease population: 1973-1983. Am J Kidney Dis. 1987; 9: 91-97.

19 Brunner FP, Brynger H, Challah S, Fassbinder W, Geerlings W, Selwood NH, Tufveson G, Wing AJ. Renal replacement therapy in patients with diabetic nephropathy, 1980-1985. Report from the European Dialysis and Transplant Association Registry. Nephrol Dial Transplant 1988; 3: 585-595.

20 Mykkänen L, Haffner SM, Kuusisto J, Pyorälä K, Laakso M. Microalbuminuria precedes the development of NIDDM. Diabetes 1994 ;43: 552-557.
21 Jarrett RJ, Viberti GC, Argyropoulos A, Hill RD, Mahmud U, Murrells TJ. Microalbuminuria predicts mortality in non-insulin-dependent diabetes. Diabetic Med 1984; 1: 17-19.
22 Mogensen CE. Microalbuminuria predicts clinical proteinuria and early mortality in maturity-onset diabetes. N Engl J Med 1984; 310: 356-360.
23 Mogensen CE, Chachati A, Christensen CK, Close CF, Deckert T, Hommel E, Kastrup J, Lefebvre P, Mathiesen ER, Feldt-Rasmussen B, Schmitz A, Viberti GC. Microalbuminuria: an early marker of renal involvement in diabetes. Uremia Invest 1985-86; 9: 85-95.
24 Mattock MB, Morrish Nj, Viberti GC, Keen H, Fitzgerald AP, Jackson G. Prospective study of microalbuminuria as predictor of mortality in NIDDM. Diabetes 1992; 41: 736-741.
25 Damsgaard EM, Frøland A, Jørgensen OD, Mogensen CE. Eight to nine year mortality in known non-insulin dependent diabetics and controls. Kidney Int 1992; 41: 731-735.
26 Dinneen SF, Gerstein HC. The association of microalbuminuria and mortality in Non-insulin-dependent diabetes mellitus. Arch Intern Med; 157: 1413-1418.
27 Neil A, Hawkins M, Potok M, Thorogood M, Cohen D, Mann J. A Prospective population-based study of microalbuminuria as a predictor of mortality in NIDDM. Diabetes Care 1993; 16: 996-1004.
28 MacLeod JM, Lutale J,Marshall SM. Albumin excretion and vascular deaths in NIDDM. Diabetologia 1995; 38: 610-616.
29 Gall M-A, Borch-Johnsen K, Hougaard P, Nielsen FS, Parving HH. Albuminuria and poor glycemic control predict mortality in NIDDM. Diabetes 1995; 44: 1303-1309.
30 Jensen JS, Borch-Johnsen K, Jensen G, Feldt-Rasmussen B. Atherosclerotic risk factors are increased in clinically healthy subjects with microalbuminuria. Atherosclerosis 1995; 112: 245-252.
31 Yudkin JS, Forrest RD, Jackson CA. Microalbuminuria as predictor of vascular disease in non-diabetic subjects. Islington diabetes survey. Lancet 1988; 2: 530-3.
32 Damsgaard EM, Mogensen CE, Microalbuminuria in elderly hyperglycaemic patients and controls. Diabetic Med 1986; 3: 430-435.
33 Hostetter TH, Rennke HG, Brenner BM. The case for intrarenal hypertension in the initiation and progression of diabetic and other glomerulopathies. Am J Med 1982; 72: 375-380.
34 Schmitz A. Increased urinary haemoglobin in diabetics with microalbuminuria – measured by an ELISA. Scand J Clin Lab Invest 1990; 50: 303-308.
35 Deckert T, Feldt-Rasmussen B, Borch-Johnsen K, Jensen T, Kofoed-Enevoldsen A. Albuminuria reflects widespread vascular damage. The Steno hypothesis. Diabetologia 1989; 32: 219-226.
36 Mattock MB, Keen H, Viberti GC, El-Gohari MR, Murrells TJ, Scott GS, Wing JR, Jackson PG. Coronary heart disease and urinary albumin excretion rate in type 2 (non-insulin-dependent) diabetic patients. Diabetologia 1988; 31: 82-87.
37 Eiskjær H, Bagger JP, Mogensen CE, Schmitz A, Pedersen EB. Enhanced urinary excretion of albumin in congestive heart failure: effect of ACE-inhibition. Scand J Clin Lab Invest 1992; 52: 193-199.
38 Kelbæk H, Jensen T, Feldt-Rasmussen B, Christensen NJ, Richter EA, Deckert T, Nielsen SL. Impaired left-ventricular function in insulin-dependent diabetic patients with increased urinary albumin excretion. Scand J Clin Lab Invest 1991; 51: 467-473.
39 Keen H. »Macrovascular disease in diabetes mellitus.« In *Diabetic Complications: Early Diagnosis and Treatment*, D. Andreani, G. Crepaldi, U. Di Mario, G. Pozza, eds. John Wiley & Sons Ltd., 1987; pp 3-12.
40 Jensen T *Albuminuria – a marker of renal and generalized vascular disease in insulin-dependent diabetes mellitus* (thesis). Copenhagen: København: Lægeforeningens Forlag, 1991.
41 Winocour PH, Durrington PN, Ishola M, Anderson DC, Cohen H. Influence of proteinuria on vascular disease, blood pressure, and lipoproteins in insulin dependent diabetes mellitus. BMJ 1987; 294: 1648-1651.
42 Niskanen L, Uusitupa M, Sarlund H, Siitonen O, Voutilainen E, Penttilä I, Pyörälä K. Microalbuminuria predicts the development of serum lipoprotein abnormalities favouring atherogenesis in newly diagnosed Type 2 (non-insulin-dependent) diabetic patients. Diabetologia 1990; 33: 237-243.

43 Strandl E, Stiegler H, Janka HU, Mehnert H. Risk profile of macrovascular disease in diabetes mellitus. Diabete Metab (Paris) 1988; 14: 505-511.

44 Schmitz A, Ingerslev J. Haemostatic measures in Type 2 diabetic patients with microalbuminuria.Diabetic Med 1990; 7: 521-525.

45 Stehouwer CDA, Nauta JJP, Zeldenrust GC, Hackeng WHL, Donker AJM, den Ottolander GJH. Urinary albumin excretion, cardiovascular disease and endothelial dysfunction in non-insulin-dependent diabetes mellitus. Lancet 1992; 340: 319-323.

46 Jensen T, Bjerre-Knudsen J, Feldt-Rasmussen B, Deckert T. Features of endothelial dysfunction in early diabetic nephropathy. Lancet 1989; i: 461-463.

47 Yudkin JS. Coronary heart disease in diabetes mellitus : three new risk factors and a unifying hypothesis. J Intern Med 1995; 238: 21-30.

48 Gellman DD, Pirani CL, Soothill JP, Muehrcke RC, Kark RM. Diabetic nephropathy, a clinical and pathologic study based on renal biopsies. Medicine 1959; 38: 321-367.

49 Thomsen AC. *The Kidney in Diabetes Mellitus* (thesis). Copenhagen: Munksgaard, 1965.

50 Schmitz A, Gundersen HJG, Østerby R. Glomerular morpology by light microscopy in non-insulin-dependent mellitus. Lack of glomerular hypertrophy. Diabetes 1988; 37: 38-43.

51 Østerby R, Gall M-A, Schmitz A, Nielsen FS, Nyberg G, Parving H-H. Glomerular structure and function in proteinuric Type 2 (non-insulin-dependent) diabetic patients. Diabetologia 1993; 36: 1064-1070.

52 Parving H-H, Gall M-A, Skøtt P, Jørgensen HE, Løkkegaard H, Jørgensen F, Nielsen B, Larsen S. Prevalence and causes of albuminuria in non-insulin-dependent diabetic patients. Kidney Int 1992; 41: 758-762.

53 Taft JL, Billson VR, Nankervis A, Kincaid-Smith P, Martin FIR. A clinical-histological study of individuals with diabetes mellitus and proteinuria. Diabetic Med 1990; 7: 215-221.

54 Olsen S, Mogensen CE. Non-diabetic renal disease in NIDDM proteinuric patients may be rare in biopsies from clinical practice (Abstract). JASN 1995; 6: 454.

55 Waldherr R, Ilkenhans C, Ritz E. How frequent is glomerulonephritis in diabetes mellitus type II ? Clin Nephrol 1992; 37: 271-273.

56 Keen H, Chlouverakis C, Fuller J, Jarrett RJ. The concomitants of raised blood sugar: studies in newly-detected hyperglycaemics II: Urinary albumin excretion, blood pressure and their relation to blood sugar levels. Guys Hosp Rep 1969; 118: 247-254.

57 Ibsen H, Hilden T. New views on the relationship between coronary heart disease and hypertension. J Intern Med 1990; 227: 77-79.

58 Jensen JS, Borch-Johnsen K, Jensen G, Feldt-Rasmussen B. Microalbuminuria reflects a generalized transvascular albumin leakiness in clinically healthy subjects. Clinical Science 1995; 88: 629-633.

59 Nannipieri M, Rizzo L, Rapuano A, Pilo A, Penno G, Navalesi R. Increased transcapillary escape rate of albumin in microalbuminuric Type II diabetic patients. Diabetes Care 1995; 18: 1-9.

60. Nielsen S, Schmitz A, Rehling M, Ingerslev J, Mogensen CE. Dissociation of urinary albumin excretion and transcapillary escape rate as markers of microvascular and/or endothelial function in NIDDM patients. Diabetes 1997; 46 (suppl. 1): 309A

61 Mogensen CE. Microalbuminuria as a predictor of clinical diabetic nephropathy. Kidney Int 1987; 31: 673-689.

62 Humphrey LL, Ballard DJ, Frohnert PP, Chu C-P, O'Fallon WM, Palumbo PJ. Chronic renal failure in non-insulin-dependent diabetes mellitus. A population based study in Rochester, Minnesota. Ann Intern Med 1989; 111: 788-796.

63 Schmitz A. Renal function changes in middle-aged and elderly Caucasian Type 1 (non-insulin-dependent) diabetic patients – a review. Diabetologia 1993; 36: 985-992.

64 Schmitz A, Væth M, Mogensen CE. Systolic blood pressure relates to the rate of progression of albuminuria in NIDDM. Diabetologia 1994; 37: 1251-1258.

65 Gall MA, Hougaard P, Borch-Johnsen K, Parving HH. Risk factors for development of incipient and overt diabetic nephropathy in patients with non-insulin dependent diabetes mellitus: prospective,observational study. BMJ 1997; 314: 783-788.

66 Kikkawa R, Haneda M. »Risk factor for progression of microalbumiuria in relatively young NIDDM-patients.« In *Kidney and Hypertension in Diabetes Mellitus, 2. ed.*, C.E. Mogensen, ed. Boston, Dordrecht, London: Kluwer Academic Publishers, 1994; pp 103-109.

67 Melbourne Diabetic Nephropathy Study Group: Comparison between peridopril and nifedipine in hypertensive and normotensive diabetic patients with microalbuminuria. BMJ 1991; 302: 210-216.
68 Lacourcière Y, Nadeau A, Poirier L, Tancrède G. Captopril or conventional therapy in hypertensive type-II diabetics – 3-year analysis. Hypertension 1993; 21: 786-794.
69 Ravid M, Lang R, Rachmani R, Lishner M. Long-term renoprotective effect of angiotensin-converting enzyme inhibition in Non-insulin-dependent diabetes mellitus. Arch Intern Med. 1996; 156: 286-289.
70 The Diabetes Control and Complications Trial Research Group. The effect of intensive treatment of diabetes on the development and progression of long-term complications in insulin-dependent diabetes mellitus. N Engl J Med 1993; 329: 977-986.
71 Hellman R, Regan J, Rosen H. Effect of intensive treatment of diabetes on the risk of death or renal failure in NIDDM and IDDM. Diabetes Care 1997; 20: 258-264.
72 Uusitupa MIJ, Niskanen LK, Siitonen O, Voutilainen E, Pyörälä K. Ten-year cardiovascular mortality in relation to risk factors and abnormalities in lipoprotein composition in Type 2 (non-insulin-dependent) diabetic and non-diabetic subjects. Diabetologia 1993; 36: 1175-1184.
73 Kuusisto J, Mykkänen L, Pyörälä K, Laakso M. NIDDM and its metabolic control predict coronary heart disease in elderly subjects. Diabetes 1994; 43: 960-967.
74 Genuth S. Exogenous insulin administration and cardiovascular risk in non-insulin-dependent and insulin-dependent diabetes mellitus. Ann Intern Med 1996; 124 (1 pt 2): 104-109.
75 U.K. Prospective Study Group. U.K. Prospective Diabetes Study 16. Overview of 6 years' therapy of type II Diabetes: A progressive disease. Diabetes 1995 ; 44: 1249-1258.
76 Wolffenbuttel BHR, van Haeften TW. Prevention of complications in non-insulin-dependent diabetes mellitus (NIDDM). Drugs 1995;50 (2): 263-288.
77 Foote EF. Prevention and treatment of diabetic nephropathy. Am J Health-Syst Pharm 1995; 52: 1781-1792.
78 Antiplatelet Trialists' Collaboration. Collaborative overview of randomized trials of antiplatelet therapy: I. Prevention of death, myocardial infarction, and stroke by prolonged antiplatelet therapy in various categories of patients. BMJ 1994; 308 : 81-106
79 Haffner SM. Editorial. The Scandinavian Simvastatin Survival Study (4S) Subgroup analyses of diabetic subjects: Implications for the prevention of coronary heart disease. Diabetes Care 1997;20: 469-471.
80 The PPP Project Investigators. Design, rationale, and baseline characteristics of the prospective Pravastatin pooling (PPP) project- A combined analyses of three large-scale randomized trials: long-term intervention with Pravastatin on ischaemic disease (LIPID), Cholesterol and recurrent events (CARE), and West of Scotland coronary prevention study (WOSCOPS). Am J Cardiol 1995; 76: 899-905.
81 Vedel P, Gæde P, Obel J, Parving H-H, Pedersen O. Intensive multifactorial intervention in NIDDM patients with persistent microalbuminuria (Abstract). Diabetologia 1996; 39: Suppl. 1: A308.

8. THE CLINICAL COURSE OF RENAL DISEASE IN CAUCASIAN NIDDM PATIENTS.

Søren Nielsen and Anita Schmitz
Medical Department M, Aarhus Kommunehospital, Aarhus, Denmark

Diabetic nephropathy is now the most prevalent cause of end-stage renal disease (ESRD) in the Western world [1], accounting for approximately 30% of all patients entering end-stage renal failure programs [2]. Albeit diabetes is the single most important cause of ESRD in the United States [3], the percentage of patients with diabetes requiring renal replacement therapy in the European population is somewhat lower [4], about 13%, leaving glomerulonephritis and renal vascular disease due to hypertension as the most frequent causes of ESRD [5]. Approximately one-half of the diabetes related ESRD occur in NIDDM patients [6,7].

Clinical monitoring of diabetic nephropathy includes consecutive determinations of glomerular filtration rate (GFR) and measurements of the urinary albumin excretion rate (UAE) in 24 hour or in overnight collections [8]. In addition to indicating the degree of renal involvement UAE also serves as a cardiovascular risk marker. Even a minor abnormality, microalbuminuria, with UAE in the range of 20-200 $\mu g\ min^{-1}$ (i.e. dipstick-negative albuminuria), predicts an increased incidence of overt diabetic nephropathy as characterised by proteinuria (i.e. UAE>200 $\mu g\ min^{-1}$) and of cardiovascular mortality [9-11]. Moreover, studies in both Caucasian subjects and the Pima Indians have shown that proteinuria is associated with a poor prognosis in terms of survival [12,13].

Measurement of the plasma clearance of an intravenously injected, single-dose of ^{51}Cr-EDTA is considered a reliable and reproducible method for routine determination of GFR, and superior to assessment of the endogenous creatinine clearance [14,15]. The coefficient of variation (CV) in an unselected group of patients with various renal disorders has been reported to be 4.1% in patients with GFR $\geq$ 30 ml min^{-1} and 11.6% in patients with a GFR<30 ml min^{-1} [15]. The reproducibility of GFR determinations in diabetic patients was recently evaluated and showed a CV of the single-shot ^{51}Cr-EDTA procedure similar to that of the afore mentioned patients and

Mogensen, C.E. (ed.), THE KIDNEY AND HYPERTENSION IN DIABETES MELLITUS.

similar to the constant ^{125}I-iothalamate infusion technique [16]. The plasma clearance technique offers an advantage in a diabetic population since it does not rely on timed urine sampling.

1. NEWLY DIAGNOSED NIDDM

Studies of Caucasian subjects have shown, that GFR is elevated by 10-20% in newly diagnosed NIDDM patients [17-19]. Moreover, renal plasma flow (RPF) [17,19] and kidney volume [18] are increased. In comparison with an age matched control group Vora et al. found, that 45% of the patients had a GFR above the mean+2 SD (=120 ml. min.$^{-1}$ 1.73 m^{-2}) of the control subjects. Frank hyperfiltration (GFR>140 ml min^{-1} 1.73 m^{-2}) was not observed by Schmitz et al. [18] in contrast to the 16% of the patients reported by Vora et al. [17]. In a population based study [20] one hour creatinine clearance was not increased in 81 subjects with fasting hyperglycaemia (i.e. previously undiagnosed diabetes) as compared to healthy sex and age matched control subjects.

2. IMPACT OF INITIAL METABOLIC TREATMENT

Schmitz et al first demonstrated that correction of glycaemic control over 3 months in 10 newly diagnosed NIDDM patients (mean(SD) age 59 (5) years) was associated with a reduction in both GFR and kidney volume to normal values as well as a decline in UAE which correlated with the fall rate of GFR [18]. Recently, Vora et al. [21] examined renal haemodynamics before and after 6 months of antidiabetic treatment in 76 newly diagnosed NIDDM patients (age 54 (10) years). GFR and albuminuria declined significantly during treatment, whereas mean values of RPF and filtration fraction were unchanged. The fall rate in GFR was significantly, but not very precisely, correlated with reductions of HBA_{1c} and RPF, but not with changes in UAE, blood pressure or lipids. The decline in GFR was more pronounced in younger patients with GFR levels above 120 ml. min.$^{-1}$ 1.73 m^{-2} before treatment. Despite the reduction after 6 months, GFR remained greater than 120 ml. min.$^{-1}$ 1.73 m^{-2} in a considerable number (32%) of patients as compared to pre-treatment level of 45%. In a very recent study Wirta et al. [22] also observed significantly higher GFR levels in 149 NIDDM patients with a disease duration of less than one year as compared with 150 healthy control subjects (117 (27) vs 103 (24) ml. min.$^{-1}$ 1.73 m^{-2}).

3. ESTABLISHED NIDDM

Cross-sectional studies of Caucasian patients with established NIDDM have shown that GFR is well preserved in patients with uncomplicated NIDDM [23] as well as in microalbuminuric patients [23-26] (Table 8-1). Glomerular hyperfiltration (e.g. GFR > mean+2 SD of a control group) has not been a consistent finding [20,23,24,27,28], but a few studies have described high levels of GFR in some of the patients [29-31]. In a follow-up of 109 NIDDM patients Wirta et al. found that the glomerular hyperfiltration observed during the first year after the diagnosis of NIDDM persisted after 6 years [26] and measurements of kidney volume of the same patients suggested that the maintenance of a high GFR level may be ascribed to an increased kidney size [29]. Recently, significantly higher GFR levels were reported by Vedel et al. in NIDDM patients with microalbuminuria as compared with normoalbuminuri patients and healthy control subjects [32]. Moreover, glomerular hyperfiltration was found in 37% of the microalbuminuric patients. The GFR of microalbuminuric patients was related to age, diabetes duration, level of glycaemic control and urinary sodium excretion. Thus, although increased glomerular filtration rate may be determined by other factors it may be regarded as a risk marker for development of diabetic nephropathy. Conversely, the presence of arterial hypertension is associated with significantly lower GFR levels in NIDDM patients without overt nephropathy as compared to normotensive NIDDM patients [33,34].

4. LONGITUDINAL STUDIES

Only a few studies studies have evaluated the rate of decline in kidney function using the direct measurements of GFR (e.g. ^{51}Cr-EDTA plasma clearance) in patients with established NIDDM with different levels of albuminuria [35-37].

Table 8-1
Glycaemic control, risk factors and kidney function in normo- and microalbuminuric NIDDM patients.

	Normoalbuminuria	Microalbuminuria
Sex (male/female)	14/5	14/5
Age (years)	64 ±4.5	64.5±4.2
Diabetes duration	7.3±5.6	8.4±6.8
Body mass index (kg. m^{-2})	27.1± 3.2	28.2±3.7
Fasting p-glucose (mmol. l^{-1})	8.5±2.5	9.1±2.7
HbA_{1c} (%)	7.7±1.5	7.7±1.3
UAE (μg. min^{-1})	7.0x/÷1.6	61.7x/÷2.3
GFR (ml. min.$^{-1}$ 1.73 m^{-2})	94±13	91±20
Kidney volume (ml. 1.73^{-2})	220±45	260±54*
Systolic blood pressure (mm Hg)	154±17	164±22
Diastolic blood pressure (mm Hg)	81±11	86±11
Retinopathy (N/B/P)	16/3/0	9/8/2*
Antidiabetic treatment (diet/oha)	6/13	4/15
Antihypertensive treatment (%)	21	37
Smokers/non-smokers	7/12	12/7

*p<0.05
Values are: UAE: geometric meanx/÷antilog SD. Other: mean ±SD or numbers.
[Data obtained from reference no. 24].

These studies describe the clinical course of renal function, not the natural history of diabetic nephropathy, since any drug therapy (e.g. antihypertensive therapy), which may influence renal function and albuminuria was continued. and adjusted during the studies.

Normo- and microalbuminuria

Recent longitudinal studies have confirmed, that NIDDM patients with normo- and microalbuminuria have preserved renal function. In a 3.4 year follow-up study of 37 patients (age 63 (5) years, known diabetes duration 7 (5) years) Nielsen et al. [35] found, that the average rate of decline in GFR in both normo- and microalbuminuric patients was similar to that reported in healthy, non-diabetic individuals (-1.0 ml. $min.^{-1}$ 1.73 m^{-2}) [38]. However, the change in GFR varied considerably between individuals: from -13.5 to +4.3 ml. $min.^{-1}$ 1.73 m^{-2} per year (patients with normoalbuminuria) and from -7.0 to +4.2 ml. $min.^{-1}$ 1.73 m^{-2} per year (patients with microalbuminuria). Multiple regression analysis revealed, that the fall rate of GFR was significantly related to the systolic blood pressure at baseline (Figure 8-1), as well as the mean systolic blood pressure during the study.

This relationship was also seen when the analysis was confined to the patients (73%) without antihypertensive treatment. The fall rate of GFR was not related to the level of albuminuria, metabolic parameters, or baseline GFR [39]. Thirty-two patients from this study population were further followed for a mean of 5.5 (range: 3.3-7.5) years, and the average fall rate of GFR did not differ from the above-mentioned results [40]. However, it was also found that poorer glycaemic control and higher level of albuminuria were independently associated with a higher fall rate of GFR in patients without antihypertensive treatment. Conversely, the relationship with systolic blood pressure was not reproduced, probably because of the patients were in relatively good blood pressure control for that age group (antihypertensive treatment: 163/86 mm Hg; no antihypertensive treatment: 148/79 mm Hg). Thus, a normal or fairly treated blood pressure may not be a primary determinant of renal function changes in this patient group, however, studying such patients may disclose factors operating beyond blood pressure. In a recent Brazilian study of normoalbuminuric NIDDM patients (age 53 (7) years, diabetes duration 7 (5) years) followed for 5 years blood pressure did not determine the fall rate of GFR [36]. However, only 6 of the 32 patients studies were characterized by hypertension at baseline. The study also provides some evidence that glomerular hyperfiltration (baseline GFR > mean+2 SD of normal control values) may be associated with an increased rate of decline of GFR although regression to the mean should be kept in mind. In another recent prospective study serum prorenin was not related to microalbuminuria, nor did prorenin predict the rate of decline of GFR or progression rate of albuminuria [41]. A relationship between the decline in renal function (estimated as the reciprocal creatinine level) and systolic blood pressure was also been found in an Israeli study of somewhat younger (age 42 (2) years, known diabetes duration<2 years), normotensive patients followed for 14 years [42].

Diabetic nephropathy

The clinical course of renal function in NIDDM patients with proteinuria was evaluated by Gall et al. in a prospective study of 26 patients (age 52 (SE 2) years, known diabetes duration 9 (1) years) followed for 5.2 (range: 1.0-7.0) years and in whom a kidney biopsy had shown diabetic glomerulosclerosis [37]. An average of 7 (range: 3-10) GFR measurements were performed in each patient. GFR decreased

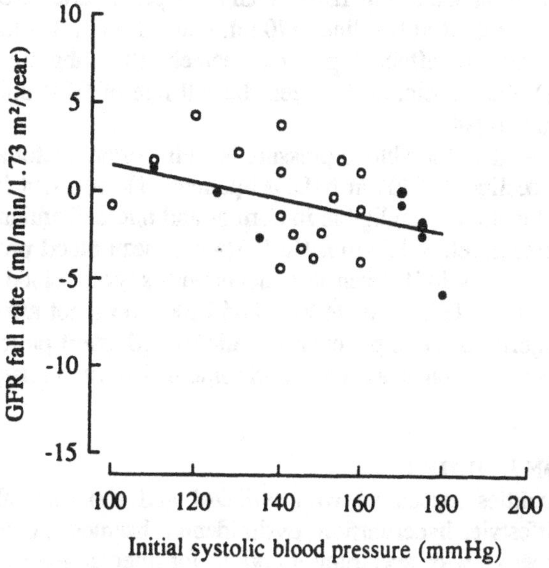

Figure 8-1

from 83 (24-146) to 58 (2-145) ml. min.$^{-1}$ 1.73 m^{-2}, with a mean reduction of 5.7 ml. min.$^{-1}$ 1.73 m^{-2} per year. Again, considerable interindividual variation was found, ranging from a decrease of 22.0 to an increase of 3.5 ml min^{-1} 1.73 m^{-2} per year. Concomitantly, albuminuria increased from 1.2 (0.3-7.2) (geometric mean (range)) to 2.3 (0.4-8.0) g/24 h ($p<0.001$). Systolic blood pressure, mean blood pressure and baseline GFR correlated significantly with the rate of decline in GFR in a univariate analysis whereas no correlations were found between the fall rate of GFR and dietary protein intake, total cholesterol, HDL-cholesterol or HbA_{1c} concentrations during the follow-up period. Multiple regression analysis revealed that the systolic blood pressure during the study was the only factor significantly determining the rate of decline in GFR. Although blood pressure was unchanged throughout the study (162/93 at entry versus 161/89 mm Hg at exit) the prevalence of arterial hypertension was quite high as judged from the substantial number of patients requiring antihypertensive medication (62% at entry versus 81% at exit). The overall mortality was 27%. Three patients died from uremia and 4 patients from cardiovascular diseases. Two patients needed renal replacement therapy at the end of the study.

Other studies have indicated that systolic blood pressure has a major impact on the progression renal function deterioration. Stornello et al. reported that normotensive NIDDM patients with persistent proteinuria treated with placebo for 12 months had stable GFR [43]. Based on measurements of creatinine clearance Biesenbach et al. recently found comparable fall rates of GFR in proteinuric IDDM and NIDDM patients who had normal GFR at baseline (>70 ml. $min.^{-1}$ 1.73 m^{-2}). Although this was a study of the most severely affected patients, namely the subgroup that eventually progressed to ESRD, the association between the fall rate of GFR and blood pressure was clearly demonstrated [44].

Thus, elevated systolic blood pressure is an important factor associated with a progressive decline decline in GFR in NIDDM patients. However, it is also clear, that the decline in renal function is negligible in normo- and microalbuminuric patients with a systolic blood pressure below 150 mm Hg [35] or a mean blood pressure around 95 mm Hg in younger subjects [45]. Even in patients with systolic blood pressures above 150 mm Hg the decline in GFR is quite low, and ESRD does not affect the long-term prognosis of the majority of these patients. In patients with overt proteinuria, however, deterioration in kidney function is accelerated in some patients and related to the systolic blood pressure [37].

5. INTERVENTION STUDIES

The list of abnormalities associated with NIDDM and abnormal albuminuria (e.g. obesity, sedentary lifestyle, hypertension, dyslipidemia, haemostatic abnormalities and insulin resistance) opens a wide spectrum of options for intervention studies focusing on the rate of progression of diabetic nephropathy.

Metabolic control

There are no long-term intervention studies of optimized metabolic control in Caucasian patients with long standing NIDDM. The large scale UK prospective study (presently in progress) will probably improve our understanding of the effects of different levels of glycaemic control on long-term complication risk (retinopathy, nephropathy, neuropathy, cardiovascular diseases, etc). The study does, however, not measure GFR, and levels of albuminuria are based on concentration measurements rather than timed excretion rates.

Non-pharmacological intervention

Currently, the influence of non-pharmacological intervention (diets, regular exercise or weight loss) on renal function in Caucasian NIDDM patients have not been reported.

Studies evaluating the renal effects of different pharmalogical treatments are sparse, mainly short-term, uncontrolled, and inconsistent in terms of the methods used for estimation of GFR.

Antihypertensive drugs

In an Australian study [46] of a mixed group of diabetic patients (62% NIDDM) with microalbuminuria, treatment with either an ACE-inhibitor or a calcium channel antagonist for 12 months significantly lowered UAE. This effect was predominantly seen in hypertensive patients (who also exhibited the greatest blood pressure reduction). Patients with GFR above 135 ml. $min.^{-1}$ 1.73 m^{-2} at baseline showed a significant decrease in GFR (from 186 to 161 ml. $min.^{-1}$ 1.73 m^{-2}), while patients with lower baseline levels displayed stable GFR values (from 96 to 92 ml. $min.^{-1}$ 1.73 m^{-2}). In an uncontrolled, long-term (36 months) study of 10 hypertensive NIDDM patients with microalbuminuria, using the single shot ^{51}Cr-EDTA procedure, treatment with Indapamide significantly reduced blood pressure from 180/100 to 140/85 mm Hg and albuminuria from (81.5 (SE 1) mg/24 h to 29.0 (4.5) mg/24 h, whereas GFR was unaffected during treatment, 95 ml. $min.^{-1}$ 1.73 m^{-2} [47]. Similar results have been described by Lacourciére et al. [48]. Ravid et al. [45] conducted a randomized, double-blind, placebo controlled trial, in which they demonstrated, that treatment of normotensive, microalbuminuric NIDDM patients (mean age 45 years, diabetes duration 7 years) with an ACE-inhibitor (Enalapril 10 mg per day) (n=49) for five years exerted a stabilizing effect on albuminuria and kidney function (estimated by the reciprocal creatinine level), while a progression was observed in the placebo group (n=45). A concomitant significant rise in mean blood pressure was noted only in the placebo treated patients, stressing the importance of blood pressure in the progression of renal disease in NIDDM. These results have now been confirmed in a further 2 year unblinded extension of the study [49]. In a recent Italian study of hypertensive normo- and microalbuminuric NIDDM patients aggressive treatment of blood pressure (<140/85 mm Hg) with cilazapril and amlodipin for 3 years was associated with an average annual fall rate of GFR of 2-2.5 ml. $min.^{-1}$ 1.73 m^{-2} [50]. In contrast, another Italian study observed increased GFR levels in a small group of microalbuminuric hypertesive patients with biopsy proven diabetic glomerulopathy treated with enalapril or nitrendipin for 27 months [51,52].

Published studies in Caucasian NIDDM patients with proteinuria are sparse and mostly short-term (6-12 months or less). In two studies of 6 months treatment with captopril a beneficial effects on GFR was observed by Stornello et al. [43], whereas a decline in GFR from 57 to 51 ml. $min.^{-1}$ 1.73 m^{-2} was found by Valvo et al. [53]. However, both studies were uncontrolled and included only 9 and 12 patients, respectively. More convincing results were reported by Nielsen et al. in a study comparing the effects of 12 months treatment with lisinopril (n=21) and atenolol (n=22) in hypertensive NIDDM patients with proteinuria [54]. Although blood pressure was markedly reduced by both treatments (from 162/85 to 136/72 mm Hg (lisinopril) and from 161/91 to 145/81 mm Hg (atenolol)) only lisinopril lowered albumin excretion rate. Importantly, however, no evidence of a stabilizing effects on GFR could be demonstrated since the annual decline in GFR was (12 (SE 2) ml. $min.^{-1}$ 1.73 m^{-2} (lisinopril) and 11 (1) ml. $min.^{-1}$ 1.73 m^{-2} (atenolol). It is to be noticed, however, that the blood pressure levels refer to 24 hour ambulatory measurements and that auscultatory clinical blood pressure values attained after 12 months treatment were rather high (158/81 mm Hg (lisinopril) and 160/83 mm Hg (atenolol). Recently, results from a 37 months follow-up of the same patients (open label treatment after the first 12 months) were published showing that the rate of decline of GFR was similar during both treatments, but that a slower progression rate could be identified after the first 6 months of treatment [55]. Conversely, in normotensive patients with persistent proteinuria, low dose administration of ß-blockers or ACE-inhibitors for 6-12 months reduce albuminuria in the absence of any effect on systemic blood pressure or GFR [43,56].

Lipid lowering agents

Chronic progressive kidney disease may be mediated by abnormal lipoprotein metabolism [57], a frequent finding in NIDDM [58,59]. A number of animal studies supporting this concept have been performed. At present published studies on long-term clinical intervention trials in Caucasian NIDDM patients is strikingly scanty. In a study by Nielsen et al. [60] 18 Caucasian patients (mean age 65 (4) years) with long-standing NIDDM (known diabetes duration 11 (6) years), moderate hypercholesterolaemia and microalbuminuria were enrolled in a randomized, double-blind, placebo controlled study of the effects of a HMG-CoA-reductase inhibitor (simvastatin 10-20 mg per day for 36 weeks) on kidney function and microalbuminuria. During simvastatin treatment total cholesterol level declined significantly (from 6.7 (0.7) to 5.1 (0.5) mmol. l^{-1}). Compared to placebo, however, this marked improvement in the hyperlipidaemia was not associated with changes in GFR (single shot ^{51}Cr-EDTA procedure), UAE or the systemic blood pressure.

Presently, studies evaluating the renal effects of intervention against haemostatic parameters and insulin resistance are not available, but in progress. General aspects of diabetic renal disease in NIDDM patients have recently been reviewed in depth [61].

REFERENCES

1. FitzSimmons SC, Agodoa L, Striker L, Conti F, Striker G. Kidney disease of diabetes mellitus: NIDDK initiatives for the comprehensive study of its natural history, pathogenesis, and prevention. Am J Kidney Dis 1989; 8: 7-10.
2. Eggers PW. Effect of transplantation on the medicare end-stage renal disease program. N Engl J Med 1993; 381: 223-229
3. Walker WG. Hypertension-related renal injury: a major contributor to end-stage renal disease. Am J Kidney Dis 1993; 22: 164-173

4. Raine AEG. Epidemiology, development and treatment of end-stage renal failure in Type 2 (non-insulin-dependent) diabetic patients in Europe. Diabetologia 1993; 36: 1099-1104
5. Brunner FP, Selwood NH. Profile of patients on RRT in Europe and death rates due to major causes of death
groups. Kidney Int 1992; 42 Suppl. 38: S4-S15
6. Rettig B, Teutsch SM. The incidence of end-stage renal disease in type II and type II diabetes mellitus. Diabetic Nephropathy 1984; 3: 26-27
7. Grenfell A, Bewick M, Parsons V, Snowden S, Taube D, Watkins PJ. Non-insulin-dependent diabetes and renal replacement therapy. Diabetic Med 1988; 5: 172-176
8. Mogensen CE, Damsgaard EM, Frøland A, Nielsen S, de Fine Olivarius N, Schmitz A. Microalbuminuria in non- insulin-dependent diabetes. Clin Nephrology 1992; 38 Suppl. 1: S28-S38
9. Mogensen CE. Microalbuminuria predicts clinical proteinuria and early mortality in maturity-onset diabetes. N Engl J Med 1984; 310: 356-360
10. Jarrett RJ, Viberti GC, Argyropoulos A, Hill RD, Mahmud U, Murrells TJ. Microalbuminuria predicts mortality in non-insulin-dependent diabetics. Diabetic Med 1984; 1: 17-19
11. Schmitz A, Vaeth M. Microalbuminuria: a major risk factor in non-insulin-dependent diabetes. A 10-year follow-up study of 503 patients. Diabetic Med 1988; 5: 126-134
12. Stephenson JM, Kenny S, Stevens LK, Fuller JH, Lee E. Proteinuria and mortality in diabetes: the WHO multinational study of vascular disease in diabetes. Diabetic Med 1995; 12: 149-155
13. Nelson RG, Pettitt DJ, Carraher MJ, Baird HR, Knowler WC. Effect of proteinuria on mortality in NIDDM. Diabetes 1988; 37: 1499-1504
14. Bröchner-Mortensen J. A simple method for the determination of glomerular filtration rate. Scand J Clin Lab Invest 1972; 30: 271-274
15. Bröchner-Mortensen J, Rødbro P. Selection of routine method for determination of glomerular filtration rate in adult patients. Scand J Clin Lab Invest 1976; 36: 35-43
16. Mogensen CE, Hansen KW, Nielsen S, Mau Pedersen M, Rehling M, Schmitz A. Monitoring diabetic nephropathy: Glomerular filtration rate and abnormal albuminuria in diabetic renal disease – reproducibility, progression, and efficacy of antihypertensive intervention. AM J Kidney Dis 1993; 22: 174-187
17. Vora JP, Dolben J, Dean JD, Thomas D, Williams JD, Owens DR, Peters JR. Renal hemodynamics in newly
presenting non-insulin dependent diabetes mellitus. Kidney Int 1992; 41: 829-835.
18. Schmitz A, Hansen HH, Christensen T. Kidney function in newly diagnosed type 2 (non-insulin-dependent) diabetic patients, before and during treatment. Diabetologia 1989; 32: 434-439.
19. Keller CK, Bergis KH, Fliser D, Ritz E. Renal findings in patients with short-term type 2 diabetes. J Am Soc
Nephrol 1996; 7: 2627-2635.
20. Damsgaard EM, Mogensen CE. Microalbuminuria in elderly hyperglycaemic patients and controls. Diabetic Med 1986; 3: 430-435.
21. Vora JP, Dolben J, Williams JD, Peters JR, Owens DR. Impact of initial treatment on renal function in newly-diagnosed Type 2 (non-insulin-dependent) diabetes mellitus. Diabetologia 1993; 36: 734-740.
22. Wirta O, Pasternack A, Mustonen J, Oksa H, Koivula T, Helin H. Albumin excretion rate and its relation to kidney disease in non-insulin-dependent diabetes mellitus. J Intern Med 1995; 237: 367-373.
23. Schmitz A, Christensen T, Jensen FT. Glomerular filtration rate and kidney volume in normoalbuminuric non-insulin-dependent diabetics - lack of glomerular hyperfiltration and renal hypertrophy in uncomplicated NIDDM. Scand J Clin Lab Invest 1989; 48: 103-108.
24. Schmitz A, Christensen T, Møller A, Mogensen CE. Kidney function and cardiovascular risk factors in non-insulin-dependent diabetics (NIDDM) with microalbuminuria. J Intern Med 1990; 228: 347-352.

25. Savage S, Nagel NJ, Estacio RO, Lukken N, Schrier RW. Clinical factors associated with urinary albumin excretion in type II diabetes. Am J Kidney Dis 1995; 25: 836-844.
26. Wirta O, Pasternack A, Laippala P, Turjanmaa V. Glomerular filtration rate and kidney size after six years disease duration in non-insulin-dependent diabetic subjects. Clin Nephrol 1996; 45: 10-17.
27. Fabre J, Balant LP, Dayer PG, Fox HM, Vernet AT. The kidney in maturity onset diabetes mellitus: A clinical study of 510 patients. Kidney Int 1982; 21: 730-738.
28. Gragnoli G, Signorini AM, Tanganelli I, Fondelli C, Borgogni P, Borgogni L, Vattimo A, Ferrari F, Guercia M. Prevalence of glomerular hyperfiltration and nephromegaly in normo- and microalbuminuric type 2 diabetic patients. Nephron 1993; 65: 206-211.
29. Wirta OR, Pasternack AI. Glomerular filtration rate and kidney size in type 2 (non-insulin-dependent) diabetes mellitus. Clin Nephrol 1995; 44: 1-7.
30. Silveiro SP, Friedman R, Gross JL. Glomerular hyperfiltration in NIDDMpatients without overt proteinuria.
Diabetes Care 1993; 16: 115-119.
31. Nowack R, Raum E, Blum W, Ritz E. Renal hemodynamics in recent-onset type II diabetes. Am J Kidney Dis 1992; 20: 342-347.
32. Vedel P, Obel J, Nielsen FS, Bang LE, Svendsen TL, Pedersen OB, Parving HH. Glomerular hyperfiltration in microalbuminuric NIDDM patients. Diabetologia 1996; 39: 1584-1589
33. Rius F, Pizarro E, Castells I, Salinas I, Sanmarti A, Romero R. Renal function changes in hypertensive patients with non-insulin-dependent diabetes mellitus. Kidney Int 1996; 55 Suppl: S88-S90.
34. Rius F, Pizaro E, Salinas I, Lucas A, Sanmarti A, Romero R. Age as a determinant of glomerular filtration rate in non-insulin-dependent diabetes mellitus. Nephrol Dial Transplant 1995; 10: 1644-1647.
35. Nielsen S, Schmitz A, Rehling M, Mogensen CE. Systolic blood pressure relates to the rate of decline of glomerular filtration rate in Type 2 diabetes mellitus. Diabetes Care 1993; 16: 1427-1432.
36. Silveiro SP, Friedman R, De Azevedo MJ, Canani LH, Gross JL. Five-year prospective study of glomerular
filtration rate and albumin excretion rate in normofiltering and hyperfiltering normoalbuminuric NIDDM patients. Diabetes Care 1996; 19: 171-174.
37. Gall M-A, Nielsen FS, Smidt UM, Parving H-H. The course of kidney function in Type 2 (non-insulin-dependent) diabetic patients with diabetic nephropathy. Diabetologia 1993; 36: 1071-1078.
38. Rowe JW, Andres R, Tobin JD, Norris AH, Shock NW. The effect of age on creatinine clearance in men: A cross-sectional and longitudinal study. J Gerontology 1976; 31: 155-163.
39. Haffner SM, Valdez RA, Hazuda HP, Mitchell BD, Morales PA, Stern MP. Prospective analysis of the insulin-resistance syndrome (Syndrome X). Diabetes 1992; 41: 715-722.
40. Nielsen S, Schmitz A, Rehling M, Mogensen CE. The clinical course of renal function in NIDDM patients with normo- and microalbuminuria. J Intern Med 1997; 241: 133-141.
41. Nielsen S, Schmitz A, Derkx FHM, Mogensen CE. Prorenin and renal function in NIDDM patients with normo- and microalbuminuria. J Intern Med 1995; 238: 499-505.
42. Ravid M, Savin H, Lang R, Jutrin I, Shoshana L, Lishner M. Proteinuria, renal impairment, metabolic control, and blood pressure in type 2 diabetes mellitus. Arch Intern Med 1992; 152: 1225-1229.
43. Stornello M, Valvo EV, Scapellato L. Angiotensin converting enzyme inhibition in normotensive type II diabetics with persistent mild proteinuria. J Hypertens 1989; 7 Suppl 6: 314-315.
44. Biesenbach G, Janko O, Zazgornik J. Similar rate of progression in the predialysis phase in type I and type II
diabetes mellitus. Nephrol Dial Transplant 1994; 9: 1097-1102.
45. Ravid M, Savin H, Jutrin I, Bental T, Katz B, Lishner M. Long-term stabilizing effect of angiotensin-converting enzyme inhibition on plasma creatinine and on proteinuria in normotensive type II diabetic patients. Ann Intern Med 1993; 118: 577-581.

46. Melbourne Diabetic Nephropathy Study Group. Comparison between perindopril and nifedipine in hypertensive and normotensive diabetic patients with microalbuminuria. BMJ 1991; 302: 210-216.
47. Gambardella S, Frontoni S, Lala A, Felici MG, Spallone V, Scoppola A, Jacoangeli F, Menzinger G. Regression of microalbuminuria in type II diabetic hypertensive patients after long-term indapamide treatment. Am Heart J 1991; 122: 1232-1238.
48. Lacourcière Y, Nadeau A, Poirier L, Tancrède G. Captopril or conventional therapy in hypertensive type II diabetics.Three-year analysis. Hypertension 1993; 21: 786-794.
49. Ravid M, Lang R, Rachmani R, Lishner M. Long-term renoprotective effect of angiotensin-converting enzyme inhibition in non-insulin-dependent diabetes mellitus. A 7-year follow-up study. Arch Intern Med 1996; 156: 286-289.
50. Velussi M, Brocco E, Frigato F, Zolli M, Muollo B, Maioli M, Carraro A, Tonolo G, Fresu P, Cernigoi AM,
Fioretto P, Nosadini R. Effects of cilazapril and amlodipine on kidney function in hypertensive NIDDM patients. Diabetes 1996; 45: 216-222.
51. Ruggenenti P, Mosconi L, Bianchi L, Cortesi L, Campana M, Pagani G, Mecca G, Remuzzi G. Long-term treatment with either enalapril or nitrendipine stabilizes albuminuria and increases glomerular filtration rate in non-insulin- dependent diabetic patients. Am J Kidney Dis 1994; 24: 753-761.
52. Mosconi L, Ruggenenti P, Perna A, Mecca G, Remuzzi G. Nitrendipine and enalapril improve albuminuria and glomerular filtration rate in non-insulin dependent diabetes. Kidney International 1996; 55 Suppl: S91-S93.
53. Valvo E, Bedogna V, Casagrande P, Antiga L, Zamboni M, Bommartini F, Oldrizzi L, Rugiu C, Maschio G.
Captopril in patients with type II diabetes and renal insufficiency: Systemic and renal hemodyna alterations. Am J Med 1988; 85: 344-348
54. Nielsen FS, Rossing P, Gall M-A, Skøtt P, Smidt UM, Parving H-H. Impact of lisinopril and atenolol on kidney function in hypertensive NIDDM subjects with diabetic nephropathy. Diabetes 1994; 43: 1108-1113
55. Nielsen FS, Rossing P, Gall MA, Skøtt P, Smidt UM, Parving HH. Long-term effect of lisinopril and atenolol on kidney function in hypertensive NIDDM subjects with diabetic nephropathy. Diabetes 1997; 46: 1182-1188.
56. Stornello M, Valvo EV, Scapellato L. Persistent albuminuria in normotensive non-insulin-dependent (type II) diabetic patients: comparative effects of angiotensin-converting enzyme inhibitors and β-adrenoceptor blockers. Clin Sci 1992; 82: 19-23
57. Moorhead JF, Chan MK, El-Nahas M, Varghese Z. Lipid nephrotoxicity in chronic progressive glomerular and tubulo-interstitial disease. Lancet 1982; 1309-1311
58. Kostner GM, Karadi I. Lipoprotein alterations in diabetes mellitus. Diabetologia 1988; 31: 717-722
59. Niskanen L, Uusitupa M, Sarlund H, Siitonen O, Voutilainen E, Penttilä I, Pyörälä K. Microalbuminuria predicts the development of serum lipoprotein abnormalities favouring atherogenesis in newly diagnosed type 2 (non-insulin-dependent) diabetic patients. Diabetologia 1990; 33: 237-43IS
60. Nielsen S, Schmitz O, Møller N, Pørksen N, Klausen IC, Alberti KGMM, Mogensen CE. Renal function and insulin sensitivity during simvastatin treatment in Type 2 (non-insulin-dependent) diabetic patients with microalbuminuria. Diabetologia 1993; 36: 1079-1086
61. Ritz E, Stefanski A. Diabetic nephropathy in type II diabetes. American Journal of Kidney Diseases 1996; 27: 167-194.

9. USE OF THE ALBUMIN/CREATININE RATIO IN PATIENT CARE AND CLINICAL STUDIES

James H. Warram, MD, ScD and Andrzej S. Krolewski, MD, PhD
Section on Genetics and Epidemiology Joslin Diabetes Center, Boston, Massachusetts, USA

INTRODUCTION

In patients with diabetes, elevated urinary albumin excretion (UAE) indicates the existence of functional as well as morphological abnormalities in the kidney [1-3]. Therefore, measurement of UAE is used for the early diagnosis of diabetic kidney disease as well as for monitoring its natural course and the effectiveness of treatment. Quantitative and semiquantitative methods are used to measure UAE.

Among quantitative methods, the albumin excretion rate (AER) determined in timed urine collections is the most direct measure of UAE [4,5]. Due to the demands of the protocol and imperfect patient adherence, however, the AER is not suitable as a screening tool if the goal is to reach the widest population possible. By contrast, a simple index determined in random urine samples, the ratio of urinary concentrations of albumin and creatinine (AC ratio), is as reliable a measurement of UAE as the AER. Its coefficient of variation is as good as any reported in literature for the UAE determined in 24-hour urine collections [6-9], and its reproducibility in serial 24-hour specimens from patients is better than that of the AER calculated for the same specimens [10]. Moreover, in paired urine specimens, one a random urine sample and the other a 3-hour urine collection immediately following the random void, we found such a close relationship, $r^2 = 0.94$, between the AC ratio in one and the AER in the other, that the two indices of UAE can be considered equivalent, differing only by an appropriate conversion formula [9]. Since random urine samples are more easily obtained than timed urine collections, a test based on them is a far more suitable screening device for measuring UAE than one based on timed samples.

UAE in the proteinuric range can be measured semiquantitatively with reagent strips (dipsticks) such as Albustix (Bayer Corporation, Diagnostics Division, Elkhart, IN). There has been a consensus that reagent strips are positive (1+) when the AER is above 300 μg/min (432 mg/24hr).However, the proportion of positive reagent strip readings (Figure 9-1) increases only gradually with increasing AER, so that urine samples in the range around 300 μg/min give positive readings barely a majority (60%) of the time.

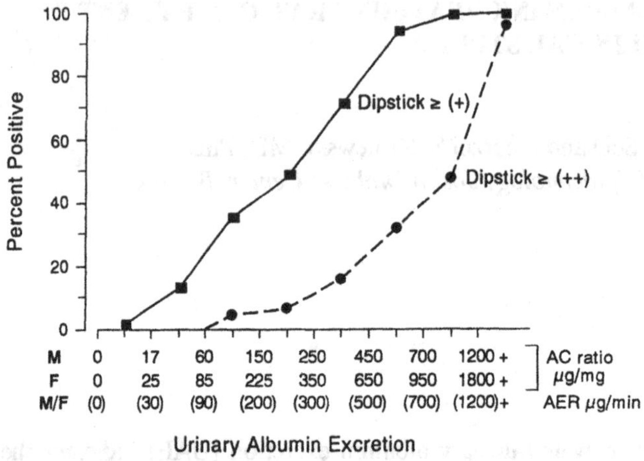

Figure 9-1 The percent of urine samples with a positive urinary albumin reagent strip (Albustix, Bayer Corporation, Diagnostics Division, Elkhart, IN.) according to the level of the albumin creatinine ratio (and equivalent albumin excretion rate) measured in the same urine. Albumin was assayed by immunonephelometry and creatinine by alkaline picric colorimetry [See ref. 9] To convert AC ratios in μg/mg to mg/mmol divide by 8.84. Adapted from Warram et al. [9].

This is because it measures albumin concentration without adjusting for hydration. Many patients with early overt proteinuria will be dipstick negative if they are well hydrated, while many patients with microalbuminuria will be dipstick positive (1+) if dehydrated [9]. In contrast, a 2+ positive dipstick is strong evidence of advanced proteinuria regardless of hydration (Figure 9-1).

Reagent strips that have also been designed to detect the lower concentrations of albumin found in patients with microalbuminuria have the same problem [11,12]. Variable hydration undermines their accuracy. A dipstick sensitive enough to detect a high proportion of microalbuminuric patients, including those who are well hydrated, will give many false positive tests in normoalbuminuric patients who are dehydrated. The patients with normal UAE who screen positive require follow up testing that causes unjustified alarm for patients and fruitless effort for healthcare providers.

In conclusion, screening methods based solely on measurements of albumin concentration are not suitable for screening for early diabetic nephropathy. The exception would be a population that has not been screened previously. The dipstick for proteinuria can be used to screen out patients with 2+ reactions whose UAE does not need further characterization. However, a 1+ reaction is not useful since it does not accurately distinguish proteinuria from microalbuminuria.

DIAGNOSIS OF EARLY NEPHROPATHY WITH THE AC RATIO

There is growing evidence that detection of the early stages of diabetic nephropathy (microalbuminuria) and appropriate treatment can prevent its progression. For example, studies have documented the importance of poor glycemic control (particularly hyperglycemia associated with a hemoglobin A1c above 8.1 %) in the progression of microalbuminuria to proteinuria [13]. Moreover, treatment with an inhibitor of angiotensin converting enzyme prevents or delays progression of early as well as late stages of nephropathy in both Type 1 and Type 2 diabetes [14-18]. The effectiveness of these programs, however, hinges on whether the methods of diagnosing the early stages of diabetic nephropathy meet the requirements of a screening procedure. At a minimum, a screening procedure must be economical and so convenient that virtually all members of the target population will participate in the detection program, not only once but repeatedly as long as they remain at risk [19]. In addition, the procedure should be accurate, i.e. lead to a high level of case detection and a reasonably low level of false positive results [19]. All of these requirements can be met by a screening protocol based on measurement of the AC ratio in random urines, and this is now reflected in the recommendations of expert committees on the screening and management of microalbuminuria [20,21].

While the expert committees agree on the utility of the AC ratio, an issue that was not fully resolved was the basis for defining microalbuminuria in terms of the AC ratio [20,21]. Therefore, we sought to develop a criterion based on the large body of empirical data from a large study of the Natural History of Microalbuminuria for which we screened over 1600 patients with IDDM between the ages of 15 and 44 years [9,22]. Since we and others have found that the relationship between the AC ratio and the AER differs for men and women, we defined criteria for men and women separately [23,24].

Definition of microalbuminuria in terms of the AC ratio: Since detectable albumin is present in the urine of most patients without any renal abnormality, it is necessary to determine a value to be considered as the upper boundary of normal. This can be approached from different perspectives. The most desirable approach is to restrict consideration to the range of AC ratio where intervention is still effective and select that value which minimizes the cost of screening and intervention [25]. However, the data required to define the lower boundary of microalbuminuria on a cost-effectiveness basis do not exist, and the various attempts to identify a predictive criterion have given discrepant results [26-30]. Lacking such data, the alternative is to set the criterion arbitrarily, for example at the 95th percentile of the distribution of UAE in non-diabetic individuals [9]. In random urine samples from non-diabetic controls, almost all AC ratios are below 1.7 mg of albumin/mmol of creatinine (15 μg/mg). The 95th percentile is 1.9 for men and 2.8 for women (17 and 25 μg/mg, respectively). These sex-specific criteria for dividing normoalbuminuria from microalbuminuria were also the values that maximized the reproducibility of positive classifications of repeat samples from individuals [9]. Interestingly, when converted to AERs by the formula developed in our comparability study [9], these cut points correspond in IDDM patients to an AER of 30 μg/min (43 mg/24hr) in timed urine collections in both men and women.

Accuracy of the AC ratio as a screening test: To evaluate the accuracy of the AC ratio in a random urine sample as a screening test for early nephropathy, we used data from our study of the Natural History of Microalbuminuria [9,22]. For this analysis, consideration was restricted to 607 patients whose nephropathy status was well documented by 4 or more determinations of the AC ratio within a two-year observation period. There were 182 patients in this group with abnormal UAE (30%), and 159 were positive on the first determination of the AC ratio. Thus, this single screening test detected 87.4% of the cases with abnormal UAE (Table 9-1).

Specificity, the proportion with negative tests among patients with normal UAE, was even higher, 92.9% (Table9-1). Note that in non-diabetics specificity would be 95%, a consequence of setting the criterion for abnormal elevation of the AC ratio at the 95th percentile of the distribution. The 7.1% prevalence of non-specific elevations of UAE in IDDM patients is similar to the 5% prevalence in non-diabetics. However, due to the fact that the majority of the target population does not have nephropathy, these false positive tests account for about one out of six positive tests. This means that a positive test has a predictive value of only 84.1%.

Improving the Accuracy of Screening: To improve accuracy of a screening test, a simple strategy is to test a second sample and, if the results are discordant, test a third in order to classify patients according to a consensus of two out of three tests. The results of such a screening algorithm are summarized in Table 9-1. Note that both sensitivity and specificity increased. The prevalence of false positives decreased from 7.1% to 1.6%, so the predictive value of a positive test increased from 84.1% to 96.0%. Therefore, this simple screening algorithm increased the predictive value of both positive and negative results to better than 95%.

The reason that a screening protocol based on the consensus of 2 out of 3 screening tests improves accuracy is because it distinguishes persistent elevation of UAE from transient elevations. Neither the natural history nor etiology of these transient elevations are understood. We have observed episodes of abnormal albumin excretion lasting up to several weeks in nondiabetics as well as patients with diabetes, so they are not peculiar to diabetes [9]. Similar episodes are observed in 24-hour urine collections, so they are not an artifact of random urine samples. They cannot be eliminated by the simple expedient of raising the upper limit of normal albumin excretion because transient elevations even into the proteinuric range are observed [31]. Thus, the most important characteristic that distinguishes microalbuminuria from these unrelated transient episodes is persistence itself. It is important, therefore, not to retest someone with a positive screening test too soon. Confirmation of a positive test after an interval of two or three months is much stronger evidence of persistence than a retest after 2 or 3 weeks, so follow up testing should be performed over a 3-6 month period [5, 20, 21].

Table 9-1 Sensitivity, Specificity and Predictive Values of Two Alternative Screening Protocols for the Detection of Microalbuminuria: Data on 607 IDDM Patients with Well Characterized Nephropathy Status Based on Two Year Follow up

	First Random Urine	Consensus of 2 out of the first 3 Random Urines*
Sensitivity	87.4% (159/182)	92.3% (168/182)
Specificity	92.9% (395/425)	98.4% (418/425)
Predictive Value of:		
Positive test	84.1% (159/189)	96.0% (168/175)
Negative test	94.5% (395/418)	96.8% (418/432)

* Collected over a 3-6 month time span. [Re-analysis of data from ref. 9.]

MONITORING THE CLINICAL COURSE OF DIABETIC NEPHROPATHY WITH THE AC RATIO

The AC ratio is useful not only in the diagnosis of early diabetic nephropathy but also for monitoring its progression and evaluating the effectiveness of treatment. Figure 9-2 traces the course of the AC ratio over intervals of 6 to 10 years in three patients with IDDM. The upper two panels are two patients who responded differently to treatment with ACE inhibitors. Although the AC ratio was measured in random urine samples obtained at intervals of several months, the response to treatment with ACE inhibition is easily recognized. It is unlikely that determination of the AER in timed urine collections, as recommended by many authors, could have provided any clearer picture.

The bottom panel of Figure 9-2 traces the natural history of the AC ratio in a patient followed for a decade, during which she was not treated with ACE inhibitors or antihypertensive agents. A curious feature of her course is the suggestion of a cyclic pattern that produces periodic elevations of her AC ratio into the microalbuminuria range. Similar cyclic patterns are recognizable in 5-10% of the IDDM patients that we are following, and they occur at any level of UAE, some cycling entirely within the normal range, others within the microalbuminuria range, and others crossing boundaries as this patient does. Note that these cycles are quite different from the episodic elevations discussed earlier in that the cycle length spans years. The physiology underlying these cycles has not been studied, presumably because frequent monitoring of UAE has been so uncommon that this phenomenon has not attracted attention. Routine use of the AC ratio in random

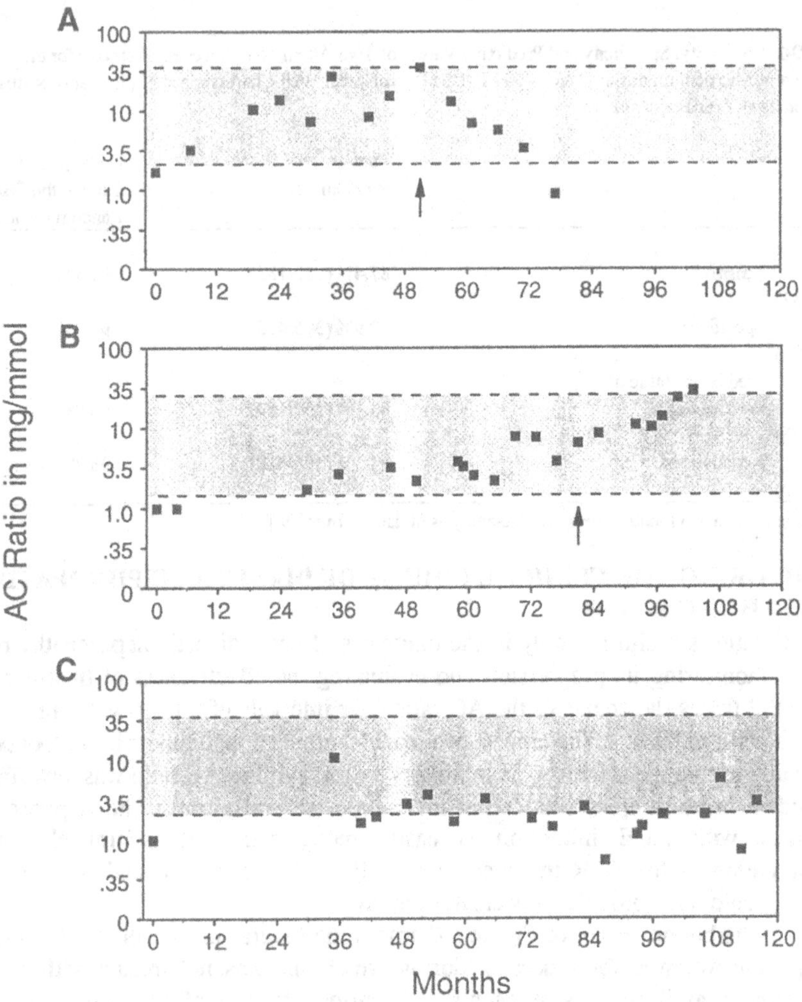

Figure 9-2 Plots of the albumin-creatinine ratio during 6 to 10 years of follow up for three patients. The shaded region represents the microalbuminuria range. Panel A illustrates a patient whose urinary albumin excretion decreased to normal levels when she was treated with an ACE inhibitor (beginning indicated by arrow). Panel B illustrates a patient whose urinary albumin excretion continued to rise despite treatment with an ACE inhibitor (beginning indicated by arrow) and the addition of other antihypertensive agents subsequently. Panel C illustrates a patient whose urinary albumin excretion seems to cycle in and out of the microalbuminuria range but appears not to have worsened during 10 years of follow up. (Warram and Krolewski, unpublished data)

urines to monitor the clinical course of patients will allow this pattern to be recognized so its underlying physiology can be studied.

APPLICATION OF THE AC RATIO IN EPIDEMIOLOGIC STUDIES

As discussed above, the easy availability of random urine samples makes the AC ratio the most practical method of screening for nephropathy in clinical practice. The same considerations make it the method best suited for use in epidemiologic studies. Two examples serve to illustrate its potential. One is its use to determine the prevalence of various stages of diabetic nephropathy according to duration of IDDM in 1613 patients of the Joslin Clinic [9]. By obtaining multiple measurements of the AC ratio over intervals of several months and applying the diagnostic criteria described above, the results shown in Figure 9-3 were obtained. Note that duration is given as post-pubertal duration. In patients with a pre-pubertal onset of IDDM, the appearance of microalbuminuria has been shown to be related to puberty [32]. Moreover, other investigators have shown that the contribution of pre-pubertal years of diabetes to the development of overt nephropathy is minimal [33]. These reports are consistent with our findings in a 35-year follow up study that the cumulative risk of endstage renal disease is more directly related to post-pubertal duration than total duration [34]. The height of the top curve represents the prevalence of all stages of diabetic nephropathy. To develop more advanced nephropathy, patients must first have developed microalbuminuria, so the prevalence of all stages of diabetic nephropathy can be considered as an estimate of the cumulative incidence of microalbuminuria according to postpubertal duration of IDDM. Similarly, the height of the lower curve indicates the prevalence (cumulative incidence) of persistent proteinuria.

In these patients with IDDM, the cumulative incidence of persistent microalbuminuria increased with duration of IDDM with distinct variations in the rate of increase.

A particularly notable feature was the very early appearance of significant numbers of patients with microalbuminuria: 6.4% of patients with IDDM for only 1 to 3 years a value eight times the 0.8% prevalence found in the sample of nondiabetics. Similar findings have been reported in other studies that determined UAE in timed urine collections, a Swedish study [35] and the EURODIAB IDDM study [36]. The cumulative incidence of microalbuminuria in our study leveled off around 20% after 10 years of diabetes and then resumed its steep climb in the second decade, reaching a new plateau around 52% after 30 years of postpubertal duration of diabetes. Overall there was no difference between men and women. The Pittsburgh Epidemiology of Diabetes Complications Study found higher prevalences of nephropathy (60 % among women and 80% among men) after 30 years of IDDM [37].

That study, however, included a very small number of individuals with a long duration of IDDM and used diagnostic methods that also included transient microalbuminuria.

The first case of overt proteinuria occurred after 7 years of post-pubertal IDDM. Beginning with the 9th year, there was an abrupt increase in the cumulative incidence of overt proteinuria as duration of diabetes increased, reaching a plateau during the third decade of IDDM, a feature similar to microalbuminuria.

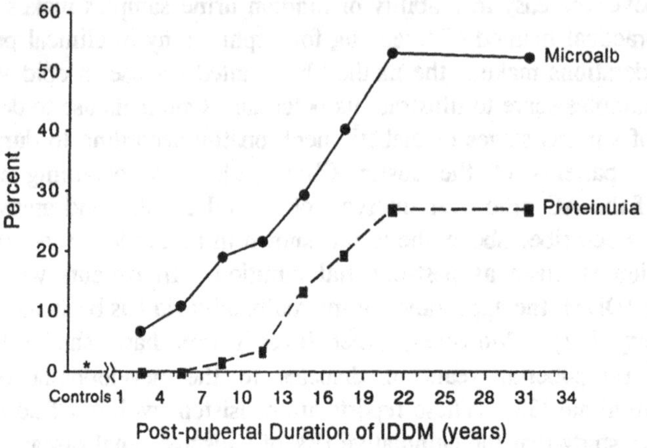

Figure 9-3 Prevalence of microalbuminuria and proteinuria according to post-pubertal duration of IDDM. See text for definitions. The solid line represents the combined prevalence of microalbuminuria and proteinuria; the broken line represents the prevalence of proteinuria. (adapted from Warram et al., ref. 9)

After 30 years of postpubertal IDDM, the cumulative incidence of overt proteinuria leveled off around 27%. The leveling off of the prevalence of proteinuria at this level is similar to the cumulative incidence of persistent proteinuria obtained in several follow-up studies [38,39].

The difference between the two cumulative incidence curves is mainly due to a rise (about 25%) in the prevalence of persistent microalbuminuria during the third decade of IDDM. It is not clear what proportion of these cases of persistent microalbuminuria represent an accumulation of cases that arose throughout the course of diabetes and did not progress (slow progressors) and what proportion are cases that occurred late in the course of diabetes and do not progress to persistent proteinuria.

The second example of the use of the AC ratio for epidemiologic studies are the comprehensive studies of the occurrence of elevated UAE in Pima Indians with NIDDM. In that population, a systematic screening for elevated UAE using the AC ratio has been conducted for almost a decade [40]. Non-diabetic Pima Indians have higher UAE then non-diabetic Caucasians. The 95th percentile of the distribution of the AC ratio in the non-diabetic Pimas equals 3.4 mg/mmol (30μg/mg). Based on this value as the cut-point for a diagnosis of nephropathy, the prevalence of nephropathy was 30% among Pima NIDDM patients with diabetes duration less then 5 years. The prevalence (cumulative incidence) of nephropathy increased with duration of diabetes to 85% after 20 years of diabetes. This is almost twice the prevalence found in the Caucasian IDDM patients of Joslin Clinic (Figure 9-3). The cumulative incidence of proteinuria was also much higher in

Pima Indians with NIDDM at each duration. After 20 years of diabetes, the prevalence of proteinuria among Pima Indians is 60% as compared to 25% in the Joslin Clinic IDDM patients. By 30 years of diabetes, however, the difference has grown much larger because the prevalence among Pimas climbs to 87%, while it levels off around 30% among Caucasian IDDM (personal communication, Dr. Robert G. Nelson).

FUTURE STUDIES, FUTURE NEEDS

As discussed above, systematic measurements of the AC ratio may be considered the best diagnostic tool for recognizing diabetic nephropathy early, as well as for monitoring its progression. In the following we outline areas for further research that would make the AC ratio an even more convenient and reliable tool for the diagnosis of diabetic nephropathy and for the investigation of the determinants of the clinical course of diabetic nephropathy.

There is a need to standardize the protocol for monitoring the AC ratio. From a pragmatic standpoint the choice is clear: a single sample is easier to obtain than timed collections of samples, and a random void demands less from patients than the collection of a first void. Moreover, it is well documented that the value in first-voided urine is 30-50% lower than the value in a random void [5, 24], so results from first voided specimens should not be intermingled with random voids since a separate set of diagnostic criteria needs to be developed for them.

Alternative laboratory methods are available for determination of both albumin and creatinine in urines; therefore, results and criteria developed at one center are not necessarily applicable elsewhere. A systematic effort to standardize determinations of the AC ratio, similar to that which is being established for assays of hemoglobin A1c as a measure of hyperglycemia, would facilitate research as well as support quality clinical care. Recently, a quantitative reagent strip (dipstick) for determining the AC ratio has been developed and is being evaluated against standard laboratory methods [41,42]. Dipsticks are particularly suited to outpatient settings, and their convenience could greatly increase the proportion of diabetic patients who are screened regularly. However, if this convenience means that the dipstick will become the predominant method in use, then its evaluation deserves as much rigor as the reference method.

Once the procedure for measuring the AC ratio is standardized, an important objective will be to develop diagnostic algorithms for diagnosing diabetic nephropathy at a stage that are optimally effective in preventing the development of advanced stages of diabetic nephropathy as well as macrovascular complications. Recognizing the heterogeneity of microalbuminuria indicated within even the small sample of patients shown in Fig. 9-2, it is likely that separate diagnostic criteria for the AC ratio will have to be developed for different circumstances. Not only will the criteria be conditioned on sex, but perhaps on duration of diabetes and age, and very importantly on race/ethnicity.

Implementation of frequent measurements of the AC ratio will allow more accurate data to be obtained about the natural history of early stages of diabetic nephropathy in IDDM as well as NIDDM. For example, it will allow a wide variety of patterns of microalbuminuria to be distinguished. This will not be just a matter of recognizing those who respond or do not respond to ACE inhibition, but also distinguishing rapid from slow progressors using the slope of the AC ratio over time. A steeply rising slope could be an indication to begin therapy early. Moreover, the ability to characterize these different patterns will also form the foundation for further studies of the etiology underlying these different subcategories of microalbuminuria.

ACKNOWLEDGEMENT

This research was supported by National Institutes of Health Grant R01-DK41526

REFERENCES

1. Hostetter TH, Rennke HG, Brenner BM. The case of intrarenal hypertension in the initiation and progression of diabetic and other glomerulopathies. Am J Med 1982; 72:375-380.
2. Chavers BM, Bilous RW, Ellis EN, Steffes MW, Mauer SM. Urinary albumin excretion as a predictor of renal structure in type I diabetic patients without overt proteinuria. N Engl J Med 1989; 320:966-970.
3. Walker JD, Close CF, Jones SL, et al. Glomerular structure in type I (insulin-dependent) diabetic patients with normo- and microalbuminuria. Kidney Int 1992; 41:741-748.
4. Mogensen CE. Urinary albumin excretion in early and long term juvenile diabetes. Scand J Clin Lab Invest 1971; 28:183-193.
5. Mogensen CE. Microalbuminuria as a predictor of clinical diabetic nephropathy. Kidney Int 1987; 31:673-89.
6. Ginsberg JM, Chang BS, Maltarese RA, Garella S. Use of single-voided urine samples to estimate quantitative proteinuria. N Engl J Med 1983; 309:1543-1546.
7. Nathan D, Rosenbaum C, Protasowiski D. Single void urine samples can be used to estimate quantitative microalbuminuria. Diabetes Care 1987; 10:414-418.
8. Dunn PJ, Jury DR. Random urine albumin:creatinine ratio measurments as a screening test for diabetic microalbuminuria-a five year follow-up. N Z Med J 1990; 103:562-564
9. Warram JH, Gearin G, Laffel L, Krolewski AS. Effect of duration of type I diabetes on the prevalence of stages of diabetic nephropathy defined by urinary albumin/creatinine ratio. J Am Soc Nephrol 1996; 7:930-937.
10. Watts GF, Kubal C, Chinn S. Long-term variability of overnight albumin excretion in insulin-dependent diabetes mellitus: Some practical recommendations for monitoring microalbuminuria. Diabetes Res Clin Pract 1990; 9:169-177.
11. Jensen JE, Nielsen SH, Foged L, Holmegaaard Sn, Magid E. The MICRAL test for diabetic microalbuminuria: predictive values as a function of prevalence. Scand J Clin Invest 1996; 56:117-122.
12. Pegoraro A, Singh A, Bakir AA, Arruda AL, Dunea G. Simplified screening for microalbuminuria. Ann Intern Med 1997; 127:817-819.
13. Cohen SE, Warram JH, Hanna LS, Laffel L, Krolewski AS. Threshold effect of hyperglycemia on the progression of microalbuminuria in type I diabetes. J Am Soc Neph 1997; 8:109A (abstract).
14. Lewis EJ, Hunsicker LG, Bain RP, Rohde RD, for the Collaborative Study Group. The effect of angiotensin-converting enzyme inhibition on diabetic nephropathy. New Engl J Med 1993; 329:1456-1462.
15. Viberti GC, Mogensen CE, Groop LC, Pauls JF, for the European Microalbuminuria Captopril Study Group. Effect of captopril on progression to clinical proteinuria in patients with insulin-dependent diabetes mellitus and microalbuminuria. JAMA 1994; 271:275-279.

16. Laffel LMB, McGill JB, Gans DJ, on behalf of the North American Microalbuminuria Study Group. The beneficial effect of angiotensin-converting enzyme inhibition with captopril on diabetic nephropathy in normotensive IDDM patients with microalbuminuria. Am J Med 1995; 99:497-504.
17. Kasiske BL, Kalil RSN, Ma JZ, Liao M, Keane WF. Effect of antihypertensive therapy on the kidney in patients with diabetes: a meta-regression analysis. Ann Intern Med 118:128-138, 1993.
18. Ravid M, Savin H, Jutrin I, Bental T, Katz B, Lishner M: Long term stabilizing effect of angiotensin converting enzyme inhibition on plasma creatinine and on proteinuria in normotensive type II diabetic patients. Ann Intern Med 1993; 118:577-581.
19. Morrison AS. Screening in chronic disease. New York, Oxford University Press, 1992, pp 1-20.
20. Bennett PH, Haffner S, Kasiske BL, Keane WF, Mogensen CE, Parving HH, Steffes MW, Striker GE. Screening and management of microalbuminuria in patients with diabetes mellitus: recommendation to the scientific advisory board of the nNational Kidney Foundation from and ad hoc committee of the Council on Diabetes Mellitus of the National Kidney Foundation. Am J Kid Dis 1995; 25:107-112.
21. Mogensen CE, Keane WF, Bennett PH, Jerums G, Parving HH, Passa P, Steffes MW, Striker GE, Viberti GC. Prevention of diabetic renal disease with special reference to microalbuminuria. Lancet 1995; 346:1080-1084.
22. Krolewski AS, Laffel LMB, Krolewski M, Quinn M, Warram JH. Glycated hemoglobin and risk of microalbuminuria in patients with insulin-dependent diabetes mellitus. New Engl J Med 1995; 332:1251-1255.
23. Connell SJ, Hollis S, Tieszen KL, McMurray JR, Dornan TL. Gender and the clinical usefulness of the albumin:creatinine ratio. Diabetic Med; 11:32-6, 1994.
24. Vestbo E, Damsgaard EM, Froland A, Mogensen CE. Urinary Albumin excretion in a population based cohort. Diabet Med 1995; 12:488-493.
25. Siegel JE, Krolewski AS, Warram JH, Weinstein MC. Cost-effectiveness of screening and early treatment of nephropathy in patients with insulin-dependent diabetes mellitus. J Am Soc Neph 1992; 3:S111-S119.
26. Viberti GC, Hill RD, Jarrett RJ, Argyropoulos A, Mahmud U, Keen H. Microalbuminuria as a predictor of clinical nephropathy in insulin-dependent diabetes mellitus. Lancet 1982; I:1430-1432.
27. Mogensen CE, Christensen CK. Predicting diabetic nephropathy in insulin-dependent patients. New Engl J Med 1984; 311:89-93.
28. Mathiesen ER, Oxenboll B, Johansen K, Svendsen PA, Deckert T. Incipient nephropathy in Type (insulin-dependent) diabetes. Diabetologia 1984; 26:406-410.
29. Bach LA, Gilbert RE, Cooper ME, Tsalamandris C, Jerums G. Prediction of persistent microalbuminuria in patients with diabetes mellitus. J Diab Comp 1993; 7:67-72.
30. Almdal T, Norgaard K, Feldt-Rasmussen B, Deckert T. The predictive value of microalbuminuria in IDDM. Diabetes Care 1994; 17:120-125.
31. Forsblom CM, Groop PH, Ekstrand A, Groop LC. Predictive value of microalbuminuria in patients with insulin-dependent diabetes of long duration. BMJ 1992; 305:1051-1053.
32. Janner M, Knill SE, Diem P, Zuppinger KA, Mullis PE. Persistent microalbuminuria in adolescents with type I (insulin-dependent) diabetes mellitus is associated to early rather than late puberty. Results of a prospective logitudinal study. Eur J Pediatr 1994; 153:403-408.
33. Kostraba JN, Dorman JS, Orchard TJ, Becker DJ, Ohki Y, Ellis D, Doft BH, Lobes LA, LaPorte RE, Drash AL. Contribution of diabetes duration before puberty to development of microvascular complications in IDDM subjects. Diabetes Care 1989; 12:686-693.
34. Krolewski M, Eggers PW, Warram JH. Magnitude of end-stage reanl disease in IDDM: a 35 year follow-up study. Kidney Int 1996; 50:2041-2046.
35. Rudberg S, Ullman E, Dahlquist G. Relationship between early metabolic control and the development of microalbuminuria - a longitudinal study in children with Type 1 (insulin-dependent) diabetes mellitus. Diabetologia 1993; 36:1309-1314.
36. Stephenson JM, Fuller JH. Microalbuminuria is not rare before 5 years of IDDM. J Diab & Comp *1994; 8:166-173.*

37. Orchard TJ, Dorman JS, Maser RE, et al. Pittsburgh epidemiology of diabetes complications study. II. Prevalence of complications in IDDM by sex and duration. Diabetes 1990; 39:1116-1124.
38. Andersen AR, Christiansen JS, Andersen JK, Kreiner S, Deckert T. Diabetic nephropathy in type I (insulin-dependent) diabetes: an epidemiological study. Diabetologia 1983; 25:496-501.
39. Krolewski AS, Warram JH, Christlieb AR, Busick EJ, Kahn CR. The changing natural history of nephropathy in Type 1 diabetes Am J Med 1989; 78:785-794.
40. Nelson RG, Kunzelman CL, Pettitt DJ, Saad MF, Bennett PH, Knowler WC. Albuminuria in Type 2 (non-insulin-dependent) diabetes mellitus and impaired glucose tolerance in Pima Indians. Diabetologia 1989; 32:870-876.
41. Pugia MJ, Lott JA, Clark LW, Parker DR, Wallace JF, Willis TW. Comparison of urine dipsticks with quantitative methods for microalbuminuria. Eur J Clin Chem CLin Biochem 1997; 35:693-700.
42. Poulsen PL, Mogensen CE. Clinical evaluation of a test for immediate and quantitative determination of urinary albumin-to-creatinine ratio. Diabetes Care 1998; 21:97-98.

10. SERUM CREATININE AND OTHER MEASURES OF GFR IN DIABETES

Peter Rossing MD
Steno Diabetes Center, Gentofte, Denmark

The measurement of renal function or the glomerular filtration rate (GFR) in diabetes can be used 1) to estimate the renal clearance of drugs to guide dosing or to identify patients at increased risk for radiocontrast-induced acute renal failure, 2) for confirming the need for treatment of end stage renal disease, or 3) to measure progression of chronic renal disease i.e. diabetic nephropathy. The evaluation of progression in renal disease is important in the clinical setting for the monitoring of development of renal insufficiency and evaluation of the effectiveness of treatment in the individual, as well as in research to evaluate the importance of putative progression promoters in observational studies or to assess and compare the rate of progression in experimental groups in clinical trials. In order to obtain a valid assessment of the rate of decline in GFR it is necessary with regular measurements of GFR over a period of at least (2)-3 years applying a method with high precision and accuracy [1]. This is due to the usually rather slow rate of decline in GFR in diabetic nephropathy. The ideal method for assessing GFR does not exist and the available methods differ regarding precision and accuracy, cost, inconvenience and safety. In general the more precise methods are being more expensive and inconvenient. Thus one has to select a method according to the clinical situation.

1. SERUM CREATININE AS A MEASURE OF GFR

The level of serum creatinine is the most widely used measure of renal function in clinical practice. Serum creatinine can be assessed at a low cost and with little inconvenience for the patient. The reciprocal relationship between serum creatinine and the creatinine clearance allows a simple estimation of renal function (Figure 10-1). When progression in renal disease is evaluated the slope of either 1/serum creatinine or log (serum creatinine) is used. This is particularly useful when serum creatinine exceeds 200 μmol/l [2].

There are however several problems related to the use of serum creatinine as a marker of renal function as reviewed by Levey [3]. Firstly there are technical difficulties with interfering substances (glucose, ketones) which can be solved by the use of a reaction kinetic principle. Secondly the level of serum creatinine is not only dependent on the GFR: creatinine does not behave like an ideal filtration marker, there is tubular secretion leading to an overestimation of GFR by a factor of at least 1.2, and the tubular secretion changes with variation in the level of GFR [4], and it is affected by several drugs (e.g. cimetidine salicylates and trimethoprim). There is extrarenal elimination particularly in patients with low GFR. Furthermore the generation of creatinine is influenced by changes in muscle mass and dietary intake of protein. In particular the ingestion of cooked meat may lead to a fast increase in serum creatinine [5]. These conditions make it difficult to use serum creatinine to correctly estimate the level of renal function.

Problems related to differences in creatinine production affecting serum creatinine as well as the influence of extrarenal creatinine elimination, can be avoided by measuring creatinine clearance which in addition to the blood sample requires a 24 hour urine collection. However this adds the problem with accuracy of timed urine collections. The problems with tubular secretion can be avoided if the tubular secretion is blocked, for instance with the use of cimetidine [6], but this further adds to the complexity of the measurement.

Because of the difficulties with urine collections, it has been attempted to solve the problems due to sex and age related changes in muscle mass with formulas like that of Cockcroft and Gault [7] using serum creatinine to estimate creatinine clearance (Cl_{crea}) taking sex, age and body weight into account: Cl_{crea}=(140-Age)*K*body weight*(1/p-creatinine), (K=1.23 for men, 1.05 for women, p-creatinine in μmol/l, weight in kg and age in years). Cross-sectional data suggest that the formula gives an accurate estimate of glomerular filtration rate in diabetic nephropathy in some [8] but not all studies [9,10]. This formula can be used to estimate the mean decline in renal function in a cohort of diabetic patients with long follow up, but it is not accurate in the individual patient [10].

In patients with declining renal function there is an increase in fractional tubular secretion and extrarenal elimination [4]. Usually there is a lowering in muscle mass and often a restriction in protein intake. All of which will tend to preserve the level of serum creatinine despite declining GFR. Accordingly Shemesh et al. [4] found that patients with a GFR as low as ~30 ml/min/1.73m^2 may have normal serum creatinine, and in their follow up study [4] reductions in GFR of 50% were not associated with increases in serum creatinine of the expected magnitude, and even a lack of increase in some patients, thus when evaluating progression in renal disease, an increase in serum creatinine is not a very sensitive measurement of a decrease in renal function. This is in particular the case in patients with normal renal function due to the reciprocal relationship between serum creatinine and GFR, large variations in GFR are only associated with small changes in serum creatinine. On the other hand an elevation in serum creatinine is very specific for a decline in GFR. Thus an elevated serum creatinine or a doubling of the baseline serum creatinine have been used as endpoints in clinical trials [11], but this is only valid if changes in serum creatinine are not due to changes in therapy, muscle mass or diet. Illustrating this problem the Modification of Diet in Renal Disease study [12] concluded, that while a significant beneficial effect of low protein diet could not be demonstrated when using a true marker of GFR (^{125}I-iothalamate), such an effect would erroneously have been found if creatinine data had been used [13].

Other endogenous markers of GFR have been evaluated including ß$_2$-

microglobulin which seems to be a more reliable method for evaluation of GFR than serum creatinine in cross sectional as well as longitudinal studies [14,15], but determination of β_2-microglobulin is expensive and not a routine method at most laboratories. In addition very high levels are found in serum in patients with certain malignant disorders or immunological diseases.

2. GLOMERULAR FILTRATION RATE

An ideal marker for determination of glomerular filtration rate should fulfil the following requirements: it should be freely filtered at the glomerulus, no tubular secretion or reabsorption, it should not be metabolized, and it should be physiologically inert without affecting renal function, distribute instantaneously and freely in the extracellular volume, and should be easily measured [16]. Such a marker does not exist. However the renal clearance of inulin during constant infusion has been considered the gold standard for determination of GFR. The clearance is corrected for body surface area and normalised to 1.73 m^2 to take into account the relationship between kidney and body size and permit comparisons between patients. The renal clearance (Cl) during constant infusion is calculated from the plasma inulin level (P), urinary inulin concentration (U) and urine flow rate (V) as Cl=UV/P. The clearance is measured in three to five 30-minute periods during an oral water load. If during a constant infusion both distribution volume and plasma inulin concentration are constant the rate of infusion equals the rate of excretion. Then inulin clearance can be calculated from inulin infusion rate and plasma inulin concentration. However it is difficult to obtain constant inulin concentrations thus this technique is rarely used. The cumbersome procedures, difficulties with measuring inulin and its limited availability and cost has encouraged the search for alternative filtration markers.

The radioisotope-labelled markers ^{125}I-Iothalamate, ^{99m}Tc-DTPA and ^{51}Cr-EDTA have been found to give accurate and precise estimates of GFR [17] when used with constant infusion renal clearance techniques. To avoid problems with incomplete urine collections, a frequent phenomenon in diabetic patients due to cystopathy [18], plasma clearance techniques can be applied. The radioactive markers have particularly been used with such techniques. With these methods the GFR is determined without urine sampling as total plasma clearance from the declining plasma concentration followed as a function of time after injection of a bolus of the marker [19]. The clearance is calculated as the ratio of the injected amount of marker (Q) and the area under the plasma curve (A) (Cl=Q/A). Determination of the entire area under the plasma curve requires the drawing of many blood samples (10 to 20) during a time period of several hours depending on the level of renal function (three to five hours in normal to moderately decreased renal function, but up to 24 hours is recommended if GFR is below 15 ml/min). The final elimination follows a monoexponential curve which is extrapolated to infinity. Simplified methods have been developed using the final slope only, determined by two to seven blood samples, the calculated area can be mathematically corrected to the total area under the curve preserving very high precision and accuracy which is necessary in longitudinal studies [20-23]. The simplified single injection technique has frequently been used in clinical studies or as a routine method for determination of GFR [19,24].

^{51}Cr-EDTA (ethylenediaminetetraacetic acid) has been extensively used for plasma clearance studies and has been found to have a renal clearance ~10% lower than clearance of inulin [25], the difference has not been explained but could be due to plasma protein binding, tubular reabsorption or dissociation of the radionuclide from EDTA. The plasma clearance is slightly higher than the renal clearance due to extrarenal elimination (~4 ml/min) [21]. The half life of the isotope is 27 days. ^{125}I-Iothalamate can be administered as subcutaneous or intravenous injection. Due to a half life of radioactive ^{125}I of 60 days samples can be stored before radioisotope counting, which makes it useful for multicenter studies with a central laboratory as demonstrated in the MDRD study [12]. ^{99m}Tc-DTPA (diethylenetriaminepenta-acetic acid) is also used for renal scans, and it is inexpensive compared to the rather expensive ^{125}I-Iothalamate. Protein binding is potentially of concern and radiochemical instability varies among DTPA kits making quality control critical [26]. The radiolabelling of DTPA has to be carried out immediately before use due to instability. The half life of ^{99m}Tc is only 6 hours thus samples must be counted soon after the procedure.

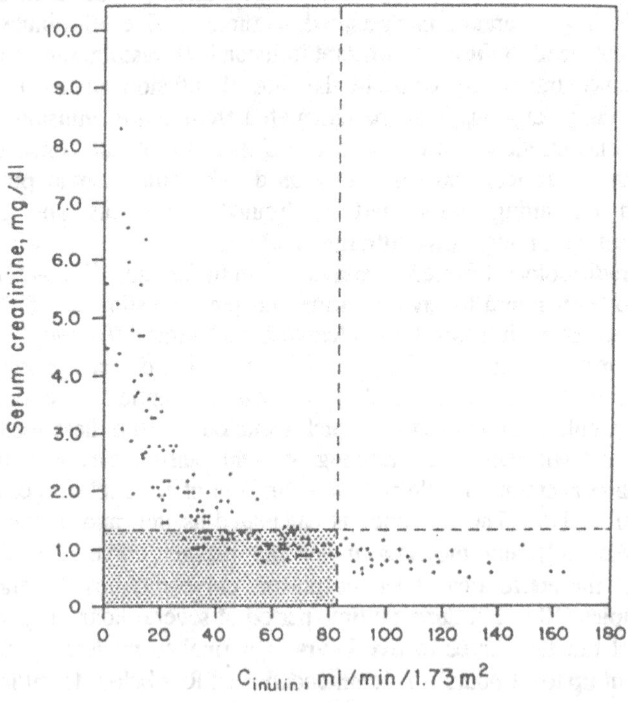

Figure 10-1. Simultaneous measurement of serum creatinine and inulin clearance in 171 patients with glomerular disease. Vertical dashed line correspond to the lower limit of inulin clearance (82 ml/min/1.73m^2), the horizontal line corresponds to the upper limit for serum creatinine (1.4 mg/dl). The shaded area include values for patients in whom inulin clearance is reduced but serum creatinine is normal. (from Shemesh et al [4]

Plasma clearance can be measured without drawing plasma samples at all, with the use of a gamma camera measuring renal elimination of a radioactive marker such as ^{99m}Tc-DTPA [27]. This technique is not as accurate as when plasma samples are collected, but it is possible to determine the contribution from each kidney, which is particularly useful when reno-vascular disease or unilateral nephrectomy is considered.

The use of radioactive markers exposes the patients to radiation, but the radiation dose is very small and for one measurement of GFR with ^{51}Cr-EDTA it is comparable to the daily background radiation dose (Effective dose equivalent <0.01 mSv.). But even if the radiation doses are small, the use of radioactive isotopes is usually avoided in children and pregnant women. As a non-radioactive alternative the radiocontrast agents such as iohexol have been suggested [28], it has also been possible to measure very small concentrations of inulin with HPLC methods making plasma clearance of inulin after a single injection a possibility [29].

3. SUMMARY

The selection of method for assessment of GFR depends on the situation. In many clinical situations the use of serum creatinine or estimated creatinine clearance based on formulas or nomograms is sufficient if the limitations are recalled. In clinical studies a more accurate and precise method is warranted. In case of severe oedema, ascites or if the renal haemodynamics are changing within hours, renal clearance methods has to be used. Apart from these special situations the simplified single injection plasma clearance methods yield sufficiently accurate and precise assessments of GFR with a minimum of inconvenience, particularly useful in long term follow-up studies.

REFERENCES:

1. Modification of Diet in Renal Disease Study group., Levey AS, Gassman J, Hall PM, Walker WG: Assessing the progression of renal disease in clinical studies: effects of duration of follow-up and regression to the mean. J Am Soc Nephrol 1991;1:1087-1094.
2. Mitch WE, Walser M, Buffington GA, Lemann J: A simple method of estimating progression of chronic renal failure. Lancet 1976;ii:1326-1328.
3. Levey AS, Perrone RD, Madias NE: Serum creatinine and renal function. Ann Rev Med 1988;39:465-490.
4 Shemesh O, Golbetz HV, Kriss JP, Myers BD: Limitations of creatinine as a filtration marker in glomerulopathic patients. Kidney Int 1985;28:830-838.
5. Jacobsen FK, Christensen CK, Mogensen CE, Andreasen F, Hejlskov NSC: Pronounced increase in serum creatinine concentration after eating cooked meat. Br Med J 1979;I:1049-1050.
6. van Acker BAC, Koome GCM, Koopman MG, de Waart DR, Arisz L: Creatinine clearance during cimetidine administration for measurement of glomerular filtration rate. Lancet 1992;340:1326-1329.
7 Cockcroft DW, Gault MH: Prediction of creatinine clearance from serum creatinine. Nephron 1976;16:31-41.
8 Sampson MJ, Drury PL: Accurate estimation of glomerular filtration rate in diabetic nephropathy from age, body weight, and serum creatinine. Diabetes Care 1992;15:609-612.
9 Waz WR, Qattrin T, Feld LG: Serum creatinine, height, and weight do not predict glomerular filtration rate in children with IDDM. Diabetes Care 1993;16:1067-1070.
10 Rossing P, Astrup A-S, Smidt UM, Parving H-H: Monitoring kidney function in diabetic nephropathy. Diabetologia 1994;37:708-712.
11 Lewis E, Hunsicker L, Bain R, Rhode R: The effect of angiotensin-converting-enzyme inhibition on diabetic nephropathy. N Engl J Med 1993;329:1456-1462.

12 Klahr S, Levey AS, Beck GJ, Caggiula AW, Hunsicker L, Kusek JW, Striker G, For The Modification Of Diet In Renal Disease Study Group: The effects of dietary protein restriction and blood-pressure control on the progression of chronic renal disease. N Engl J Med 1994;330:877-884.

13 Levey AS, Bosch JP, Coggins CH, Greene T, Mitch WE, Schluchter MD, Schwab SJ, The Modification of Diet in Renal Disease Study: Effects of diet and blood pressure on creatinine clearance (C_{Cr}) and serum creatinine (P_{Cr}) in the MDRD study. J Am Soc Nephrol 1993;4:253(Abstract)

14 Parving H-H, Andersen AR, Smidt UM: Monitoring progression of diabetic nephropathy. Upsala J Med Sci 1985;90:15-23.

15 Viberti GC, Bilous RW, Mackintosh D, Keen H: Monitoring glomerular function in diabetic nephropathy. Am J Med 1983;74:256-264.

16 Kasiske BL, Keane WF: Laboratory assessment of renal disease: clearance, urinalysis, and renal biopsy; in Brenner BM (ed): The kidney. Philadelphia, Saunders, 1997, pp 1137-1174.

17 Levey AS: Assessing the effectiveness of therapy to prevent the progression of renal disease. Am J Kidney Dis 1993;22:207-214.

18 Frimondt-Møller C: Diabetic cystopathy. Dan Med Bull 1978;25:49-60.

19 Bröchner-Mortensen J: Current status on assessment and measurement of glomerular filtration rate. Clin Physiol 1985;5:1-17.

20 Bröchner-Mortensen J: Routine methods and their reliability for assessment of glomerular filtration rate in adults with special reference to total [^{51}Cr]EDTA plasma clearance. Dan Med Bull 1978;25:181-202.

21 Bröchner-Mortensen J, Rödbro P: Selection of routine method for determination of glomerular filtration rate in adult patients. Scand J Clin Lab Invest 1976;36:35-45.

22 Bröchner-Mortensen J: A simple method for the determination of glomerular filtration rate. Scand J Clin Lab Invest 1972;30:271-274.

23 Sambataro M, Thomaseth K, Pacini G, Robaudo C, Carraro A, Bruseghin M, Brocco E, Abaterusso C, DeFerrari G, Fioretto P, Maioli M, Tonolo G, Crepaldi G, Nosadini R: Plasma clearance rate of 51Cr-EDTA provides a precise and convenient technique for measurement of glomerular filtration rate in diabetic humans.J Am Soc Nephrol 1996;7:118-127.

24 Parving H-H, Smidt UM, Hommel E, Mathiesen ER, Rossing P, Nielsen FS, Gall M-A: Effective Antihypertensive Treatment Postpones Renal Insufficiency in Diabetic Nephropathy. Am J Kidney Dis 1993;22:188-195.

25 Chantler C, Garnett ES, Parsons V, Veall N: Glomerular filtration rate measurement in man by the single injection method using ^{51}Cr-EDTA. Clin Sci 1969;37:169-180.

26 Carlsen;J.E., Lehd Møller M, Lund JO, Trap-Jensen J: Comparison of four commercial Tc-99 (sn) DTPA preparations used for the measurement of glomerular filtration rate: concise communication. J Nucl Med 1980;126-129.

27 Rodby RA, Ali A, Rohde RD, Lewis E: Renal scanning ^{99m}Tc diethylene-triamine pentaacetic acid glomerular filtration rate (GFR) determination compared with iothalamate clearance GFR in diabetics. Am J Kidney Dis 1992;20:569-573.

28 Stake G, Monn E, Rootwell IT, Monclair T: The clearance of iohexol as a measure of glomerular filtration rate in children with chronic renal failure. Scand J Clin Lab Invest 1991;51:729-734.

29 Mantini G, Dalton RN, Tomlinson PA: The estimation of glomerular filtration rate from single injection plasma inulin measurements using numerical analysis. Abst Paeditr 1989;c128 (Abstract).

11. FAMILIAL FACTORS IN DIABETIC NEPHROPATHY

David J. Pettitt, William C. Knowler and Robert G. Nelson
Phoenix Epidemiology and Clinical Research Branch, NIDDK, Phoenix, Arizona, USA

Reports of nephropathy developing in some patients with apparently well controlled diabetes and not developing in some patients even after years of severe hyperglycemia lead to the conclusion, expressed by several researchers [1-5], that some, but not all, individuals are predisposed to the development of diabetic renal disease. This chapter reviews some of the data that indicate that there are familial differences in the predisposition to diabetic renal disease. If this familial predisposition is genetic, there must be an interaction between the genes and the environment, and it is often impossible to differentiate between genetic inheritance and the effect of a common environment shared by family members.

1. RACIAL DIFFERENCES IN PREVALENCE OF RENAL DISEASE

Some familial clustering of diabetic nephropathy may be accounted for by racial background, as diabetic nephropathy occurs at different rates in different racial groups. Several inter-racial comparisons have been made [6-10]. Rostand et al. [6] and Cowie et al. [9] both reported higher rates of end-stage renal disease in American Blacks than Whites, and Pugh et al. [7] reported higher rates in Mexican Americans than in Non-Hispanic Whites. Diabetes duration, which is a strong risk factor for end-stage renal disease, may account for some of the racial differences in these studies. However, with diabetes duration accounted for, Haffner et al. [8]found higher rates of proteinuria among Mexican Americans, and there are several reports of very high rates of renal disease among the Pima Indians [11-14], a population which has high rates of type 2 diabetes [15,16]. The incidence of end-stage renal disease in Pima Indians was similar to that in subjects with type 1 diabetes in Boston, Massachusetts [11], but almost four times as high as in Caucasians with type 2 diabetes in Rochester, Minnesota [14].

The reasons for inter-population differences in rates of renal disease are unclear. Rostand [10] has argued that barriers to medical care for Black and Mexican Americans may impede early detection, and therefore control, of microalbuminuria and hypertension with a consequent adverse effect on the prevalence of renal disease. However, the cost, one of the major barriers to medical care, is not a factor for the Pima Indians, who have access to free medical care by providers who are well aware of the high risk of diabetic renal disease in this population. Thus, cost of medical care cannot be the only reason for racial differences. However, other aspects of access to medical care, such as transportation or cultural barriers, could be important.

Genes predisposing to renal disease might well exist at different rates in different races resulting in differences in susceptibility. Thus, if renal disease is genetic its prevalence would be expected to differ by race. However, finding different rates in different races is consistent not only with genetic inheritance but also with differing environmental exposures or with differences in competing causes of death.

2. SIBLINGS OF AFFECTED INDIVIDUALS

Seaquist et al. [17] reported familial clustering of nephropathy among diabetic siblings of diabetic probands recruited from either the University of Minnesota kidney transplant registry or from a family diabetes study. Nephropathy was found among 83% of the diabetic siblings of diabetic probands with nephropathy but among only 17% of siblings of probands without nephropathy (figure 11-1). Furthermore, 41% of the siblings of probands with nephropathy had end-stage renal disease. Clustering of diabetic nephropathy among siblings was confirmed by Borch-Johnsen et al. [18], and higher albumin exretion was found in the nondiabetic siblings of probands with type 2 diabetes than of those without [19]. These data, which are consistent with the hypothesis that genetic heredity is a major determinant of diabetic nephropathy, are also consistent with the hypothesis that an environmental factor or factors shared by siblings is responsible for the development of nephropathy in some families.

3. OFFSPRING OF AFFECTED INDIVIDUALS

Proteinuria and elevated serum creatinine concentrations were studied in Pima Indian families with diabetes in two generations [20]. Proteinuria occurred among 14% of the diabetic offspring of diabetic parents if neither parent had proteinuria, 23% if one parent had proteinuria, and 46% if both parents had diabetes with proteinuria (figure 11-2). The familial occurrence of an elevated creatinine was limited to male offspring, among whom 11.7% had a high creatinine if the parent had a high creatinine but only 1.5% did so if the diabetic parent had a normal creatinine. These data demonstrate that proteinuria and elevated creatinine aggregate in Pima families and suggest that the susceptibility to renal disease is inherited independently of the diabetes. As with the sibling concordance described above, the inheritance could be a shared environment, but since the environments of parents and of their children are very likely to differ more than those of siblings, a genetic inheritance is a strong possibility.

More recent data from the Pima Indians indicate that diabetic nephropathy in parents is a risk factor for diabetes in the offspring [21]. The prevalence of diabetes at 25 to 34 years of age was 46% among the offspring of two diabetic parents if one had proteinuria and only 18% if neither had proteinuria. Corresponding rates among subjects with one diabetic and one nondiabetic parent were 29% if the diabetic parent had proteinuria and 11% if not. Thus, multiple loci or homozygosity at a single locus may determine susceptibility to both diabetes and renal disease. In other words, parents with diabetes and renal disease may have a higher genetic load which increases the risk of diabetes in the offspring as well as increasing the risk of nephropathy once the diabetes develops.

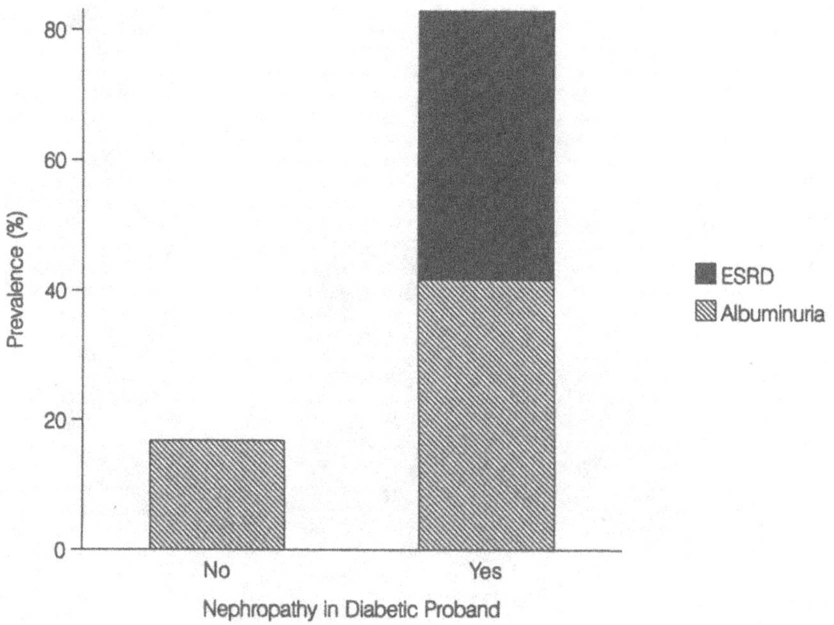

Figure 11-1 Prevalences of albuminuria and end-stage renal disease (ESRD) in diabetic siblings of diabetic probands with or without nephropathy. Adapted from Seaquist et al [17].

4. FAMILIAL HYPERTENSION AND RENAL DISEASE

The frequent association of renal disease with hypertension has led to the examination of blood pressure in nondiabetic family members of persons with diabetes and in individuals thought to be at high risk of developing diabetes in the future. Viberti et al. found that both systolic and diastolic blood pressures were significantly higher in the parents of diabetic subjects with proteinuria than in the parents of diabetic subjects without proteinuria [22]. The difference between the mean blood pressures averaged 15 mm Hg. Similarly, Krolewski et al. [23] reported that the risk of nephropathy among subjects with type 1 diabetes was three times as high in those having a parent with a history of hypertension as in those whose parents had no such history, and Takeda et al. [24] found evidence suggesting that paternal hypertension might be related to the development of nephropathy in patients with type 2 diabetes. Beatty et al. [25] have recently found more insulin resistance as well as higher blood pressures in the offspring of hypertensive than of normotensive parents. These offspring, therefore, are presumably at increased risk of developing diabetes. Since they already have significantly higher blood pressures, they may be at particular risk of renal disease if they do develop diabetes.

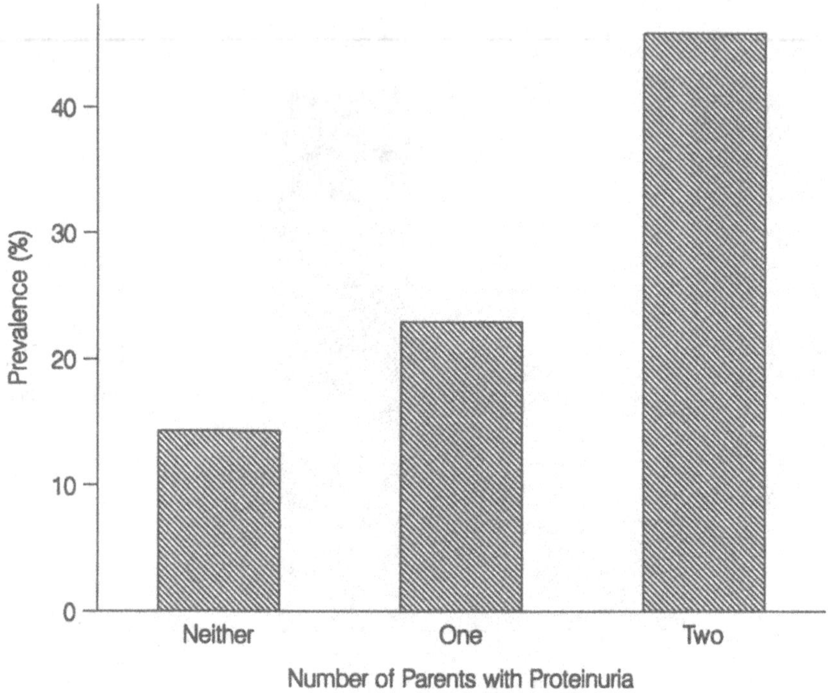

Figure 11-2 Prevalence of proteinuria by number of parents with proteinuria adjusted for age, sex, blood pressure, diabetes duration and glucose concentration. Adapted from Pettitt et al [20].

Among diabetic Pima Indians whose parents did not have proteinuria, those with hypertensive parents had a higher prevalence of proteinuria than those with normotensive parents [26]. This finding was observed even among those with nondiabetic parents (figure 11-3).

Sodium-lithium countertransport activity in red cells, a genetically transmitted trait, is reported in some studies to be abnormal in subjects at risk of essential hypertension [27-30]. Rates of countertransport activity are higher in diabetic subjects with renal disease than in those with diabetes alone [23,31]. Kelleher et al. [32] reported more hypertension among the siblings of hypertensive than of normotensive subjects with type 1 diabetes. However, hypertension among siblings of subjects with type 2 diabetes was more prevalent than among siblings of subjects with type 1 diabetes and was not related to hypertension in the diabetic proband. Given the association between hypertension and nephropathy, it is reasonable to assume that these hypertensive diabetic patients may be at risk for developing nephropathy, or may already have some nephropathy, and the hypertensive siblings might be at risk themselves if they were to develop diabetes.

Among Pima Indians, higher mean blood pressure measured at least one year prior to the onset of diabetes predicted an abnormal urinary excretion of albumin determined after the diagnosis of diabetes [33]. Thus, the hypertension so often associated with diabetic nephropathy cross-sectionally does not appear to be entirely a result of the renal disease. This hypertension, which appears to be familial in several studies, may precede and contribute to the renal disease seen after several years of diabetes in some subjects.

5. GENETIC MARKERS

The possibility of genetic causes for diabetic microvascular complications has stimulated the search for a disease gene or for linkage between the disease and a genetic marker. The data for type 1 diabetes have been reviewed extensively [34]. Several reports of associations between markers and retinopathy are encouraging [35,36], but the findings of associations with renal disease are mixed [35,37,38]. Among patients with type 1 diabetes, Barbosa [35] found similar frequencies of HLA-A and HLA-B antigens, but Christy et al. [37] found a different distribution of

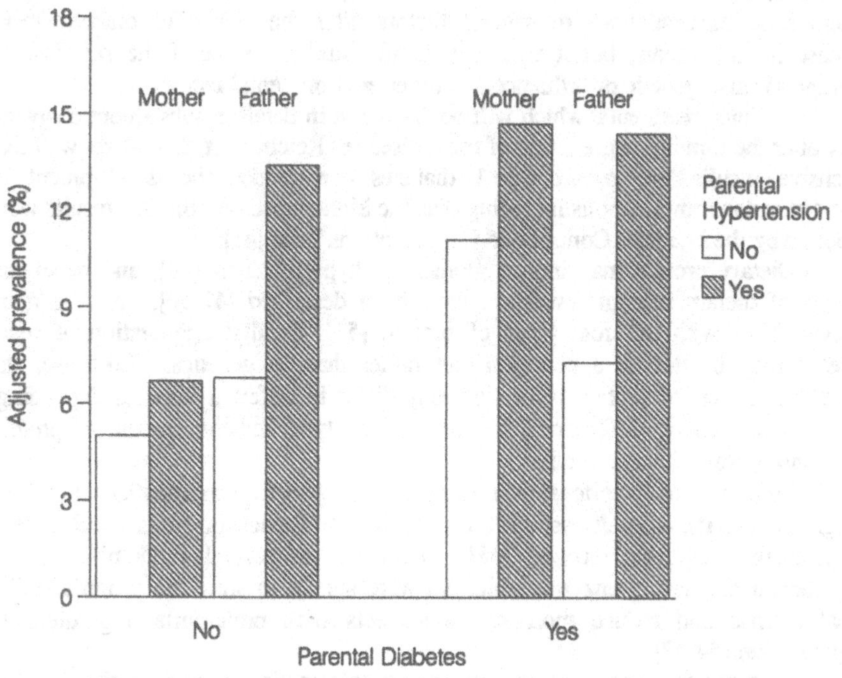

Figure 11-3 Prevalance of proteinuria according to parental hypertension and diabetes, adjusted for age, sex, diabetes duration and post-load plasma glucose. Adapted from Nelson et al. [26].

HLA/DR markers in those with and in those without nephropathy. Walton et al. [38], in a very small sample, also found no evidence of an HLA association with nephropathy. Mijovic's [39] findings suggest that microangiopathy (not limited to renal disease) was influenced by genes in linkage disequilibrium with both the major histocompatibility complex and the Gm loci. Doria et al. reported that, among subjects with type 1 diabetes, an uncommon DNA sequence for the angiotensin I converting enzyme was more common in those with nephropathy than in those without [40]. Among Pima Indians with type 2 diabetes, Imperatore et al. [41] found suggestive linkage for nephropathy on chromosome 7, and for hypertension on chromosomes 5 and 6.

Reviews of the subject by Barbosa and Saner [42] and by Barnett and Pyke [43] concluded that there is no convincing evidence that genetic factors play a role in the pathogenesis of diabetic renal disease. Twin studies, which suggest a genetic component in the pathogenesis of retinopathy, have had too few twin pairs to provide any evidence for the genetics of nephropathy [43].

6. MODIFICATION OF DISEASE

Environmental factors, most of which probably remain unknown, which influence the development or progression of renal disease in subjects with diabetes are likely to be shared with other family members resulting in concordance of renal disease. Therapeutic manipulations of several factors alter the course of diabetic renal disease in individuals, but it will take family studies to see if the response to therapies is also genetic or influenced by other environmental factors.

Various treatments, which will be discussed in detail in subsequent chapters, may alter the familial aggregation of renal disease. Reichard et al. [44] showed that intensive insulin therapy in type 1 diabetes can reduce the development of microvascular complications including diabetic kidney disease. Similar results were reported by the Diabetes Control and Complications Trial [45].

Dietary protein may induce glomerular hyperfiltration [46], and beneficial effects of dietary protein restriction have been described [47-50]. As the renal effects differ with different types of protein [51], familial aggregation of renal disease may be due to a common diet rather than to genetics. Likewise, the beneficial effects of protein restriction may differ in different families depending, not only on genetic differences, but also on the type and the amount of protein consumed before the intervention.

Treatment of hypertension in subjects with diabetic nephropathy retards the progression of the renal disease [52], especially with the use of drugs which inhibit angiotensin converting enzyme [53]. Recently, in several randomized trials, angiotensin converting enzyme inhibitors were shown to slow the progression of renal disease and reduce mortality in subjects with proteinuria, regardless of hypertension [54-57].

In summary, much of the intriguing information regarding the familial occurrence of diabetic renal disease suggests a genetic component for this disorder but is also consistent with environmental effects. The epidemiology of renal disease is complicated by the fact that several forms of therapy currently employed to treat hyperglycemia, proteinuria and hypertension can alter the progression of renal disease and may, in some cases, even prevent its development. Selective prevention of renal disease will likely alter the familial aggregation of the disease. If there are important genes providing susceptibility to renal disease or influencing the response to treatment, even if the contribution is small, their identification could increase the clinician's knowledge about the risk for a given patient and help identify those for whom intensive therapy may be most beneficial [58,59].

REFERENCES

1. Deckert T, Poulsen JE: Diabetic nephropathy: fault or destiny? Diabetologia 21:178-183, 1981.
2. Moloney A, Tunbridge WMG, Ireland JT, Watkins PJ: Mortality from diabetic nephropathy in the United Kingdom. Diabetologia 25:26-30, 1983.
3. Krolewski AS, Warram JH, Christlieb AR, Busick EJ, Kahn CR: The changing natural history of nephropathy in type I diabetes. Am J Med 78:785-794, 1985.
4. Seaquist ER, Goetz FC, Povey S: Diabetic nephropathy: an hypothesis regarding genetic susceptibility for the disorder. Minnesota Med 69:457-459, 1986.
5. What causes diabetic renal failure? [Editorial] Lancet 1:1433-1434, 1988.
6. Rostand SG, Kirk KA, Rutsky EA, Pate BA: Racial differences in the incidence of treatment for end-stage renal disease. N Engl J Med 306:1276-1279, 1982.
7. Pugh JA, Stern MP, Haffner SM, Eifler CW, Zapata M: Excess incidence of treatment of end-stage renal disease in Mexican Americans. Am J Epidemiol 127:135-144, 1988.
8. Haffner SM, Mitchell BD, Pugh JA, Stern MP, Kozlowski MK, Hazuda HP, Patterson JK, Klein R: Proteinuria in Mexican Americans and non-Hispanic Whites with NIDDM. Diabetes Care 12:530-536, 1989.
9. Cowie CC, Port FK, Wolfe RA, Savage PJ, Moll PP, Hawthorne VM: Disparities in incidence of diabetic end-stage renal disease according to race and type of diabetes. N Engl J Med 321:1074-1079, 1989.
10. Rostand SG: Diabetic renal disease in blacks — inevitable or preventable? [Editorial] N Engl J Med 321:1121-1122, 1989.
11. Nelson RG, Newman JM, Knowler WC, Sievers ML, Kunzelman CL, Pettitt DJ, Moffett CD, Teutch SM, Bennett PH: Incidence of end-stage renal disease in type 2 (non-insulin-dependent) diabetes mellitus in Pima Indians. Diabetologia 31:730-736, 1988.
12. Kunzelman CL, Knowler WC, Pettitt DJ, Bennett PH: Incidence of proteinuria in type 2 diabetes mellitus in the Pima Indians. Kidney Int 35:681-687, 1989.
13 Nelson RG, Knowler WC, Pettitt DJ, Saad MF, Bennett PH: Diabetic kidney disease in Pima Indians. Diabetes Care [Suppl 1] 16:335-341, 1993.
14. Nelson RG, Knowler WC, McCance DR, Sievers ML, Pettitt DJ, Charles MA, Hanson RL, Liu QZ, Bennett PH: Determinants of end-stage renal disease in Pima Indians with Type 2 (non-insulin-dependent) diabetes mellitus and proteinuria. Diabetologia 36:1087-1093, 1993.
15. Bennett PH, Burch TA, Miller M. Diabetes mellitus in American (Pima) Indians. Lancet 2:125-128, 1971.
16. Knowler WC, Pettitt DJ, Saad MF, Bennett PH: Diabetes mellitus in the Pima Indians: incidence, risk factors and pathogenesis. Diabetes Metab Rev 6:1-27, 1990.
17. Seaquist ER, Goetz FC, Rich S, Barbosa J: Familial clustering of diabetic kidney disease: evidence for genetic susceptibility to diabetic nephropathy. N Engl J Med 320:1161-1165, 1989.
18. Borch-Johnsen K, Nørgaard, Hommel E, Mathiesen ER, Jensen JS, Deckert T, Parving H-H: Is diabetic nephropathy an inherited complication? Kidney Int 41:719-722, 1992.
19. Faronato PP, Maioli M, Tonolo G, Brocco E, Noventa E, Piarulli F, Abaterusso C, Modena F, de Bigontina G, Velussi M, Inchiostro S, Santeusanio F, Bueti kA, Nosadini R. Clustering of albumin excretion rate abnormalities in Caucasian patients with NIDDM. Diabetologia 1997;40:816-823.
20. Pettitt DJ, Saad MF, Bennett PH, Nelson RG, Knowler WC: Familial predisposition to renal disease in two generations of Pima Indians with type 2 (non-insulin-dependent) diabetes mellitus. Diabetologia 33:438-443, 1990.

21. McCance DR, Hanson RL, Pettitt DJ, Jacobsson LTH, Bennett PH, Bishop DT, Knowler WC. Diabetic nephropathy: a risk factor for diabetes mellitus in offspring. Diabetologia 38:221-226, 1995.
22. Viberti GC, Keen H, Wiseman MJ: Raised arterial pressure in parents of proteinuric insulin dependent diabetics. Br Med J 295:515-517, 1987.
23. Krolewski AS, Canessa M, Warram JH, Laffel LMB, Christlieb AR, Knowler WC, Rand LI: Predisposition to hypertension and susceptibility to renal disease in insulin-dependent diabetes mellitus. N Engl J Med 318:140-145, 1988.
24. Takeda H, Ohta K, Hagiwara M, Hori K, Watanabe K, Suzuki D, Tanaka K, Machimura H, Ya-Game M, Kaneshige H, Sakai H. Genetic predisposing factors in non-insulin-dependent diabetes with persistent albuminuria. Tokai J Exp Clin Med. 17:199-203, 1992
25. Beatty OL, Harper R, Sheridan B, Atkinson AB, Bell PM: Insulin resistance in offspring of hypertensive parents. Br Med J 307:92-96, 1993.
26. Nelson RG, Pettitt DJ, de Courten MP, Hanson RL, Knowler WC, Bennett PH. Parental hypertension and proteinuria in Pima Indians with NIDDM. Diabetologia 39:433-438, 1996
27. Canessa M, Adragna N, Solomon HS, Connolly TM, Tosteson DC: Increased sodium-lithium countertransport in red cells of patients with essential hypertension. N Engl J Med 302:772-776, 1980.
28. Woods JW, Falk RJ, Pittman AW, Klemmer PJ, Watson BS, Namboodiri K: Increased red-cell sodium-lithium countertransport in normotensive sons of hypertensive parents. N Engl J Med 306:593-595, 1982.
29. Clegg G, Morgan DB, Davidson C: The heterogeneity of essential hypertension: relation between lithium efflux and sodium content of erythrocytes and a family history of hypertension. Lancet 2:891-894, 1982.
30. Cooper R, LeGrady D, Nanas S, Trevisan M, Mansour M, Histand P, Ostrow D, Stamler J: Increased sodium-lithium countertransport in college students with elevated blood pressure. JAMA 249:1030-1034, 1983.
31. Mangili R, Bending JJ, Scott G, Li LK, Gupta A, Viberti GC: Increased sodium-lithium countertransport activity in red cells of patients with insulin-dependent diabetes and nephropathy. N Engl J Med 318:146-150, 1988.
32. Kelleher C, Kingston SM, Barry DG, Cole MM, Ferriss JB, Grealy G, Joyce C, O'Sullivan DJ: Hypertension in diabetic clinic patients and their siblings. Diabetologia 31:76-81, 1988.
33. Nelson RG, Pettitt DJ, Baird HR, Charles MA, Liu QZ, Bennett PH, Knowler WC: Pre-diabetic blood pressure predicts urinary albumin excretion after the onset of type 2 (non-insulin-dependent) diabetes mellitus in Pima Indians. Diabetologia 36:998-1001, 1993.
34. Doria A, Warram JH, Krolewski AS. Genetic susceptibility to nephropathy in insulin-dependent diabetes: from epidemiology to molecular genetics. Diabetes/Metab Rev 1995;11:287-314.
35. Barbosa J: Is diabetic microangiopathy genetically heterogeneous? HLA and diabetic nephropathy. Horm Metab Res Suppl 11:77-80, 1981.
36. Scaldaferri E, Devidè A: Microangiopatia diabetica: esiste una suscettibilità genetica HLA-correlata? Minerva Endocrinol 10:115-124, 1985.
37. Christy M, Anderson AR, Nerup J, Platz P, Ryder L, Thomsen M, Morling M, Svejgaard A: HLA/DR in longstanding IDDM with and without nephropathy — evidence for heterogeneity? [abstr] Diabetologia 21:259, 1981.
38. Walton C, Dyer PA, Davidson JA, Harris R, Mallick NP, Oleesky S: HLA antigens and risk factors for nephropathy in type 1 (insulin-dependent) diabetes mellitus. Diabetologia 27:3-7, 1984.
39. Mijovic C, Fletcher JA, Bradwell AR, Barnett AH: Phenotypes of the heavy chains of immunoglobulins in patients with diabetic microangiopathy: evidence for an immunogenetic predisposition. Br Med J 292:433-435, 1986.
40. Doria A, Warram JH, Krolewski AS. Genetic predisposition to diabetic nephropathy: evidence for a role of the angiotensin I-converting enzyme gene. Diabetes 43:690-695, 1994.
41. Imperatore G, Hanson RL, Bennett PH, Knowler WC. Genome-wide search for susceptibility genes for nephropathy and hypertension among diabetic Pima Indians. (Abstract). Am J Hum Gen 1996;59:A45.
42. Barbosa J, Saner B: Do genetic factors play a role in the pathogenesis of diabetic microangiopathy? Diabetologia 27:487-492, 1984.

43. Barnett AH, Pyke DA: The genetics of diabetic complications. Clinics Endocrinol and Metab 15:715-726, 1986.
44. Reichard P, Nilsson B-Y, Rosenqvist U: The effect of long-term intensified insulin treatment on the development of microvascular complications of diabetes mellitus. N Engl J Med 329:304-309, 1993.
45. The Diabetes Control and Complications Trial Research Group: The effect of intensive treatment of diabetes on the development and progression of long-term complications in insulin-dependent diabetes mellitus. N Engl J Med 329:977-986, 1993.
46. Krishna GP, Newell G, Miller E, Heeger P, Smith R, Polansky M, Kapoor S, Hoeldtke R: Protein-induced glomerular hyperfiltration: role of hormonal factors. Kidney Int 33:578-583, 1988.
47. Wiseman MJ, Dodds R, Bending JJ, Viberti GC: Dietary protein and the diabetic kidney. Diabetic Med 4:144-146, 1987.
48. Walker JD, Dodds RA, Murrells TJ, Bending JJ, Mattock MB, Keen H, Viberti GC: Restriction of dietary protein and progression of renal failure in diabetic nephropathy. Lancet 2:1411-1415, 1989.
49. Mitch WE: Dietary protein restriction in chronic renal failure: nutritional efficacy, compliance, and progression of renal insufficiency. J Am Soc Nephrol 2:823-831, 1991.
50. Zeller K, Whittaker E, Sullivan L, Raskin P, Jacobson HR: Effect of restricting dietary protein on the progression of renal failure in patients with insulin-dependent diabetes mellitus. N Engl J Med 324:78-84, 1991.
51. Nakamura H, Ito S, Ebe N, Shibata A: Renal effects of different types of protein in healthy volunteer subjects and diabetic patients. Diabetes Care 16:1071-1075, 1993.
52. Mogensen CE: Long-term antihypertensive treatment inhibiting progression of diabetic nephropathy. Br Med J 285:685-688, 1982.
53. Parving H-H, Hommel E, Smidt UM: Protection of kidney function and decrease in albuminuria by captopril in insulin dependent diabetics with nephropathy. Br Med J 297:1086-1091, 1988.
54. Marre M, Chatellier G, Leblanc H, Guyene TT, Menard J, Passa P: Prevention of diabetic nephropathy with enalapril in normotensive diabetics with microalbuminuria. Br Med J 297:1092-1095, 1988.
55. Mathiesen ER, Hommel E, Giese J, Parving H-H: Efficacy of captopril in postponing nephropathy in normotensive insulin dependent diabetic patients with microalbuminuria. Br Med J 303:81-87, 1991.
56. Ravid M, Savin H, Jutrin I, Bental T, Katz B, Lishner M: Long-term stabilizing effect of angiotensin-converting enzyme inhibition on plasma creatinine and on proteinuria in normotensive type II diabetic patients. Ann Int Med 118, 577-581, 1993.
57. Lewis EJ, Hunsicker LG, Bain RP, Rohde RD. The effect of angiotensin-converting-enzyme inhibition on diabetic nephropathy. N Engl J Med 329:1456-1462, 1993
58. Stattin EL, Rudberg S, Dahlquist G. Hereditary risk determinants of micro- and macroalbuminuria in young IDDM patients (Abstract). Diabetologia 1996;39: Suppl. 1:A299.
59. Quinn M, Angelico MC, Warram JH, Krolewski AS. Familial factors determine the development of diabetic nephropathy in patients with IDDM. Diabetologia 1996;39:940-945.

12. GENETICS AND DIABETIC NEPHROPATHY

Michel Marre, Béatrice Bouhanick
Centre Hospitalier Universitaire, Angers, France.

INTRODUCTION

Both genetic determinants and environmental conditions can affect enzyme activity. As all IDDM complications are secondary to long lasting hyperglycemia, the search for a genetic basis to diabetic nephropathy represents a typical example of search for gene-environment interaction. Furthermore, gene-gene interactions must be expected, as determinants for IDDM complications are multifactorial. Lastly, the level of evidence for one given gene polymorphism is currently low to account for diabetic nephropathy. Thus, practical implications for this type of investigation in patient care are currently premature.

EPIDEMIOLOGICAL EVIDENCES FOR A GENETIC BASIS TO DIABETIC NEPHROPATHY:

One study published by SIPERSTEIN et al in 1968 suggested that capillary basement membrane enlargement (a typical sign for diabetic microangiopathy) preceded diabetes, and consequently that IDDM complications could be genetically determined independently of glycemic level [1]. However, large amounts of experimental and clinical data have accumulated to contradict this possibility, which established that anatomical and functional signs of diabetic nephropathy are acquired and secondary to hyperglycemia and its consequent disorders [2, 3]. In diabetic patients, Jean PIRART produced a large, 25-yr, prospective, follow-up study, establishing that the development of diabetic complications (including diabetic nephropathy) was proportional to the duration of diabetes and to diabetes control (as assessed by the amount of glycosuria and by random blood glucose measurements) [4]. Last, but not the least, intervention studies (the DCCT trial [5] being the most important quantitatively) indicated that reduction of hyperglycemia reduced the risk of diabetic nephropathy, as assessed by the incidence of microalbuminuria and proteinuria. However, prospective, follow-up studies suggest that long-term, uncontrolled IDDM is a necessary, but not sufficient conditional for diabetic nephropathy to develop. For instance, Jean PIRART [4] noticed that concordance was not perfect between onset of each of the 3 specific complications (retinopathy, neuropathy, and nephropathy), as illustrated in Figure 12-1 : hardly one fourth of the patients developing retinopathy, or neuropathy, displayed nephropathy. Diabetic nephropathy occurs in hardly half of IDDM patients, and presents with a peak of onset between the 10th and 25th year of IDDM duration, as documented by follow-up studies in the Joslin Clinic in Boston and in the Steno Memorial Hospital in Copenhagen [6, 7, 8].

The concept of a genetic basis for diabetic nephropathy is also supported by familial aggregation of this complication within families with several members affected by IDDM [9, 10, 11]. Moreover, phenotypes attached to diabetic

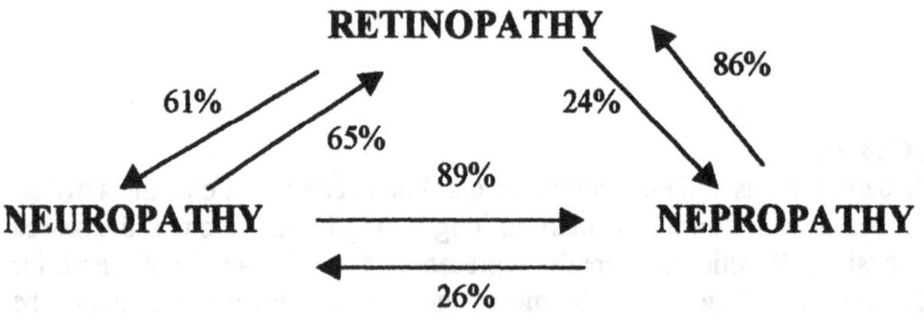

Figure 12-1. Concordance between diabetic complications in the follow-up study by Jean PIRART [4]. For each new case of one given complication, the probability to display another complication is indicated by the percentage attached to the arrow directed to this complication (e.g., among new cases of retinopathy, 61% already had neuropathy, and 24% nephropathy).

nephropathy like high blood pressure seem to segregate with diabetic nephropathy in families of IDDM patients [12]. The major drawback of family studies is that members of families can share the same environmental conditions, in addition to the same genes, and this remark was applied to the study of families with several IDDM patients [13]. However, studies in Pima Indians are of importance in this respect, because families share similar environmental conditions. The fact that familial aggregation for proteinuria was found among diabetic siblings of this ethnic group is an important argument for a genetic basis to diabetic nephropathy, eventhough these patients are mostly NIDDM [14].

CANDIDATE GENE VERSUS WHOLE GENOME SCREENING APPROACH

The whole genome screening approach is a promising strategy currently applied to monogenic diseases. In multifactorial diseases, this strategy may be less effective, and no clear-cut result was obtained with diabetic nephropathy to date. However, this strategy was already used to study the determinants of blood pressure, a variable tightly linked to glomerular disease. For instance, an original methodological approach indicated recently that a genetic region at or near the lipoprotein lipase gene locus was related to blood pressure in humans [15]. Also, the techniques of reverse genetics lead to the discovery of a link between severe, familial hypertension, and angiotensinogen gene polymorphisms, and then angiotensinogen plasma levels [16].

However, the candidate-gene approach has been the most fruitful approach in the domain of cardiovascular risk to date [17, 18, 19].

WHICH CANDIDATE GENES TO BE TESTED FOR DIABETIC NEPHROPATHY ?

Target tissues/organs susceptible to diabetic complications are those for which insulin is not required for glucose to be trapped and/or metabolized, i.e., nerves, lens, kidneys, blood cells, epithelial and endothelial cells. Glucose metabolism is altered in these tissues/organs through a few biochemical pathways, e.g., polyol pathway or non-enzymatic glycation of proteins. On the other hand, the vascular (and especially the renal) complications encountered in IDDM can be explained by hemodynamic factors [20] : increased arteriolar vasodilatation due to high glucose [3] creates high hydraustatic capillary pressure [21] resulting into arteriosclerosis and glomerulosclerosis [22, 23]. In this context, search for candidate genes able to modulate the risk of renal complications due to long-term hyperglycemia can be divided into two avenues : first, to search gene polymorphism of enzymes driving glucose metabolism in tissue/target organs ; second, to test gene polymorphism affecting background vascular risk in general population. Using the first strategy, a dinucleotide repeat polymorphism was found at the 5'end of the aldose reductase gene to be associated with early onset of retinopathy in Chinese, NIDDM patients [24]. Later on, another group found this polymorphism to be associated with diabetic nephropathy in Caucasian IDDM patients, although the interaction with presence or absence of retinopathy was not clearly delineated [25]. Thus, it is possible that aldose reductase, an enzyme able to affect glucose metabolism within target tissues/organs of diabetic microangiopathy, may affect vascular prognosis of IDDM patients, including nephropathy through variable, genetically determined, levels of its activity.

A second strategy consists of applying candidate genes for cardiovascular risk (especially those for alterations in microcirculation) to the risk for diabetic nephropathy. The working hypothesis relies on the assumption that global capillary vasodilatation provoked by hyperglycemia and/or insulinopenia in IDDM [3,21] also affects renal circulation, and that glomerular capillary hypertension (a universal cause for progression towards glomerulosclerosis and renal failure [26]) is due to an imbalance between hyperglycemia-induced afferent glomerular vasodilatation and constitutive, efferent, glomerular relative vasoconstriction (Figure 12-2).

There are a serie of regulatory systems able to affect glomerular hemodynamics. Within each of these systems, enhanced or reduced activity of one of its components can lead to high/low glomerular hydraulic pressure. Indeed, pharmacological alterations in these systems can affect glomerular hemodynamics, as indicated by changes in albuminuria. For instance, angiotensin I converting enzyme inhibitors can block the renin-angiotensin and kallikrein-kinins systems and reduce micro- or macroalbuminuria [27, 28]. However, reduction in urinary albumin can also be obtained through blockade of prostanoïds with indomethacin [29], or alterations of hemostasis and proteoglycans with heparin [30]. Thus, new polymorphisms within each component of these various regulatory systems are worth being tested for their roles in the development of IDDM complications, especially diabetic nephropathy [31, 32]. This is especially true, if gene polymorphisms are associated with variable levels of expression of the concerned protein.

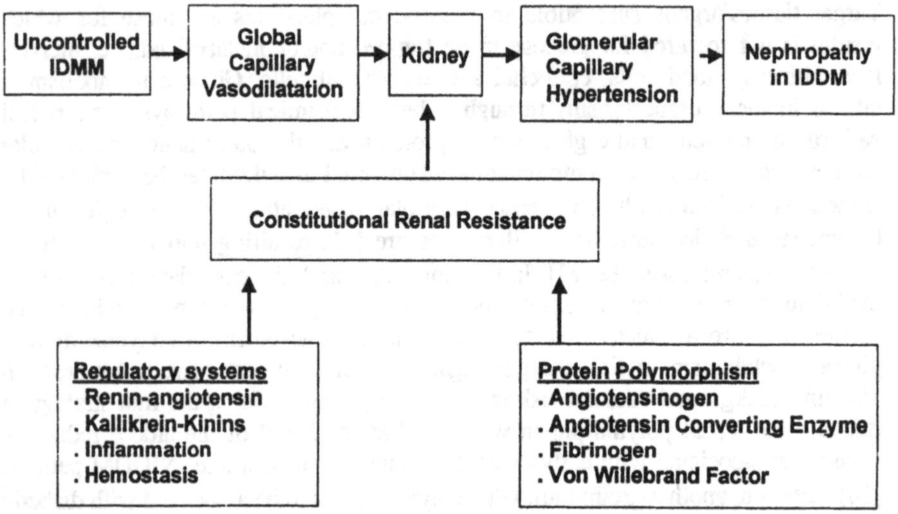

Figure 12-2. Working hypothesis to study susceptibility to nephropathy in IDDM. Glomerular capillary hypertension, a universal cause for glomerulosclerosis and renal failure, is due to an imbalance between pre-glomerular vasodilatation produced by IDDM, and constitutional renal assistance. Renal resistances result from several regulatory systems, among them several proteins can display polymorphisms affecting the activity of the considered systems.

WORKING HYPOTHESIS : POLYMORPHISM OF THE RENIN-ANGIOTENSIN SYSTEM AND RISK FOR DIABETIC NEPHROPATHY

Background hypothesis

As depicted in Figure 12-3, angiotensin II (AII) generation is consequent to a serie of enzymatic reactions, and AII interacts with a well-defined membrane receptor, of which the sub-type 1 AII receptor (AT1R) is of interest.

Several of these components displayed genetic polymorphisms, but only two of them displayed polymorphisms related to variable expressions of the protein : the renin substrate angiotensinogen (AGT) through the M235T and T174M polymorphisms [16], and the Angiotensin I Converting Enzyme (ACE) through an Insertion/Deletion (I/D) polymorphism located in intron 16 of the gene [33]. The effect of diabetes on glomerular circulation ressembles that of AII [34, 35].

Protein	Polymorphism	Association with	References
Angiotensiogen	M235T, T174M	Essential Hypertension	[16]
↓ ← Renin			
Angiotensin I			
↓←ACE*	I/D	Myocardial Infarction Renal Failure	[18] [40]
Angiotensin II			
↓			
AT1R	A1166C	Essential Hypertension	[39]

Figure 12-3. Schematic diagram of the renin-angiotensin system. Only two proteins (angiotensinogen, ACE) display variable levels of protein expression according to genetic polymorphisms. Numbers between parentheses indicate reference numbers* ; ACE : angiotensin converting enzyme.

Furthermore, ACE inhibition prevents diabetic nephropathy [36], or halts its progression [37]. If we accept the ancient hypothesis proposed by VANE that the ACE availability can limit transformation of angiotensin I into AII within the glomerular circulation [38], it was tempting to test the hypothesis of a role for ACE I/D polymorphism in the risk of diabetic nephropathy for IDDM patients. Also, genetically determined AGT levels could effect AII, in that the amount of substrate for renin (an enzyme without relevant genetic polymorphism) may limit angiotensin I production [16], although the proportion of the inter-subject variance of AGT due to genetic factors is relatively low (10-15 %), compared to that of ACE accounted for by genetic factors (~ 75 %), of which the I/D polymorphism makes ~ 50 % minimally [19]. Finally, a A1166C AT1R polymorphism was described in relation to essential hypertension [39], but no study has demonstrated to date, that it affects AII sensitivity.

Case-control studies on Diabetic Nephropathy and ACE I/D polymorphism in IDDM patients

Using the hypothesis depicted in Figure 12-2, we produced a case-control study indicating that IDDM subjects homozygotes for the ACE I allele seemed protected against diabetic nephropathy through low circulating ACE levels [40]. In this study, controls of nephropathy were carefully matched with cases for short-and long-term glycemic control (as assessed by HbA1c and the severity of retinopathy), and not only for age, sex, and IDDM duration. This result was challenged by some other, apparently negative, case-control studies, although bia due to a better glycemic control of controls than of cases was observable in these studies [41, 42, 43, 44].

In order to reduce the uncertainty due to the variable IDMM control and duration on the role for one given protein polymorphism in the kidney prognosis of

IDDM patients, we organized a multi-center, cross-sectional study of IDDM patients having expressed their risk of kidney disease due to IDDM : those who developed proliferative retinopathy, a clear hallmark for uncontrolled IDDM [45]. Then, we found that the severity of renal involvement was dependent of ACE I/D polymorphism with a dominant effect of ACE D allele [adjusted odds ratio for renal involvement attributable to the D allele 1.889 (95 % CI 1.209-2.952)]. There was no independent effect of AGT, or AT1R polymorphisms on the risk for diabetic nephropathy, but a significant interaction between ACE I/D and AGT M235T polymorphisms, suggesting that genetically determined AGT levels can affect risk for diabetic nephropathy through angiotensin I generation, if angiotensin I transformation into AII is not restrained by ACE availability (i.e., the patients with the ACE II genotype) [45].

Finally, some meta-analysis of all currently available studies on ACE I/D polymorphism and diabetic nephropathy support that the II genotype may confer a relative protection against diabetic nephropathy [46,47].

Clinical investigations on renal haemodynamics and ACE I/D polymorphism

Recently, J. MILLER et al reported that IDDM patients with the II genotype displayed higher glomerular filtration rate and effective renal plasma flow during normoglycemia than IDDM patients within the ID or DD genotypes [48]. These results are consistent with the effect of ACE inhibition on renal hemodynamics reported in normoalbuminuric [49] and microalbuminuric [28] subjects and consistent with a global, systemic vasodilatation due to low circulating AII levels. These alterations make protection against diabetic nephropathy [36]. Conversely, we studied recently the effect of acute hyperglycaemia in normotensive normoalbuminuric IDDM patients, and found that those with the ID or DD genotypes displayed alterations in glomerular haemodynamics consistent with a rise in glomerular capillary hydraulic pressure, while this was not observed in the pathients with the II genotype [50]. Thus, these investigations are arguments to support that ACE I/D polymorphism and related ACE levels can affect constitution and progression of diabetic nephropathy.

Follow-up studies and intervention studies according to ACE I/D genotypes

One follow-up study in Austria indicated that ACE I/D polymorphism can affect the course of kidney disease in IDDM patients [51]. Also, Parving et al reported that ACE I/D polymorphism can affect the course of glomerular filtration rate, once diabetic nephropathy is established [52]. Moreover, these authors [52] suggested that ACE inhibition was less effective to prevent the evolution towards renal failure, if the IDDM patients displayed the DD genotype, than if they did not [52]. However, these studies must be cautiously examined, because of the possible survival bia and other unidentified, hidden bias. Thus, prospective follow-up of kidney function must be organized according to ACE genotypes and other possibly important polymorphisms. Intervention studies (especially with ACE inhibitors) must be designed according to ACE I/D polymorphism with an appropriate method, probably using surrogate end-point like urinary albumin excretion as main outcome in a first step.

ACE I/D polymorphism and diabetic nephropathy in NIDDM patients

ACE I/D polymorphism was reported to be associated with risk for coronary heart disease in NIDDM [53]. As microalbuminuria or proteinuria predicts or is associated with coronary heart disease in NIDDM [54, 55, 56], it was worth looking for an association between urinary albumin and ACE I/D polymorphism in NIDDM. This association was reported to be positive in the UKPDS study [57]. Also, positive studies on the association between ACE I/D polymorphism and diabetic nephropathy were reported in Japanese NIDDM patients by most [58, 59, 60], if not all studies [61]. A study performed in Caucasian patients was negative [62]. Thus, the issue of an association between ACE I/D polymorphism remains debatable, because microalbuminuria or proteinuria is attributable to diabetic nephropathy in only a portion of cases with NIDDM [63] and because the interaction between elevated urinary albumin, coronary heart disease and ACE I/D polymorphism must be clarified. Lastly, the frequency of ACE II genotype is higher among Asian (~ 40-45%) than among Caucasian (~ 20-25%) subjects, and the clinical characteristics and age at onset of NIDDM are not similar in Japanese and Caucasian patients. Thus, the portion of the risk for (protection against) diabetic nephropathy / coronary heart disease may be different among Asian and Caucasian NIDDM patients.

ACKNOWLEDGEMENTS

The author thank Mrs Line GODIVEAU for her excellent secretarial assistance.

REFERENCES

1. Siperstein M.D., Unger R.H., madison L.L.Studies of muscle capillary basement membranes in normal subjects, diabetic and prediabetic patients. J. Clin. Invest., 1968, 47: 1973-1999
2. Mauer S., Steffes M.W., Sutherland D.E.R., Najarian J.S., Michael A.F., Brownd M. Studies of the rate of regression of the glomerular lesions in diabetic rats treated with pancreatic islet transplantation. Diabetes, 1975, 24: 250-255
3. Williamson J.R., Chang K., Frangos M., Hasan K.S., Ido Y., Kawamura F., Nyengaard J.R., Van Den Enden M., Kilo C., Tilton R.G. Hyperglycemic pseudohypoxia and diabetic complications. Diabetes, 1993, 42: 801-813
4. Pirart J. Diabète et complications dégénératives. Présentation d'une étude prospective portant sur 4400 cas observés entre 1947 et 1973. Diabete Metab., 1977, 3: 97-107, 3: 173-182, 3: 245-256
5. The Diabetes Control and Complications Trial Research Group.The effect of intensive treatment of diabetes on the development and progression of long-term complications in insulin-dependent diabetes mellitus. N. Engl. J. Med., 1993, 329: 977-986
6. Krolewski A.J., Warram J.H., Rand L.I., Kahn C.R. Epidemiologic approach to the etiology of type I diabetes mellitus and its Complications. N. Engl. J. Med, 1987, 317: 1390-1398
7. Andersen A.R., Christiansen J.S., Andersen J.K., Kreiner S., Deckert T. Diabetic nephropathy in type 1 (insulin-dependent) diabetes: an epidemiological Study. Diabetologia, 1983, 2: 496-501.
8. Borch-Johnsen K., Andersen P.K., Deckert T. The effect of proteinuria on relative mortality in type 1 (insulin-dependent) diabetes mellitus. Diabetologia, 1985, 28: 590-596
9. Seaquist E.R., Goetz F.C., Rich S., Barbosa J. Familial clustering ofdiabetic kidney disease : evidence for genetic susceptibility to diabetic nephropathy. N. Engl. J. Med, 1989, 320: 1161-1165
10. Earle K., Walker J., Hill C., Viberti G.C. Familial clustering of cardiovascular disease in patients with insulin-dependent diabetes and nephropathy. N. Engl. J. Med, 1992, 326: 673-677

11. Quinn M., Angelico M.C., Warram J.H., Krolewski A.S. Familial factors determine the development of diabetic nephropathy in patients with IDDM. Diabetologia, 1996, 39: 940-945
12. Viberti G.C., Keen H., Wiseman M.J. Raised arterial pressure in parents of proteinuric insulin-dependent diabetics. B.M.J, 1987, 295: 515-517
13. Borch-Johnsen K., Norgaard K., Hommel E., Mathiesen E.R., Jensen J.S., Deckert T., Parving H.H. Is diabetic nephropathy an inherited complication? Kidney Int, 1992, 41: 719-722
14. Pettit D.J., Saad M.F., Bennett P.H., Nelson R.G., Knowler W.C. Familial predisposition to renal disease in two generations of Pima Indians with 2 (non-insulin-dependent) diabetes mellitus. Diabetologia, 1990, 33: 438-443
15. Wu D.A., Bu X., Harden C.H., Shen D.D.C., Jeng C.Y., Sheu W.H.H., Fuh M.M.T., Katsuya T., Dzau V.J., Reaven G.M., Lusis A.J., Rotter J.I, Chen D.I. Quantitative trait locus mapping of human blood pressure to a genetic region at or near the Lipoprotein lipase gene locus on chromosome 8p22.J. Clin. Invest, 1996, 97: 2111-2118
16. Jeunemaitre X., Soubrier F., Kotelevtsev Y., Lifton R., Williams C., Charru A., Hunt S., Hopkins P., Williams R., Lalouel J.M., Corvol P. Molecular basis of human hypertension: role of angiotensinogen. Cell, 1992, 71: 169-180
17. Cambien F., Alhenc-Gelas F., Herberth B., Andre J.L., Rakotovao R., Gonzales M.F., Allegrini J., Bloch C. Familial ressemblance of plasma angiotensin converting enzyme level: the Nancy study. Am. J. Hum. Genet, 1988, 43: 774-780
18. Cambien F., Poirier O., Lecerf L., Evans A., Cambou J.P., Arveiler D., Luc G., Bard J.M., Bara L., Ricard S., Tiret L., Amouyel Ph., Alhenc-Gelas F., Soubrier F. Deletion polymorphism in the gene for angiotensin converting enzyme is a potent risk factor for myocardial infarction. Nature, 1992, 359: 641-644
19. Cambien F., Costerousse O., Tiret L., Poirier O., Lecerf L., Gonzales M.F., Evans A., Arveiler D., Cambou J.P., Luc G., Rakotovao R., Ducimetiere P., Soubrier F., Alheno-Gelas F. Plasma level and gene polymorphism of angiotensin concerting enzyme in relation to myocardial infarction. Circulation, 1994, 90: 669-676
20. Parving H.H., Viberti G.C., Keen H., Christiansen J.S., Lassen N.A. Hemodynamic factors in the genesis of diabetic microangiopathy. Metabolism, 1983, 32: 943-949
21. Tooke J.E. Microvascular function in human diabetes. A physiological perspective. Diabetes, 1995, 44: 721-726
22. Zatz R., Dunn B.R., Meyer T.W., Anderson S., Rennke H.G., Brenner B.M. Prevention of diabetic glomerulopathy by pharmacological of glomerular capillary hypertension. J. Clin. Invest, 1986,
77: 1925 –1930
23. Deckert T., Feldt-Rasmussen B., Borch-Johnsen K., Jensen T., Kofoed-Enevoldsen A. Albuminuria reflects widespread vascular damage: the Steno hypothesis. Diabetologia, 1989, 32: 219-226
24. Ko B.C.B., Lam K.S.L., Wat N.M.S., Chung S.S.M. An (A-C)n dinucleotide repeat polymorphic marker at the 5' end of the aldose reductase gene is associated with early-onset diabetic retinopathy in NIDDM patients. Diabetes, 1995, 44: 727-732
25. Heesom A.E., Hibberd M.L., Millward A., Demaine A.G. Polymorphism in the 5'-end of the aldose reductase gene is strongly associated with the development of diabetic nephropathy in type I diabetes. Diabetes, 1997, 46 : 287-291
26. Brenner B.M. Hemodynamicaly mediated glomerular injury and the progressive nature of kidney disease. Kidney Intern, 1983, 23: 617-655.,
27. Taguma Y., Kitamoto Y., Futaki G., Ueda H., Monma H., Ishizaki M., Takahashi H., Sekino H., Sasaky Y. Effect of Captopril on heavy proteinuria in azotemic diabetics. N. Engl. J. Med, 1985, 313: 1617-1620
28. Marre M., Leblanc H., Suarez L., Guyenne T.T., Menard J., Passa P. Converting enzyme inhibition and kidney function in normotensive diabetic patients with persistent microalbuminuria. B.M.J, 1987, 294: 1448-1452
29. Hommel E., Mathiesen E., Olsen U.B., Parving H.H. Effects of indomethacin on kidney function in type 1 (insulin-dependent) diabetic patients with nephropathy. Diabetologia, 1987, 30: 78-81
30. Myrup B., Hansen P.M., Jensen J., Kofoed-Enevoldsen A., Feldt-Rasmussen B., Gram J., Kluft C., Jespersen J., Deckert T. Effect of low-dose heparin on urinary albumin excretion in insulin-dependent diabetes mellitus. Lancet, 1995, 345: 421-422

31. Torremocha F, Marechaud R, Marre M., Passa Ph., Rodier M., Alhenc-Gelas F., Jeunemaitre X. for the GENEDIAB group Lack of relation between renal kallidrein gene polymorphism and diabetic nephropathy. Diabetologia, 1997, 40, A520 (abstract)
32. Gaucher C., Lacquemant C., Delorme C., Ruiz J., Mazurier C., Rodier M., Bauduceau B., Gallois Y., Passa Ph., Marre M., Froguel P., et le groupe GENEDIAB Polymorphisme THR/ALA789 du facteur Von Willebrand et maladie coronarienne chez les diabétiques insulino-dépendants. Diabète et Métabolisme, 1997, Vol. 23, p. XXII
33. Rigat B., Hubert C., Alhenc-Gelas F., Cambien F., Corvol P., Soubrier F. An insertion deletion polymorphism in angiotensin I convertion enzyme gene accounting for half of the variance of serum enzyme levels. J. Clin. Invest, 1990, 86: 1343-1346
34. Hostetter T.H., Troy J.L., Brenner B.M. Glomerular hemodynamics in experimental diabetes mellitus. Kidney Int., 1981, 19: 410-415
35. Hall J.E., Guyton A.C., Jackson T.E., Coleman T.G., Lohmeier T.E., Tripoddo N.C. Control of glomerular filtration rate by renin-angiotensin system. Am. J. Physiol., 1977, 233: F366-F372
36. Marre M., Chatellier G., Leblanc H., Guyenne Tt, Menard J., Passa P. Prevention of diabetic nephropathy with enalapril in normotensive diabetics with microalbuminuria. B.M.J., 1988, 297: 1092-1095
37. Lewis E.J., Hunsiker L.G., Bain R.P., Rohde R.D., for the Collaborative Study Group. The effect of angiotensin-converting-enzyme inhibition on diabetic nephropathy. N. Engl. J. Med., 1993, 329: 1456-1462
38. Vane J.R. Sites of conversion of angiotensin I. In Hypertension. Genest J., Koine E., eds Berlin, Springer Verlag, 1972, p 523-532
39. Bonnardeaux A., Davies E., Jeunemaitre X., Fery I., Charru A., Clauser E., Tiret L., Cambien F., Corvol P., Soubrier F. Angiotensin II type 1 receptor gene polymorphisms in human essential hypertension. Hypertension, 1994, 24: 63-69
40. Marre M., Bernadet P., Gallois Y., Savagner F., Guyene T.T., Hallab M., Cambien F., Passa Ph., Alhenc-Gelas F. Relationships between angiotensin I converting enzyme gene polymorphism, plasma levels, and diabetic retinal and renal complications. Diabetes, 1994, 43: 384-388
41. Tarnow L., Cambien F., Rossing P., Nielsen F.S., Hansen B.V., Lecerf L., Poirier O., Danilov S., Parving H.H. Lack of relationship between an insertion / deletion polymorphism in the I-converting enzyme gene and diabetic nephropathy and proliferative retinopathy in IDDM patients. Diabetes, 1995, 44: 489-494
42. Schmidt S., Schone N., Ritz E., and the Diabetic Nephropathy Study Group: Association of ACE gene polymorphism and diabetic nephropathy ? Kidney Int., 1995, 47: 1176-1181
43. Powrie J.K., Watts G.F., Ingham J.N., Taub N.A., Talmud P.J., Shaw K.M. Role of glycæmic control in development of microalbuminuria in patients with insulin-dependent diabetes. B.M.J., 1994, 309: 1608-1612
44. Chowdhury T.A., Dronsfield M.J., Kumar S., Gough S.L.C., Gibson S.P., Khatoon A., Macdonald F., Rowe B.R., Dunger D.B., Dean J.D., Davies S.J., Webber J., Smith P.R., Macrin P., Marshall S.M., Adu D., Morris P.J.M., Todd J.A., Barnett A.H., Boulton A.J.M., Bain S.C. Examination of two genetic polymorphisms within the renin-angiotensin system : no evidence for an association with nephropathy in IDDM. Diabetologia, 1996, 39 : 1108-1114
45. Marre M., Jeunemaitre X., Gallois Y., Rodier M., Chatellier G., Sert C., Dusselier L., Kahal Z., Chaillous L., Halimi S., Muller A., Sackmann H., Bauduceau B., Bled F., Passa Ph., Alhenc-Gelas F. Contribution of Genetic polymorphism in the Renin-Angiotensin System to the development of renal complications in insulin-dependent diabetes. J. Clin. Invest., 1997, 99, 1585-1595
46. Staessen JA, Wang JG, Ginocchio G, Petrov V, Saavedra AP, Soubrier F, Vlietinck R, Fagard R. The delation/insertion polymorphism of the angiotension converting enzyme gene and cardiovascular-renal risk. J Hypertension, 1997, 15 :1575-1592.
47. Fujisawa T, Ikegemi H, Kawaguchi Y, Hamada Y, Ueda H, Shintani M, Fakuda M, Ogihara T. Meta-analysis of association of insertion/deletion polymorphism of angiotensin I-converting enzyme gene with diabetic nephropathy and retinopathy. Diabetologia, 1998, 41 : 47-53.
48. Miller J.A., Scholey J.W., Thai K., Pei Y.P.C. Angiotensin converting enzyme gene polymorphism and renal hemodynamic function in early diabetes. Kidney International, 1997, 51: 119-124

49. Mau-Pedersen M., Schmitz A., Pedersen E.B., Danielsen H., Christiansen J.S. Acute and long-term renal effects of angiotensin converting enzyme inhibition in normotensive, normoalbuminuric insulin-dependent diabetic patients. Diabetic Med, 1988, 5: 562-569

50. Marre M., Gallois Y., Bled F., Pean F., Bouhanick B., Le Jeune J.J., Alhenc-Gelas F. Renal response to hyperglycemia and angiotensin I converting enzyme deletion (D) allele in IDDM (abstract). Diabetologia, 1997, 40 (suppl 1) : A521

51. Barnas U., Schmidt A., Illievich A., Kiener H.P., Rabensteiner D., Kaider A., Prager R., Abrahamian H., Irsigler K., Mayer G. Evaluation of risk factors for the development of nephropathy in patients with IDDM : insertion/deletion angiotensin converting enzyme gene polymorphism, hypertension and metabolic control. Diabetologia, 1997, 40 : 327-331

52. Parving H.H., Jacobsen P., Tarnow L., Rossing P., Lecerf L., Poirier O., Cambien F. Effect of deletion polymorphism of angiotensin enzyme gene on progression of diabetic nephropathy during inhibition of angiotensin converting enzyme, observational follow-up study. B.M.J., 1996, 313: 591-594

53. Ruiz J., Blanche H., Cohen N., Velho G., Cambien F., Cohen D., Passa Ph., Froguel Ph. Insertion / Deletion polymorphism of the angiotensin converting enzyme gene is strongly associated with coronary heart disease in non-insulin-dependent diabetes mellitus Proc. Natl. Acad. Sci. USA, 1994, 91: 3662-3665

54. Mogensen C.E. Microalbuminuria predicts clinical proteinuria and early mortality in maturity-onset diabetes. N. Engl. J. Med., 1984, 310: 356-360

55. Jarrett R.J., Viberti G.C., Argyropoulos A., Hill R.D., Mahmud U., Murrels T.J. Microalbuminuria predicts mortality in non insulin-dependent diabetics. Diabetic Med., 1984, 1: 17-19

56. Mattock M.B., Morrish N.J., Viberti G.C., Keen H., Fitzerald A.P., Jackson G. Prospective study of microalbuminuria as predictor of mortality in NIDDM. Diabetes 1992, 41: 736-741

57. Dubley C.R.K., Keavney B., Stratton I.M., Turner R.C., Ratcliffe P.J. U.K. prospective diabetes study XV: relationship of renin-angiotensin system gene polymorphisms with microalbuminuria in NIDDM.Kidney Int., 1995, 48: 1907-1911

58. Mizuiri S., Hemmi H., Inoue A., Yoshikawa H., Tanegashima M., Fushimi T., Ishigami M., Amagasaki Y., Ohara T., Shimatake H., Hasegawa A. Angiotensin-converting-enzyme polymorphism and development of diabetic nephropathy in non-insulin-dependent diabetes mellitus. Nephron., 1995, 70: 455-459

59. Doi Y., Yoshizumi H., Lino K., Yamamoto M., Ichikawa K., Iwase M., Fujishima M. Association between a polymorphism in the angiotensin-converting-enzyme gene and microavascular complications in Japanese patients with NIDDM. Diabetologia, 1996, 39: 97-102

60. Ohno T., Kawazu S., Tomono S. Association analyse of the polymorphisms of angiotensin-converting enzyme and angiotensinogen genes with diabetic nephropathy in Japanese non-insulin-dependent diabetics. Metabolism, 1996, 45 : 218-222

61. Fujisawa T., Ikegami H., Shen G.Q., Yamato E., Takekawa K., Nakagawa Y., Hamada Y.,Ueda H., Rakugi H., Higaki J., Ohishi M., Fujii K., Fukuda M., Ogihara T. Angiotensin I converting enzyme gene polymorphism is associated with myocardial infarction, but not with retinopathy or nephropathy, in NIDDM. Diabetes Care, 1995, 18: July

62. Schmidt S., Schone N., Ritz E., and the Diabetic Nephropathy Study Group: Association of ACE gene polymorphism and diabetic nephropathy ? Kidney Int., 1995, 47: 1176-1181

63. Gambara V., Mecca G., Remuzzi G., Bertani T. Heterogeneous nature of renal lesions in type II diabetes. J. Am. Soc. Nephrol., 1993, 3: 1458-1466

13. THE CONCEPT OF LOW BIRTH WEIGHT AND RENAL DISEASE

J.R. Nyengaard, E. Vestbo
Stereological Research Laboratory, University of Aarhus and Department of Medicine M, Aarhus Kommunehospital, Aarhus, Denmark

Much attention has been focused on the lack of nutrition in the early environment of human beings, in order to explain the development of disease in adult life [1,2]. Nutrition in an inadequately nourished foetus may be reserved for the developing brain, at the expense of other less important organs such as the pancreas and the kidney. These organs may then in later life suffer from diseases because they have been deprived of nutrition at a crucial stage in their development. In the kidney, for instance, the embryological development is very tightly controlled [3]. In vitro studies have shown that manipulation of the matrix of glomerular morphogenesis may generate less developed nephrons [4], and in vivo studies have shown that protein restriction in pregnant rats results in new-born rats with fewer and a smaller number of glomeruli [5, 6].

BARKER HYPOTHESIS

The result of malnutrition in early pregnancy may be symmetrically small babies with low birth weight. In mid-pregnancy, the placenta grows faster than the foetus and mild malnutrition in this period of time may result in a child with low birth weight and a small or hypertrophied placenta. Late in pregnancy, malnutrition may result in thin babies, as the foetus may loose weight [7]. Retarded foetal growth can be characterised by low birth weight, low birth weight relative to placental weight or low ponderal index (birth weight/height) [8].

Barker and co-workers have found an association between low birth weight and the development of cardiovascular disease [7, 9, 10], and between low birth weight and the development of death from coronary heart disease [9, 10, 11] in adult human subjects. There is an association between low birth weight (in combination with a big placenta) and the development of hypertension in mature human beings [12, 13]. Impaired maternal nutrition in pregnancy has been linked to development of hypertension in the offspring's [14, 15]. Low birth weight has also been associated with an increased risk for the development of insulin resistance [16], impaired beta cell function [17], and impaired glucose tolerance [18, 19, 20, 21]. In

Pima Indians, who have a very high prevalence of Non-Insulin Dependent Diabetes Mellitus (NIDDM), the association between birth weight and the prevalence of NIDDM is U-formed [22]. In the Health Professionals Follow-up study including 22,846 US men, self-reported low birth weight was associated to higher frequency of hypertension and diabetes whereas high birth weight was associated to adult obesity [23]. In the Nurses' Health study 92,940 women with high birth weight were more obese than subjects with low birth weight whereas the prevalence of hypertension was higher in subjects with low birth weight compared to subjects with high birth weight [24]. All these associations between low birth weight and the development of key determinants of coronary heart disease, like hypertension and glucose intolerance in adult human life, have been named the "Barker hypothesis".

Several different changes in foetal life [25], primarily focusing upon changes in maternal glucocorticoids [8, 26], have been brought into light in order to explain the association between low birth weight and hypertension. Persistent changes in the secretion of foetal hormones and the altered sensitivity of different kinds of tissue to the maternal glucocorticoids may result in the development of hypertension. Dysfunction of placental glucocorticoid barrier may result in increased maternal glucocorticoids in the foetus, resulting in impaired foetal growth. The maternal glucocorticoids, which are exposed to the foetus, may effect the development of the foetal vessels, thus increasing the risk of developing hypertension in adult life [8].

There have been several arguments raised in opposition to the Barker hypothesis. The Barker hypothesis is challenged by data showing that plasma insulin concentration is more strongly associated with current body mass index than with birth weight because Barker et al. cancel out the positive effect of birth weight on the current body mass index and the development of glucose intolerance [27]. Secondly, one would expect that the growth retardation in twins would lead to an increased risk of developing cardiovascular death, according to the Barker hypothesis, because twins have greatly restricted growth in the third trimester. Apparently, the mortality of twins after the age of 6 does not differ from the background population [28]. Thirdly, in Great Britain, the initial and current place of residence contribute equally to the risk of coronary heart disease and migrants seem to acquire the mortality risk from stroke of the area to which they move [29]. Fourth, the Barker hypothesis predicts a link between a high ratio of placental weight to foetal weight and adult hypertension, but a recent study including 2,507 pregnant women concluded that the ratio of placental weight to birth weight is an inaccurate marker of foetal growth [30]. Other factors than birth weight may carry greater importance: these factors are maternal obesity [31], maternal smoking [32], maternal diabetes [33], and gestation age [34]. Fifth, both maternal smoking and social class are well recognised as having a significant impact on birth weight in many other studies [27]. Barker and colleagues have never taken maternal smoking into account and the social class of the mothers did not associate with birth weight in their studies. Finally, in 33,545 and 10,883 subjects from Israel, factors reflecting poor intrauterine nutrition, e.g. low birth weight, were poorly or not associated with higher blood pressure in late adolescence [35, 36] as shown in other studies [37, 38].

Thus, the inverse correlation between birth weight and blood pressure is inconsistently found, and when found, is weak.

BRENNER HYPOTHESIS

Brenner et al. postulated in 1988 [39] that essential hypertension may be the result of an inborn reduction in the total glomerular filtration surface area, due to a low number of glomeruli and/or small glomeruli (a low filtration surface area per glomerulus). This hypothesis was based both on clinical and experimental evidence. During the growth phase of a human being, the hypertension may result in glomerular capillary hypertension and later on in glomerular sclerosis, which will further reduce the total glomerular filtration surface area, thus perpetuating a vicious cycle [40].

The variation in expression of renal disease among, for example, diabetic patients was explained by the big variation in glomerular number and glomerular size within these patients [41, 42]. Those persons borne with a greater total glomerular filtration surface area would be less prone to develop diabetic nephropathy than those with a small total glomerular filtration surface area, due to a reduced haemodynamic burden on individual glomeruli.

It is beyond the scope of this chapter to discuss pros and cons for the Brenner hypothesis and interested readers can refer to other chapters in this book.

BARKER AND BRENNER

With relation to the kidney in diabetic patients, it is possible to make a unification of the Barker hypothesis and Brenner hypothesis [25, 40]: Intrauterine growth retardation, caused by any kind of mechanism, generates babies with a low birth weight. These smaller babies have smaller kidneys with fewer and/or smaller glomeruli. Fewer and/or smaller glomeruli result in a decreased total glomerular filtration surface area, giving rise to individual glomerular hypertension due to a reduced renal functional reserve. The diabetic patients with the fewest and/or smallest glomeruli will then be more prone to develop irreversible renal failure when exposed to a renal insult in later life.

The unification of Brenner and Barker's hypothesis has had support from five studies: 1) 23 young women with scarred kidneys but stable renal function weighed more at birth than 17 similar patients with progressive renal failure [43;] 2) birth weights correlated with the gradients of reciprocal serum creatinine regression lines in 12 patients with idiopathic membranous nephropathy [44] 3) in 45 patients with Insulin Dependent Diabetes Mellitus for more than 20 years, the patients without proteinuria had a greater birth weight than those with microalbuminuria or proteinuria [45] 4) infants with a low birth weight below the 10th percentile had a lower kidney weight and a reduced number of glomeruli per optical field covering the entire height of the cortex, than infants with a normal birth weight [46] 5) eight type II intrauterine growth retarded infants with birth weights below the 10th percentile for the accurately determined gestation age, had 65% of the number of glomeruli when compared with seven infants with birth weights above the 10th percentile [47].

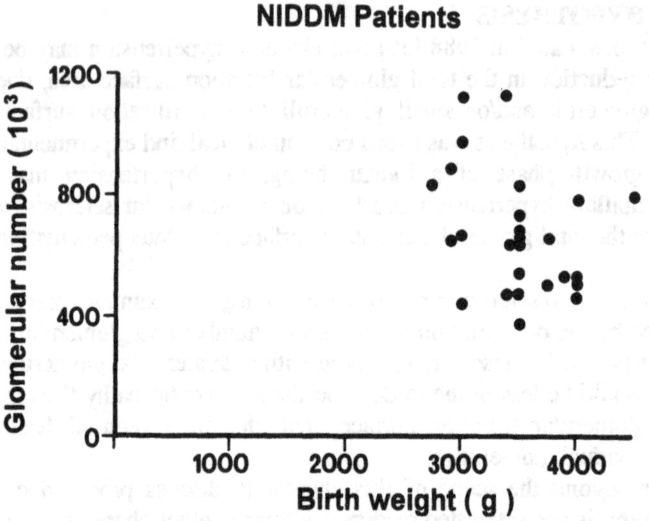

Figure 13-1. There is no significant correlation (r=-0.33; 2*p*=0.10) between birth weight and total glomerular number in 26 NIDDM patients (from ref. 41 with permission).

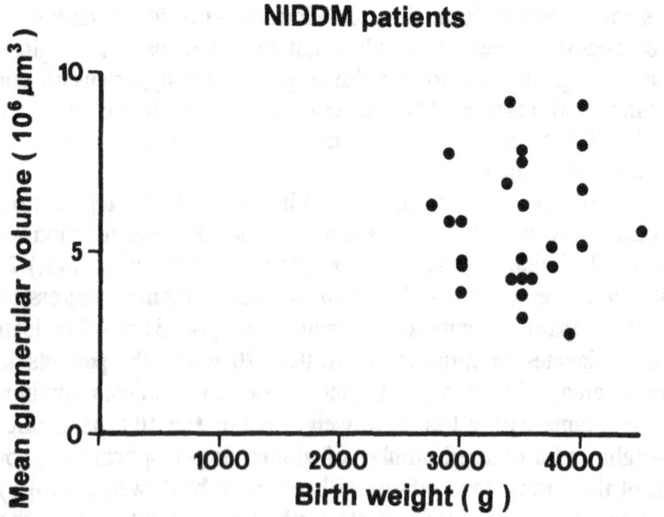

Figure 13-2. There is no significant correlation (r=0.06; 2*p*=0.78) between birth weight and mean glomerular volume in 26 NIDDM patients (from ref. 41 with permission).

The unification of Brenner and Barker's hypothesis has been challenged by four recent studies: 1) there was no difference in birth weight between 25 type 1 diabetic patients without diabetic nephropathy and 22 patients with diabetic nephropathy [48; 2] there was no correlation between low birth weight, few and/or small glomeruli or low kidney weight and there was no difference between the four parameters in 19 control subjects and 26 NIDDM patients (See figures 13-1 + 13-2 and table 13-1) [49; 3] in an epidemiological study of 620 Caucasian non-diabetic subjects, there was no correlation between birth weight and blood pressure or between birth weight and urinary albumin excretion rate [50, 4] eleven non-diabetic subjects with microalbuminuria did not have significantly lower birth weight when compared to 225 controls and subjects exposed to intrauterine starvation did not have higher urinary albumin excretion than controls [51].

It is important to emphasise that the number of patients included in the above-mentioned studies is relatively limited.

Table 13-1. The sex, age, kidney weight, glomerular number and size, and birth weight on 19 normal persons (C) and 26 NIDDM patients. Mean, (SD) and [range] are shown [from ref. 41].

	C	NIDDM
Sex (f = females, m = males)	8m/11f	14m/12f
Age (years)	59 (16) [34; 87]	63 (11) [35; 85]
Kidney weight (g)	137 (36) [91; 206]	150 (38) [82; 228]
glomerular number (10^3)	670 (176) [393; 1056]	673 (200) [379; 1124]
Mean glomerular volume (10^6 μm^3)	6.25 (1.48) [3.95; 8.97]	5.71 (1.74) [2.81; 9.18]
Birth weight (g)	3577 (400) [2900; 4250]	3489 (429) [2750; 4500]

CONCLUSION

The unification of Brenner and Barker's hypothesis is deduced from observations suggesting; that low birth weight results in high blood pressure and impaired glucose tolerance in adult life; that low birth weight results in a low nephron number; and that a low nephron number results in high blood pressure. In our opinion, it is likely that infants with very low birth weight (< 2750 g) may have fewer and/or smaller glomeruli. Recent data suggests that in normal persons and in NIDDM patients, this association is of very limited importance, where many other factors may carry a far greater importance in a population where so few people have a very low birth weight. Thus the hypothesis that low birth weight in a population of human beings should have a significant effect on the development of NIDDM and smaller kidneys with few and/or small glomeruli seems relatively unimportant. It is therefore difficult to support the unification of Brenner and Barker's hypothesis with regards to diabetic kidneys, at this point in time.

ACKNOWLEDGEMENTS

The skilful technical assistance of Ms. A.M. Funder and Ms. A. Larsen is thankfully acknowledged. The study was supported by the Danish Heart Association, the Danish Medical Research Council, Fonden til Lægevidenskabens Fremme, NOVO Foundation, and Aarhus University Research Foundation.

REFERENCES

1. Barker DJP: Fetal and infant origins of adult disease. London: BMJ Publications; 1992.
2. Barker DJP: Mothers, babies, and disease in later life. London: BMJ Publications; 1994.
3. Bard JB, Wolf AS: Nephrogenesis and the development of renal disease. Nephrol Dial Transplant 1992; 7: 563-572.
4. Bard JB: Traction and the formation of mesenchymal condensations *in vivo.* BioEssays 1990; 12: 389-393.
5. Zeman FJ: Effects of maternel protein restriction on the kidney of the newborn young of rats. J Nutr 1968; 94: 111-116.
6. Merlet-Benichou C, Lelievre-Pegorier M, Gilbert T, Muffat-Joly M, Leroy B: Intrauterine growth retardation (IUGR) and inborn nephron deficit in the rat. J Am Soc Nephrol 1992; 3: 49P.
7. Barker DJP, Gluckman PD, Godfrey KM, Harding JE, Owens JA, Robinson JS: Fetal nutrition and cardiovascular disease in adult life. Lancet 1993; 341: 938-941.
8. Edwards CRW, Benediktsson R, Lindsay RS, Seckl JR: Dysfunction of placental glucocorticoid barrier: link between fetal environment and adult hypertension? Lancet 1993; 341: 355-357.
9. Osmond C, Barker DJP, Winter PD, Fall CHD, Simmonds SJ: Early growth and death from cardiovascular disease in women. BMJ 1993; 307: 1519-1524.
10. Fall CHD, Vijayakumar M, Barker DJP, Osmond C, Duggleby C: Weight in infancy and prevalence of coronary herat disease in adult life. BMJ 1995; 310: 17-19.
11. Barker DJP, Winter PD, Osmond C, Margetts B, Simmonds SJ: Weight in infancy and death from ischaemic heart disease. Lancet 1989; i: 578-580.
12. Barker DJP, Bull AR, Osmond C, Simmonds SJ: Fetal and placental size and risk of hypertension in adult life. BMJ 1990; 301: 259-262.
13. Holland FJ, Stark O, Ades AE, Peckman CS: Birth weight and body mass index in childhood, adolescence, and adulthood as predictors of blood pressure at age 36. J Epidemiol Community Health 1993; 47: 432-435.
14. Godfrey KM, Forrester T, Jackson AA, Landman JP, Hall JS, Cox V, Osmond C: Maternal nutritional status in pregnancy and blood pressure in childhood. Brit J Obstet Gynecol 1994; 101: 398-403.
15. Campbell DM, Hall MH, Barker DJ, Cross J, Shiell AW, Godfrey KM: Diet in pregnancy and the offspring's blood pressure 40 years later. Brit J Obstet Gynecol 1996; 103: 273-280.
16. Phillips DJ, Barker DJP, Hales CN, Hirst S, Osmond C: Thinness at birth and insulin resistance in adult life. Diabetologia 1994; 37: 150-154.
17. Cook JTE, Levy JC, Page RCL, Shaw JAG, Hattersley AT, Turner RC: Association of low birth weight with β cell function in the adult first degree relatives of non-insulin dependent diabetic subjects. BMJ 1993; 306: 302-306.
18. Hales CN, Barker DJP, Clark PMS, Cox LJ, Fall C, Osmond C, Winther PD: Fetal and infant growth and impaired glucose intolerance at age 64. BMJ 1991; 303: 1019-1022.
19. Phipps K, Barker DJP, Hales CN, Fall CHD, Osmond C, Clark PMS: fetal growth and impaired glucose intolerance in men and women. Diabetologia 1993; 36: 225-228.
20. Robinson S, Walton RJ, Clark PM, Barker DJP, Hales CN, Osmond C: The relation of fetal growth to plasma glucose in young men. Diabetologia 1992; 35: 444-446.
21. Fall CHD, Osmond C, Barker DJP, Clark PMS, Hales CN, Stirling Y, Meade TW: Fetal and infant growth and cardiovascular risk factors in women. BMJ 1995; 310: 428-432.
22. McCance DR, Pettitt DJ, Hanson RL, Jacobsson LT, Knowler WC, Bennett PH: Birth weight and non-insulin dependent diabetes: thrifty genotype, thrifty phenotype, or surviving small baby genotype? BMJ 1994; 308: 942-945.
23. Curhan GC, Willett WC, Rimm EB, Spiegelman D, Ascherio AL, Stampfer MJ: Birth weight and adult hypertension, diabetes mellitus, and obesity in US men. Circulation 1996; 94: 3246-3250.

24. Curhan GC, Chetow GM, Willett WC, Spiegelman D, Coldiz GA, Manson JAE, Speizer FE, Stampfer MJ: Birth weight and adult hypertension, and obesity in US women. Circulation 1996; 94: 1310-1315.
25. Garrett PJ, Bass PS, Sandeman DD: Barker, Brenner, and babies - early environment and renal disease in adulthood. J Pathol 1994; 173: 299-300.
26. Benediktsson R, Lindsay RS, Noble J, Seckl JR, Edwards CRW: Glucocorticoid exposure in utero: new model for adult hypertension. Lancet 1993; 341: 339-341.
27. Paneth N, Susser M: Early origin of coronary heart disease ("the Barker Hypothesis"). BMJ 1995; 310: 411-412.
28. Christensen K, Vaupel JW, Holm NW, Yashin AI: Mortality among twins after age 6: fetal origins hypothesis versus twin method. BMJ 1995; 310: 432-436.
29. Strachan DP, Leon DA, Dodgeon B: Mortality from cardiovascular disease among interregional migrants in England and Wales. BMJ 1995; 310: 423-427.
30. Williams LA, Evans SF, Newnham JP: Prospective cohort study of factors influencing the relative weights of the placenta and the newborn infant. BMJ 1997; 314: 1864-1868.
31. Perry IJ, Beevers DG, Whincup PH, Beresford D: Predictors of ratio of placental weight to fetal weight in multiethnic community. BMJ 1995; 310: 436-439.
32. Beaulac-Baillargeon L, Desrosiers C: Caffeine-cigarette interaction on fetal growth. Am J Obstet Gynecol 1987; 157: 1236-1240.
33. Clarson C, Tevaarweek GJM, Harding PGR, Chance GW, Haust MD: Placental weight in diabetic pregnancies. Placenta 1989; 10: 275-281.
34. Dombrowski MP, Berry SM, Johnson MP, Saleh AAA, Sokol RJ: Birth weight-length ratios, ponderal indexes, placental weights and birth weight-placenta ratios in a large population. Arch Pediatr Adoles Med 1994; 148: 508-512.
35. Seidman DS, Laor A, Gale R, Stevenson DK, Mashiach S, Danon YI: Birth weight, current body weight and blood pressure in late adolescence. BMJ 1991; 302: 1235-1237.
36. Laor A, Stevenson DK, Shemer J, Gale R, Seidman DS: Size at birth, maternal nutritional status in pregnancy, and blood pressure at age 17: population based analysis. BMJ 1997; 315: 449-453.
37. Williams S, St. George IM, Silva PA: Intrauterine growth retardation and blood pressure at age seven and eighteen. J Clin Epidemiol 1992; 45: 1257-1267.
38. Macintyre S, Watt G, West P, Ecob R: Correlates of blood pressure in 15 year olds in the west of Scotland. J Epidemiol Community Health 1991; 45: 143-147.
39. Brenner BM, Garcoa DL, Anderson S: Glomeruli and blood pressure: Less of one, more the other? Am J Hypertens 1988; 1: 335-347.
40. Brenner BM, Chertow GM: Congenital oligonephropathy and the etiology of adult hypertension and progressive renal injury. Am J Kid Dis 1994; 23: 171-175.
41. Nyengaard JR, Bendtsen TF: Glomerular number and size in relation to age, kidney weight, and body surface in normal man. Anat Rec 1992; 232: 194-201.
42. Bendtsen TF, Nyengaard JR: The number of glomeruli in Type I (insulin-dependent) and Type II (non-insulin-dependent) diabetic patients. Diabetologia 1992; 35: 844-850.
43. Garrett PJ, Sandeman DD, Reza M, Rogerson ME, Bass PS, Duncan RC, Dathan JR: Weight at birth and renal disease in adulthood. Nephrol. Dial. Transplant 1993; 8: 920.
44. Duncan RC, Bass PS, Garrett PJ, Dathan JR: Weight at birth and other factors influencing progression of idiopathic membranous nephropathy. Nephrol Dial Transplant 1994; 9: 871-880.
45. Sandeman DD, Reza M, Phillips DD, Barker DJP, Osmond C, Leatherdale BA: Why do some type 1 diabetics develop nephropathy? A possible role of birthweight. Diab Med 1992; 9(Suppl.1): 36A.
46. Leroy B, Josset P, Morgan G, Costil J, Merlet-Benichou C: Intrauterine growth retardation (IUGR) and nephron deficit: Preliminary study in man. Pediatr. Nephrol. 1992; 6: 3.
47. Hinchliffe SA, Lynch MRJ, Sargent PH, Howard CV, Van Velzen V: The effect of intrauterine growth retardation on the development of renal nephrons. Brit J Obstet Gynecol 1992; 99: 296-301.
48. Eshøj O, Vaag A, Feldt-Rasmussen B, Borch-Johnsen K, Beck-Nielsen H: No evidence of low birth weight as a risk factor for diabetic nephropathy in type 1 diabetic patients. Diabetologia 1995; 38 (Suppl. 1): A222.
49. Nyengaard JR, Bendtsen TF, Mogensen CE: Low birth weight - is it associated with few and small glomeruli in normal persons and NIDDM (non-insulin-dependent diabetes mellitus) patients? Diabetologia 1996; 39: 1634-1637.

50. Vestbo E, Damsgaard EM, Frøland A, Mogensen CE: Birth weight and cardiovascular factors in an epidemiological study. Diabetologia 1996; 39: 1598-1602.
51. Yudkin JS, Phillips DIW, Stanner S: Proteinuria and progressive renal disease:birth weight and microalbuminuria. Nephrol. Dial. Transplant 1997; 12(Suppl. 2): 10-13.

14. EFFECTS OF INSULIN ON THE KIDNEY AND THE CARDIOVASCULAR SYSTEM

Ele Ferrannini, MD
Department of Internal Medicine and Metabolism Unit, C N R Institute of Clinical Physiology at the University of Pisa, Italy

THE CARDIOVASCULAR SYSTEM

The concept that exogenous insulin administration may be associated with haemodynamic changes has appeared in the literature soon after the purified hormone became available for use in humans (*e.g.* [1]). Subsequently, however, these changes have mostly been ascribed to the counter-regulatory hormone response to the attendant hypoglycaemia. It has not been until the introduction of the glucose clamp technique, by which hyperinsulinaemia can be uncoupled from hypoglycaemia, that the existence of specific vascular actions of the hormone has been recognised. Interest has initially focussed on insulin-induced vasodilatation [2]; more recently, a wider range of haemodynamic effects of insulin has been characterised, and their possible physiological significance is beginning to be appreciated.

BLOOD FLOW

Against a background of mostly negative reports, the careful studies of Baron and his co-workers [3] have established that insulin infusion with maintenance of glycaemia is followed by an increase in leg blood flow in healthy, young volunteers. Typically in these studies [3,4], following a few hours of euglycaemic hyperinsulinaemia (in the range of 300-700 pmol/l) leg blood flow, as measured by thermodilution, rose approximately 2-fold above baseline values in resting subjects under controlled experimental conditions. As this effect was found to be blunted in patients with insulin resistance of glucose uptake (obese [3], hypertensive [5] or diabetic [6,7]), Baron [8] pioneered the interpretation that insulin-induced vasodilatation, by increasing substrate and hormone delivery to target tissues such as skeletal muscle, is a physiological determinant of insulin action on glucose uptake.

Both the basic observation and its interpretation have been challenged, and still are a subject of controversy. Discrepancies have been imputed to the technique for measuring blood flow (indicator dilution, thermodilution, venous occlusion plethysmography, Doppler ultrasound, positron-emitting tomography [PET]), the limb tested (forearm *vs* calf), the dose and duration of insulin administration, and the selection of study subjects. As recently reviewed [9], insulin exposure (*i.e.* dose *x* time) and limb muscularity appear to be more important factors than the anatomical site or the experimental technique in contributing to the variability of insulin-induced vasodilatation. By compiling a vast amount of data in the literature, the relationship between insulin exposure (with the hormone infused locally through the brachial or femoral artery or systemically through a forearm vein) and changes in blood flow (forearm or calf) can be schematised as depicted in fig.. 14-1: within the physiological range of insulin exposure (the darker shade), limb blood flow may rise up to 30% of its baseline value, with a rather wide scatter depending on the experimental circumstances.

Thus, insulin does have intrinsic, if weak, vasoactive properties. The physiological impact of insulin-induced vasodilatation on glucose metabolism is, however, marginal on several accounts. Firstly, resting skeletal muscle has a low extraction coefficient for glucose, and is therefore little sensitive to changes in blood flow. Recent PET studies [10] have demonstrated that leg muscle blood flow is distributed in a heterogeneous pattern, and that glucose uptake co-localises with higher perfusion rates in response to strong insulin stimulation. These findings, however, may simply reflect regional differences in muscle fibre composition, as oxidative type I fibres are both more sensitive to insulin and more richly capillarised [11]. By itself, co-localisation of flow and metabolism does not prove that insulin actually recruits previously unperfused areas, thereby exposing more tissue to its metabolic action. In addition, relative to the time-course of insulin action on glucose extraction, insulin vasodilatation is a late phenomenon [12,13]. Finally, in the forearm of insulin resistant subjects, insulin-mediated glucose extraction is impaired but the exchange of other substrates (lactate, pyruvate, and fats) is superimposable on that of insulin sensitive individuals [14]. This observation argues against significant flow-limitation of glucose uptake during insulin stimulation. In keeping with this, insulin vasodilatation has been reported to be unaltered in native states of insulin resistance (insulin-dependent diabetes [15], non-insulin-dependent diabetes [10,16], essential hypertension [17], and familial hypertension [18]). Moreover, in insulin resistant patients with essential hypertension the intra-arterial infusion of an endogenous vasodilator, adenosine [19], or of a direct nitric oxide donor, sodium nitroprusside [20], fails to overcome the insulin resistance. Collectively, these observations indicate that pharmacological exposure to acute insulinisation is followed by some increase in limb blood flow, but this haemodynamic effect is of limited consequence for insulin stimulation of glucose uptake.

The mechanism by which insulin increases blood flow is interesting. Neither adrenergic nor cholinergic blockade abolishes insulin-induced stimulation of calf blood flow [21], whilst both N^G-monomethyl-L-arginine (L-NMMA), a competitive inhibitor of nitric oxide (NO) synthase, and ouabain, which blocks the

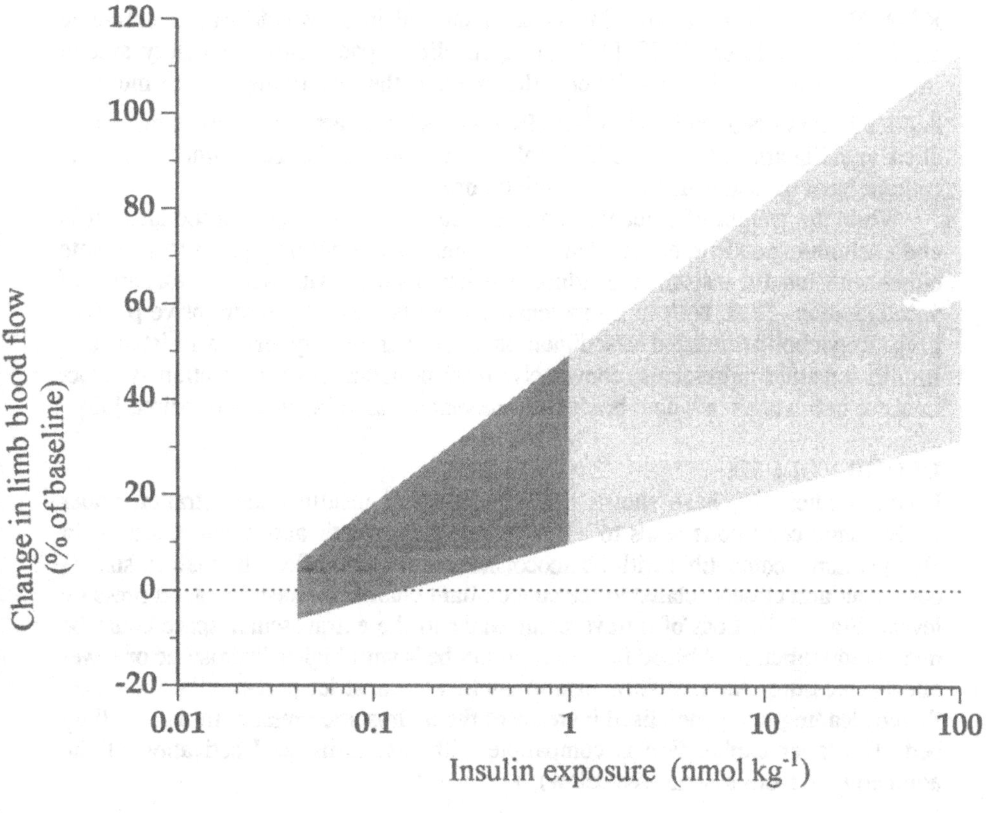

Fig.14-1 Relationship between insulin exposure (expressed as total amount infused per kilogram of body weight or per 10 kg of forearm muscle, for systemic intravenous and local intra-arterial administration, respectively) and percent change in limb blood flow [re-calculated from ref. 8].

insulin-stimulatable sodium potassium pump [22], have been shown to antagonise insulin-induced vasodilatation [23-25]. Furthermore, in both normal subjects and patients with essential hypertension local insulin infusion in physiological amounts potentiates acetylcholine-induced vasodilatation [26]. The exact site of this action of insulin, whether endothelial or smooth muscle cells, is not known. Both cell types carry insulin receptors as well as Na^+-K^+-ATPase activity in their plasma membrane [27,28], and can synthesise and release NO. In cultured smooth muscle [29], insulin attenuates agonist-induced increases in intracellular calcium concentrations, thereby causing relaxation. This effect may be due to antagonism of inositol-triphosphate-sensitive calcium release from intracellular stores. As L-

NMMA blocks the insulin-induced decrease in cytosolic calcium in smooth muscle cells, NO-mediated increases in cyclic nucleotides (both cAMP and cGMP) appear to be involved [30]. In turn, NO can activate Na^+-K^+-ATPase in a cGMP-independent fashion [31]. In endothelial cells, on the other hand, activation of Na^+-K^+-ATPase leads to a rise in intracellular calcium, which would stimulate synthesis and release of NO [32]. Thus, insulin impacts on a regulatory system involving at least 2 tissues - the endothelium and the underlying smooth muscle - and 2 effectors - NO, and Na^+-K^+-ATPase - which interact in a complex fashion to elicit vasodilatation. Clearly, additional investigation is needed to understand the cellular basis of insulin-induced vasodilatation.

While the weight of evidence indicates that insulin-mediated vasodilatation is endothelium-dependent, endothelial dysfunction *per se* does not appear to segregate either with insulin resistance of glucose metabolism or with insulin resistance of vasodilatation. Thus, both in normotensive subjects [33] and hypertensive patients [34], acetylcholine-induced vasodilatation is similar in very insulin-resistant and insulin sensitive individuals; conversely, insulin-mediated vasodilatation is intact in obese individuals in whom bradykinin-mediated vasodilatation is impaired [35].

BLOOD VOLUME

Recent studies [36] have shown that physiological insulin administration under euglycaemic conditions leads to a 3% rise in haematocrit and a 7% reduction in blood volume, compatible with haemoconcentration. This effect, if small in size, is consistent and closely related to the concomitant change in diastolic blood pressure levels (Fig. 14-2). Loss of intravascular water to the extravascular space could be due to redistribution of blood flow to capillary beds with higher hydrostatic or lower oncotic pressure. Alternatively, insulin could vasoconstrict post-capillary venules, thereby leading to a generalised increase of the hydrostatic pressure in the capillary bed. The latter explanation is compatible with insulin-induced activation of the adrenergic nervous system (see below).

CARDIAC OUTPUT AND BLOOD PRESSURE

During systemic insulin administration at physiological doses, cardiac output increases by 10-15% as a result of a small but consistent acceleration of heart rate (2 bpm on average) coupled with an increase in stroke volume [37]. These haemodynamic responses are mediated by adrenergic activation, as documented by a rise in circulating noradrenaline concentrations [38], an enhanced firing rate in the peroneal nerve, as measured by microneurography [4], and an upward shift in the sympathetic/vagal activity ratio, as measured by spectral analysis of heart rate variability [37].

The overall effect of simultaneous changes in cardiac output, blood volume, and peripheral vascular resistance in response to euglycaemic hyperinsulinaemia is maintenance of mean arterial blood pressure [37]. This, however, is a compound of opposite changes in systolic and diastolic blood pressure. The former, in fact, tends to increase as cardiac dynamics are excited by enhanced adrenergic discharge, while the latter decreases due to the drop in peripheral vascular resistances.

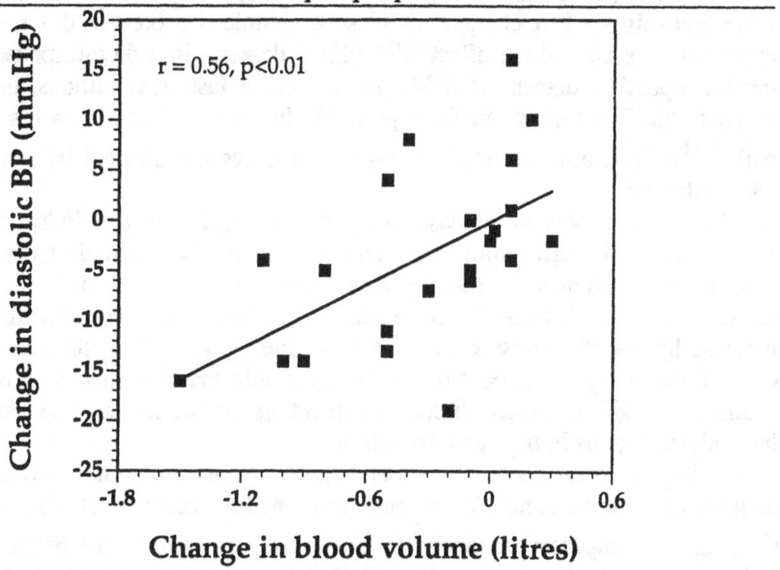

Fig. 14- 2. Direct relationship between concomitant changes in blood volume and diastolic blood pressure induced by physiological hyperinsulinaemia (~600 pmol/l) under euglycaemic conditions. Note that the regression line predicts a 1 mmHg fall in blood pressure for each 0.1 litre decrease in blood volume.

It is interesting to note that the effects of insulin on the cardiovascular system are mediated by both peripheral reflexes and direct central neural influences. Thus, direct relaxation of resistance arteries by insulin evokes tachycardia through the unloading of arterial baroreceptors, a reflex arch that involves central relays. In addition, insulin appears to directly desensitise the sinoatrial node to the baroreflex control of heart rate [37]. Mounting evidence [39], however, indicates that insulin, by trespassing the blood-brain barrier in the periventricular area, binds to neurons in the arcuate and paraventricular nuclei, which then send inhibitory impulses to the vagus and excitatory impulses to the sympathetic nuclei. This reaction is completed by the release of corticotropin releasing hormone (CRH), which orchestrates a response including stimulation of cortisol and prolactin release and depression of growth hormone and thyroid stimulating hormone [37,40]. Overall, even in the absence of hypoglycaemia the cardiovascular system responds to acute insulin administration with a moderate stress reaction. The full physiological significance and the possible pathophysiological implications of this response in states of chronic hyperinsulinaemia and insulin resistance remain to be established.

THE KIDNEY

Insulin and glomerular function

With regard to the effect of insulin on glomerular filtration rate (GFR), observations in the isolated kidney, in experimental animals, and in humans have yielded contradictory results, as decreased, increased or unchanged GFRs have all been reported (reviewed in [41]). In healthy subjects under conditions of forced water diuresis - when changes in plasma volume are prevented - euglycaemic hyperinsulinaemia did not affect GFR [42]. Likewise, in a dose-response study in insulin-dependent diabetic (IDDM) patients under fasting conditions, insulin was without significant effect on GFR [43]. Neither renal plasma flow (as measured with ^{131}I-hippuran) nor renal vascular resistances are affected by acute insulin administration.

The role of plasma glucose concentration itself in the induction and/or maintenance of hyperfiltration has been controversial. During oral glucose loading, if large fluid volumes are administered, plasma volume and, in turn, GFR will increase. On the other hand, a large glucose delivery to the proximal tubule could increase hydrostatic pressure in the tubular lumen, thereby leading to decreased GFR. Collectively, it appears that hyperglycaemia may be associated with small changes in GFR in either direction depending on factors such as duration of hyperglycaemia, hydration, and urine flow.

An important question is whether insulin affects glomerular permeability to albumin and other proteins. We recently examined the acute effect of insulin on the systemic transcapillary escape rate (measured by the ^{131}I-labelled albumin technique) and the urinary excretion of albumin under time-controlled, steady-state conditions of glucose concentrations, urine output, blood pressure, and creatinine clearance. While no significant change in albumin exit from the vascular compartment was found, physiological hyperinsulinaemia increased urinary albumin excretion by 50% in normoalbuminuric patients with NIDDM but not in healthy subjects [36]. Though small, this interaction between insulin and hyperglycaemia on glomerulo-tubular function deserves further investigation as it may be an early sign of renal involvement in diabetes.

Insulin and tubular function

Specific binding of insulin is greatest in the thick ascending limb and distal convoluted tubules [44]. Insulin has been found to stimulate sodium transport in proximal tubules in the rabbit [45], and to increase chloride reabsorption by the loop segment in the rat [46]. Human studies, however, have suggested that the antinatriuretic action of insulin takes place in the distal tubule [47,48]. Whether insulin affects sodium absorption by a direct effect on the renal tubules or through modulation of local or systemic factors that control sodium chloride reabsorption is still uncertain. Friedberg *et al.* [47], for example, reported that the antinatriuretic effect of insulin was no longer observed when insulin-induced hypokalaemia was prevented by a simultaneous potassium administration. To test this hypothesis, we performed oral glucose tolerance tests with or without potassium replacement in a group of healthy subjects [48]. Moreover, to determine whether the antinatriuretic effect of insulin is preserved in patients with impaired insulin action on glucose metabolism, a group of non-diabetic patients with essential hypertension was also studied. We found that healthy individuals and hypertensive patients exhibited similar antinatriuresis whether or not exogenous potassium was given to clamp serum potassium at basal levels. Also, insulin antinatriuresis was independent of the presence of metabolic insulin resistance. The discordance with the results of Friedberg *et al.* [47] may depend on the differences between their experimental conditions (forced water diuresis, euglycaemic hyperinsulinaemia) and ours (maintenance of basal urine output, hyperglycaemic hyperinsulinaemia). In fact, *in vitro* studies have shown that glucose increases antinatriuresis due to enhanced glucose-sodium co-transport at the level of the convoluted proximal tubule [45]. *In vivo* studies using lithium clearance have demonstrated that proximal sodium reabsorption is stimulated by hyperglycaemia in rats [49], and is higher in diabetics under hyperglycaemic than euglycaemic conditions [50]. At least in part, the effect of hyperglycaemia can be ascribed to the brush-border sodium co-transport, where the glucose:sodium stoichiometry is 1:2 ([51]. In a series of elegant studies, Nosadini *et al.* [52] found that NIDDM patients with insulin resistance of glucose metabolism retained more sodium than non-diabetic subjects at similar plasma glucose concentrations and filtered glucose. Moreover, at comparable degrees of hyperglycaemia the more insulin resistant diabetic patients exhibited more sodium retention, suggesting that insulin resistance reflects an intrinsic renal abnormality.

In summary, both insulin alone and hyperglycaemia reduce renal sodium excretion; the most probable sites of action are the proximal tubule for hyperglycaemia, the distal portions of the nephron for insulin, though the latter is still somewhat uncertain. These two actions are combined in the physiological response to feeding [48]. Most importantly, in patients with insulin resistance of glucose metabolism - diabetic [52], hypertensive [53], or obese [54] - insulin antinatriuresis is preserved. Thus, the compensatory hyperinsulinaemia of insulin resistant patients imposes a chronic antinatriuretic pressure on the kidney, which may play a role in the development or maintenance of high blood pressure.

Insulin has a major role in potassium homeostasis. In dose-response studies in humans [55], euglycaemic hyperinsulinaemia stimulated potassium uptake by both liver and peripheral tissues. Insulin-induced hypokalaemia is accompanied by a reduction in urinary potassium excretion. Insulin does not appear to have a direct effect on renal potassium handling, however. Thus, in our own studies [48] the antikaliuretic response to oral glucose was abolished when insulin-induced hypokalaemia was prevented. Interestingly, when plasma potassium concentrations were clamped at their basal levels, glucose-induced insulin secretion was significantly heightened [48]. Thus, insulin modulates renal potassium excretion *and* its own release by the ß-cell through the same signal, *i.e.* hypokalaemia. This constitutes a dual feedback loop, or glucose-potassium cycle, which serves the function of storing glucose and potassium in cells while limiting the risk of hypoglycaemia.

Sodium and uric acid excretion parallel one another under many physiological conditions [57,58]. During euglycaemic hyperinsulinaemia, serum uric acid levels and creatinine clearance do not change, whereas the clearance rate and fractional excretion of uric acid decrease by 30%. The change in uric acid excretion is significantly related to the concomitant fall in urinary sodium excretion [59]. In patients with essential hypertension [53] and in obese subjects (unpublished observations), we have found that the anti-uricosuric effect of insulin is maintained, and thus is independent of metabolic insulin resistance. The finding that uric acid and sodium urinary excretion are both restrained by physiological hyperinsulinaemia provides an explanation for the clustering of hyperuricaemia with insulin resistant states such as hypertension, obesity, and diabetes mellitus [60,61].

REFERENCES

1. Zierler KL. Theory of the use of arteriovenous concentration differences for measuring metabolism in steady state and non-steady states. J Clin Invest 1961;40:2111-2125
2. Steinberg HO, Chaker H, Leaming R, Johnson A, Brechtel G, Baron AD. Obesity/insulin resistance is associated with endothelial dysfunction. Implications for the syndrome of insulin resistance. J Clin Invest 1996;97:2601-2610
3. Laakso M, Edelman SV, Brechtel G, Baron AD. Decreased effect of insulin to stimulate skeletal muscle blood flow in obese man. J Clin Invest 1990;85:1844-1852
4. Anderson EA, Hoffman RP, Balon TW, Sinkey CA, Mark AL. Hyperinsulinemia produces both sympathetic neural activation and vasodilatation in normal humans. J Clin Invest 1991;87:2246-2252
5. Baron AD, Brechtel-Hook G, Johnson A, Hardin D. Skeletal muscle blood flow. A possible link between insulin resistance and blood pressure. Hypertension 1993;21:129-135
6. Baron AD, Laakso M, Brechtel G, Edelman SV. Mechanism of insulin resistance in insulin-dependent diabetes mellitus: a major role for reduced skeletal muscle blood flow. J Clin Endocrinol Metab 1991;73:637-643
7. Laakso M, Edelman SV, Brechtel G, Baron AD. Impaired insulin-mediatede skeletal muscle blood flow in patients with NIDDM. Diabetes 1992;41:1076-1083
8. Baron AD, Steinberg HO, Chaker H, Leaming R, Johnson A, Brechtel G. Insulin-mediated skeletal muscle vasodilatation contributes to both insulin sensitivity and responsiveness in lean humans. J Clin Invest 1995;96:786-792
9. Yki-Järvinen H, Utriainen T. Insulin-induced vasodilatation: physiology or pharmacology? Diabetologia (*in press*)
10. Utriainen T, Nuutila P, Takala T, Vicini P, Ruotsalainen U, Rönnemaa T, Tolvanen T, Raitakari M, Haaparanta M, Kirvelä O, Cobelli C, Yki-Järvinen H. Intact insulin stimulation of skeletal muscle blood flow, its heterogeneity and redistribution but not of glucose uptake in non-insulin-dependent diabetezs mellitus. J Clin Invest 1997;100:777-785
11. Utriainen T, Holmäng A, Björntorp P, Mäkimattila S, Sovijärvi A, Lindholm H, Yki-Järvinen H. Physical fitness, muscle morphology and insulin-stimulated limb blood flow in normal subjects. Am J Physiol 1996;270:E905-E911
12. Utriainen T, Malmström R, Mäkimattila S, Yki-Järvinen H. Methodological aspects, dose-response characetristics and causes of inter-individual variation in insulin stimulation of limb blood flow in normal subjects. Diabetologia 1995;38:555-564
13. Tack CJJ, Schefman AEP, Willems JL, Thien T, Lutterman JA, Smits P. Direct vasodilator effects of physiological hyperinsulinaemia in human skeletal muscle. Eur J Clin Invest 1996;26:772-778
14. Natali A, Santoro D, Palombo C, Cerri M, Ghione S, Ferrannini E. Impaired insulin action on skeletal muscle metabolism in essential hypertension. Hypertension 1991;17:170-178
15. Mättimakila S, Virtamäki A, Malmström R, Utriainen T, Yki-Järvinen H. Insulin resistance in type I diabetes mellitus: a major role for reduced glucose extraction. J Clin Endocrinol Metab 1996;81:707-712
16. Tack CJJ, Smits P, Willemsen JJ, Lenders JWM, Thien T, Lutterman JA. Effects of insulin on vascular tone and sympathetic nervous system in NIDDM. Diabetes 1996;45:15-22
17. Hunter SJ, Harper R, Ennis CN, Sheridan B, Atkinson AB, Bell PM. Skeletal muscle blood flow is not a determinant of insulin resistance in essential hypertension. J Hypertens 1997;15:73-77
18. Hulten UL, Endre T, Mattiasson I, Berglund G. Insulin and forearm vasodilatation in hypertension-prone men. Hypertension 1995;25:214-218
19. Natali A, Bonadonna R, Santoro D, Quiñones Galvan A, Baldi S, Frascerra S, Palombo C, Ghione S, Ferrannini E. Insulin resistance and vasodilatation in essential hypertension. Studies with adenosine. J Clin Invest 1994;94:1570-1576

20. Natali A, Quiñones Galvan A, Toschi E, Pecori N, Sanna G, Ferrannini E. Vasodilation with sodium nitroprusside does not improve insulin action in essential hypertension. Hypertension (*in press*)
21. Randin D, Vollenweider P, Tappy L, Jequier E, Nicod P, Scherrer U. Effects of adrenergic and cholinergic blockade on insulin-induced stimulation of calf blood flow in humans. Am J Physiol 1994;266:R809-R816
22. Ferrannini E, Taddei S, Santoro D, Natali A, Boni C, Del Chiaro D, Buzzigoli G. Independent stimulation of glucose metabolism and Na^+-K^+ exchange by insulin in the human forearm. Am J Physiol 1988;266:E953-E958
23. Steinberg HO, Brechtel G, Johson A, Fireberg N, Baron AD. Insulin-mediated skeletal muscle vasodilatation is nitric oxide dependent. A novel action of insulin to increase nitric oxide release. J Clin Invest 1994;94:1172-1179
24. Scherrer U, Randin D, Vollenweider P, Vollenweider L, Nicod P. Nitric oxide release accounts for insulin's vascular effects in humans. J Clin Invest 1994;94:2511-2615
25. Tack CJJ, Lutterman JA, Vervoot G, Thien T, Smits P. Activation of the sodium-potassium pump contributes to insulin-induced vasodilatation in humans. Hypertension 1996;28:426-432
26. Taddei S, Virdis A, Mattei P, Natali A, Ferrannini E, Salvetti A. Effect of insulin on acetylcholine-induced vasodilatation in normotensive subjects and patients with essential hypertension. Circulation 1995;92:2911-2918
27. Meharg JV, McGowan-Jordan J, Charles A, Parmelee JT, Cutaia MV, Rounds S. Hydrogen peroxide stimulates sodium-potassium pump activity in cultured pulmonary arterial endothelial cells. Am J Physiol 1993;265:L613-L621
28. Tirupattur PR, Ram JL, Tandley PR, Sowers JR. Regulation of Na^+-K^+-ATPase gene expression by insulin in vascular smooth muscle cells. Am J Hypertens 1993;6:626-629
29. Kahn AM, Seidel CL, Allen JC, O'Neil G, Shelat H, Song T. Insulin reduces contraction and intracellular calcium concentration in vascular smooth muscle. Hypertension 1993;22:735-742
30. Trovati M, Anfossi G. Insulin, insulin resistance and platelet function: similarities with the insulin effects on cultured smooth muscle cells. Diabetologia (*in press*)
31. Gupta S, McArthur C, Grady C, Ruderman NB. Stimulation of vascular Na^+-K^+-ATPase activity by nitric oxide: a cGMP-independent effect. Am J Physiol 1994;266:H2146-2151
32. Moncada S, Palmer RMJ. The L-arginine-nitric oxide pathway in the vessel wall. In: Moncada S, Higgs B, eds. Nitric Oxide from L-arginine: a Bioregulatory System. Amsterdam, Elsevier, 1990, pp 19-33
33. Utriainen T, Mäkimattila S, Virkamäki A, Bergholm R, Yki-Järvinen H. Dissociation between insulin sensitivity of glucose uptake and endothelial function in normal subjects. Diabetologia 1996;39:1477-1482
34. Natali A, Taddei S, Quiñones Galvan A, Camastra S, Baldi S, Frascerra S, Virdis A, Sudano I, Salvetti A, Ferrannini E. Insulin sensitivity, vascular reactivity, and clamp-induced vasodilatation in essential hypertension. Circulation 1997;96:849-855
35. Laine H, Yki-Järvinen H, Kirvela O, Tolvanen T, Raitakari M, Solin O, Haaparanta M, Knuuti J, Nuutila P. Insulin resistance of glucose uptake in skeletal muscle cannot be ameliorated by enhancing endothelium-dependent blood flow in obesity. J Clin Invest (*in press*)
36. Catalano C, Muscelli E, Quiñones Galvan A, Baldi S, Masoni A, Gibb I, Torffvit O, Seghieri G, Ferrannini E. Effect of insulin on systemic and renal handling of albumin in nondiabetic and NIDDM subjects. Diabetes 1997;46:868-875
37. Muscelli E, Emdin M, Natali A, Pratali L, Camastra S, Baldi S, Carpeggiani C, Ferrannini E. Cardiac responses to insulin in vivo: influence of obesity. J Clin Endocrinol Metab (in press)
38. Rowe JW, Young JB, Minaker KL, Stevens AL, Pallotta J, Landsberg L. Effect of insulin and glucose infusions on sympathetic nervous system activity in normal man. Diabetes 1981;30: 219-225.
39. Davis SN, Colburn C, Robbins R, Nadeau S, Neal D, Williams P, Cherrington AD. Evidence that the brain of the conscious dog is insulin sensitive. J Clin Invest 1995;95:593-602
40. Schwartz MW, Figlewicz DP, Baskin DB, Woods SC, Porte D, Jr. Insulin in the brain: a hormonal regulator of energy balance. Endocr Rev 1992;13:81-113
41. Quiñones-Galvan A, Ferrannini E. Renal effects of insulin in man. J Nephrol 1997;10:188-191
42. DeFronzo RA, Cooke CR, Andres R, Faloona GR, Davis PJ. The effect of insulin on renal handling of sodium, potassium, calcium, and phosphate in man. J Clin Invest 1975;55:845-855.

43. Christiansen JS, Frandsen M, Parving H-H. The effect of intravenous insulin infusion on kidney function in insulin-dependent diabetes mellitus. Diabetologia 1981;20:199-204.
44. Butlen D, Vadrot S, Roseau S, Model F. Insulin receptors along the rat nephron: [^{125}I] insulin binding in microdissected glomeruli and tubules. Pflugers Arch 1988;412:604-612.
45. Baum M. Insulin stimulates sodium transport in rabbit proximal convoluted tubule. J Clin Invest 1987;79:1104-1109.
46. Kirchner KA. Insulin increases loop segment chloride reabsorption in the euglycemic rat. Am J Physiol 1988;24:F1206-F1213.
47. DeFronzo RA, Goldberg M, Agus Z. The effects of glucose and insulin on renal electrolyte transport. J Clin Invest 1976;58:83-90.
48. Skott P, Vaag A, Bruun NE, Hother-Nielsen O, Gall MA, Beck-Nielsen H, Parving H-H. Effect of insulin on renal sodium handling in hyperinsulinemic Type 2 (non-insulin-dependendent) diabetic patients with peripheral insulin resistance. Diabetologia 1991;34:275-281.
47. Friedberg CE, Buren MW, Bijisma JA, Koomans HA. Insulin increases sodium reabsorption in diluting segments in humans: evidence for indirect mediation through hypokalemia. Kidney Int 1991;40:251-256.
48. Natali A, Quiñones-Galvan A, Santoro D, Pecori N, Taddei S, Salvetti A, Ferrannini E. Relationship between insulin release, antinatriuresis and hypokalemia after glucose ingestion in normal and hypertensive man. Clin Sci 1993;85;327-335.
49. Bank N, Anynedjan HS. Progressive increases in luminal glucose stimulate proximal tubular reabsorption in normal and diabetic rats. J Clin Invest 1990;86:309-316.
50. Hannedouche JP, Delgado AG, Guionshade DA, Boitard C, Lacour B, Grunfeld JP. Renal hemodynamics and segmental tubular reabsorption in early type I diabetes. Kidney Int 1989;37:1126-1133.
51. Turner RJ, Moran A. Further studies of proximal tubular brush border membrane D-glucose heterogeneity. J Membr Biol 1982;70:37-45.
52. Nosadini R, Sambataro M, Tomaseth K, Pacini G, Cipollina MR, Solini A, Carraro A, Velussi M, Frigato F, Crepaldi G. Role of hyperglycemia and insulin resistance in determining sodium retention in non-insulin dependent diabetes. Kidney Int 1993;44:139-146.
53. Muscelli E, Natali A, Bianchi S, Bigazzi R, Quiñones-Galvan A, Sironi AM, Frascerra S, Ciociaro D, Ferrannini E. Effect of insulin on renal sodium and uric acid handling in essential hypertension. Am J Hypertens 1996;9:746-752
54. Rocchini AP, Katch V, Kveselis D, Moorehead C, Martin M, Lampman R, Gregory M. Insulin and renal sodium retention in obese adolescents. Hypertension 1989;14:367-374
55. DeFronzo RA, Felig P, Ferrannini E, Wahren J. Effect of graded doses of insulin on splanchnic and peripheral potassium metabolism in man. Am J Physiol 1980;238:E421-E427.
57. Cannon PJ, Svahn DS, Demartini FE. The influence of hypertonic saline infusion upon the fractional reabsorption of urate and other ions in normal and hypertensive man. Circulation 1970;41:97-108.
58. Holmes WE, Kelley NW, Wyngaarden JB. The kidney and uric acid excretion in man. Kidney Int 1972;2:115-118.
59. Quiñones-Galvan A, Natali A, Baldi S, Frascerra S, Sanna G, Ciociaro D, Ferrannini E. Effect of insulin on uric acid excretion in humans. Am J Physiol 1995;268:E1-E5.
60. Cannon PJ, Stason WB, Demartini FE, Sommers SC, Laragh JH. Hyperuricemia in primary and renal hypertension. N Engl J Med 1966;275:457-464..
61. Modan M, Halkin H, Karasik A, Lusky A. Elevated serum uric acid - a facet of hyperinsulinaemia. Diabetologia 1987;30:713-718.

15. DIABETES, HYPERTENSION, AND KIDNEY DISEASE IN THE PIMA INDIANS.

William C. Knowler, Robert G. Nelson, David J. Pettitt
National Institute of Diabetes and Digestive and Kidney Diseases, Phoenix, Arizona, USA

Hypertension and kidney disease are well-known concomitants of both type 1 and type 2 diabetes mellitus. Hypertension, kidney disease, and diabetes are associated with each other, but the associations vary between populations, and the causal interpretations, especially regarding hypertension and diabetic nephropathy, are controversial. The complications of diabetes have been studied extensively among the Pima Indians of Arizona, U.S.A. In this chapter, we describe the epidemiology of diabetic renal disease and its relationship with hypertension in the Pima Indians.

1. THE PIMA INDIAN DIABETES STUDY

The Pima Indians have the world's highest reported incidence and prevalence of diabetes [1]. Since 1965, this population has participated in a longitudinal epidemiologic study of diabetes and its complications [2]. At each examination, conducted at about two-year intervals, an oral glucose tolerance test is performed and classified according to the World Health Organization criteria [3]. Throughout the study, urine samples with at least a trace of protein on dipstick have been assayed for total protein, and the urine protein-to-creatinine ratio has been used as an estimate of the protein excretion rate [4]. Since 1982, the urine samples have been assayed for albumin, and a urine albumin-to-creatinine ratio has been used as an estimate of the urinary albumin excretion rate [5]. Blood pressure is measured at each examination with the subject at rest in the supine position [6].

Renal function has been studied in more detail in a subset of nondiabetic and diabetic Pima Indians. These studies include serial measurements of glomerular filtration rate (GFR), renal plasma flow, albumin and IgG excretion, and glomerular capillarypermeability to dextran particles of different sizes [7].

The prevalence of diabetes in Pima Indians is almost 13 times as high as in the mostly white population of Rochester, Minnesota [1]. Diabetes occurs in

Mogensen, C.E. (ed.), THE KIDNEY AND HYPERTENSION IN DIABETES MELLITUS.

over one-third of Pima Indians aged 35-44 years and in over 60% of those ≥45 years old [2]. Many cases develop before the age of 25 years. Pima Indians develop only type 2 diabetes [8], and they differ from other populations in that the disease develops at younger ages [1,2]. Diabetic complications also develop at rates similar to those of other populations. In contrast to populations in which type 2 diabetes usually develops later in life, many Pima Indians have diabetes of sufficient duration for nephropathy to develop.

2. THE COURSE OF DIABETIC NEPHROPATHY IN PIMA INDIANS

The onset of type 2 diabetes in Pima Indians is characterized, on average, by an elevated GFR and a modest size-selective abnormality of the glomerular capillary wall [9]. Abnormally elevated albuminuria is another characteristic early sign of diabetic nephropathy. In a cross-sectional study of albuminuria in Pima Indians ≥15 years of age, abnormal albuminuria was defined by a urine albumin-to-creatinine ratio ≥ 30 mg/g [5]. A ratio of 30-299 mg/g corresponds approximately to the definition of incipient nephropathy of Mogensen et al [10]. Abnormal albuminuria was found in 8% of those with normal glucose tolerance, 15% of those with impaired glucose tolerance, and 47% of those with diabetes [5]. The prevalence was also related to the duration of diabetes, varying from 29% within five years of diagnosis to 86% after 20 years of diabetes. The high prevalence in diabetes and the relationship with diabetes duration indicate that albuminuria is a complication of diabetes, but there is also a substantial prevalence in those with normal or impaired glucose tolerance, indicating that diabetes is not the sole cause of abnormal albuminuria in this population. Abnormal albuminuria is often followed by more serious renal disease. Among diabetic Pimas, the degree of albuminuria over the range of values < 300 mg/g predicts the subsequent incidence of overt nephropathy, defined by a protein-to-creatinine ratio ≤ 1.0 g/g [11].

Among diabetic Pima Indians with normal albumin excretion (albuminuria < 30 mg/g), the incidence rate of elevated albuminuria (≥30 mg/g) is similar to that previously reported in type 1 diabetes [12]. Incidence rates, shown in figure 15-1, increase with duration of diabetes at least past 15 years. Thus there is no evidence that beyond a certain duration of diabetes, diabetic Pimas with normal albumin excretion have passed a period of susceptibility to abnormal albuminuria.

The incidence of overt diabetic nephropathy, defined by urine protein/creatinine ≥ 1.0 g/g, is shown in figure 15-2. Again there was no suggestion of a duration of diabetes after which the incidence of nephropathy declines. Such a decline, observed after about 20 years of type 1 diabetes, has been interpreted as an exhaustion of susceptible persons [13].

GFR was measured in Pimas with diabetes of ≥ 5 years duration with normal albuminuria (n=20) or with macroalbuminuria (n=34) [14]. At baseline, those with macroalbuminuria had, on average, lower GFR and higher blood pressure. During 48 months of follow-up of 30 of those with macroalbuminuria, the GFR declined by an average of 9 ml/min per year, higher than the rate of decline reported for similar patients with type 1 diabetes. The slope of GFR over time was highly correlated with the increase in albumin or IgG clearance. Dextran sieving studies suggested that the progressive decline in GFR is caused by a decline in average density of glomerular pores, which is accompanied by a widening of the pore size distribution, allowing greater permeability to albumin and IgG through the increased number of larger pores.

Figure 15-3 summarizes the degree of albuminuria, expressed as an albumin-to-creatinine ratio, in five groups of subjects followed for up to four years [7]. On average, those with impaired glucose tolerance, newly diagnosed diabetes, or longstanding diabetes with normo-albuminuria (by definition) had normal urine albumin excretion at baseline. There was little change, on average, during follow-up of those in the first two groups. The degree of albuminuria tended to increase, however, in all three groups with long-standing diabetes, whether they had normo-, micro-, or macro-albuminuria at baseline. During this time, GFR increased in persons with impaired glucose tolerance or newly diagnosed diabetes, was relatively stable in those with longstanding diabetes with normo- or micro-albuminuria, and declined in those with macro-albuminuria at baseline (figure 15-3). The major predictor of declining GFR was the degree of albuminuria. By contrast, baseline GFR did not predict change in GFR or in albuminuria. Thus the degree of elevation in albumin excretion is the major predictor of worsening diabetic nephropathy.

In diabetic persons, the onset of clinical proteinuria, defined by the urinary excretion of at least 500 mg protein per day, heralds a progressive decline of renal function that often leads to end-stage renal disease (ESRD) [15].

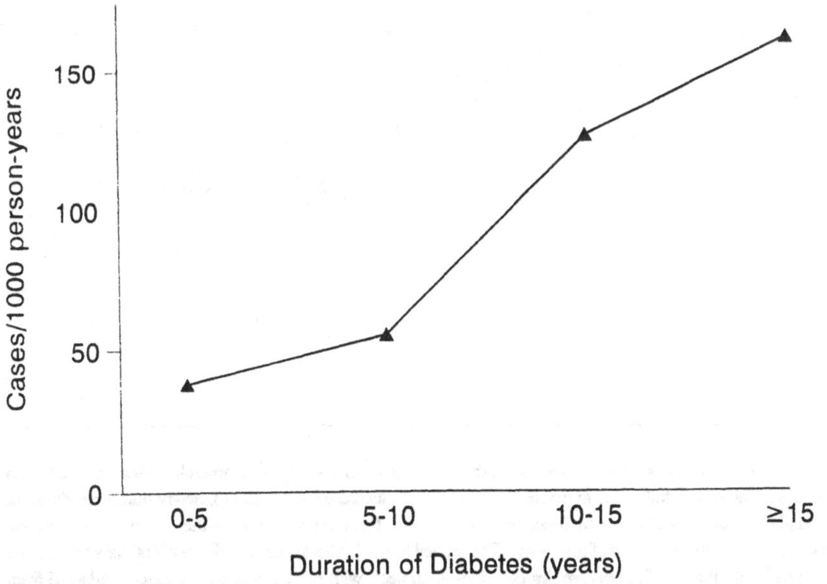

Figure 15-1 Incidence rates of elevated albuminuria (urine albumin-to-creatinine ratio ≥ 30 mg/g) by duration of diabetes in Pima Indians. Adapted from Nelson, et al [12].

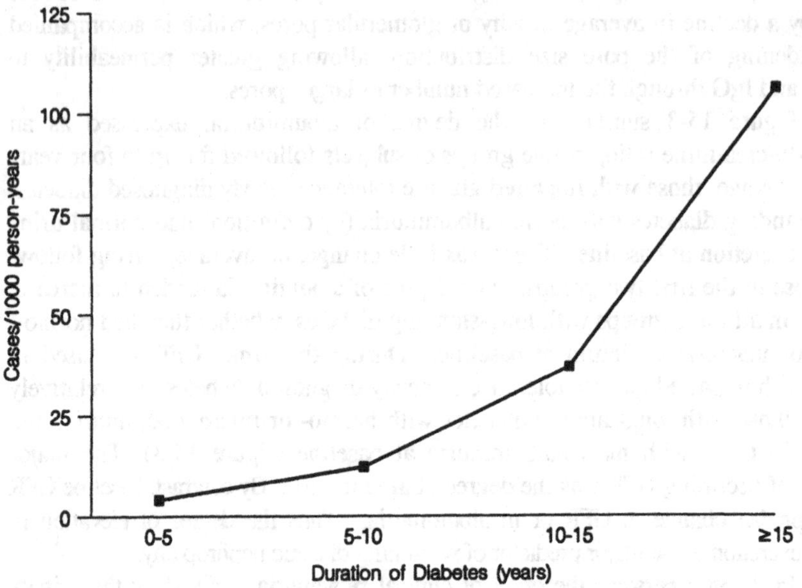

Figure 15-2 Incidence rates of overt nephropathy (urine protein-to-creatinine ratio ≥1.0 g/g) by duration of diabetes in Pima Indians. Adapted from Kunzelman et al [4].

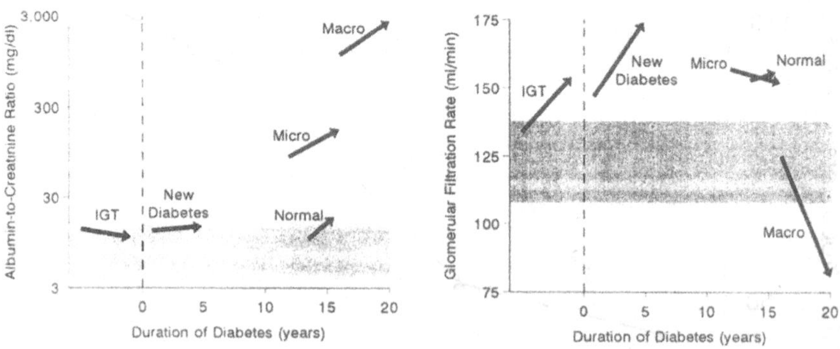

Figure 15-3 Changes in median urinary albumin-to-creatinine ratio (left) and mean glomerular filtration rate (right) from baseline to the end of follow-up in persons with impaired glucose tolerance (IGT), newly diagnosed diabetes, and longstanding diabetes according to baseline albuminuria. Each arrow connects the value at the baseline examination and the value at the end of follow-up. The dashed line indicates the time of diagnosis of diabetes, and the shaded area the 25th through 75th percentiles of values in subjects with normal glucose tolerance. Adapted from Nelson et al. [7].

Figure 15-4 shows the cumulative incidence of ESRD as a function of the duration of proteinuria in Pima Indians and, using similar definitions of proteinuria, in whites with type 1 [16] or type 2 diabetes [17]. Coronary heart disease is a frequent cause of death in older persons with diabetes and proteinuria and may, in part, account for the lower incidence of ESRD in whites with type 2 diabetes. Due to the relatively young age at onset of diabetes in Pima Indians and their lower death rate from coronary heart disease [18], the cumulative incidence of ESRD in this population more closely resembles that of whites with type 1 diabetes than those with type 2 diabetes.

When expressed as a function of duration of diabetes, the cumulative incidence of ESRD is also nearly identical in the Pimas with type 2 diabetes and the whites with type 1 diabetes [19]. Other studies comparing persons with type 1 diabetes and type 2 diabetes in the same populations have concluded that the duration-specific risk of ESRD is similar in the two types of diabetes [17,20].

The incidence of ESRD is also very high among other American Indians [reviewed in 21], but diabetes is apparently not responsible for as great a proportion of cases of ESRD in some of the other American Indian tribes. The degree of albuminuria was higher in Pima Indians than in several other American Indian tribes, even when controlled for differences in age, sex, fasting plasma glucose, blood pressure, and fibrinogen [22].

The greater degree of albuminuria in Pima Indians compared with the other American Indian tribes, as well as the increased risk of diabetic nephropathy in Pima Indians whose parents have nephropathy [23] or hypertension [24], and the familial aggregation of diabetic nephropathy in other populations suggests that susceptibility to this disease may be genetically transmitted, as reviewed in Chapter 11. Further evidence for genetic susceptibility to diabetic nephropathy comes from a genetic linkage study in which 98 diabetic sibling pairs affected with nephropathy were included in a genome-wide scan. A DNA marker on chromosome 7 was tentatively linked to nephropathy (LOD = 2.73), suggesting that a genetic element in the region of this marker influences susceptibility to diabetic nephropathy [25]. Other factors, including duration of diabetes, blood pressure, level of glycemia, and pharmacologic treatment of diabetes are associated with the development of renal disease in Pima Indians [4,15,19]. There was no evidence for a role of hantavirus infection, which has been implicated in renal disease in other populations [26].

Nearly all of the excess mortality associated with diabetes in this population occurs in persons with clinically detectable proteinuria, and the age-sex-adjusted death rate in diabetic subjects without proteinuria is no greater than the rate in nondiabetic subjects [27]. Thus, proteinuria is a marker not only for diabetic renal disease, but identifies those with diabetes who are at increased risk for a number of macro- and microvascular complications and for death. Similar findings have been observed in persons with type 1 diabetes and suggest a common underlying cause for albuminuria and the other associated diabetic complications, both renal and extrarenal [28]. Autopsy studies indicate that intercapillary glomerular sclerosis, typical of diabetic nephropathy in other ethnic groups, is the predominant renal disease in the Pimas [29], although other glomerular lesions were found in some nondiabetic Pimas [30]. In kidney biopsies from 51 diabetic Pima Indians, total glomerular volume and mesangial volume were positively correlated with stage of diabetic nephropathy. Clinical nephropathy was associated with widening of epithelial cell foot processes and thickening of the glomerular basement membrane [31].

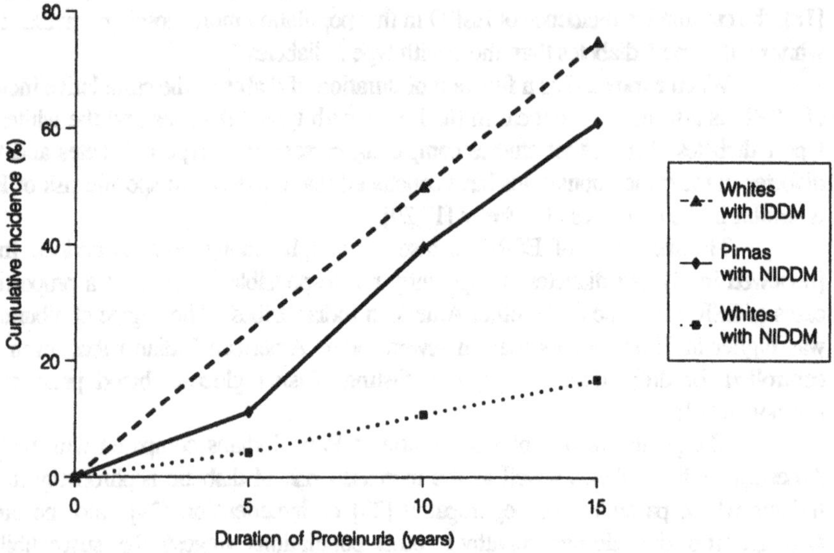

Figure 15-4 Cumulative incidence of end stage renal disease by duration of proteinuria. Adapted from Nelson et al. [15], Krolewski et al. [16], and Humphrey et al. [17].

3. RELATIONSHIP OF BLOOD PRESSURE TO DIABETES AND KIDNEY DISEASE

The relationships of blood pressure to glucose tolerance, hyperinsulinemia, and insulin resistance have been examined in many populations. A difficulty in examining these relationships is that many drugs used in treating high blood pressure may also affect insulin resistance or glycemia. Thus, correlations of these variables are difficult to interpret if studies include subjects taking antihypertensive drugs; yet if such subjects are excluded, the associations might be underestimated because of exclusion of those with the most severe hypertension. One approach is to divide blood pressure into two categories, hypertension or not, and include those treated with antihypertensive drugs as hypertensive regardless of their measured blood pressure. Even this approach may not be satisfactory, however, as many diabetic patients are treated with antihypertensive drugs for reno-protection rather than because of hypertension.

Blood pressure (or hypertension) is related to glucose tolerance in Pima Indians. The age-sex-adjusted prevalence rates of hypertension (systolic blood pressure ≥160 mm Hg, diastolic blood pressure ≥ 95 mm Hg, or receiving antihypertensive drugs) among those with normal glucose tolerance, impaired glucose tolerance, or diabetes were

7%, 13%, and 20%, respectively, an almost three-fold difference [6]. Similarly, as continuous variables, blood pressure and two-hour plasma glucose concentrations were correlated among subjects who were not treated with either antihypertensive or hypoglycemic drugs. It has been proposed that this relationship, also observed in other populations, is explained by hyperinsulinemia, as serum insulin concentrations tend to be higher in persons with impaired glucose tolerance and in some persons with diabetes than in those with normal glucose tolerance. Yet in the Pimas blood pressure has a much stronger correlation with plasma glucose than with serum insulin concentrations, and the partial correlation of blood pressure with fasting insulin, controlled for age, sex, BMI, and glucose, is practically zero [6]. Thus the relationship, at least among the Pimas, is primarily with glucose, and the correlation with insulin may be secondary.

In addition to studies of blood pressure and serum insulin concentrations, the correlation of blood pressure with insulin resistance was assessed by the euglycemic clamp. In a study of three racial groups, among nondiabetic, normotensive subjects not taking any medicines, blood pressure and insulin resistance were correlated only among whites, but not among blacks or Pima Indians [32]. While this study confirmed previous reports of a correlation of blood pressure with insulin resistance in whites, it suggests that such a relationship is race-specific, and hence does not indicate that insulin resistance is an important or consistent cause of hypertension.

Although blood pressure and plasma glucose concentrations are correlated and the prevalence of hypertension is related to 2-hr glucose, even among nondiabetic subjects, hyperglycemia is not the only factor of importance for blood pressure in diabetes. Blood pressure and kidney disease are clearly related, although the causes of this relationship are not clear and have been debated extensively, with some arguing that the elevated blood pressure in diabetes is only secondary to diabetic nephropathy [28,33], and others that elevated blood pressure due to a genetic predisposition that contributes to the development of diabetic nephropathy [34,35].

Among adult Pima Indians, urinary albumin-to-creatinine ratios were higher with progressively worse glucose tolerance or longer duration of diabetes, and among diabetic patients were higher in those treated with insulin [36]. Regardless of the degree of hyperglycemia and duration of diabetes, those with hypertension had greater albuminuria. The associations of each of these variables with albuminuria were highly significant, but the causal directions underlying them have not been determined. The relationship of insulin treatment with albuminuria is similar to that of insulin treatment with many complications of diabetes [4,5,18,37,38] and might reflect more severe diabetes (i.e. those with greater hyperglycemia or more complications have a greater need for insulin treatment).

The relationship between blood pressure and renal disease, however, is problematic since elevated blood pressure is both a cause and a consequence of renal disease. In the Pima Indians, higher blood pressure *before* the onset of diabetes confers a greater risk of renal disease *after* diabetes develops (figure 15-5), and among the diabetic subjects with normo- or micro-albuminuria, higher blood pressure predicts increasing urinary albumin excretion rates [7]. On the other hand, higher blood pressure does not predict ESRD in diabetic Pima Indians who already have proteinuria [15]. This suggests that blood pressure may contribute to the initiation of diabetic nephropathy [39], but not to its progression once proteinuria has developed [15]. The higher pre-diabetic blood pressure in those destined to have elevated albuminuria after the onset of diabetes

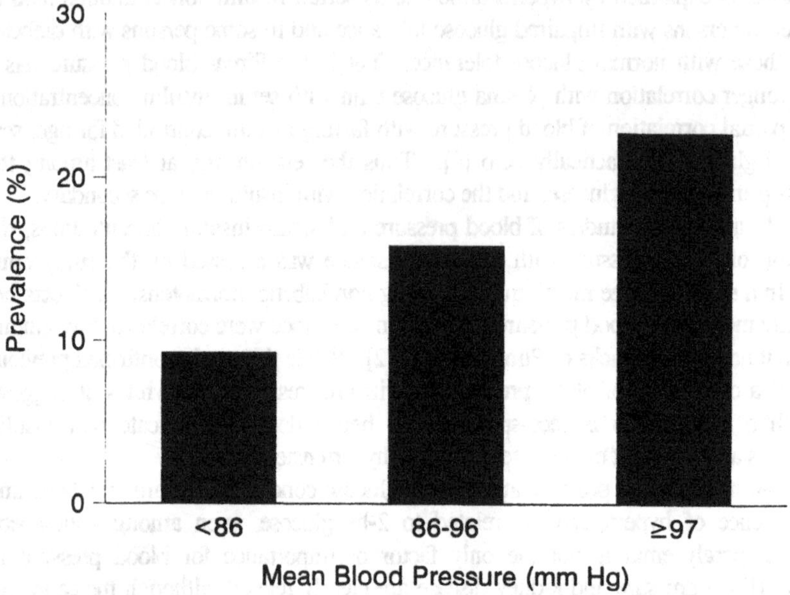

Figure 15-5 Prevalence of elevated albuminuria (urine albumin-to-creatinine ratio ≥100 mg/g) after the diagnosis of diabetes by prediabetic blood pressure. Adapted from Nelson et al. [39].

may be an early manifestation of an underlying susceptibility to renal disease which develops only in the presence of diabetes. This susceptibility factor for nephropathy may also be a risk factor for diabetes [40].

4. CONCLUSIONS

Hypertension and kidney disease are common complications of diabetes in the Pima Indians, as they are in other populations, and patients with these conditions have a particularly bad prognosis. Almost all of the excess mortality in diabetic Pimas is associated with nephropathy. Albuminuria is associated with hypertension, insulin treatment, and duration of diabetes. The higher prevalence of abnormal albumin excretion in diabetic subjects who had higher blood pressures before the onset of diabetes suggests that the hypertension of diabetes is not entirely secondary to diabetic nephropathy, but that higher blood pressure contributes to this complication.

REFERENCES

1. Knowler WC, Bennett PH, Hamman RF, Miller M: Diabetes incidence and prevalence in Pima Indians: a 19-fold greater incidence than in Rochester, Minnesota. Am J Epidemiol 108:497-505, 1978.

2. Knowler WC, Pettitt DJ, Saad MF, Bennett PH: Diabetes mellitus in the Pima Indians: incidence, risk factors, and pathogenesis. Diabetes/Metabolism Reviews 6:1-27, 1990.
3. Diabetes mellitus: report of a WHO study group. WHO Technical Report Series 727. Geneva, World Health Organization, 1985.
4. Kunzelman CL, Knowler WC, Pettitt DJ, Bennett PH: Incidence of nephropathy in type 2 diabetes mellitus in the Pima Indians. Kidney Int 35:681-687, 1989.
5. Nelson RG, Kunzelman CL, Pettitt DJ, Saad MF, Bennett PH, Knowler WC: Albuminuria in Type 2 (non-insulin-dependent) diabetes mellitus and impaired glucose tolerance in Pima Indians. Diabetologia 32:870-876, 1989.
6. Saad MF, Knowler WC, Pettitt DJ, Nelson RG, Mott DM, Bennett PH: Insulin and hypertension: relationship to obesity and glucose intolerance in Pima Indians. Diabetes 39:1430-1435, 1990.
7. Nelson RG, Bennett PH, Beck GJ, Tan M, Knowler WC, Mitch WE, Hirschman GH, Myers BD, for the Diabetic Renal Disease Study: Development and progression of renal disease in Pima Indians with non-insulin-dependent diabetes mellitus. N Engl J Med 335: 1636-1642, 1996.
8. Knowler WC, Bennett PH, Bottazzo GF, Doniach D: Islet cell antibodies and diabetes mellitus in Pima Indians. Diabetologia 17:161-164, 1979.
9. Myers BD, Nelson RG, Williams GW, Bennett PH, Hardy SA, Berg RL, Loon N, Knowler WC, Mitch WE: Glomerular function in Pima Indians with non-insulin-dependent diabetes mellitus of recent onset. J Clin Invest 88:524-530, 1991.
10. Mogensen CE, Christensen CK, Vittinghus E: The stages in diabetic renal disease: with emphasis on the stage of incipient diabetic nephropathy. Diabetes [suppl 2] 32:64-78, 1983.
11. Nelson RG, Knowler WC, Pettitt DJ, Saad MF, Charles MA, Bennett PH: Assessment of risk of overt nephropathy in diabetic patients from albumin excretion in untimed urine specimens. Arch Int Med 151:1761-1765, 1991.
12. Nelson RG, Knowler WC, Pettitt DJ, Hanson RL, Bennett PH: Incidence and determinants of elevated urinary albumin excretion in Pima Indians with NIDDM. Diabetes Care 18:182-187, 1995.
13. Andersen AR, Christiansen JS, Andersen JK, Kreiner S, Deckert T: Diabetic nephropathy in Type 1 (insulin-dependent) diabetes: an epidemiological study. Diabetologia 25:496-501, 1983.
14. Myers BD, Nelson RG, Tan M, Beck GJ, Bennett PH, Knowler WC, Blouch K, Mitch WE: Progression of overt nephropathy in non-insulin-dependent diabetes. Kidney Int 47:1781-1789, 1995.
15. Nelson RG, Knowler WC, McCance DR, Sievers ML, Pettitt DJ, Charles MA, Hanson RL, Liu QZ, Bennett PH: Determinants of end-stage renal disease in Pima Indians with type 2 (non-insulin-dependent) diabetes mellitus and proteinuria. Diabetologia 36:1087-1093, 1993.
16. Krolewski AS, Warram JH, Cristlieb AR, Busick EJ, Kahn C: The changing natural history of nephropathy in Type 1 diabetes. Am J Med 78:785-793, 1985.
17. Humphrey LL, Ballard DJ, Frohnert PP, Chu C-P, O'Fallon WM, Palumbo PJ: Chronic renal failure in non-insulin-dependent diabetes mellitus: a population-based study in Rochester, Minnesota. Ann Intern Med 111:788-796, 1989.
18. Nelson RG, Sievers ML, Knowler WC, Swinburn BA, Pettitt DJ, Saad MF, Garrison R, Liebow IM, Howard BV, Bennett PH: Low incidence of fatal coronary heart disease in Pima Indians despite high prevalence of non-insulin-dependent diabetes. Circulation 81:987-995, 1990.
19. Nelson RG, Newman JM, Knowler WC, Sievers ML, Kunzelman CL, Pettitt DJ, Moffett CD, Teutsch SM, Bennett PH: Incidence of end-stage renal disease in Type 2 (non-insulin-dependent) diabetes mellitus in Pima Indians. Diabetologia 31:730-736, 1988.
20. Hasslacher C, Ritz E, Wahl P, Michael C: Similar risks of nephropathy in patients with type I and type II diabetes mellitus. Nephrol Dial Transplant 4:859-863, 1989.
21. Nelson RG, Knowler WC, Pettitt DJ, Saad MF, Bennett PH: Diabetic kidney disease in Pima Indians. Diabetes Care 16:335-341, 1993.
22. Robbins DC, Knowler WC, Lee ET, Yeh J, Go OT, Welty T, Fabsitz R, Howard BV: Regional differences in albuminuria among American Indians: an epidemic of renal disease. Kidney Int 49:557-563, 1996.
23. Pettitt DJ, Saad MF, Bennett PH, Nelson RG, Knowler WC: Familial predisposition to renal disease in two generations of Pima Indians with Type 2 (non-insulin-dependent) diabetes mellitus. Diabetologia 33:438-443, 1990.

24. Nelson RG, Pettitt DJ, de Courten MP, Hanson RL, Knowler WC, Bennett PH: Parental hypertension and proteinuria in Pima Indians with NIDDM. Diabetologia 39:433-438, 1996.
25. Imperatore G, Hanson RL, Pettitt DJ, Kobes S, Bennett PH, Knowler WC, and the Pima Diabetes Genes Group: Sib-pair linkage analysis for susceptibility genes for microvascular complications among Pima Indians with type 2 diabetes mellitus. Diabetes (in press)
26. de Courten MP, Ksiazek TG, Rollin PE, Kahn AS, Daily PJ, Knowler WC: Sero-prevalence study of hantavirus antibodies in Pima Indians with renal disease. J Infectious Dis 171:762-763, 1995.
27. Nelson RG, Pettitt DJ, Carraher MJ, Baird HR, Knowler WC: Effect of proteinuria on mortality in NIDDM. Diabetes 37:1499-1504, 1988.
28. Deckert T, Feldt-Rasmussen B, Borch-Johnsen K, Jensen T, Kofoed-Enevoldsen A: Albuminuria reflects widespread vascular damage. The Steno hypothesis. Diabetologia 32:219-226, 1989.
29. Kamenetzky SA, Bennett PH, Dippe SE, Miller M, LeCompte PM: A clinical and histologic study of diabetic nephropathy in the Pima Indians. Diabetes 23:61-68, 1974.
30. Schmidt K, Pesce C, Liu Q, Nelson RG, Bennett PH, Karnitschnig H, Striker LJ, Striker GE: Large glomerular size in Pima Indians: lack of change with diabetic nephropathy. J Am Soc Nephrol 3:229-235, 1992.
31. Pagtalunan ME, Miller PL, Jumping-Eagle S, Nelson RG, Myers BD, Rennke HG, Coplon NS, Sun L, Meyer TW: Podocyte loss and progressive glomerular injury in type II diabetes. J Clin Invest 99: 342-348, 1997.
32. Saad MF, Lillioja S, Nyomba BL, Castillo C, Ferraro R, DeGregoria M, Ravussin E, Knowler WC, Bennett PH, Howard BV, Bogardus C: Racial differences in the relation between blood pressure and insulin resistance. N Engl J Med 324:733-739, 1991.
33. Mathiesen ER, R□nn B, Jensen T, Storm B, Deckert T: Relationship between blood pressure and urinary albumin excretion in development of microalbuminuria. Diabetes 39:245-249, 1990.
34. Viberti CG, Keen H, Wiseman MJ: Raised arterial pressure in parents of proteinuric insulin-dependent diabetics. Br Med J 295:551-517, 1987.
35. Krolewski AS, Canessa M, Warram JH, Laffel LMB, Christlieb AR, Knowler WC, Rand LI: Predisposition to hypertension and susceptibility to renal disease in insulin-dependent diabetes mellitus. N Engl J Med 318:140-145, 1988.
36. Knowler WC, Nelson RG, Pettitt DJ: Diabetes, hypertension, and kidney disease in the Pima Indians compared with other populations. In Mogensen CE, ed: The Kidney and Hypertension in Diabetes Mellitus, 2nd ed., Kluwer Academic Publishers, Boston, 1994, pp. 53-62.
37. Knowler WC, Bennett PH, Ballintine EJ: Increased incidence of retinopathy in diabetics with elevated blood pressure: a six-year followup study in Pima Indians. N Eng J Med 302:645-650, 1980.
38. Liu QZ, Knowler WC, Nelson RG, Saad MF, Charles MA, Liebow IM, Bennett PH, Pettitt DJ: Insulin treatment, endogenous insulin concentration, and ECG abnormalities in diabetic Pima Indians: cross-sectional and prospective analyses. Diabetes 41:1141-1150, 1992.
39. Nelson RG, Pettitt DJ, Baird HR, Charles MA, Liu QZ, Bennett PH, Knowler WC: Prediabetic blood pressure predicts urinary albumin excretion after the onset of type 2 (non-insulin-dependent) diabetes mellitus in Pima Indians. Diabetologia 36:998-1001, 1993.
40. McCance DR, Hanson RL, Pettitt DJ, Jacobsson LTH, Bennett PH, Bishop DT, Knowler WC: Diabetic nephropathy: a risk factor for diabetes in offspring. Diabetologia 38:221-226, 1995.

16. VALUE OF SCREENING FOR MICROALBUMINURIA IN PEOPLE WITH DIABETES AS WELL AS IN THE GENERAL POPULATION

Bo Feldt-Rasmussen, Jan Skov Jensen and Knut Borch-Johnsen
Rigshospitalet University Hospital, Department of Nephrology, Copenhagen, and Steno Diabetes Center, Gentofte, Denmark

The concept of microalbuminuria was first introduced among diabetologists [1,2]. It is diagnosed when the urinary albumin excretion rate (UAER) is slightly elevated compared with a normal reference range but lower than what is seen when the classical dipstix are positive for protein or albumin. Microalbuminuria is a marker of an increased risk of diabetic nephropathy and of cardiovascular disease in patients with insulin-dependent (IDDM) as well as with non-insulin-dependent (NIDDM) diabetes mellitus [1-18]. A high number of studies of the pathophysiology and of interventional measures in these patients have been published as reviewed in a number of dissertations and reviews since 1989 [19-27] and seven sets of recommendations on the prevention of diabetic nephropathy, with special reference to microalbuminuria have been published [28-34]. More recently microalbuminuria has been brought into a wider perspective because it has been found to be associated with cardiovascular disease also in the non-diabetic population. In fact microalbuminuria may show to be a *risk factor* of cardiovascular disease among otherwise apparently healthy persons [35-49].

Defining microalbuminuria

Microalbuminuria has been defined using different units of measurement. According to the Gentofte-Montecatini convention [50] microalbuminuria is present when the UAER in a 24-hour urine or a short time collected urine during daytime is in the range of 30 to 300 mg/24h (20 to 200 μg/min) equivalent to 0.46 to 4.6 μmol/24h [50,51]. The upper level is corresponding to a total urinary protein concentration of approximately 0.5 g/l which was previously considered to be the first marker of clinical diabetic nephropathy. The lower limit predicting nephropathy was defined on the basis of the results of four prospective studies in IDDM patients [1-4] (table 16-1). As shown in the table the studies have used different sampling periods, number of urine samples, reference range and they differed with respect to the length of the follow up periods. Nevertheless an international agreement was made on a lower predictive level of 30 mg/24h (20 μ g/min) in order to make it possible to compare the outcome of studies from the various international study groups [50].

In the non-diabetic population clinical cardiovascular disease is often present in subjects with an UAER in the range of 30 to 300 mg/24h [35-49] (table 16-2). Therefore the level of microalbuminuria must be lower if the measuring of UAER also should *predict* cardiovascular disease in the population. This will be discussed at the end of this chapter.

Methodological problems

The concentration of albumin in the urine can be assayed using a number of immunoassays [20]. The major problem is the day to day variation of 23 to 52 %.

Table 16-1. Four prospective studies demonstrating that an increased urinary albumin excretion rate (UAER) is a predictor of nephropathy in IDDM patients.

	Gentofte (1)*	London (2)	Aarhus (3)	Gentofte 2 (4)
Number of patients	23	63	44	71
Method for collecting urine	24 hours			24 hours
UAER Predictive Value for nephropathy (μg/min)	30	30	15	70
Observation (years)	6	14	10	6
Number of patients with UAER above the predictive value who progressed to nephropathy	5/8	7/8	12/14	7/7

*)the patients from this study were also included as a part of Gentofte 2.

This variation is similar regardless of the urine collection procedure used: 24h, overnight collection, timed collection at daytime, during water diureses or by calculating an albumin/creatinine-ratio [4,20,22,51]. It is therefore recommended that presence of microalbuminuria is confirmed in at least two more urine collections [50].

The UAER is increased in the presence of urinary tract infections, menstrual bleedings, nephrological diseases other than diabetic nephropathy, severe hypertension and severe cardiac disease which all have to be excluded. It is also elevated during heavy physical exercise but not significantly affected in healthy subjects during normal daily life activities [20,22].

The UAER is elevated in diabetic patients in very poor glycaemic control with ketonuria and during episodes of ketoacidoses [20].

The collection period is also of importance. The level is similar in urines collected over 24-h and in timed daytime urine collections but reduced by 25% in urines collected overnight. Therefore the range of microalbuminuria in overnight urines should be an UAER of 23 to 230 mg/24h (15 to 150 μg/min) [20,23].

The pathophysiology of development of microalbuminuria is not yet clarified [52-57]. If a timed collection cannot be obtained, an index of albumin/creatinine (μg/μmol) can be calculated. Microalbuminuria is present at an index >3.5 (sensitivity > 95%, specificity >65%) [58]. A close time-relationship between increase in UAER and increase in blood pressure has been demonstrated. The increase in UAER may precede the increase in blood pressure [58].

MICROALBUMINURIA AS A RISK FACTOR

Insulin-dependent diabetes mellitus (IDDM)

The prevalence of microalbuminuria is 16 to 22% [27,59]. Normally no other signs of micro- or macroangiopathy are present at the first diagnosis of microalbuminuria. Later on with higher levels of microalbuminuria retinopathy will become much more frequent, and in fact microalbuminuria is a strong risk marker of severe retinopathy [20,22,23]. The blood-pressure is usually below 160/95 mmHg, but the mean blood-pressure is increasing by 3 mmHg per year [20,22,60]. The kidney function in terms of S-creatinine and glomerular filtration rate (GFR) are normal. The loss of kidney function is observed only in patients with the highest levels of UAER in the microalbuminuric range in whom a decline rate of GFR of 3 to 4 ml/(min*year) has been described [20,22,60]. The risk of clinical diabetic nephropathy is the highest among patients with an UAER in the range of 100 to 300 mg/24h (70 to 200 μg/min) [16,18,53]. The classical definition of clinical diabetic nephropathy at levels of UAER above 300 mg/24h therefore seems to be historical and dictated by the low sensitivity of the older methods for determining protein in urine.

IDDM patients with classical proteinuria >0.5g/l are carrying almost the entire burden of the overmortality of diabetic patients [19]. This overmortality is only to a small extent caused by end stage renal failure. By far most of the patients are dying from cardiovascular diseases [19]. It is therefore widely accepted that microalbuminuria in the IDDM patient should be a valuable diagnostic parameter being highly predictive of excess mortality and cardiovascular morbidity [7-10]. The predictive value of microalbuminuria for cardiovascular diseases seems to be independent of conventional atherosclerotic risk factors, diabetic nephropathy, and diabetes duration and control [7].

It is important to identify all IDDM patients with microalbuminuria because the progression of their disease can be delayed. Antihypertensive treatment reduces the fall rate of GFR by 50 % from 10 to less than 5 ml/(min*year) as observed in patients with clinical nephropathy[61-65]. The effect may be even more impressive when treatment is started at the first signs of an increasing blood-pressure but before development of overt hypertension [23,64,65].

The effect of antihypertensive treatment is further emphasized by the important observation in Denmark of an increased patient survival following the implementation of early antihypertensive treatment [23,66].

Optimizing the glycaemic control has also shown to be effective in arresting the progression of diabetic renal disease in its early stages i.e. delaying development and in some cases also the progression of microalbuminuria [60,67-71].

Non-insulin-dependent diabetes mellitus (NIDDM)

The prevalence of microalbuminuria is also high in NIDDM patients : 30 to 40 % [24,25,72]. Microalbuminuria is often present at diagnosis of the diabetic state. It is primarily associated to cardiovascular disease and NIDDM patients with microalbuminuria are at an increased risk of cardiovascular death compared with NIDDM patients with a normal UAER [5,6,11-24,25].

End stage renal failure only occurs in 3 to 8 % of NIDDM patients despite the high prevalence of microalbuminuria. On the other hand microalbuminuria is a predictor of increasing levels of very low density lipoprotein cholesterol and a decrease of high density lipoprotein cholesterol [73]. Microalbuminuria therefore seems to be a *risk factor* of generalized disease to an even higher extent than in IDDM patients.

Also in NIDDM patients the causal link between microalbuminuria and generalized vascular disease is speculative. It is likely that a link should be found in alterations in the composition of the basal membranes of the capillaries and of the extracellular matrices as also hypothesized in IDDM patients. In any case presence of the well-known risk factors is not sufficient to explain the entire overmortality of patients with NIDDM: hypertension, dyslipidaemia, atherogenic changes in the haemostatic system (increased von Willebrand factor and plasma fibrinogen) [24,25]. In contrast microalbuminuria appears to be an independent risk factor as is the case in IDDM patients.

The diabetic state per se and its associated syndrome of insulin resistance is also likely to be an important risk factor.

Treating normotensive NIDDM patients with microalbuminuria with ACE inhibitors delays the progression to diabetic nephropathy [74].

Non-diabetics

Microalbuminuria is also present in the non-diabetic population. This has now been described in a number of studies [35-49]. Whenever mentioned, the reference range of the UAER seems to be rather low in relation to the classical definition of

Author	Haffner	Winocour	Woo	Metcalf	Gould	Dimmitt	Beatty	Mykkänen	Jensen
Publication year	1990	1992	1992	1992 & 1993	1993	1993	1993	1994	1997
Microalbuminura	U_{alb}>30 mg/l	U_{alb}>20 mg/l	U_{alb}/U_{Creat}> 90%-ile	U_{alb} continuous variable	UAER 20-200μg/min	U_{alb}>me dial	UAER 20-200μg/min	U_{alb}/U_{create}>2	UAER> 90%-ile
Sample size	316	447	1.333	5.349	959	474	264	1.068	2.613
Male sex					↑	↑			↑
Age					↑	↓		↑	
Blood pressure	↑	↑	↑	↑	↑			↑	↑
S-insulin	↑		↑					↑	
P-lipids	↑			↑		↑	↑	↑	
Body mass index				↑					↑
Smoking				↑					↑
Height					↓				
B-glucose					↑		↑		

↑, microalbuminuria is assoiated with increased levels of the risk factor; ↓, microalbuminuria is assoiated with increased levels of the risk factor. U_{alb}, urinary albumin concentretion; U_{creat}, urinary creatinine concentretion; UAER, urinary albumin excretion rate.

Table 16-2. Associations between microalbuminuria and atherosclerotic risk factors.

microalbuminuria. In table 16-3 is shown the reference range of UAER in 10 different studies. Except for one study with a higher level, the median or mean value of UAER is given from 2.6 to 8 μg/min and the upper 95% percentile in more than 50% of the studies as 15 μg/min or below [36,40,43,45,47,49,54,75-77]. Microalbuminuria in its classical definition therefore seems to represent a relatively high UAER among non-diabetics. In an English 4-year follow-up study microalbuminuria, however, increased the mortality rate 24 times [35]. In a Danish study UAER was measured in 216 non-diabetic subjects, 60 to 74 years of age [36]. The median UAER was 7.52 μg/min (25 and 75 percentiles were 4.77 and 14.85 μ g/min). The subjects were reexamined 7 years later. Among the 107 subjects with an initial UAER above the median value 23 had died in contrast to 8 out of 107 below the median UAER ($p<0.008$). In both studies the predictive effect of microalbuminuria was independent of the conventional atherosclerotic risk factors [35,36] which are usually increased among non-diabetic subjects with microalbuminuria (table 16-2).

More recently two larger scaled population based studies have confirmed that a UAER above a certain level is predictive of developing ischaemic heart disease and increased mortality (48, Borch-Johnsen et al unpublished results). In a Finnisch study of Kuusisto et al, 1.069 elderly inhabitants were followed for 3-4 years. Those who at baseline had an A/C ratio above the upper quintile (>3.2 mg albumin/mmol creatinine) had a higher morbidity and mortality from ischaemic heart disease (odds ratio 2.2) (48). In our own study of 2.181 participants of the 1st Monica Population Study, Glostrup, Copenhagen County, an A/C ratio above the upper decile (>0.65 mg albumin/mmol creatinine) was significantly associated with an increased relative risk of 2.3 for development of ischaemic heart disease (Borch-Johnsen et al unpublished results). Also in the two latter studies, the predictive effect of microalbuminuria was independent of the conventional atherosclerotic risk factors.

Therefore, the link between microalbuminuria and cardiovascular disease may be explained by other pathophysiologic mechanisms, e.g. an universally increased transvascular albumin leakage [78,79] as well as other signs of endothelial dysfunction (Clausen et al, unpublished results).

Prospective population studies including our own are in progress aiming to further clarify the role of UAER as a predictor of premature death of cardiovascular disease in apparently healthy subjects.

CONCLUSIONS AND REÇOMMENDATIONS

Measuring the UAER is a well documented and a well established part of monitoring *IDDM patients*. The most simple urine sampling procedures can be

Study (author, contry, publication year)	Urine collection	Sampel size (numbers)	Age (years)	Sex (M/F)	Urinary albumin excretion
Marre et al., France (1987)	Timed overnight	60	40±13	28/32	4.2 ±4.1 μ/min[a] [a]
Marre et al., France (1987)	Timed daytime	60	40±13	28/32	6.6 ±7.7 μ/min[a] [a]
Marre et al., France (1987)	Timed 24-hours	60	40±13	28/32	8.0 ± 8.1 μ/min[a] [a]
Watts et al., UK (1988)	Morning spot	127	33±12	59/68	3.9 (0.9-16.2)[a] mg/l [f]
Watts et al., UK (1988)	Timed overnight	127	33±12	59/68	3.2(1.2-8.6) μg/[a]min [f]
Watts et al., UK (1988)	Timed daytime	127	33±12	59/68	4.5 (1.0-9.1)μg/[a]min [f]
Yudkin et al., UK (1988)	Timed daytime	184	60±12	68/116	2.8(0.09-154.6)[a] μg/min [c]
Gosling & Beevers, UK (1989)	Timed 24-hours	199	40±11	99/100	3.7(0.1-22.9)μg[a]/min [c]
Damsgaard et al., Denmark (1990)	Timed daytime	223	68(64-71)	89/134	7.5(4.8-14.9) μg/[b]min [b]
Metcalf et al., New Zealand (1992)	Morning spot	5.670	49(40-78)	4.106/1.564	5.2(5.1-5.4)mg/l[c] [g]
Dimmitt et al., Australia (1993)	Morning spot	474	34(17-64)	241/233	5.3mg/ [ch]
Mykkänen et al., Finland (1994)	Morning spot	826	69.0±0.1	312/514	23.7±2.5 mg/l[d] [d]
Gould et al., UK (1994)	Timed overnight	812	40-75	359/453	2.6(0.1-148.8)[e] μg/min [c]
Gould et al., UK (1994)	Timed daytime	913	40-75	411/502	4.1(0.1-165.6) μg/min [c]
Jensen et al., Denmark (1997)	Timed overnight	2.613	30-70	1.340/1.273	2.8(1.2-7.0) μg/[a]min [i]

[a]Mean±SD [b]Median (1.-3. interquartile range) [c]median (range) [d]mean ±SE [e]range [f]mean (95% C.I) [g]geometric mean (95% C.I.) [h]median [i]median (10-90 interpercentile range)

Table 16-3. Reference values of urinary excretion in non-diabetic individuals

used as long as the UAER is not significantly elevated i.e. as long as the albumin/creatinine index is below 3.5 μg/μmol. It should be examined at least once a year. When microalbuminuria is suspected, a method of quantitating the UAER should be used at all subsequent visits in the out-patient clinic or until it is found normal at three consecutive visits. Presence of microalbuminuria warrants intensified follow up in order to diagnose and to intervene against retinopathy, nephropathy, hypertension and, if necessary to optimize the glycaemic control [80].

In *patients with NIDDM* the UAER should be measured at diagnosis and once a year. Measuring the UAER is part of the general description of the cardiovascular risk profile of the individual patient. If the UAER is elevated the indications are that treatment with ACE inhibitors may be beneficial. Presence of microalbuminuria will emphasize the need for intervention against any other risk factor present (hypertension, dyslipidaemia, tobacco smoking and obesity).

Among non-diabetic subjects an increased UAER is a marker of cardiovascular disease as well as a risk factor of premature death. Examining the UAER is recommended as part of the routine medical check up of the adult and to replace the less sensitive examination for protein in the urine which after all only serves to disclose diseases of the kidneys and the urinary tract. As was the case in NIDDM patients precense of increased values will reinforce the need to intervene against any other risk factor present. Values of UAER above the microalbuminuric range should obviously lead to routine examinations to exclude nephro-urological diseases. The significance of an increased UAER on development of cardiovascular disease is to some extent clarified but so far no direct clinical consequences should be drawn of microalbuminuria per se.

Among non-diabetic subjects the present indications are that UAER is significantly elevated and predictive of disease at a much lower level than in diabetic patients i.e. at a level below the classical definition of microalbuminuria. Further research is needed for this clarification as well as for the investigation of interventional measures. Microalbuminuria is therefore at present in focus in numerous epidemiological and pathophysiological studies. Measurement is also relevant in relation races, because hypertension and diabetes seem very prevalent in several areas of the world, e.g. among Africans in Cameroon [81].

REFERENCES

1. Parving H-H, Oxenbøll B, Svendsen PAa, Christiansen JS, Andersen AR. Early detection of patients at risk of developing diabetic nephropathy. Acta Endocrinol (Copenh) 1982; 100: 550-555.
2. Viberti GC, Hill RD, Jarret RJ, Argyropoulos A, Mahmud U, Keen H. Microalbuminuria as a predictor of clinical nephropathy in insulin-dependent diabetes mellitus. Lancet 1982; i: 1430-1432.
3. Mogensen CE, Christensen CK. Predicting diabetic nephropathy in insulin-dependent patients. N Engl J Med 1984; 311: 89-93.
4. Mathiesen ER, Oxenbøll B, Johansen K, Svendsen PAa, Deckert T. Incipient nephropathy in Type 1 (insulin-dependent) diabetes. Diabetologia 1984; 26: 406-410.
5. Mogensen CE. Microalbuminuria predicts clinical proteinuria and early mortality in maturity onset diabetes. N Engl J Med 1984; 310: 356-360.
6. Jarrett RJ, Viberti GC, Argyropoulos A, Hill RD, Mahmud U, Murrels TJ. Microalbuminuria predicts mortality in non-insulin-dependent diabetes. Diabetic Med 1984; 1: 17-19.

7. Deckert T, Yokoyama H, Mathiesen ER, Rønn B, Jensen T, Feldt-Rasmussen B, Borch-Johnsen K, Jensen JS. Cohort study of predictive value of urinary albumin excretion for atherosclerotic vascular disease in patients with insulin dependent diabetes. BMJ 1996; 312: 871-874.
8. Messent JWC, Elliot TG, Hill RD, Jarrett RJ, Keen H, Viberti GC. Prognostic significance of microalbuminuria in insulin-dependent diabetes mellitus: A tventy-three year follow-up study. Kidney Int 1992; 41: 836-839.
9. Torffvit O, Agardh C-D. The predictive value of albuminuria for cardiovascular and renal disease. A 5-year follow-up study of 476 patients with type 1 diabetes mellitus. J Diabetic Compl 1993; 7: 49-56.
10. Jensen T, Borch-Johnsen K, Kofoed-Enevoldsen A, Deckert T. Coronary heart disease in young type 1 (insulin-depedent) diabetic patients with and without diabetic nephropathy: Incidence and risk factors. Diabetologia 1987; 30: 144-148.
11. Schmitz A, Vaeth M. Microalbuminuria: A major risk factor in non-insulin-dependent diabetes. A 10-year follow-up study of 503 patients. Diabetic Med 1988; 5: 1126-1134.
12. Mattock MB, Morrish NJ, Viberti GC, Keen H, Fitzgerald AP, Jackson G. Prospective study of microalbuminuria as predictor of mortality in NIDDM. Diabetes 1992; 41: 736-741.
13. Neil A, Hawkins M, Potok M, Thororgood M, Cohen D, Mann J. A prospective population-based study of microalbuminuria as a predictor of mortality in NIDDM. Diabetes Care 1993; 16: 996-1003.
14. Gall M-A, Borch-Johnsen K, Hougaard P, Nielsen FS, Parving H-H. Albuminuria and poor glycemic control predict mortality in NIDDM. Diabetes 1995; 44: 1303-1309.
15. Rossing P, Hougaard P, Borch-Johnsen K, Parving H-H. Predictors of mortality in insulin dependent diabetes: 10 year observational follow up study. BMJ 1996; 313: 779-784.
16. Damsgaard EM, Frøland A, Jørgensen OD, Mogensen CE. Eight to nine year mortality in known non-insulin dependent diabetics and controls. Kidney Internat 1992; 41: 731-735.
17. MacLeod JM, Lutale J, Marshall SM. Albumin excretion and vascular deaths in NIDDM. Diabetologia 1995; 38: 610-616.
18. Beilin J, Stanton KG, McCann VJ, Knuiman MW, Divitini ML. Microalbuminuria in type 2 diabetes: an independent predictor of cardiovascular mortality. Aust Nz J Med 1996; 26: 519-525.
19. Borch-Johnsen K. The prognosis of insulin-dependent diabetes - an epidemiological approach (Thesis). Dan Med Bull 1989; 36: 336-348.
20. Feldt-Rasmussen B. Microalbuminuria and clinical nephropathy in Type 1 (insulin-dependent) diabetes mellitus: Pathophysiological mechanisms and intervention studies (Thesis). Dan Med Bull 1989; 36: 405-415.
21. Jensen T. Albuminuria - a marker of renal and general vascular disease in IDDM (Thesis). Dan Med Bull 1991; 38: 134-144.
22. Christensen CK. The pre-proteinuric phase of diabetic nephropathy (Thesis). Dan Med Bull 1991; 38: 145-159.
23. Mathiesen ER. Prevention of diabetic nephropathy: Microalbuminuria and perspectives for intervention in insulin-dependent diabetes (Thesis). Dan Med Bull 1993; 40: 273-285.
24. Schmitz A. The kidney in non-insulin-dependent diabetes. Studies on glomerular structure and function and the relationship between microalbuminuria and mortality. Acta Diabetologica 1992; 29: 47-69.
25. Gall M. Albuminuria in non-insulin-dependent diabetes mellitus: prevalence, causes and consequences (Thesis). Dan Med Bull 1997: 44: 465-485.
26. Deckert T, Feldt-Rasmussen B, Borch-Johnsen K, Jensen T, Kofoed-Enevoldsen A. Albuminuria reflects widespread vascular damage. The Steno hypothesis. Diabetologia 1989; 32: 219-226.
27. Mogensen CE, Hansen KW, Sommer S et al. »Microalbuminuria: studies in diabetes, essential hypertension and renal disease as compared with the background population.« In *Advances in Nephrology*. Grunfeld JP, ed. Mosby Year Book, 1991; vol 20: 191-228.
28. Viberti GC, Mogensen CE, Passa P, Bilous R, Mangili R. »St Vincent Declaration, 1994: Guidelines for the prevention of diabetic renal failure.« In *The Kidney and Hypertension in Diabetes Mellitus*, 2nd ed. Mogensen CE, ed. Boston, Dordrecht, London: Kluwer Academic Publishers, 1994; pp 515-527.
29. Anon. Prevention of diabetes mellitus: report of a WHO study group. WHO Tech Rep Ser 844. Geneva: WHO, 1994: 55-59.
30. Jerums G, Cooper M, Gilbert R, O'Brien R, Taft J. Microalbuminuria in diabetes. Med J Aust 1994; 161: 265-268.

31. Consensus development conference on the diagnosis and management of nephropathy in patients with diabetes mellitus. Diabetes Care 1994; 17: 1357-1361.

32. Bennett PH, Haffner S, Kaiske BL, et al. Screening and management of microalbuminuria in patients with diabetes mellitus: recommendations to the scientific advisory board of the National Kidney Foundation from an ad hoc committee of the council on diabetes mellitus of the National Kidney Foundation. Am J Kidney Dis 1995; 25: 107-112.

33. Striker GE. Report on a workshop to develop management recommendations for the prevention of progression in chronic renal disease (Bethesda, April, 1994). Nephrol Dial Transplant 1995; 10: 290-292.

34. Mogensen CE, Keane WF, Bennett PH, Jerums G, Parving H-H, Passa P, Steffes MW, Striker GE, Viberti GC. Prevention of diabetic renal disease with special reference to microalbuminuria. Lancet 1995; 346: 1080-1084.

35. Yudkin JS, Forrest RD, Jackson CA. Microalbuminuria as predictor of vascular disease in non-diabetic subjects: Islington diabetes survey. Lancet 1988; ii: 530-533.

36. Damsgaard EM, Frøland A, Jørgensen OD, Mogensen CE. Microalbuminuria as predictor of increased mortality in elderly people. BMJ 1990; 300: 297-300.

37. Haffner SM, Stern MP, Gruber KK, Hazuda HP, Mitchell BD, Patterson JK. Microalbuminuria. Potential marker for increased cardiovascular risk factors in non-diabetic subjects. Arteriosclerosis 1990; 10: 727-731.

38. Winocour PH, Harland JOE, Millar JP, Laker MF, Alberti KGMM. Microalbuminuria and associated cardiovascular risk factors in the community. Atherosclerosis 1992; 93: 71-81.

39. Woo J, Cockram CS, Swaminathan R, Lau E, Chan E, Cheung R. Microalbuminuria and other cardiovascular risk factors in non-diabetic subjects. Int J Cardiol 1992; 37: 345-350.

40. Metcalff P, Baker J, Scott A, Wild C, Scragg R, Dryson E. Albuminuria in people at least 40 years old: Effect of obesity, hypertension and hyperlipidemia. Clin Chem 1992; 38: 1802-1808.

41. Metcalff PA, Baker JR, Scragg RKR, Dryson E, Scott AJ, Wild CJ. Albuminuria in people at least 40 years old. Effect of alcohol consumption, regular exercise, and cigarette smoking. Clin Chem 1993; 39: 1793-1797.

42. Gould MM, Mohamed-Ali V, Goubet SA, Yudkin JS, Haines AP. Microalbuminuria: associations with height and sex in non-diabetic subjects. BMJ 1993; 306: 240-242.

43. Dimmitt SB, Lindquist TL, Mamotte CDS, Burke V, Beilin LJ. Urine albumin excretion in healthy subjects. J Human Hypertens 1993; 7: 239-243.

44. Beatty OL, Atkinson AB, Browne J, Clarke K, Sheridan B, Bell PM. Microalbuminuria does not predict cardiovascular disease in a normal general practice population. Ir J Med Sci 1993; 163: 140-142.

45. Mykkänen L, Haffner SM, Kuusisto J, Pyorälä K, Laakso M. Microalbuminuria precedes the development of NIDDM. Diabetes 1994; 43: 552-557.

46. Jensen JS, Borch-Johnsen K, Feldt-Rasmussen B, Jensen G, Feldt-Rasmussen B. Atherosclerotic risk factors are increased in clinically healthy subjects with microalbuminuria. Atherosclerosis 1995; 112: 245-252.

47. Gould MM, Mohamed-Ali V, Goubet SA, Yudkin JS, Haines AP. Associations of urinary albumin excretion rate with vascular disease in Europid nondiabetic subjects. J Diabetic Compl 1994; 8: 180-188.

48. Kuusisto J, Mykkänin L, Pyörälä K, Laakso M. Hyperinsulinemic microalbuminuria. A new risk indicator for coronary heart disease. Ciculation 1995: 91: 831-837.

49. Jensen JS, Borch-Johnsen K, Feldt-Rasmussen B, Appleyard M, Jensen G. Urinary albumin excretion and history of acute myocardial infarction in a cross-sectional population study of 2613 individuals. Journal of Cardiovascular Risk 1997; 4: 121-125.

50. Mogensen CE, Chachati A, Christensen CK, Close CF, Deckert T, Hommel E, Kastrup J, Lefebvre P, Mathiesen ER, Feldt-Rasmussen B, Schmitz A, Viberti GC. Microalbuminuria: an early marker of renal involvement in diabetes. Uremia Invest 1985-86; 9: 85-95.

51. Feldt-Rasmussen B, Dinesen B, Deckert M. Enzyme immuno assay. an improved determination of urinary albumin in diabetics with incipient nephropathy. Scand J Clin Lab Invest 1985; 45: 539-544.

52. Christiansen JS. Glomerular hyperfiltration in diabetes mellitus. Diabetic Med 1985; 2: 235-239.

53. Parving H-H, Mogensen CE, Jensen HÆ et al. Increased urinary albumin excretion rate in benign essential hypertension. Lancet 1974; i: 1190-1192.

54. Gosling P, Beevers DG. Urinary albumin excretion and blood pressure in the general population. Clin Sci 1989; 76: 39-42.
55. Hommel E, Mathiesen ER, Edsberg B, Bahnsen M, Parving H-H. Acute reduction of arterial blood pressure reduces urinary albumin excretion in type 1 (insulin-dependent) diabetic patients with incipient nephropathy. Diabetologia 1986; 29: 211-215.
56. Deckert T, Kofoed-Enevoldsen A, Vidal P, Nørgaard K, Andreassen HB, Feldt-Rasmussen B. Size and charge selectivity of glomerular filtration in insulin-dependent diabetic patients with and without albuminuria. Diabetologia 1993; 36: 244-251.
57. Feldt-Rasmussen B. Increased transcapillary escape rate of albumin in insulin-dependent diabetic patients with microalbuminuria. Diabetologia 1986; 29: 282-286.
58. Mathiesen ER, Rønn B, Jensen T, Storm B, Deckert T. The relationship between blood pressure and urinary albumin excretion in the development of microalbuminuria. Diabetes 1990; 39: 245-249.
59. Parving H-H, Hommel E, Mathiesen ER, Skøtt P, Edsberg B, Bahnsen M et al. Prevalence of microalbuminuria, arterial hypertension, retinopathy and neuropathy in patients with insulin dependent diabetes. BMJ 1988; 296: 157-160.
60. Feldt-Rasmussen B, Mathiesen ER, Jensen T, Lauritzen T, Deckert T. Effect of improved metabolic control on loss of kidney function in insulin-dependent diabetic patients. Diabetologia 1991; 34: 164-170.
61. Bjorck S, Mulec H, Johnsen SA et al. Renal protective effect of Enalapril in diabetic nephropathy. BMJ 1992; 304: 339-343.
62. Lewis EJ, Hunsicker LG, Bain RP, Rohde RD, for the Collaborative Study Group. The effect of angiotensin-converting-enzyme inhibition on diabetic nephropathy. N Engl J Med 1993; 329: 1456-1462.
63. Parving H-H, Andersen AR, Schmidt UM, Hommel E, Mathiesen ER, Svendsen PAa. Effect of antihypertensive treatment on kidney function in diabetic nephropathy. BMJ 1987; 294: 1443-1447.
64. Mathiesen ER, Hommel E, Giese J, Parving H-H. Efficacy of captopril in postponing nephropathy in normotensive insulin-dependent diabetic patients with microalbuminuria. BMJ 1991; 303: 81-87.
65. Viberti GC, Mogensen CE, Groop L, Pauls JF, for the European Microalbuminuria Captopril Study Group. Effect of captopril on progression to clinical proteinuria in patients with insulin-dependent diabetes mellitus and microalbuminuria. JAMA 1994; 271: 275-279.
66. Parving H-H, Hommel E. Prognosis in diabetic nephropathy. BMJ 1989; 299: 230-233.
67. Dahl-Jørgensen K, Hanssen KF, Kierulf P, Bjøro T, Sandvik L, Aagenaess Ø. Reduction of urinary albumin excretion after 4 years of continuous subcutaneous insulin infusion in insulin-dependent diabetes mellitus. Acta Endocrinol (Copenh) 1988; 117: 19-25.
68. Reichard P, Berglund B, Britz A, Cars I, Nilsson BY, Rosenqvist U. Intensified conventional insulin treatment retards the microvascular complications of insulin-dependent diabetes mellitus (IDDM). The Stockholm Diabetes Intervention Study after five years. J Intern Med 1991; 230: 101-108.
69. The Diabetes Control and Complications Trial Research Group. The effect of intensive treatment of diabetes on the development and progression of long-term complications in insulin-dependent diabetes mellitus. N Engl J Med 1993; 329: 977-986.
70. Diabetes Control and Complications (DCCT) Research Group. Effect of intensive therapy on the development and progression of diabetic nephropathy in the diabetes control and complications trial. Kidney Int 1995; 42: 1703-1720.
71. Microalbuminuria Collaborative Study Group, United Kingdom. Intensive therapy and progression to clinical albuminuria in patients with insulin dependent diabetes mellitus and microalbuminuria. BMJ 1995; 311: 973-977.
72. Gall M, Rossing P, Skøtt P, Damsbo P, Vaag A, Bech K et al. Prevalence of micro- and macro-albuminuria, arterial hypertension, retinopathy and large vessel disease in European Type 2 (non-insulin-dependent) diabetic patients. Diabetologia 1991; 34: 655-661.
73. Niskanen L, Uusitupa M, Sarlund H, Siitonen O, Voutilainen E, Penttila I et al. Microalbuminuria predicts the development of serum lipoprotein abnormalities favouring atherogenesis in newly diagnosed Type 2 (non-insulin-dependent) diabetic patients. Diabetologia 1990; 33: 237-243.
74. Ravid M, Savin H, Jutrin I, Bental T, Katz B, Lishner M. Long-term stabilizing effect of angiotensin-converting enzyme inhibition on plasma creatinine and on proteinuria in normotensive type II diabetic patients. Ann Intern Med 1993; 118: 577-581.
75. Marre M, Claudel J-P, Ciret P, Luis N, Suarez L, Passa P. Laser immunonephelometry for routine quantification of urinary albumin excretion. Clin Chem 1987; 33: 209-213.

76. Watts GF, Morris RW, Khan K, Polak A. Urinary albumin excretion in healthy adult subjects: reference values and some factors affectin their interpretation. Clin Chim Acta 1988; 172: 191-198.
77. Jensen JS, Feldt-Rasmussen B, Borch-Johnsen K, Jensen G and the Copenhagen City Heart Study Group. Urinary albumin excretion in a population based sample of 1011 middle aged non-diabetic subjects. Scand J Clin Lab Invest 1993; 53: 867-872
78. Jensen JS, Borch-Johnsen K, Jensen G, Feldt-Rasmussen B. Microalbuminuria reflects a generalized transvascular albumin leakiness in clinically healthy subjects. Clin Sci 1995; 88: 629-33.
79. Jensen JS, Borch-Johnsen K, Deckert T, Deckert M, Jensen G, Feldt-Rasmussen B. Reduced glomerular size- and charge-selectivity in clinically healthy individuals with microalbuminuria. Eur J Clin Invest 1995; 25: 608-614.
80. Borch-Johnsen K, Wenzel H, Viberti GC, Mogensen CE. Is screening and intervention for Microalbuminuria worthwhile in patients with insulin dependent diabetes? BMJ 1993; 306: 1722-1725.
81. Ducorps M, Bauduceau B, Poirier JM, Cosson E, Belmejdoub G, Mayaudon H. Hypertension in black African diabetics (Abstract). Diabetologia 1996; 39: Suppl. 1: A287.

17. INCIDENCE OF NEPHROPATHY IN IDDM AS RELATED TO MORTALITY. COSTS AND BENEFITS OF EARLY INTERVENTION.

Knut Borch-Johnsen,
Steno Diabetes Centre, Gentofte Denmark

Development of persistent proteinuria - the clinical manifestation of diabetic nephropathy - is a strong prognostic marker in IDDM-patients. Not only does it precede the development of end stage renal failure, it is also associated with an increased risk of proliferative retinopathy, visual impairment and blindness, and with an increased risk of atherosclerosis leading to peripheral vascular disease and amputations, coronary artery disease, myocardial infarction, sudden death and cerebrovascular disease and stroke.

As discussed elsewhere in this book, effective antihypertensive treatment has improved the prognosis of patients with diabetic nephropathy, but in many countries diabetic nephropathy is still the most frequent condition, leading to dialysis and transplantation. Thus, the focus of this chapter is:

- the epidemiological pattern of diabetic nephropathy
- mortality in patients with and without nephropathy
- mortality and microalbuminuria
- prospects for prevention, including health economical aspects

1. EPIDEMIOLOGICAL PATTERN OF DIABETIC NEPHROPATHY

Clinical diabetic nephropathy (i.e. persistent proteinuria ≥ 0.5 g/24 h or ≥ 300 mg albumin/24 h) is rare in the first 10 years of diabetes duration, but thereafter the incidence increases to a maximum of 2-3 %/year after 13-20 years of duration. Thereafter, the incidence decreases and remains at a level of < 0.5 %/year. This incidence pattern has been demonstrated in several studies [1-4] and it has remained remarkably constant over time [1, 2]. The incidence of nephropathy has, however, decreased markedly during the last 50 years, and in Denmark [1, 2] as well as in USA [3], and the life time of nephropathy decreased from 50 % to 25 %. In Sweden an even more dramatic reduction was observed in cohorts of children with IDDM, an in the youngest cohort no cases of nephropathy was observed at all [5]. These result were obtained in a paediatric clinic which has proven to be able to maintain remarkably low HbA_{1C} values in their patients. This result is encouraging and demonstrates the importance of strict metabolic control, but unfortunately the same level of HbA_{1C} has not been obtainable in other countries [6] and that may well explain why a similar decline in the incidence has not been found in other countries [7].

The reason why the life time risk of nephropathy has decreased from 50% to 25 % is only partly known. Improved metabolic regulation is likely to be the most important single factor. It is likely that the modifications in care, therapeutic strategies and introduction of the "self care" principle has lead to improved metabolic control. Furthermore, the DCCT-study has not only demonstrated a beneficial effect of good metabolic control, it also showed that the most dramatic absolute risk reduction was obtained in the high range of HbA_{1C} values. Other factors like antihypertensive treatment and dietary changes may have contributed to a lesser degree to the decrease in incidence of nephropathy by reducing the risk of progression from microalbuminuria to overt nephropathy.

2. MORTALITY AND PROTEINURIA

Studies from different parts of the world consistently show, that IDDM-patients have an excess mortality compared with the non-diabetic population. The excess mortality varies with age and diabetes duration [1], and also shows considerable variation between countries [2]. As shown in table 17-1, the distribution of causes of death varies according to diabetes duration.

Table 17-1. Cause of death according to diabetes duration in a cohort of 2,900 Danish IDDM-patients diagnosed 1932-1972, before the age of 31 years [17]

Cause of death	Diabetes Duration		
	0-15 years (n=124)	16-30 years (n=513)	> 30 years (n=199)
Vascular			
Acute myocardial infarction	9%	17%	36%
Other cardiovascular	4%	3%	11%
Cerebrovascular	2%	4%	10%
Diabetic nephropathy	17%	52%	15%
Ketoacidosis	18%	2%	3%
Hypoglycaemia	6%	3%	2%
Diabetes NOD	2%	1%	1%
Infections	14%	5%	10%
Suicide	8%	3%	3%
Cancer	2%	3%	4%
Other	19%	7%	9%

While acute, metabolic complications and infections dominates in patients with short diabetes duration, diabetic nephropathy and cardiovascular diseases account for 70-80 % of all deaths in patients with longer diabetes duration.

In 1972 Watkins et al suggested, that development of proteinuria was a strong prognostic marker in diabetes, and probably even stronger than grading of nephropathy on the basis of histo-pathological findings [11]. In our study of excess mortality in 1030 IDDM patients followed for 30 to 50 years we found [12], (figures 17-1) that the very high excess mortality of IDDM-patients was found only in patients who developed persistent proteinuria (clinical diabetic nephropathy), while patients not developing clinical nephropathy had a low and rather constant excess mortality. The high mortality of patients with nephropathy has been confirmed by several other studies [13, 14]. In patients with nephropathy the leading causes of death are uraemia/end stage renal failure and macrovascular disease. Myocardial infarction and stroke is 10 times more frequent in patients with than in patients without nephropathy [15] and below the age of 50 years the excess mortality from macrovascular disease is almost entirely confined to patients with diabetic nephropathy [16]. Thus, in conclusion from these studies, the most effective way of improving the prognosis of IDDM would be to prevent development of diabetic nephropathy. As already mentioned the incidence of nephropathy has decreased, and thus it is not surprising, that in a study of the relative mortality of IDDM-patients in Denmark during the period from 1930 to 1981 we found [17] that the excess mortality decreased by nearly 40 %. The study included nearly three thousand patients diagnosed before the age of 31 years, diagnosed during the period 1933 to 1972 and admitted to the Steno Memorial Hospital (Steno Diabetes Centre). All patients were followed up from their first admission to the hospital until death, emigration or January 1st 1982.

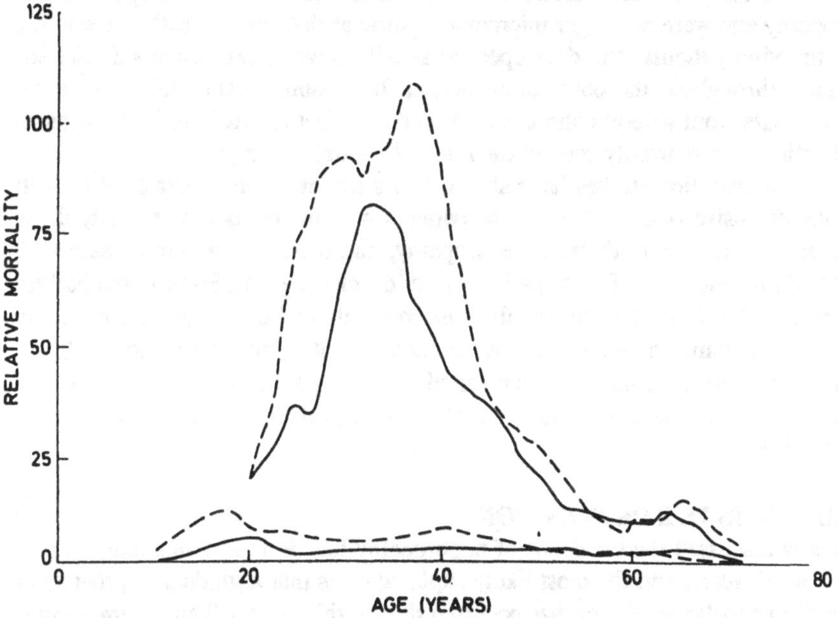

Figure 17-1 Age adjusted relative mortality of IDDM-patients with proteinuria (upper curves) and without proteinuria (lower curves) in a cohort of 1003 Danish IDDM-patients: - - - - Women, — Men. (Reproduced with permission from Diabetologia and Springer Verlag [12]).

The major decrease in the excess mortality took place in patients diagnosed from 1940 to 1955, but a constant and gradual decline was found over the entire period.

3. MORTALITY AND MICROALBUMINURIA

Patients with microalbuminuria i.e. urinary albumin excretion rate from 30 to 300 mg/24 h (also known as incipient nephropathy) have long been known as a high risk group for development of diabetic nephropathy [18-20]. Dyslipidaemia and changes in other cardiovascular risk factors including blood pressure and rheological factors are well established characteristics of patients with microalbuminuria [21, 22], and in NIDDM patient's microalbuminuria is associated with increased cardiovascular morbidity and mortality [23, 24]. Thus, the question is whether microalbuminuria predicts increased mortality - particularly from cardiovascular disease, even in IDDM patients. In non-insulin dependent diabetic patient [25, 26] as well as in non-diabetic individuals [27, 28] microalbuminuria is associated with a marked excess mortality particularly from cardiovascular disease. Very few studies have been performed in IDDM patients, and methodologically these studies are difficult to perform, as patients developing nephropathy should be excluded (censored) from the cohort at onset of nephropathy. The magnitude of this problem is illustrated in a study by Messent [30] where they followed microalbuminuric IDDM patients for more than twenty years, this group of patients had a significant excess mortality. Among the eight patients with microalbuminuria originally included in the study five died. However, all deceased patients had developed clinical nephropathy and were no longer microalbuminuric at the time of death. Among the three surviving patients, one developed renal failure while two remained microalbuminuric throughout the observation period. In a more recent study, where we combined data from several cohorts we showed [31] that microalbuminuria is associated with excess mortality even in the microalbuminuric range.

Intervention studies have shown that strict metabolic control [8] as well as antihypertensive treatment of IDDM patients with microalbuminuria may delay or prevent progression to diabetic nephropathy, and it must therefore be assumed, that it will prevent some of these patients from developing End Stage Renal Failure and uraemia. The impact of this on all cause mortality and cardiovascular mortality in particular remains unknown, at strict metabolic control may not be able to bring mortality rates down to the same controlled clinical trials have been so small and running for so short periods of time [32-35] that an evaluation of this has been impossible so far.

4. PROSPECTS FOR PREVENTION

As already discussed the incidence of nephropathy has decreased markedly during the last 30-50 years, and the most likely explanation is that a gradual improvement in overall metabolic regulation has occurred during this period. Thus, primary prevention of nephropathy in IDDM patients is possible. Secondary prevention, i.e. prevention of progression from microalbuminuria to overt nephropathy is also possible by antihypertensive treatment [32-35], but other factors like smoking [36] and dietary factors [37] may also be important risk factors for progression to nephropathy. All of these factors will be dealt with in details in other chapters of this book and will not be discussed further here. The main lesson is that primary and secondary prevention is possible. Secondary prevention is, however, possible only if patients developing microalbuminuria are identified at an early stage of the condition, where there is room for early intervention. For this reason all patients with IDDM should be screened annually for microalbuminuria. This could not only contribute to an improvement of the prognosis of the individual, but, as discussed below, even lead to considerable savings in the health care system.

5. SCREENING, INTERVENTION AND COST EFFECTIVENESS

As trials aiming at early intervention in the microalbuminuric stage are relatively small and few, it is difficult to estimate the cost effectiveness of different regimens for screening for and early intervention in microalbuminuria. On the other hand, treatment of end stage renal failure with dialysis or renal transplantation is so expensive (costs approximately 25 to 40.000 US $ per year) [38], that if intervention programmes are effective, then they are also likely to be cost-beneficial. Furthermore, screening for microalbuminuria is becoming increasingly simple, fast and cheap with the availability of methods described elsewhere in this book.

Two independent groups have tried to estimate the likely cost-benefit and cost effectiveness of different regimens for screening and intervention. In the study of Siegel et al [39], the authors compared the likely costs and savings related to four different programmes: 1: No screening for microalbuminuria or proteinuria, antihypertensive treatment at BP 140/90, 2: Screening for proteinuria (0.5 g/24 h) and ACE-inhibitor treatment in case of proteinuria, 3: Screening for microalbuminuria, treatment with ACE-inhibitor if UAER 100 µg/min and 4: Screening for microalbuminuria and ACE-inhibitor if UAER 20 µg/min. The authors used previously published epidemiological data regarding the natural history of diabetic nephropathy to estimate the time of progression from norm-to microalbuminuria, from microalbuminuria to proteinuria and from proteinuria to end stage renal failure. They then assumed two different potential effects of antihypertensive treatment, 50 % increase in progression time (called conservative estimate) and 75 % increased progression time (called optimistic estimate).

The second study [40], used a rather similar design including annual testing for microalbuminuria in all IDDM patients from five to 30 years of diabetes duration. Antihypertensive treatment using an ACE-inhibitor would be initiated in all patients with microalbuminuria (30 mg/24 h). The study used data from a previously published Danish epidemiological study [41] of the incidence of nephropathy and the mortality in patients with and without proteinuria to estimate mortality rates and transmission times without intervention. Based on the results from controlled clinical trials [32-35, 42] they estimated that the increase rate in UAER could be decreased by 33 or 67 per cent.

Both studies conclude, that if antihypertensive treatment can lower the annual increase rate in UAER in microalbuminuric patients, then screening- and intervention programmes will save money for the providers of the health care system. In our own study, we found [40] that even when taking discounting into consideration, a treatment effect of the antihypertensive treatment of 8 to 12 % would be sufficient to out-balance costs and savings. In patients with nephropathy, antihypertensive treatment has been shown to decrease the decline-rate in GFR and to decrease the mortality rates by 67 % [43, 44]. If this was the case also in patients with microalbuminuria, then screening and intervention for microalbuminuria would increase the median life-expectancy of IDDM patients by more than 10 years, and the life-time risk of developing end stage renal failure would decrease by more than 60 %.

The conclusions drawn in the studies by Siegel et al. [39] and Borch-Johnsen et al [40] have recently been disputed by Kiberd and Jindal [46]. Like the two previous studies they performed a cost-effectiveness study, but compared a scenario with screening for microalbuminuria with a scenario screening for hypertension. They concluded that screening for hypertension would be more cost effective than screening for microalbuminuria. In their paper they, however, never defined hypertension, making it difficult to take recommendations from their study. Furthermore, their analysis was based on a set of critical assumptions, including that: i) Insulin dependent diabetic patients with microalbuminuria usually develop hypertension before they develop nephropathy. Ii) A diagnosis of hypertension can be made precisely without false positive and false negative cases of hypertension and iii) prevention of nephropathy is the only reason for surveillance and intervention. The premises for assumptions i) and ii) are discussed elsewhere in this book, but it is likely that microalbuminuria and increasing blood pressure develops in parallel [46]. Furthermore, it is well known that there is a huge variability in blood pressure, particularly when measured in routine clinical settings [47]. Finally, microalbuminuria is a marker, not only of early renal disease, but also of generalised micro-and macrovascular disease [21, 31]. Thus, it is a marker of high risk individuals that should be screened regularly for other complications, and therefore premise iii) is not valid.

CONCLUSION

Proteinuria and microalbuminuria are both not only well established risk factors for end stage renal failure but also the strongest prognostic markers even identified in diabetic individuals. Fifteen years ago we would have measured them first of all for scientific purposes, but now they will have therapeutic implications (e.g. strict metabolic control, antihypertensive treatment etc.) and they will indicate that this is a high risk patient who needs intensified care to prevent macroangiopathy (i.e. focus on the entire cardiovascular risk profile) and to prevent proliferative retinopathy and visual impairment. As neither microalbuminuria nor proteinuria causes any subjective symptoms to the patient, they reflect the large group of clinically silent but life threatening conditions that can only be detected by screening.

REFERENCES

1. Andersen AR, Christiansen JS, Andersen JK, Kreiner S & Deckert T. Diabetic nephropathy in Type 1 (insulin-dependent) diabetes: and epidemiological study. Diabetologia 1983;25:496-501.
2. Kofoed-Enevoldsen A, Borch-Johnsen K, Kreiner S, Nerup J, Deckert T. Declining incidence of persistent proteinuria in Type 1 (insulin-dependent) diabetic patients in Denmark. Diabetes 1987;36:205-209.
3. Krolewski AS, Warram JH, Christlieb ARE, Busick EJ, Kahn CR. The changing natural history of nephropathy in Type 1 diabetes. Am J Med 1985;78:785-794.
4. Tchobroutsky G. Relation of diabetic control to development of microvascular complications. Diabetologia 1978;15:143-153.
5. Bojestig M, Arnqvist HJ, Hermansson G, Karlberg BE, Ludvigsson J. Declining incidence of nephropathy in insulin-dependent diabetes mellitus. N Engl J Med 1994;330:15-18.
6. Mortensen HB, Hougaard P. Comparison of metabolic control in a cross-sectional study of 2,873 children and adolescents with IDDM from 18 countries. Diabetes Care 1997;20:714.
7. Rossing P, Rossing K, Jacobsen P, Parving HH. Unchanged incidence of diabetic nephropathy in IDDM patients. Diabetes 1995;44:739-743.
8. The Diabetes Control and Complications Trial Research Group. The effect of intensive treatment of diabetes on the development and progression of long-term complications in insulin-dependent diabetes mellitus. N Engl J Med 1993;329:977-986.
9. Borch-Johnsen K. The prognosis of insulin-dependent diabetes mellitus. Dan Med Bull 1989;36:336-348.
10. Diabetes Epidemiology Research International (DERI) Mortality Study Group. Major Cross-Country differences in risk of dying for people with IDDM. Diabetes Care 1991;14:49-54.
11. Watson PJ, Blainey JD, Brewer DB, Fitzgerald MG, Malins JM, O'Sullivan DJ, Pinto JA. The natural history of diabetic renal disease. Q J Med 1972;164:437-456.
12. Borch-Johnsen K, Andersen PK, Deckert T. The effect of proteinuria on relative mortality in Type 1 (insulin-dependent) diabetes mellitus. Diabetologia 1985;28:590-596.
13. Parving HH, Hommel E. Prognosis in diabetic nephropathy. BMJ 1989;299:230-233.
14. Rossing P, Hougaard P, Borch-Johnsen K, Parving HH. Predictors of mortality in insulin dependent diabetes: 10 year observational follow up study. BMJ 1996;313:779-784.
15. Jensen T, Borch-Johnsen K, Deckert T. Coronary heart disease in young Type 1 (insulin-dependent) diabetic patients with diabetic nephropathy: Incidence and risk factors. Diabetologia 1987;30:144-148.
16. Borch-Johnsen K, Kreiner S. Proteinuria: value as predictor of cardio-vascular mortality in insulin-dependent diabetes mellitus. Br Med J 1987;294:1651-1654.
17. Borch-Johnsen K, Kreiner S, Deckert T. Mortality of Type 1 (insulin-dependent) diabetes mellitus in Denmark. Diabetologia 1986;29:767-772.
18. Viberti GC, Jarrett RJ, Mahmud U, Hill RD, Argyropoulos A, Keen H. Microalbuminuria as a predictor of clinical nephropathy in insulin dependent diabetes mellitus. Lancet 1982;i:1430-1432.
19. Mogensen CE, Christensen CK. Predicting diabetic nephropathy in insulin-dependent patients. N Engl J Med 1984;311:89-93.
20. Mathiesen ER, Oxenbøll B, Johansen K, Svendsen PAa, Deckert T. incipient nephropathy in Type 1 (insulin-dependent) diabetes. Diabetologia 1984;26:406-410.
21. Jensen T. Albuminuria - a marker of renal and generalized vascular disease in insulin-dependent diabetes mellitus. Dan Med Bull 1991;38:134-144.
22. Feldt-Rasmussen B. Microalbuminuria and clinical nephropathy in Type 1 (insulin-dependent) diabetes mellitus: pathophysiological mechanisms and intervention studies. Dan Med Bull 1989;36:405-415.
23. Gall M-A, Borch-Johnsen K, Hougaard P, Nielsen FS, and Parving H-H. Albuminuria and poor glycemic control predict mortality in NIDDM. Diabetes 1995;44:1303-1309.
24. Agewall S, Wikstrand J, Ljungman S, Herlitz H, and Fagerberg B. Does microalbuminuria predict cardiovascular events in nondiabetic men with treated hypertension? AJH 1995;8:337-342.
25. Mogensen CE. Microalbuminuria predicts clinical proteinuria and early mortality in maturity onset diabetes. N Engl J Med 1984;310:356-360.
26. Jarrett RJ, Viberti GC, Argyropoulos A, Hill RD, Mahmud U, Murrells TJ. Microalbuminuria predicts mortality in non-insulin-dependent diabetes. Diabetic Med 1984;I:17-19.

27. Yudkin JS, Forrest RD, Jackson CA. Microalbuminuria as predictor of vascular disease in non-diabetic subjects. Lancet 1988;ii:530-533.
28. Damsgaard EM, Frøland A, Jørgensen OD, Mogensen CE. Micro-albuminuria as predictor of increased mortality in elderly people. BMJ 1990;300:297-300.
29. Borch-Johnsen K, Feldt-Rasmussen B, Strandgaard S, Schroll M, Jensen JS. Microalbuminuria: a novel independent risk factor for ischemic heart disease. Submitted BMJ 1997.
30. Messent JWC, Elliott TG, Hill RD, Jarrett RJ, Keen H, Viberti GC. Prognostic significance of microalbuminuria in insulin-dependent diabetes mellitus: a twenty year follow-up study. Kidney Int 1992;41:836-839.
31. Deckert T, Yokoyama H, Mathiesen ER, Rønn B, Jansen T, Feldt-Rasmussen B, Borch-Johnsen K, Jensen JS. Cohort study of predictive value of urinary albumin excretion for atherosclerotic vascular disease in insulin dependent diabetes. BMJ 1996;312:871-874.
32. Marre M, Chatellier G, Leblanc H, Guyene TT, Menard J, Passa P. Prevention of diabetic nephropathy with enalapril in normotensive diabetics with microalbuminuria. BMJ 1988;297:1092-1095.
33. Mathiesen ER, Hommel E, Giese J, Parving H-H. Efficacy of captopril in postponing nephropathy in normotensive insulin-dependent diabetic patients with microalbuminuria. BMJ 1991;303:81-87.
34. Melbourne Diabetic nephropathy study group. Comparison between perindopril and nifedipine in hypertensive and normotensive diabetic patients with microalbuminuria. BMJ 1991;302:210-216.
35. Viberti GC, Mogensen CE, Groop L, Pauls JF for the European Microalbuminuria Captopril Study Group. Effect of captopril on progression to clinical proteinuria in patients with insulin-dependent diabetes mellitus and microalbuminuria. JAMA 1994;271:275-279.
36. Sawicki PT, Mühlhaser I, Bender R, Pethke W, Heinemann L, Berger M. Effects of smoking on blood pressure and proteinuria in patients with diabetic nephropathy. J Intern Med 1996;239:345-352.
37. Pedrini MT, Levey AS, Lau J, Chalmers TC, Wang PH. The effect of dietary protein restriction on the progression of diabetic and non-diabetic renal disease: a meta-analysis. Ann Intern Med 1996;124:627-632.
38. Eggers PW. Health Care Policies/economics of the geriatric renal population. Am J Kidney Dis 1990;16:384-391.
39. Siegel JE, Krolewski AS, Warram JH, Weinstein MC. Cost-effectiveness of screening and early treatment of nephropathy in patients with insulin-dependent diabetes mellitus. J AM Soc Nephrol 1992;3:3111-3119.
40. Borch-Johnsen K, Wenzel H, Viberti GC, Mogensen CE. Is screening and intervention for Microalbuminuria worthwhile in patients with insulin dependent diabetes? BMJ 1993;306:1722-1725.
41. Ramlau-Hansen H, Bang Jespersen NC, Andersen PK, Borch-Johnsen K, Deckert T. Life insurance for insulin-dependent diabetics. Scand Actuarial J 1987;19-36.
42. Feldt-Rasmussen B, Mathiesen ER, Jensen T, Lauritzen T, Deckert T. Effect of improved metabolic control on loss of kidney function in Type 1 (insulin-dependent) diabetic patients: an update of the Steno studies. Diabetologia 1991;34:164-170.
43. Parving H-H, Andersen ARE, Smidt UM, Svendsen PAA. Early aggressive antihypertensive treatment reduces the rate of decline in kidney function in diabetic nephropathy. Lancet 1983;i:1175-1179.
44. Mathiesen ER, Borch-Johnsen K, Jensen DV, Deckert T. Improved survival in patients with diabetic nephropathy. Diabetologia 1989;32:884-886.
45. Kiberd BA, Jindal KK. Screening to prevent renal failure in insulin dependent diabetic patients: an economical evaluation: BMJ 1995;311:595-599.
46. Microalbuminuria Collaborative Study Group, UK. Risk factors for development of microalbuminuria in insulin dependent diabetic patients: a cohort study. BMJ 1993;306:1235-1239.
47. Hansen KW, Christensen CK, Andersen PH, Mau Pedersen M, Christiansen JS, Mogensen CE. Ambulatory blood pressure in microalbuminuric type 1 diabetic patients. Kidney Int 1992;41:847-854.

18. MEASUREMENT OF ALBUMIN AND OTHER URINARY PROTEINS IN LOW CONCENTRATION IN DIABETES MELLITUS: TECHNIQUES AND CLINICAL SIGNIFICANCE

Rowe DJF and Gatling W,
Department of Chemical Pathology, Southampton University Hospitals NHS Trust and Department of Diabetes, Poole Hospital NHS Trust

MICROALBUMINURIA

Independent clinical studies have indicated that urinary albumin excretion increased above normal but below the level of detection by Albustix ("microalbuminuria") predicts accurately the development of clinical nephropathy and end-stage renal failure in adults with insulin-dependent diabetes (IDD) [1-3].

Following these studies, measurement of urinary albumin has been used to investigate changes in renal function in children with IDD [4-6], in non-insulin dependent diabetic subjects [7,8], in non-diabetics with heart failure and/or hypertension [9,10] and in pregnancy [11]. The measurement may also predict mortality as well as morbidity from non-renal causes [7,8,12,13].

The clinical significance of the excretion of other urinary proteins has also been investigated. Conclusions that the excretion of B2-microglobulin was not increased in early diabetic renal disease have been shown to be flawed due to the instability of this protein in urine under normal collection conditions [14].

Does microalbuminuria predict progression of renal disease?

Recent studies have challenged the belief that microalbuminuria is a strong predictor of progression to diabetic nephropathy.

In adult IDD with duration of diabetes >15 years there was only limited evidence of progression of microalbuminuria to clinical nephropathy (5/18 subjects) or of progression of clinical nephropathy to end-stage renal failure over a 10 year follow-up.[15] Young insulin dependent and adult insulin-requiring diabetic subjects showed no significant change in urinary albumin/creatinine ratio (ACR) in random samples over 8-15 years follow-up, nor was there any consistent change in ACR in those subjects with microalbuminuria (20% and 28% of the respective clinic populations) (figure 18-1) [16].

Histological studies have demonstrated that structural abnormalities in glomerular basement membrane thickness and in mesangial volume are present in some diabetic patients without apparent abnormalities in urinary albumin excretion [17]. The relationship between the pathological features and functional abnormalities in diabetic renal disease have always been difficult to correlate. All diabetic patients with duration over 10 years have histological features of kidney disease yet only a proportion of these will have functional abnormalities such as increased protein excretion.

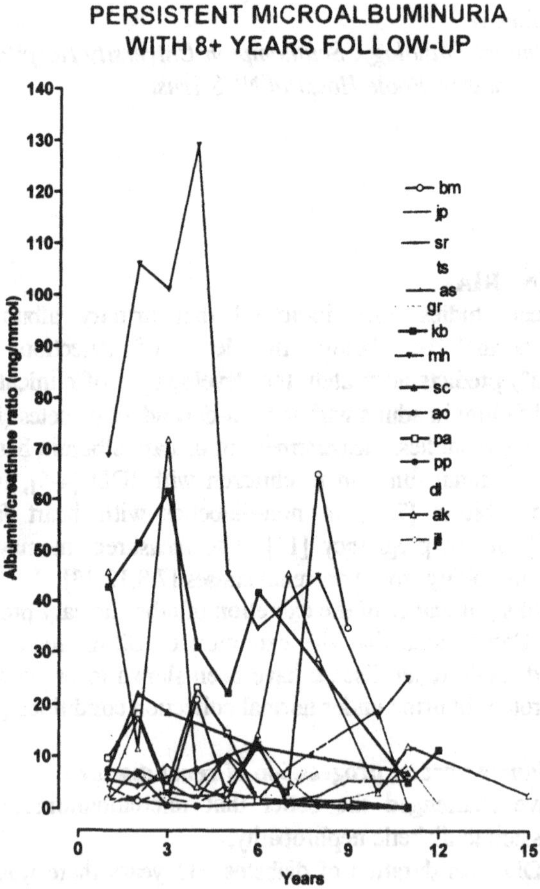

Figure 18-1 longitudinal data from individual diabetic children with persistent microalbuminuria over 8-15 years. Follow up.

Other urinary proteins

The excretion of many enzymes and small-molecular weight proteins are increased early in the diabetic process, in many cases independent of the excretion of albumin.

Conclusions that the excretion of B2-microglobulin was not increased in early diabetic renal disease were flawed due to the instability of this protein in normally acid urine. This was shown by Bernard [14] and confirmed independently by Watts et al [18]. These workers measured B2-microglobulin and retinol-binding protein (RBP), which are both considered to reflect changes in renal tubular function, in non-diabetic and diabetic subjects. A weak correlation was shown between the excretion of the two proteins accompanied by a lower mass excretion of B2-microglobulin. The experiment was repeated after *in vivo* alkalinisation prior to urine collection. The correlation between the proteins increased to r=0.8 and the mass excretion of B2-microglobulin increased to equivalence with that of RBP. The excretion of RBP did not increase significantly after alkalinisation.

The excretion of enzymes such as n-acetyl B-D-glucosaminidase (NAG), gamma-glutamyl transferase and alkaline phosphatase and other proteins such as a1-microglobulin, RBP, immunoglobulin light chains and transferrin may be increased early in the diabetic process and independent of the excretion of albumin [4,20-29,31]. One study demonstrated that the excretion of a1-microglobulin and gamma light chains was significantly increased and correlated with HbA1 in young people with IDD without significant change in the excretion of albumin [22]. Pontuch also showed a correlation between RBP excretion and HbA1c but not with albumin excretion [20]. Others showed a correlation between RBP excretion and albumin but not HbA1 [30]. Neither study could relate RBP to duration of disease. Elsewhere, the excretion of NAG and RBP correlated with albumin excretion and with HbA1c [4]. Holm and others showed the increased excretion of RBP in IDD with no correlation to HbA1, fructosamine or urinary albumin [23,24].

The excretion of NAG has been shown to be the most sensitive tubular function marker in terms of increased excretion in diabetic subjects [27]. No study has yet shown a predictive value for tubular markers indicating progression of renal disease although none of them have been studied for as long as albumin.

The increased urinary excretion of haemoglobin has also been demonstrated in both IDD and NIDD. In the former group 12.5% of a group of patients with clinical proteinuria also had microscopic hematuria; in most attributed to a non-diabetic glomerulopathy [47]. In NIDD, Schmitz detected a positive correlation between urinary albumin and hemoglobin excretion (measured by an ELISA method) and proposed that occult hematuria and/or hemoglobinuria may often be present in diabetic patients with microalbuminuria [48].

More recently, the prevalence of increased excretion of hemoglobin has been investigated in juvenile and adult IDD and in NIDD after adequate stabilisation of the urine sample. Urinary hemoglobin concentration was increased above the upper limit of the adult non-diabetic reference range (8.8ug/mmol creatinine) in 32 and 33% of diabetic children and adults respectively with normal urinary albumin excretion (<3.3mg/mmol creatinine). There was no statistically significant relationship between the excretion of hemoglobin and of albumin, retinol-binding protein or NAG in normoalbuminuric adult diabetic subjects (unpublished observations).

Tubular markers and glycemic control

The increased excretion of these markers may be related particularly to changes in acute glycaemic control. In 1985, Miltenyi showed that NAG excretion was increased in diabetic children with ketoacidosis and glycosuria compared to well-controlled diabetic children and non-diabetic subjects. Excretion of the enzyme decreased with the establishment of diabetic control over eight days. However, NAG excretion continued to remain higher than in the non-diabetic controls suggesting than an abnormality in tubular function persisted [31].

One study has demonstrated the increased excretion of RBP in response to acute glucose and insulin infusion in subjects undergoing euglycaemic clamping [32]. There was no clamping of blood glucose in the non-diabetic controls in this study and the results could not be confirmed by others [33]. In a third study, acute hyperglycemia was shown to increase the excretion of albumin and of B2-microglobulin but not of kappa light-chains in normal subjects [25]. RBP excretion has also been shown to be increased in chronic heart disease [10].

Physiological variability in the excretion of these tubular proteins occurs as for albumin. Thus, normal volunteers show an acute increase in the excretion of tubular proteins in response to exercise and in the day-to day variability of pre-exercise samples [34].

METHODS FOR MEASUREMENT OF SPECIFIC URINARY PROTEINS

Albumin

Immunoassay techniques for the measurement of urinary albumin have been reviewed [35-37]. Approximately 70% of UK health service laboratories use immunoturbidimetry, approximately 20% use immunonephelometry and the remainder of laboratories a mixture of radio- or enzyme-immunoassays. Commercial kits for urinary albumin measurement are available although in-house methods are easy to establish and maintain. Overall, the between-laboratory agreement of the different assay types is similar; results from the UK External Quality Assessment Scheme for urinary albumin are shown in Fig 18-2.

Immunoturbidimetry lacks the sensitivity to detect reliably normal albumin excretion which is frequently less than 5mg/L. It is therefore less suitable than the more sensitive immunoassays for use in research applications. Immunonephelometric methods have adequate sensitivity to measure urinary albumin excretion within the normal range and can be automated onto platforms such as the Behring BN range of analysers. Accuracy and precision appear good compared to immunoturbidimetric methods. The more sensitive RIA and ELISA methods require assay desensitisation or sample dilution before use.

A common problem with many of the competitive immunoassays for urinary albumin is that of "antigen-excess" detection. In a recent return of United Kingdom EQA reports approximately 17 percent of laboratories failed to detect a high concentration of albumin in one sample. It should be standard practice to test using dip-sticks each sample before analysis for microalbuminuria, unless the analyser has an adequate protocol for the detection of "antigen-excess".

An alternative non-immunassay dye-binding method has been published. The method has adequate sensitivity (detection limit 1mg/L) to detect albumin concentrations into the normal range, correlates well with immunonephelometry and does not produce false-negative results at high albumin concentrations [52].

"Tubular" proteins

High sensitivity immunoassays using ELISA [4], RIA [30]and latex-agglutination [14] methods have been described for the detection of proteins such as RBP and B2-microglobulin into the normal range. Most methods for the analysis of NAG use p-nitrophenyl-N-acetyl-B-D- glucosamide as substrate [4,26]. Such enzymic methods are easily automated on modern laboratory analysers.

Haemoglobin

Measurement of haemoglobin in urine by immunoassay requires preservation of the sample. There are large and variable losses of hemoglobin immunoreactivity with time after urine collection which are not avoided by immediate freezing and storage of the sample at -20oC. Voiding of the sample into a buffer/serum albumin solution is necessary for adequate sample preservation [49].

Type of urine sample for measurement of albumin

Although urine can be stored at +4o for at least 7 days before analysis and for longer if sodium azide is added as preservative [37], storage at -20oC may result in losses of albumin from urine and from standard solutions, particularly at low concentration. Two studies have investigated the loss of albumin following 2 months, 6 months and 2 years at -20oC and have shown variable but marked losses of 28 and 39% a nd 27 and 50% at 6 months and at 2 years for albumin/creatinine (ACR) and NAG/creatinine ratios respectively [19,38]. Creatinine concentration also decreased over 2 years. In contrast to these reports another study found no effect of storage for up to 6 months at -20oC nor the type of storage container nor the presence or lack of centrifugation on urinary albumin concentration [46]. Two recent studies show the importance of adequate mixing of samples before analysis after frozen storage and conclude that in most samples the original albumin concentration is retained after this treatment. However, the albumin concentration is truly decreased in a small proportion of samples [53,54].

There is little deterioration in RBP levels in urine samples stored at -20oC for 12 months (unpublished observations).

Near-patient testing

Several dipstick and tablet screening methods have been developed for the detection of microalbuminuria in clinics and are reviewed elsewhere in this book. They may provide a useful screen but positive cases need to be followed up by quantitative measurement of urinary albumin in the laboratory and by correction of the concentration by time or by creatinine concentration.

Recently, the Bayer Corporation has produced a modification of the DCA 2000™ HbA1c analyser to also provide a quantitative urinary albumin and creatinine result and a calculated albumin/creatinine ratio. The DCA 2000+ analyser is self-calibrating and its immunoturbidimetric assay for albumin correlates closely with an established laboratory method (Dr D Newman, unpublished observations). A result is available within 8 minutes and the assay would appear to offer a significant advantage over existing methods in providing an accurate result at the diabetic clinic.

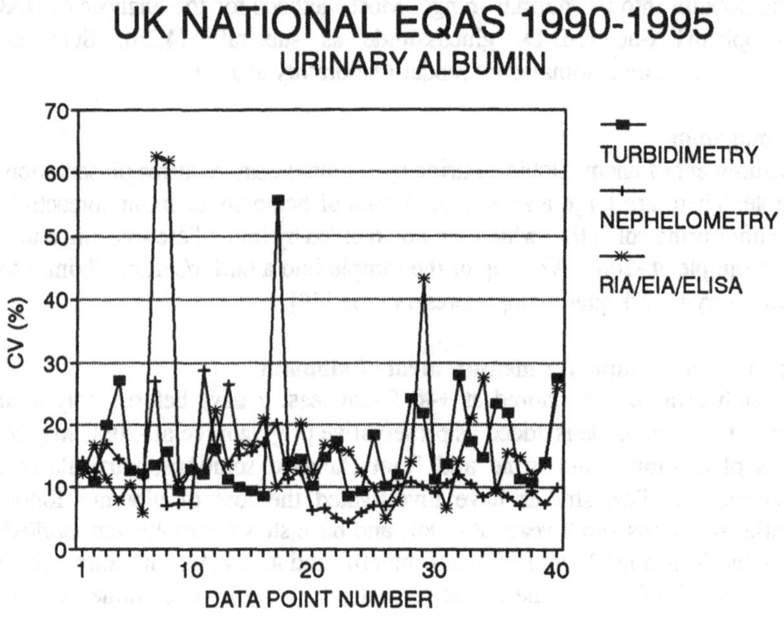

Figure 18-2 United Kingdom National External Quality Assurance data

Which urine sample to screen for microalbuminuria?

Gatling assessed the ability of an overnight ACR, an overnight albumin concentration or a random ACR to predict a timed overnight albumin excretion rate (AER) of >30 ug/min. An overnight ACR was found to be the optimal screening test. A random ACR >3 mg/mmol had only 12% predictive value for AER >30 ug/min [39].

Marshall has recommended an early morning sample as being the best compromise to predict a "gold standard" overnight AER or ACR [40]. She reported sensitivity and specificity between 82-100% and between 74-100% respectively from several independent studies depending on the cutoffs set for ACR and for microalbuminuria. The data for random clinic samples indicated sensitivities between 56-100% and specificities between 81-96% respectively. She suggested that if early morning ACR was <3.5 mg/mmol then the patient be considered normal and be rescreened annually. If >10 mg/mmol then active treatment is indicated. If 3.6-10 mg/mmol then the patient be rescreened at the next clinic visit. Others have argued that there may be unacceptable delay clinically with a cutoff of 3.5 mg/mmol and annual retesting. THey recommend a lower cutoff of 2 mg/mmol in this situation [39]. Both authors suggest that attempts to assess microalbuminuria on the basis of concentration alone are not valid. Kouri concluded that the false positive and false negative rates incurred with testing random clinic samples were unacceptable clinically and placed unnecessary work upon hospital laboratories [41]. Bouhanick however, stated that a single random clinic sample uncorrected for creatinine or for time could predict persistent microalbuminuria or clinical proteinuria in 24 hour samples (sensitivity 83%, specificity 82%, positive predictive value 69%, concordance 80%) [42]. Importantly there are differences between men and women in ACR because of lower excretion of creatinine in women (~50% higher in men). This results in a higher ratio in women [43]. The most appropriate sample to screen for developing microalbuminuria in young diabetics has also been studied. In 104 young diabetics an albumin/creatinine ratio >1.9mg/mmol was found to predict microalbuminuria defined on the basis of timed overnight collections with a specificity of 93% and sensitivity of 97%. 12.5% of the population had microalbuminuria [50]. Although young diabetics have a lower prevalence of microalbuminuria than do their adult counterparts, it is important to recognise and treat the condition early through improved metabolic control and the possible use of angiotensin-converting enzyme inhibitors [51].

There is no long-term study available to suggest that strictly normoalbuminuric patients (at baseline) with exercise-induced microalbuminuria progress more readily than patients with only a small response in albuminuria to exercise.

Variability of urinary albumin

Variability in assay methods is relatively small in comparison to physiological variation. This creates major difficulties in the interpretation of changes in urinary albumin excretion in adult and juvenile diabetics and non-diabetics. Urinary albumin excretion may fluctuate by more than 100% and indicates the need to average multiple measurements on an individual before deciding on intervention. In addition, upright posture and exercise may both increase the excretion of albumin [43]. These factors may explain the variability in reference ranges between 24-hour, overnight and random daytime samples [44].

CONCLUSIONS

Techniques for the measurement of urinary albumin are routine in many laboratories. The type of technique should be dictated by the sensitivity required for the population under study.

Storage of urine samples deep-frozen may result in variable losses of albumin and of NAG. RBP appears to be stable at -20oC for at least 6 months.

Measurement of an albumin/creatinine ratio on an early morning sample is recommended for screening purposes.

Multiple samples are needed to confirm persistent microalbuminuria.

Excretion of tubular proteins may reflect changes in acute glycaemic control more clearly than that of albumin.

Excretion of hemoglobin appears to be increased in both young and adult IDD and NIDD, irrespective of the presence or absence of microalbuminuria or clinical proteinuria

No studies have yet shown a relation between tubular proteinuria and progression of renal disease.

B2-microglobulin measurement should only be used as a marker of renal tubular function after prior alkalinisation of the subject.

REFERENCES

1. Mogensen CE Christensen CK Predicting diabetic nephropathy in insulin-dependent patients. New Eng J Med 1984; 311: 89-93
2. Viberti GC, Jarrett RJ, Mahmud et al. Microalbuminuria as a predictor of clinical nephropathy in insulin-dependent diabetes mellitus. Lancet 1982;1: 1430-2.
3. Mathiesen ER Oxenboll B, Johansen K et al Incipient nephropathy in type 1 (insulin-dependent) diabetes Diabetologia 1984; 26: 406-10
4. Gibb DM, Tomlinson PA, Dalton NR et al Renal tubular proteinuria and microalbuminuria in diabetic patients. Arch Dis Child 1989; 64: 129-134
5. Davies AG, Price DA, Postlethwaite RJ et al. Renal function in diabetes mellitus. Arch Dis Child 1985; 60: 299-304
6. Rowe DJF, Hayward M, Bagga H, Betts P Effect of glycaemic control and duration of disease on overnight albumin excretion in diabetic children. Brit Med J 1984;289: 957-959
7. Mogensen CE Microalbuminuria predicts clinical proteinuria and early mortality in maturity-onset diabetes.
New Eng J Med 1984;310:356-60
8. Marshall SM Alberti KGMM Comparison of the prevalence and associated features of abnormal albumin excretion in insulin-dependent and non-insulin-dependent diabetes. Quart J Med 1989;261:61-71
9. Christensen CK The pre-proteinuric phase of diabetic nephropathy. Danish Med Bull 1991;38:145-59
10. Ellekilde G, Holm J, von Eyben FE, Hemmingsen L. Above-normal urinary excretion of albumin and retinol-binding protein in chronic heart failure. Clin Chem 1992; 38: 593-4
11. Gero G, Anthony F, Davis M et al Retinol binding protein, albumin and total protein excretion patterns during normal pregnancy. J Obst and Gyn 1987; 8: 104-108
12. Damsgaard EM, Froland A, Jorgensen OD, Mogensen CE. Microalbuminuria as predictor of increased mortality in elderly people. Brit Med J 1990; 300: 297-300
13. Yudkin JS, Forrest RD, Jackson CA. Microalbuminuria as predictor of vascular disease in non-diabetic subjects. Lancet 1988; ii: 530-3.
14. Bernard AM, Moreau D, Lauwreys R Comparison of retinol-binding protein and B2-microglobulin determination in urine for the early detection of tubular proteinuria. Clin Chim Acta 1982; 126:1-7
15. Forsblom CM, Groop P-H, Ekstrand A, Groop LC. Predictive value of microalbuminuria in patients with insulin-dependent diabetes of long duration. Brit Med J 1992; 305: 1051-1053
16. Mansell P, Twyman SJ, Rowe DJF et al Urinary albumin excretion in longitudinal samples in a young diabetic population. British Diabetic Association meeting; Spring 1993, University of Liverpool: A15
17. Chavers BM, Bilous RW, Ellis EN et al Glomerular lesions and urinary albumin excretion in type 1 diabetes without overt proteinuria. New Eng J Med 1989;320:966-70

18. Watts GF, Powell M, Rowe DJF, Shaw KM. Low molecular weight proteinuria in insulin-dependent diabetes mellitus: a study of the urinary excretion of B2-microglobulin and retinol-binding protein in alkalinised patients with and without microalbuminuria.
Diabetes Res 1989;12:31-36
19. Elving LD, Bakkeren JAJM, Jansen MJH et al. Screening for microalbuminuria in patients with diabetes mellitus: frozen storage of urine samples decreases their albumin content.
Clin Chem 1989; 35: 308-10
20. Pontuch P, Jensen T, Deckert T et al. Urinary excretion of retinol-binding protein in type 1 (insulin-dependent) diabetic patients with microalbuminuria and clinical diabetic nephropathy. Acta Diabetologia 1992; 28: 206-10
21. Lervang H-H, Jensen S, Brochner-Mortensen J, Ditzel J. Does increased glomerular filtration rate or disturbed tubular function early in the course of childhood type 1 diabetes predict the development of nephropathy. Diab Med 1992; 9:635-40.
22. Walton C, Bodansky HJ, Wales JK et al Tubular dysfunction and microalbuminuria in insulin dependent diabetes.
Arch Dis Child 1988;63:244-9
23. Holm J, Hemmingsen L, Neilsen NV Thomsen M Increased urinary excretion of the retinol-binding protein in insulin-dependent diabetes mellitus in the absence of microalbuminuria.
Clin Chim Acta 1987;170:345-50
24. Holm J, Hemmingsen L, Neilsen NV Relationship between the urinary excretion of albumin and retinol-binding protein in insulin-dependent diabetics. Clin Chim Acta 1988;177:101-6
25. Groop L, Makipernaa A, Stenman S et al Urinary excretion of kappa light chains in patients with diabetes mellitus.
Kidney Int 1990;37:1120-5
26. Skrha J, Haas T, Sperl M et al A six-year follow-up of the relationship between n-acetyl B-D glucosaminidase and albuminuria in relation to retinopathy. Diab Med 1991;8:817-21
27. Jung K, Pergande M, Schimke E et al Urinary enzymes and low-molecular-mass proteins as indicators of diabetic nephropathy.
Clin Chem 1988;34 544-547
28. Twyman SJ, Rowe DJF Relationship of n-acetyl B-D-glucosaminidase, retinol-binding protein and albumin to glycaemic control in young diabetic subjects.
Ann Clin Biochem 1993; Proceedings of National Meeting C53
29. Twyman SJ, Rowe DJF The reduction in excretion of a tubular protein and albumin by improved glycaemic control in diabetics.
Annales de Biologie Clinique 1993;51:Eur Cong of Clin Chem Abstr 175
30. Rowe DJF, Anthony F, Polak A, et al. Retinol binding protein as a small molecular weight marker of renal tubular function in diabetes mellitus. Ann Clin Biochem. 1987; 24: 477-82
31. Miltenyi M, Korner A, Tulassay T, Szabo A. Tubular dysfunction in type 1 diabetes mellitus. Arch Dis Child. 1985; 60: 929-31
32. Catalano et al Effect of posture and acute glycemic control on the excretion of retinol-binding protein in normoalbuminuric insulin-dependent diabetic patients. Clin Sci 1993;84:461-467
33. Rowe DJF, Twyman SJ, Mansell P, Bisson D Excretion of retinol-binding protein in non-diabetic subjects undergoing a glucose and insulin clamp. British Diabetic Association, Autumn meeting, September 1993.
34. Cooper T, Davies R, Linton D, Rowe DJF. The effect of strenuous exercise on urinary excretion of albumin and retinol-binding protein. Ann Clin Biochem 1989; Proceedings of National Meeting: No 204
35. Gatling W, Rowe DJF, Hill RD Microalbuminuria: an appraisal of assay techniques and urine collection procedures for measuring urinary albumin at low concentrations *in* THE KIDNEY AND HYPERTENSION IN DIABETES MELLITUS Mogensen CE (ed) 1988 Martinus Nijhoff Publishing, Boston
36. Watts GF, Bennett JE, Rowe DJ et al Assessment of immunochemical methods for determining low concentrations of albumin in urine.
Clin Chem 1986;32:1544-8
37. Rowe DJF, Dawnay A, Watts GF Microalbuminuria in diabetes mellitus: review and recommendations for the measurement of albumin in urine. Ann Clin Biochem 1990; 27: 297-312

38. Manley SE, Burton ME, Fisher KE et al. Decreases in albumin/creatinine and N-Acetylglucosaminidase/creatinine ratios in urines samples stored at -20oC. Clin Chem 1992; 38: 2294-2299
39. Gatling W, Knight C, Mullee MA, Hill RD. Microalbuminuria in diabetes: a population study of the prevalence and an assessment of three screening tests. Diab Med 1988; 5: 343-47
40. Marshall SM Screening for microalbuminuria: which measurement. Diab Med 1991; 8: 706-11
41. Kouri TT, Viikari JS, Mattila KS, Irjala KM Microalbuminuria: Invalidity of simple concentration-based screening tests for early nephropathy due to urinary volumes of diabetic patients. Diabetes Care 1991; 14: 591-3
42. Bouhanick B, Berrut G, Chameau AM, et al. Predictive value of testing random urine sample to detect microalbuminuria in diabetic subjects during outpatient visit. Diabete et Metabolisme 1992; 18: 54-58
43. Connell SJ, Hollis S, Teiszen KL, McMurray JR, Dornan TL. Gender and the clinical usefulness of the albumin:creatinine ratio. Diabetic Med 1994;11:32-36
44. Rowe DJF, Bagga H, Betts P. Normal variation in the rate of albumin excretion and albumin to creatinine ratios in overnight and daytime urine collections in non-diabetic children. Brit Med J 1985; 291: 693-694
45. Watts GF, Morris RW, Khan K, Polak A Urinary albumin excretion in healthy adult subjects: reference values and some factors affecting their interpretation. Clin Chim Acta 1988;172:191-8
46. Collins AC, Sethi M, MacDonald FA et al Storage temperature and differing methods of sample preparation in the measurement of urinary albumin. Diabetologia 1993;36:993-7
47. Hommel E, Carstensen H, Skott P, Larsen S, Parving H-H Prevalence and causes of microscopic hematuria in Type I1 (insulin-dependent) diabetic patients with persistent proteinuria. Diabetologia 1987;30:627-30.
48. Schmitz A Increased urinary hemoglobin in diabetics with microalbuminuria - measured by an ELISA. Scand J Clin Lab Invest 1990;50:303-8
49. Twyman S, Rowe DJF A sensitive radioimmunoassay for the determination of haemoglobin in urine Ann Clin Biochem 1995;32:506-508
50. Shield JP, Hunt LP, Baum JD, Pennock CA Screening for diabetic microalbuminuria in routine clinical care: which method? Arch Dis Child 1995;72:524-525
51. Campbell FM Microalbuminuria and nephropathy in insulin dependent diabetes mellitus. Arch Dis Child 1995;73:4-7
52. Kessler MA, Meinitzer A, Petek W, Wolfbeis OS Microalbuminuria and borderline-increased albumin excretion determined with a centrifugal analyser and the Albumin Blue 580 fluorescence assay Clin Chem 1997; 43:996-1002.
53. Townsend JR, Sadler WA, Shanks GM The effect of storage pH on the precipitation of proteins and deep-frozen urine samples J Clin Biochem 1987;24:111-2
54. Innanen VT, Groom BM, de Campos FM Microalbumin and Freezing Clin Chem 1997;43:1093-4

19. OFFICE TESTS FOR MICROALBUMINURIA

Per Løgstrup Poulsen
Medical Department M, Aarhus Kommunehospital, Aarhus, Denmark

INTRODUCTION

Microalbuminuria defined as an increase in urinary albumin excretion rate to the range 20-200 μg/min not only predicts later development of nephropathy in diabetic subjects [1-4] but may also guide the detection or prediction of other complications e.g. proliferative retinopathy [5,6]. In addition, microalbuminuria is also strongly associated with cardiovascular risk factors and coronary heart disease in diabetic as well as non-diabetic patients [7,8].

The clinical usefulness of the versatile and strong predictive power of microalbuminuria has been further augmented as it has now been shown that effective intervention modalities exist. Several studies have shown that antihypertensive treatment of normotensive (maybe certainly a debatable concept) microalbuminuric IDDM patients reduces urinary albumin excretion rate considerably and probably postpones or prevents clinical nephropathy [9-14]. Furthermore, it is now established that achievement of good glycemic control has similar beneficial effects [15-17].

The strong predictive power in combination with effective treatment modalities clearly indicates that screening for microalbuminuria should be an essential part of the care for IDDM patients [18].

THE INTRA-INDIVIDUAL VARIATION OF URINARY ALBUMIN EXCRETION - SCREENING AS A CONTINUOUS PROCESS

There is considerable intra-individual variation in urinary albumin excretion, up to 40-50% [19] or even greater when measuring albumin concentrations or albumin:creatinine ratios under routine clinical conditions [20]. Thus, several samples should be taken in order to avoid misclassification of patients and screening should be a continuous process.

There is now a consensus e.g. in the St. Vincent document that persons with IDDM should be screened at least once every year and more often if microalbuminuria is detected. As the prevalence of microalbuminuria in IDDM is very low before five years diabetes duration [21] annual screening could be initiated at this point.

HOW TO SCREEN - TIMED COLLECTIONS OR ALBUMIN CONCENTRATION?

Timed urinary collections (24 h or overnight) remains the 'gold standard'. However, they are cumbersome to the patient, and in repeated large scale screening this may become a significant problem [22]. In one large study a patient compliance of only 59% was reported [23]. It should be emphasized that these figures are obtained under study conditions and that compliance may well turn out to be further reduced with repeated screening in clinical practice.

Aggravating this problem is the fact that diabetic nephropathy is often seen in 'non attenders' to diabetic care [24] who presumably have even less patience with cumbersome screening tests.

In addition, timed urinary collections are subject to collection errors or timing errors which can make the interpretation of results difficult, though creatinine concentration measurements and calculation of albumin:creatinine ratio may be helpful. As women excrete less creatinine than males, sex specific cut of points for albumine/creatinine ratios are recommended: 2.5 mg/mmol for men and 3.5 mg/mmol for women [25].

In order to assure good compliance it is crucial that screening procedures are acceptable to the patients.

OFFICE TEST: ADVANTAGES AND DISADVANTAGES

In general, office tests for detecting abnormal albuminuria should be simple in use, robust, quick, inexpensive and have sufficient specificity and sensibility. Several tests have now been evaluated [26-41]. They all share the advantage of bringing the result of test closer to the patient. It is possible to get the result before the patient leaves the outpatient clinic or the general practitioner. On the basis of the result, immediately action can be taken, whether it is arrangement of annual rescreening (negative test) or in the case of a positive test e.g. arrange collection of timed urinary samples to assess urinary albumin excretion rate.

Several office tests seem to fulfil the requirements of adequate sensitivity, specificity and reproducibility. However, it should be noted, that all the tests are critically dependent on correct handling. Thus, training in the use of the stick must have high priority and continuous monitoring of results is recommendable.

As to costs analysis regarding quantitative lab methods vs. semiquantitative office tests the result will depend on the local organization of the health system: If a majority of diabetic patients are seen in large outpatients clinics automated laboratory procedures (e.g. turbimetric methods) can be set up permitting a large number of samples to be processed in a minimum of time, at a very low cost -- probably below the price of the office tests. If, on the other hand, the care for diabetic patients is mainly in the hands of general practitioners costs of sending the samples to the laboratory should be taken into account and economy may point towards office tests.

EVALUATION OF THE PERFORMANCE OF OFFICE TESTS FOR MICROALBUMINURIA

The Micral-Test®II test-strip (Boehringer Mannheim GmbH, Mannheim) is a gold labelled optically read immuno-assay to detect albumin in urine samples. By dipping the test strip into a urine sample urine passes via a wick fleece into the conjugate fleece. Any albumin present in the sample binds itself specifically to the gold labelled antibodies. Excess antibodies are bound by immobilized albumin in the capture matrix. Only antibodies bound to albumin from the urine can pass through. These gold labelled antibodies flow to the detection pad and turn it red. The reaction time is one minute. The colour is visually compared to colour blocks on a chart attached to the vial with colours representing 0 mg/l, 20 mg/l, 50 mg/l and 100 mg/l albumin. In our evaluation of this second generation strip[39], 263 urinary samples representing a broad spectrum of albumin concentrations (0-200 mg/l) were tested blindly by 5 laboratory technicians and compared with a nephelometric method. With cut off point for abnormal albumin concentration of ≥ 15 mg/l (respectively ≥ 20 mg/l), sensitivity was 95% (97%), specificity 93% (72 %), predictive value of positive test 97% (84%), and predictive value of negative test 88% (94%). The percentage of correctly classified samples was 95% (87%). The distribution of nephelometric values for strips assigned to each of the four test-strip colour bands (0. 20, 50 and 100 mg/l) is depicted in Figures 19-1 and 19-2.

The stability of the reaction colour over time was tested as this was a crucial point for the predecessor, making the exactly correct reading time absolutely necessary. Five laboratory technicians tested each 20 urinary samples with readings after 2, 15, and 60 min, and 24 hour. Results are given in table 19-1. Readings after 2, 15, and 60 min. gave results identical to reading after 1 min, whereas reading after 24 h became increasingly difficult with deviations from baseline values.

In a recent large multicenter evaluation of the Micral-Test®II strip in eight European study sites[40], 2228 urine samples from diabetic patients were investigated. For a cutoff concentration of 20 mg/l with respect to the routine methods, a sensitivity of 96.7% and a specificity of 71% were calculated for the Micral-Test®II test-strip. The negative predictive value was 0.95 and the positive predictive value 0.78 with a prevalence of positive samples (laboratory method) of 52%. The interperson variability of colour interpretation showed 93% concordant readings.

These data indicates that Micral-Test®II provides an accurate tool for the detection of microalbuminuria. The stability of the reaction colour over time constitutes a significant advantage compared to previous strips.

As previously mentioned, the spot urine albumin-to-creatinine ratio accounts for possible errors in urine concentration. Immediate albumin-to-creatinine assays have not been available until now.

We have recently evaluated a new test for immediate and quantitative determination of urinary albumin-to-creatinine ratio[41]. The DCA 2000® microalbumin/creatinine assay system detects albumin by a immunoturbidimetric direct antibody-antigen aggregation and measures creatinine colorimetrically using the Benedict-Behre reaction. Results are available in 7 minutes without sample dilution, reagent preparation, or wet calibration. Specimens from diabetic patients were screened consequtively in our outpatient clinic using a dipstick test. Specimens which were negative for proteinuria (n=195) were tested blindly by three nurses and the DCA 2000 results were compared to those of our routine method (a immunoturbidimetric essay). Of those specimens 40.5% were classified as positive for microalbuminuria using our routine laboratory method with cutoff albumin-to-creatinine ratios of 2.5 mg/mmol for males and 3.5 mg/mmol for females. Results are depicted in figure 19-3 and in table 19-2.

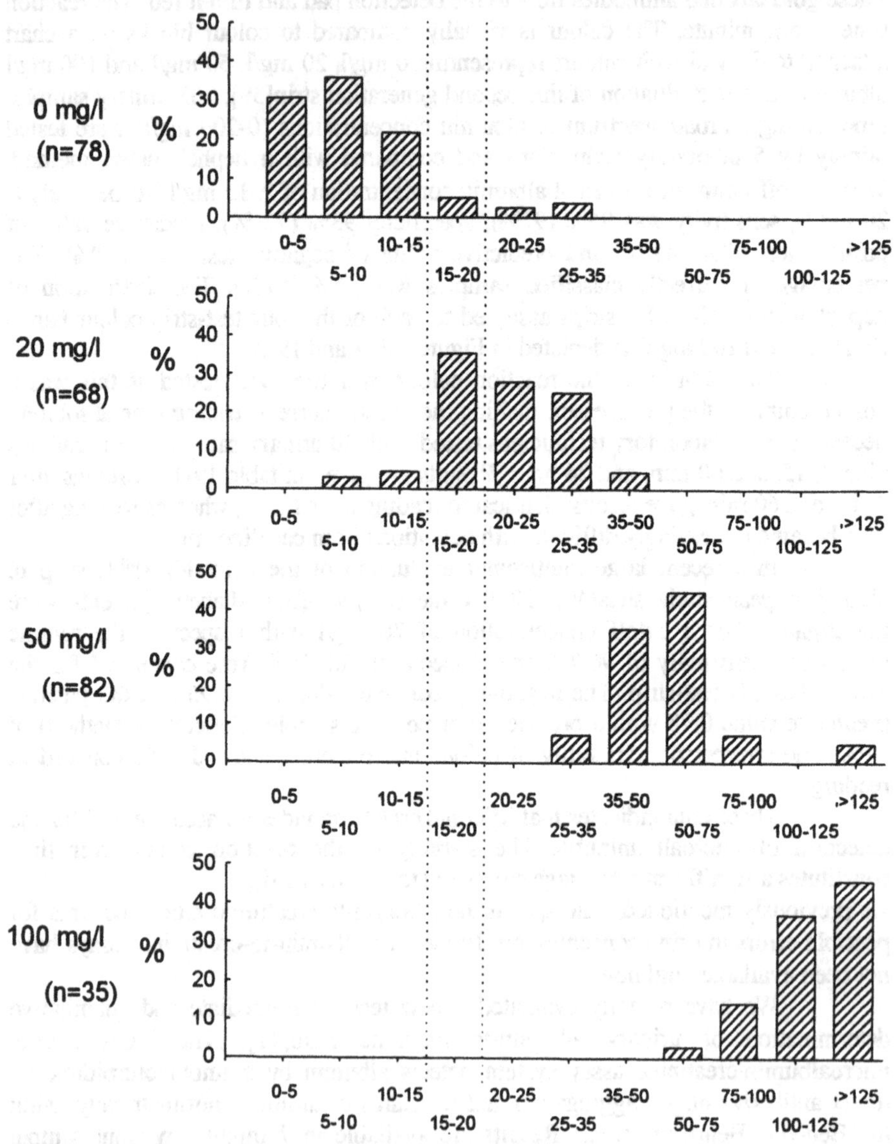

Figure 19-1. Micral-Test® II. Each histogram describes the distribution of nephelometric values for strips assigned to one of the four test-strip colour bands: 0, 20, 50 and 100 mg/l. Published by permission [39].

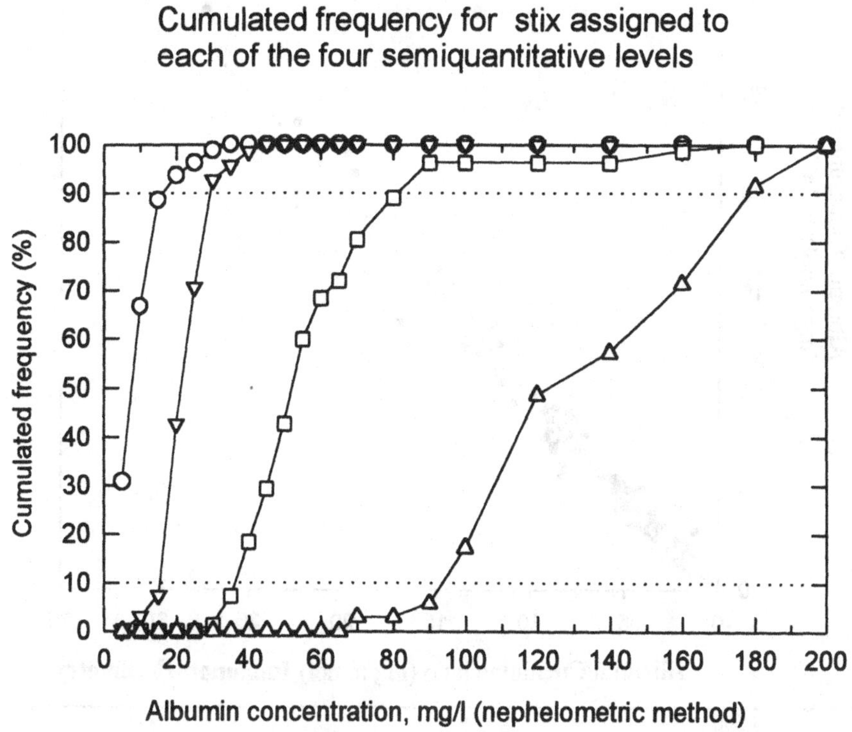

Figure 19-2. Micral-Test® II. Each curve describes the cumulated frequency for stix assigned to each of the four semiquantitative levels (0, 20, 50 and 100 mg/l). Stix read as: o: 0 mg/l, n=78; v: 20 mg/l, n=68; □: 50 mg/l, n=82; ∇: 100 mg/l, n=35.

Observer	2 min	15 min	60 min	24 hour
A	20	20	19 (1↑)	20
B	20	20	20	20
C	20	18 (2↑)	19 (1↑)	18(2↑)
D	19(1↑)	19(1↑)	18 (2↑)	14(6↑)
E	20	20	18(2↑)	12(2↓,1↑.5?)

Table 19-1. Micral-Test® II. The stability of the reaction colour over time: Five observers (A, B, C, D and E) each read 20 stix. The figures indicate # of stix identical to initial readings and deviations (↑: One step higher, ↓: One step lower, ?: Unable to determine).

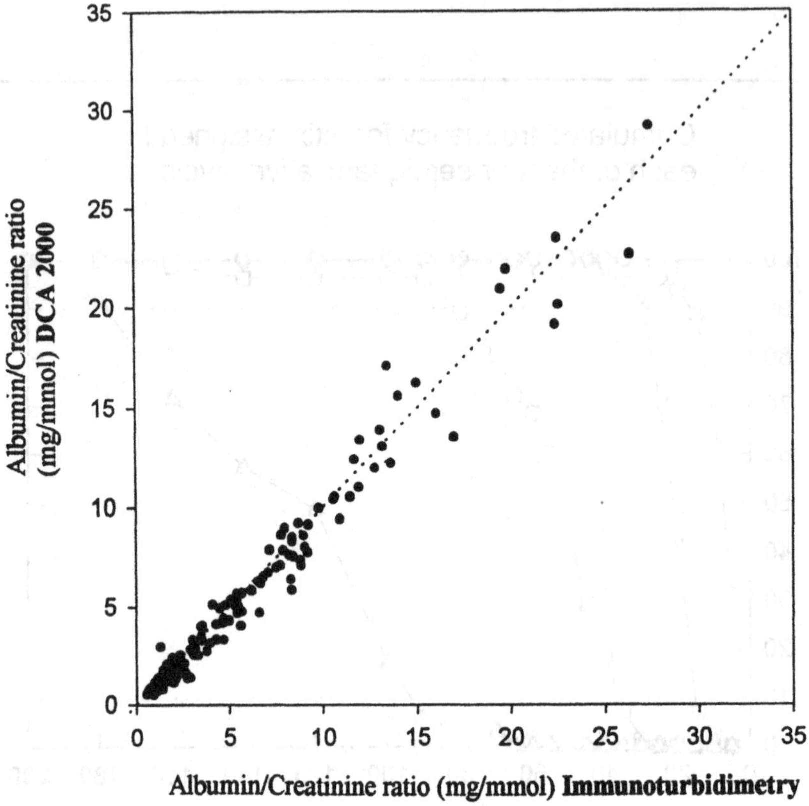

Figure 19-3. Albumin/creatinine ratios from non-proteinuric diabetic patients tested with DCA2000 and immunoturbudimetry (n=195, r=0.987, $p<10^{-5}$). (Published by permission)[41].

	A/C ratio by routine test Normal		Total
A/C ratio by DCA 2000® Normal	114	7	121
Abnormal	2	72	74
Total	116	79	195

Table 19-2 Cut-off for abnormal A/C ratio: 2.5 mg/mmol for males and 3.5 mg/mmol for females

The sensitivity was 91.1%, specificity 98.3%, the predictive value of a positive test 97.3%, and the predictive value of a negative test 94.2%. Our data indicate that the DCA 2000® microalbumin/creatinine assay provides an immediate, quantitative, and accurate tool for the detection of microalbuminuria. It complements the DCA 2000® hemoglobin A_{1c} assay in the care of diabetes.

SUMMARY

Several reliable office tests for detecting microalbuminuria exist. They share the advantage of providing results before the patient leaves the outpatients clinic or the general practitioner. Whether the tests are economically attractive will depend on the local organization of the health system. The tests are critically dependent on correct handling although second generation tests have improved in this respect. Training in the use of the tests is important and continuous monitoring of results is recommendable.

REFERENCES

1. Viberti GC, Hill RD, Jarrett RJ, Argyropoulos A, Mahmud U, Keen H. Microalbuminuria as a predictor of clinical nephropathy in insulin-dependent diabetes mellitus. Lancet 1982; i: 1430-1432.
2. Parving H-H, Oxenbøll B, Johansen K, Svendsen PA, Christiansen JS, Andersen AR. Early detection of patients at risk of developing diabetic nephropathy: a longitudinal study of urinary albumin excretion. Acta Endocrinol (Copenh) 1982; 100: 500-505.
3. Mogensen CE, Christensen CK. Predicting diabetic nephropathy in insulin-dependent patients. N Engl J Med 1984; 311: 89-93.
4. Mathiesen ER, Oxenbøll B, Johansen K, Svendsen PA, Deckert T. Incipient nephropathy in type 1 (insulin-dependent) diabetes. Diabetologia 1984; 26: 406-410.
5. Vigstrup J, Mogensen CE. Proliferative diabetic retinopathy: at risk patients identified by early detection of microalbuminuria. Acta Ophthalmol (Copenh) 1985; 63: 530-534.
6. Parving H-H, Hommel E, Mathiesen E. Prevalence of microalbuminuria, arterial hypertension, retinopathy and neuropathy in patients with insulin dependent diabetes mellitus. BMJ 1988; 296: 156-160.
7. Damsgaard EM, Frøland A, Jørgensen OD, Mogensen CE. Microalbuminuria as a predictor of increased mortality in elderly people. BMJ 1990; 300: 297-300.
8. Yudkin JS, Forrest RD, Jackson CA. Microalbuminuria as a predictor of vascular disease in non-diabetic subjects. Lancet 1988; ii: 530-533.
9. Marre M, Chatellier G, Leblanc H, Guyene TT, Menard J, Passa P. Prevention of diabetic nephropathy with enalapril in normotensive diabetics with microalbuminuria. BMJ 1988; 297: 1092-1095.
10. Mathiesen ER, Hommel E, Giese J, Parving H-H. Efficacy of captopril in postponing nephropathy in normotensive insulin dependent diabetic patients with microalbuminuria. BMJ 1991; 303: 81-87.
11. Hallab M, Gallois Y, Chatellier G, Rohmer V, Fressinaud P, Marre M. Comparison of reduction in microalbuminuria by enalapril and hydrochlorothiazide in normotensive patients with insulin dependent diabetes. BMJ 1993; 306: 175-182.
12. Viberti GC, Mogensen CE, Groop L, Pauls JF for the European Microalbuminuria Captopril Study Group. Effect of captopril on progression to clinical proteinuria in patients with insulin-dependent diabetes mellitus and microalbuminuria. JAMA 1994; 271: 275-279.
13. The Microalbuminuria Captopril Study Group. Captopril reduces the risk of nephropathy in IDDM patients with microalbuminuria. Diabetologia 1996;39(5): 587-593.
14. The EUCLID Study Group : Randomised placebo-controlled trial of lisinopril in normotensive patients with insulin-dependent diabetes and normoalbuminuria or microalbuminuria. Lancet 1997; 349: 1787-1792.
15. The Kroc Collaborative Study Group. Blood glucose control and the evolution of diabetic retinopathy and albuminuria. N Engl J Med 1984; 311: 365-372.
16. Reichard P, Nilsson BY, Rosenqvist U. The effect of long-term intensified insulin treatment on the development of microvascular complications of diabetes mellitus. N Engl J Med 1993; 329: 304-309.

17. Feldt-Rasmussen B, Mathiesen ER, Jensen T, Lauritzen T, Deckert T. Effect of improved metabolic control on loss of kidney function in type 1 (insulin-dependent) diabetic patients: an update of the Steno studies. Diabetologia 1991; 34: 164-170.
18. Borch-Johnsen K, Wenzel H, Viberti GC, Mogensen CE. Is screening and intervention for microalbuminuria worthwhile in patients with insulin dependent diabetes? BMJ 1993; 306: 1722-1723.
19. Feldt-Rasmussen B, Mathiesen ER. Variability of urinary excretion in incipient diabetic nephropathy. Diabetic Nephropathy 1984; 3: 101-103.
20. Johnston J, Paterson KR, O'Reilly D. Estimating urinary albumin excretion rate of diabetic patients in clinical practice. BMJ 1993; 306: 493-494.
21. Marshall SM, Alberti KG. Comparison of the prevalence and associated features of abnormal albumin excretion in insulin-dependent and non-insulin-dependent diabetes. Q J Med 1989; 70: 61-71.
22. Hutchison AS, Paterson KR. Collecting urine for microalbumin assay. Diabetic Med 1988; 5: 527-532.
23. Gatling W, Knight C, Hill RD. Screening for early diabetic nephropathy: Which sample to detect microalbuminuria? Diabetic Med 1985; 2: 451-455.
24. Krolewski AS, Warram JH, Christlieb AR. The changing natural history of nephropathy in type I diabetes. Am J Med 1985; 78: 785-794.
25. Mogensen CE, Keane WF, Bennett PH, Jerums G, Parving H-H, Passa P, Steffes MW, Striker GE, Viberti CG: Prevention of diabetic renal disease with special reference to microalbuminuria. *Lancet* 346:1080-1084, 1995
26. Poulsen PL, Mogensen CE: Evaluation of a New Semiquantitative Stix for Microalbuminuria. Diabetes Care 8:732-733, 1995.
27. Schmitz A. Microalbutest: A new screening method for detection of microalbuminuria in diabetes mellitus. Uremia Invest 1985; 9: 79-84.
28. Leedman PJ, Nankervis A, Goodwin M, Ratnaike S. Assessment of the albuscreen microalbuminuria kit in diabetic outpatients. Med J Aust 1987; 147: 285-286.
29. Collins V, Zimmet P, Dowse GK, Finch CF. Performance of Micro-Bumintest tablets for detection of microalbuminuria in Nauruaans. Diabetes Res Clin Pract 1989; 6: 271-277.
30. Coonrod BA, Ellis D, Becker DJ, et al. Assessment of AlbuSure and its usefulness in identifying IDDM subjects at increased risk for developing clinical diabetic nephropathy. Diabetes Care 1989; 12: 389-393.
31. Bangstad HJ, Try K, Dahl Jørgensen K, Hanssen KF. New semiquantitative dipstick test for microalbuminuria. Diabetes Care 1991; 14: 1094-1097.
32. Jury DR, Mikkelsen DJ, Glen D, Dunn PJ. Assessment of Micral-Test microalbuminuria test strip in the laboratory and in diabetic outpatients. Ann Clin Biochem 1992; 29: 96-100.
33. Poulsen PL, Hansen B, Amby T, Terkelsen T, Mogensen CE. Evaluation of a dipstick test for microalbuminuria in three different clinical settings, including the correlation with urinary albumin excretion rate. Diabete Metab 1992; 18: 395-400.
34. Marshall SM, Shearing PA, Alberti KG. Micral-Test strips evaluated for screening for albuminuria. Clin Chem 1992; 38: 588-591.
35. Agardh CD. A new semiquantitative rapid test for screening for microalbuminuria. Pract Diabetes 1993; 10: 146-147.
36. Adamson CL, Kumar S, Sutcliffe H, France MW, Boulton AJM. Screening for strategies in the detection of microalbuminuria in insulin-dependent diabetic patients. Pract Diabetes 1993; 10: 142-144.
37. Jensen J-EB, Nielsen SH, Foged L, Holmegaard SN, Magid E. The Micral® test for diabetic microalbuminuria: predictive values as a function of prevalence. Scand J Clin Lab Invest 1996; 56: 117-122.
38. Pugia MJ, Lott JA, Clark LW, Parker DR, WallaceJF, Willis TW. Comparison of urine dipsticks with quantitative methods for microlbuminuria. Eur J Clin Biochem 1997; 35(9):693-700.
39. Poulsen PL., and Mogensen CE. Evaluation of a new semiquantitative stix for microalbuminuria *Diabetes Care*1995; 18:732-733.

40. Mogensen, C. E., G. C. Viberti, E. Peheim, D. Kutter, C. Hasslacher, W. Hofmann, R. Renner, M. Bojestig, P. L. Poulsen, G. Scott, J. Thoma, J. Kuefer, B. Nilsson, B. Gambke, P. Mueller, J. Steinbiss, and K. D. Willamovski. 1997. Multicenter evaluation of the Micral-testII test-strip, an immunological rapid test for the detection of microalbuminuria. *Diabetes Care* 1997; 20:1642-1646.

41. Poulsen PL. and CE. Mogensen. 1998. Clinical evaluation of a test for immediate and quantitative determination of urinary albumin-to-creatinine ratio. *Diabetes Care* 1998; 21:97-98.

20. EXERCISE AND THE KIDNEY IN DIABETES

Carl Erik Mogensen
Medical Department M, Aarhus Kommunehospital, Aarhus, Denmark

Exercise proteinuria has been known in many years. There are early descriptions of the phenomenon, but the first published reports of exercise-induced albuminuria is given by Collier in 1907, describing »functional albuminuria« in athletes [1]. Since then many papers on this topic related to normal renal physiology have been published [2-19]. The first to describe comprehensively haemodynamic effect of exercise in diabetes was the Swedish investigator T. Karlefors. He studied exercise tests in male diabetics and looked for instance at heart rate and systolic blood pressure raises [20]. A new era started around 1970 after the introduction of exact measurement of urinary albumin excretion rate, for instance by radioimmunoassay or other immuno-based techniques [21,22].

Regular physical exercise is usually recommended as part of the clinical care of diabetic patients of both categories of diabetes. However, exercise may also have important interaction in relation to vascular function and disease. It is well-known that diabetic nephropathy eventually may develop in about 1/3 of IDDM-patients [23,24] and also in a considerable of the number of NIDDM-patients. Patients with incipient and overt diabetic nephropathy are known to manifest generalized vascular complications, which could be exaggerated or complicated by the impact of exercise. Antihypertensive treatment and good metabolic control seems to be the most effective intervention measure in postponing progression of early and late renal disease [15,23]. It is important in this respect that exercise-induced blood pressure elevation is also reduced during antihypertensive treatment [15,25-29].

1. RENAL AND BLOOD PRESSURE RESPONSE TO EXERCISE IN HEALTHY INDIVIDUALS

Numerous studies have explored the acute and prolonged effects of exercise on renal haemodynamics, albuminuria and blood pressure. It is well-known that exercise, (e.g. on a bicycle ergometer), considerably increases blood pressure in direct relation to the exercise-load [11,30,31]. At the same time it can cause pronounced changes in renal function [32]. With severe acute exercise some decline in the glomerular filtration rate (GFR) and an even more pronounced reduction in renal plasma flow occurs. Thus the filtration fraction is considerably increased [32], and filtration pressure over the glomerular membrane is very likely increased. The latter may lead to an increase in urinary albumin excretion rate, especially with severe or prolonged exercise, even in normal individuals [31]. Such exercise induced changes in renal function are transient and usually after one hour at rest the haemodynamic pattern is again reversed [31,32]. There are no reports indicating that in otherwise healthy individuals, exercise-induced changes in renal function are deleterious in the long run. In other words, healthy individuals exposed to long-term exercise, by their jobs or their sport activities, do not appear to be more likely to develop renal disease.

2. RENAL AND BLOOD PRESSURE RESPONSE TO EXERCISE IN DIABETIC (IDDM) INDIVIDUALS

Karlefors, many years ago, examined the haemodynamic response to exercise in diabetic individuals with complications [20]. Since then, numerous studies have been performed to explore the renal and BP response to exercise in diabetic individuals [10-13,16,27,28,30-50], especially after it became possible to measure urinary proteins in small concentrations [21,22]. This review will focus on type 1 diabetes, since only little information is available on patients with type 2 diabetes [12,51,52].

Usually the baseline urinary albumin excretion rate is increased in newly diagnosed IDDM-patients, at least in those with very poor glycemic control [31]. This increase in albumin excretion rate is amplified by light and moderate physical exercise [31]. Beta-2-microglobulin excretion, a marker of tubular proteinuria, is normal suggesting that the changes are of glomerular origin [10]. It is also clear that glomerular hyperfiltration is often found at the time hyperglycemia is first diagnosed. With proper insulin treatment for a few weeks these renal abnormalities are normalized although some degree of glomerular hyperfiltration usually persists. Most IDDM-patients exhibit a normal baseline albumin excretion rate for the first five years after diagnosis [24], although new studies suggests that this is not universally the case [23].

3. NORMOALBUMINURIC DIABETIC INDIVIDUALS

In normoalbuminuric IDDM-individuals changes in GFR and RPF are observed in response to exercise, corresponding the responses in healthy persons. As in controls, there is a slight reduction in GFR during exercise and a more pronounced reduction in plasma flow resulting in an increased filtration fraction. Usually, filtration fraction is increased already at baseline in IDDM and this abnormality is amplified by exercise. Thus, an already abnormal filtration fraction is further increased [32]. It is therefore not surprising that exercise may lead to increased albumin excretion rate in a considerable proportion in diabetic individuals. Exercise-induced microalbuminuria in diabetes was first described in 1975 [11]. It soon became clear to us that the greatest increase in fact occurred immediately after exercise [10]. It should be stressed that this increase in albumin excretion is clearly of glomerular origin, since in beta-2-microglobulin excretion is not increased by exercise in these patients. Therefore, the exercise test reveals early glomerular changes or abnormalities [10].

In some studies exercise induced albuminuria was not different in normoalbuminuric patients with IDDM and healthy controls [36]. This may reflect differences in diabetes duration and also the nature of exercise test. Some investigators used a fixed exercise load, others a submaximal exercise load related to a calculated maximal exercise level [36].

It has been suggested that exercise-induced albuminuria (in normoalbuminuric individuals) could be a predictor of the later development of microalbuminuria in IDDM-patients, as suggested in a recent report [53]. However, no proper prospective long-term study with several follow-up examinations has been conducted to clarify completely this issue. Since there is a considerable variability in exercise-induced albuminuria in patients with normal baseline value, a priori, this test may not be very valid due to the variability of the response. Resting baseline values, (e.g. overnight collections or early morning urines) show a quite gradual increase in albumin excretion with time in patients progressing to microalbuminuria or overt renal disease. Therefore many longitudinal measurements of baseline values may be more useful than the exercise test, both in the clinical setting and in research projects. It should be remembered that baseline values for albumin excretion at rest also show considerable variability, but it is easy to do many repeated measurements. Another potential use of the exercise test would be to study the response to antihypertensive treatment. It may be considered beneficial if administration of a drug protects not only against an exercise-induced blood pressure elevation, but also ameliorated exercise-induced albuminuria [26-29].

Since exercise may induce microalbuminuria in normoalbuminuric individuals, care should be taken that urine samples after exercise are not used in the clinical follow-up of patients. In this context it be recommended that early morning urine is used in the follow-up of patients [23].

4. MICROALBUMINURIC DIABETIC INDIVIDUALS

IDDM-patients with microalbuminuria or incipient diabetic nephropathy usually show some increase in blood pressure in the baseline resting situation. This increase is further aggravated by physical exercise, and usually there is a correlation between the exercise-induced albuminuria and the blood pressure increase, induced by exercise [30]. As in patients with normoalbuminuria, the exercise-induced albuminuria in patients with microalbuminuria at rest is of glomerular origin [10,30,31]. It is likely that the increased systemic blood pressure response in microalbuminuric individuals is to some extent transmitted to the glomerulus, inducing a stretching effect on the glomerular structure and thus producing an increased glomerular passage of plasma protein molecules, in particular albumin. Whether the increased albuminuria caused by this mechanism promotes further renal damage is so far unknown, although it has been proposed that albuminuria in its own right may contribute to renal structural damage [23]. In diabetics, so far, there is no evidence that short-term periods of exercise, by provoking proteinuria, cause renal damage. However, this possibility can by no means be excluded.

5. OVERT PROTEINURIA

Overt proteinuria is characterized by large increases in urinary albumin excretion to rates, higher than 200 μg/min. With the development of proteinuria the decline in

GFR usually starts. It has been shown that exercise increases blood pressure abnormally in proteinuric diabetic individuals [20]. The clearance of large molecular dextran is also enhanced by exercise in these individuals [33]. This has been attributed to depletion of negative charges on the glomerular capillary wall; however, whether this phenomenon influences exercise-induced proteinuria is unknown. The influence of exercise on the clinical status of patients with overt nephropathy has been poorly investigated and warrants further studies.

6. THE DAILY LIFE EXERCISE SITUATION AND RENAL PROGNOSIS

As indicated, there may be a potential risk of more rapid progression of nephropathy in individuals who exercise intensively on a regular basis and thus have more exercise induced albuminuria and blood pressure rises during their daily life situation. There are definitive studies that address this important clinical issue. A study from Japan in a small series of patients, suggests that there is no difference in clinical outcome between individuals who exercised to a limited extent and heavily in their daily life situation [54]. Less questionable is the potential risk of severe exercise in patients with nephropathy who also have proliferative retinopathy, that could be adversely affected by a substantial blood pressure elevation.

7. EFFECT OF INTERVENTION PROGRAMMES ON EXERCISE-INDUCED ALBUMINURIA

It has been documented that exercise-induced albuminuria can be reduced by good metabolic control in patients with IDDM [31,43,48]. Exercise-induced albuminuria in IDDM patients can also be reduced short-term as well as long-term by antihypertensive treatment [26-28]. A similar effect of antihypertensive agents has also been observed in patients with essential hypertension [15,25,29]. Exercise induced albuminuria may be reduced by aspirin and dipyridamole, but further studies are needed [40]. Similar results were obtained by Giustina et al. [55] using Picotamide in NIDDM-patients.

8. PRAGMATIC EXERCISE RECOMMENDATIONS IN IDDM-PATIENTS

It is questionable if it is necessarily to implement specific exercise recommendations in the care of far most patients with incipient or overt nephropathy. Usually in patients with overt nephropathy, there is a self-limitation, because exercise capacity is usually limited in these individuals and thus the patients may be left on their own in the management of exercise. However, clearly it would not be prudent to recommend severe exercise or exorbitant sport activities in these individuals, even in the lack of clinical trials in this area. If specific types of exercise is recommended, is also uncertain. Obviously, it would be prudent to recommend light to moderate exercise, maybe on a daily life basis, to be included in the patients usual diabetes programme. This may also be useful for other reasons and such a proposal is unlikely to have any harmful effect on renal function. Severe and very severe exercise should be avoided.

Also, it is not known if daily life activities implicating severe exercise from the diagnosis of diabetes implies a poor prognosis. However, usually severe exercise at least irregular exercise is certainly not recommended, due to rapid changes in glycemic control, where as regular and limited exercise programmes on a daily basis may be useful.

9. NOTES REGARDING NIDDM

There are only few studies about exercise-induced albuminuria in type 2 diabetes [12,51,52]. Light to moderate exercise may also induce microalbuminuria in this disease entity and good control may ameliorate the abnormality [12]. Moderate exercise is of importance in the clinical management of NIDDM-patients, and there is no evidence that such a moderate degree of exercise has any adverse effect on renal prognosis, rather it should be encouraged. Such an exercise programme may also in the long run reduce the associated hypertension, although there are no clinical trials in this area. It is important to note that usually patients with type 2 diabetes are quite sedentary, and in the clinical management it is usually more advisable to propose exercise than the opposite.

REFERENCES

1. Collier W. Functional albuminuria in athletes. BMJ 1907; I: 4-6.
2. Campanacci L, Faccini L, Englaro E, Rustia R, Guarnieri GF, Barat R, Carraro M, De Zotti R, Micheli W. Exercise-induced proteinuria. Contr Nephrol 1981; 26: 31-41.
3. Castenfors J. Renal function during exercise. With special reference to exercise proteinuria and the release of renin. Acta Physiol Scand 1967; 70: Suppl. 293.
4. Clerico A, Giammattei C, Cecchini L, Lucchetti A, Cruschelli L, Penno G, Gregori G, Giampietro O. Exercise-induced proteinuria in well-trained athletes. Clin Chem 1990; 36: 562-564.
5. Houser MT, Jahn MF, Kobayashi A, Walburn J. Assessment of urinary protein excretion in the adolescent: Effect of body position and exercise. J Pediatr 1986; 109: 556-561.
6. Houser MT. Characterization of recumbent, ambulatory, and postexercise proteinuria in the adolescent. Pediatr Res 1987; 21: 442-446.
7. Huttunen N-P, Käär M-L, Pietiläinen M, Vierikko P, Reinilä M. Exercise-induced proteinuria in children and adolescents. Scand J Clin Lab Invest 1981; 41: 583-587.
8. Kachadorian WA, Johnson RE. Renal responses to various rates of exercise. J Appl Physiol 1970; 28: 748-752.
9. Krämer BK, Kernz M, Ress KM, Pfohl M, Müller GA, Schmülling R-M, Risler T. Influence of strenuous exercise on albumin excretion Clin Chem 1988; 34: 2516-2518.
10. Mogensen CE, Vittinghus E, Sølling E. Abnormal albumin excretion after two provocative renal tests in diabetes: Physical exercise and lysine injection. Kidney Int 1979; 16: 385-393.
11. Mogensen CE, Vittinghus E. Urinary albumin excretion during exercise in juvenile diabetes. A provocative test for early abnormalities. Scand J Clin Lab Invest 1975; 35: 295-300.
12. Mohamed A, Wilkin T, Leatherdale BA, Rowe D. Response of urinary albumin to submaximal exercise in newly diagnosed non-insulin dependent diabetes. BMJ 1984; 288: 1342-1343.
13. Nordgren H, Freyschuss U, Persson B. Blood pressure response to physical exercise in healthy adolescents and adolescents with insulin-dependent diabetes mellitus. Clin Sci 1994; 86: 425-432.
14. Osei K. Ambulatory and exercise-induced blood pressure responses in type I diabetic patients and normal subjects. Diabetes Res Clin Pract 1987; 3: 125-134.
15. Pedersen EB, Mogensen CE, Larsen JS. Effects of exercise on urinary excretion of albumin and beta-2-microglobulin in young patients with mild essential hypertension without treatment and during long-term propranolol treatment. Scand J Clin Lab Invest 1981; 41: 493-498.
16. Poortmans J, Dorchy H, Toussaint D. Urinary excretion of total proteins, albumin, and β_2-microglobulin during rest and exercise in diabetic adolescents with and without retinopathy. Diabetes Care 1982; 5: 617-623.
17. Poortmans JR. Postexercise proteinuria in humans. Facts and mechanisms. JAMA 1985; 253: 236-240.

18. Robertshaw M, Cheung CK, Fairly I, Swaminathan R. Protein excretion after prolonged exercise. Ann Clin Biochem 1993; 30: 34-37.

19. Taylor A. Some characteristics of exercise proteinuria. Clin Sci 1960; 19: 209-217.
45.Torffvit O, Castenfors J, Bengtsson U, Agardh CD. Exercise stimulation in insulin-dependent diabetics, normal increase in albuminuria with abnormal blood pressure response. Scand J Clin Lab Invest 1987; 47: 253-259.

20. Karlefors T. Circulatory studies during exercise with particular reference to diabetics. Acta Med Scand 1966; 180: Suppl. 449.

21. Keen H, Chlouverakis C. Urinary albumin excretion and diabetes mellitus. Lancet 1964; ii: 1155-1156.

22. Miles DW, Mogensen CE, Gundersen HJG. Radioimmunoassay for urinary albumin using a single antibody. Scand J Clin Lab Invest 1970; 26: 5-11.

23. Mogensen CE, Vestbo E, Poulsen PL, Christiansen C, Damsgaard EM, Eiskjær H, Frøland A, Hansen KW, Nielsen S, Mau Pedersen M. Microalbuminuria and potential confounders. A review and some observations on variability of urinary albumin excretion. Diabetes Care 1995; 18: 572-581.

24. Mogensen CE. Microalbuminuria, early blood pressure elevation, and diabetic renal disease. Current Opinion in Endocrinology and Diabetes 1994; 1: 239-247.

25. Christensen CK, Krusell LR. Acute and long-term effect of antihypertensive treatment on exercise induced microalbuminuria in essential hypertension. J Clin Hypertension 1987; 3: 704-712.

26. Christensen CK, Mogensen CE. Acute and long-term effect of antihypertensive treatment on exercise-induced albuminuria in incipient diabetic nephropathy. Scand J Clin Lab Invest 1986; 46: 553-559.

27. Romanelli G, Giustina A, Bossoni S, Caldonaxxo A, Cimino A, Cravarezza P, Giustina G. Short-term administration of captopril and nifedipine and exercise-induced albuminuria in normotensive diabetic patients with early-stage nephropathy. Diabetes 1990; 39: 1333-1338.

28. Romanelli G, Giustina A, Cimino A. Short term effect of captopril on microalbuminuria induced by exercise in normotensive diabetics. BMJ 1989; 298: 284-288.

29. Rångemark C, Lind H, Lindholm L, Hedner T, Samuelsson O. Lisinopril reduces postexercise albuminuria more effectively than atenolol in primary hypertension. Eur J Clin Pharmacol 1996; 49: 267-271.

30. Christensen CK. Abnormal albuminuria and blood pressure rise in incipient diabetic nephropathy induced by exercise. Kidney Int 1984; 25: 819-823.

31. Vittinghus E, Mogensen CE. Graded exercise and protein excretion in diabetic man and the effect of insulin treatment. Kidney Int 1982; 21: 725-729.

32. Vittinghus E, Mogensen CE. Albumin excretion and renal haemodynamic response to physical exercise in normal and diabetic man. Scand J Clin Lab Invest 1981; 41: 627-632.

33. Ala-Houhala I. Effects of exercise on glomerular passage of macromolecules in patients with diabetic nephropathy and in healthy subjects. Scand J Clin Lab Invest 1990; 50: 27-33.

34. Brouhard BH, Allen K, Sapire D, Travis LB. Effect of exercise on urinary N-acetyl-beta-D-glucosaminidase activity and albumin excretion in children with type I diabetes mellitus. Diabetes Care 1985; 8: 466-472.

35. Chase HP, Garg SK, Harris S, Marshall G, Hoops S. Elevation of resting and exercise blood pressures in subjects with type I diabetes and relation to albuminuria. J Diabetic Compl 1992; 6: 138-142.

36. Feldt-Rasmussen B, Baker L, Deckert T. Exercise as a provocative test in early renal disease in Type 1 (insulin-dependent) diabetes: albuminuric, systemic and renal haemodynamic responses. Diabetologia 1985; 28: 389-396.

37. Garg SK, Chase HP, Harris S, Marshall G, Hoops S, Osberg I. Glycemic control and longitudinal testing for exercise microalbuminuria in subjects with type I diabetes. J Diabetic Compl 1990; 4: 154-158.

38. Groop L, Stenman S, Groop PH, Mäkipernaa A, Teppo AM. The effect of exercise on urinary excretion of different size proteins in patients with insulin-dependent diabetes mellitus. Scand J Clin Lab Invest 1990; 50: 525-532.

39. Hermansson G, Ludvigsson J. Renal function and blood-pressure reaction during exercise in diabetic and non-diabetic children and adolescents. Acta Paediatr Scand 1980;Suppl. 283: 89-94.

40. Hopper AH, Tindall H, Urquhart S, Davies JA. Reduction of exercise-induced albuminuria by aspirin-dipyridamole in patients with diabetes mellitus. Horm Metab Res 1987; 19: 210-213.
41. Huttunen N-P, Käär M-L, Puukka R, Åkerblom HK. Exercise-induced proteinuria in children and adolescents with type 1 (insulin dependent) diabetes. Diabetologia 1981; 21: 495-497.
42. Jefferson JG, Greene SA, Smith MA, Smith RF, Griffin NKG, Baum JD. Urine albumin to creatinine ratio response to exercise in diabetes. Arch Dis Child 1985; 60: 305.
43. Koivisto VA, Huttunen N-P, Vierikko P. Continuous subcutaneous insulin infusion corrects exercise-induced albuminuria in juvenile diabetes. BMJ 1981; 282: 778-779.
44. Rubler S, Arvan SB. Exercise testing in young asymptomatic diabetic patients. Angiology 1976; 27: 539-548.
45. Mogensen CE. Renal function changes in diabetes. Diabetes 1976; 25: suppl. 2: 872-879.
46. Townsend JC. Increased albumin excretion in diabetes. J Clin Path 1990; 43: 3-8.
47. Viberti GC, Jarrett RJ, McCartney M, Keen M. Increased glomerular permeability to albumin induced by exercise in diabetic subjects. Diabetologia 1978; 14: 293-300.
48. Viberti GC, Pickup JC, Bilous RW, Keen H, Mackintosh D. Correction of exercise-induced microalbuminuria in insulin-dependent diabetics after 3 weeks of subcutaneous insulin infusion. Diabetes 1981; 30: 818-823.
49. Watts GF, Williams I, Morris RW, Mandalia S, Shaw KM, Polak A. An acceptable exercise test to study microalbuminuria in Type 1 diabetes. Diabetic Med 1989; 6: 787-792.
50. Dahlquist G, Aperia A, Carlsson L, Linne T, Persson B, Thoren C, Wilton P. Effect of metabolic control and duration on exercise-induced albuminuria in diabetic teen-agers. Acta Paediatr Scand 1983; 72: 895-902.
51. Fujita Y, Matoba K, Takeuchi H, Ishii K, Yajima Y. Anaerobic threshold can provoke microalbuminuria in non-insulin-dependent diabetics. Diabetes Res Clin Pract 1994; 22: 155-162.
52. Inomata S, Oosawa Y, Itoh M, Inoue M, Masamune O. Analysis of urinary proteins in diabetes mellitus - with reference to the relationship between microalbuminuria and diabetic renal lesions. J Japan Diabetic Soc 1987; 30: 429-435.
53. O'Brien SF, Watts GF, Powrie JK, Shaw KM. Exercise testing as a long-term predictor of the development of microalbuminuria in normoalbuminuric IDDM patients. Diabetes Care 1995; 18: 1602-1605.
54. Matsuoka K, Nakao T, Atsumi Y, Takekoshi H. Exercise regimen for patients with diabetic nephropathy. J Diabetic Compl 1991; 5: 98-100.
55. Giustina A, Perini P, Desenzani P, Bossoni S, Ianniello P, Milani M, Davi G, Romanelli G. Long-term treatment with the dual antithromboxane agent picotamide decreases microalbuminuria in normotensive type 2 diabetic patients. Diabetes 47: 423-430, 1998

21. VON WILLEBRAND FACTOR, DYSFUNCTION OF THE VASCULAR ENDOTHELIUM, AND THE DEVELOPMENT OF RENAL AND VASCULAR COMPLICATIONS IN DIABETES.

Coen D.A. Stehouwer
Department of Medicine, Free University Hospital, Amsterdam, The Netherlands

Both in IDDM [1-4] and in NIDDM [5-11], the presence of microalbuminuria or clinical proteinuria identifies a group of patients at very high risk of developing severe vascular complications, i.e. proliferative retinopathy, renal insufficiency, and cardiovascular disease. Several hypotheses have been advanced to explain why an increased urinary albumin excretion rate should be associated with an excess of *extrarenal* complications [1,12-14]. This chapter will discuss the role of *von Willebrand factor* (vWF), a haemostatic glycoprotein synthesised by endothelial cells and megakaryocytes, and of dysfunction of the vascular endothelium.

It has long been known that the plasma vWF level is often elevated in diabetes [reviewed in ref. 13]. Recent studies have shown such elevated plasma (or serum) levels to be closely related to an elevated urinary albumin excretion rate [10,15-20] and cardiovascular disease [10], but not to the diabetic state *per se*, nor to early retinopathy [13,15,21].

This brief review will focus on the association of elevated vWF levels and endothelial dysfunction with microalbuminuria [10,13-16,18,20] and the use of plasma vWF level as an estimate of endothelial function.

1. WHAT IS VON WILLEBRAND FACTOR?

vWF has a key role in platelet adhesion, thrombus formation and coagulation. It facilitates platelet adhesion to the subendothelium by binding to the subendothelial matrix and to platelet glycoprotein Ib; this process exposes glycoprotein IIb-IIIa at the platelet surface, which in turn enhances platelet adhesion and promotes aggregation. In addition, vWF binds and stabilises factor VIII, thus protecting this crucial coagulation cofactor from inactivation. vWF is a polymer of variable molecular weight (MW, 0.5-20mDa), which consists of a series of dimer subunits (MW ≈ 260 kDa). It is secreted by endothelial cells, both constitutively and, under certain circumstances, acutely, the latter by release from a storage compartment, the so-called Weibel-Palade bodies. In addition, it is released from platelet α-granules during platelet aggregation [22,23]. Normal plasma values of vWF antigen are 50-150% (0.5-1.5U/ml).

2. HIGH PLASMA vWF: MARKER OF ENDOTHELIAL INJURY

Injury to endohelial cells is associated with increased secretion of vWF, both *in vitro* and *in vivo*. Thus plasma levels are elevated in vasculitis and atherosclerosis [reviewed in ref. 13]. By analogy, high vWF levels in diabetic patients with microalbuminuria probably reflect endothelial injury. This contention is supported by the fact that microalbuminuria is also associated with other markers of vascular or endothelial damage. Thus, in IDDM, microalbuminuria is accompanied by increased plasma concentration of angiotensin-converting enzyme, plasminogen activator inhibitor-1 (PAI-1), endothelin and fibronectin, a high urinary excretion of type IV collagen fragments, a decreased basal release of nitric oxide, and an increased transcapillary escape rate of albumin [1,13,24-26]. In NIDDM, microalbuminuria has been shown to be related to elevated levels of plasma fibronectin, thrombomodulin, tissue plasminogen activator, PAI-1 and serum type IV collagen [13,18,26]. Studied in isolation, these markers are not specific for *endothelial* injury. But their clustering points to the endothelium as the most likely common source. Similarly, it cannot be entirely excluded that platelet activation and/or decreased vWF clearance, rather than increased endothelial secretion, contribute to high vWF levels. But direct evidence to support these possibilities is lacking, whereas the indirect evidence cited above is consistent with the endothelium as the origin of elevated plasma vWF.

3. ENDOTHELIAL INJURY: CAUSE OF DYSFUNCTION

The close linkage between microalbuminuria and endothelial injury in diabetes is an attractive explanation for the fact that microalbuminuria seems to be a risk marker for atherosclerotic cardiovascular disease, because endothelial *injury*, which leads to endothelial *dysfunction*, is a central feature of current models of atherogenesis [27]. Furthermore, endothelial dysfunction may be important in the pathogenesis of albuminuria [28]. Endothelial dysfunction might directly cause microalbuminuria both by contributing to the synthesis of a leaky glomerular basement membrane and by influencing glomerular mesangial and epithelial cell function in a paracrine fashion. Alternatively, both generalised endothelial dysfunction and microalbuminuria might develop in parallel as a result of some common underlying pathophysiological process, for which there is no lack of contenders but no definite proof [14,26].

The vascular endothelium has extensive regulatory capacities. First, it controls vascular permeability to macromolecules by modulating the biochemical and biophysical properties of the extracellular matrix. Second, it affects vascular smooth muscle and renal mesangial cell function by producing mediators such as nitric oxide and endothelin. Endothelin, a 21-amino acid polypeptide, stimulates contraction and proliferation of smooth muscle and mesangial cells; nitric oxide has opposite effects. Third, endothelial cells normally inhibit platelet adhesion and aggregation by producing prostacyclin and nitric oxide, limit activation of the coagulation cascade by the thrombomodulin-protein C and the heparan sulphate-antithrombin III pathways, and regulate fibrinolysis by producing tissue plasminogen activator and its inhibitor, PAI-1.

Endothelial injury alters these functions. The extent to which this occurs depends on the nature of the injury and on the intrinsic properties of the endothelium. In diabetes, the proximate causes of endothelial injury are not known but are likely to include hyperglycaemia, advanced glycosylation products, and the components of the insulin resistance syndrome (see 4). Various biochemical mechanisms have been proposed to be at the heart of the pathogenesis of endothelial dysfunction in diabetes. As reviewed elsewhere [26], there is good experimental evidence for important roles for hyperglycaemic pseudohypoxia, activation of protein kinase C (Chapter 35), increased expression of transforming growth factor-β (Chapter 38) and vascular endothelial growth factor, non-enzymatic glycation (Chapter 33) and oxidative stress. Yet the relevance of these biochemical mechanisms for the development of endothelial dysfunction in diabetes in man has only just begun to be investigated. Moreover, differences in the intrinsic vulnerability of the endothelium probably contribute to the variation in susceptibility to these factors that is clinically apparent.

Endothelial dysfunction in human diabetes takes various forms [26]. First, it contributes to basement membrane thickening; high levels of plama fibronectin and serum or urine type IV collagen may be markers of this process. Second, vascular permeability is increased. In IDDM, this may be specifically due to loss of heparan sulphate proteoglycan, which may explain the increased transcapillary escape rate of albumin in microalbuminuric patients [1]. Third, vascular smooth muscle cell contraction is enhanced, predisposing to the development of hypertension. Fourth, platelet adhesion and aggregation are no longer inhibited but may actually be stimulated through increased vWF secretion. Fifth, the endothelium loses its anticoagulant and profibrinolytic nature, and may instead acquire procoagulatory and antifibrinolytic properties, a transition marked by high plasma levels of thrombomodulin and PAI-1. Sixth, endothelium-dependent, nitric oxide-mediated vasodilation decreases [25,29-31], which, in view of nitric oxide's widespread actions, signifies impaired vasodilative, antiproliferative, anticoagulant and permeability-decreasing endothelial properties.

From the foregoing it is clear that endothelial dysfunction is *not* a discrete entity, nor does a gold standard exist. Endothelial dysfunction, in its various manifestations, is closely linked to an increased urinary albumin excretion rate. Disturbances in endothelial functions are involved in the pathogenesis of both microalbuminuria and cardiovascular disease, and may thus explain their association. High plasma vWF levels represent one particular type of endothelial dysfunction. Importantly, such dysfunction has been shown to precede and predict the development of microalbuminuria both in IDDM [19; figure 21-1] and in NIDDM [10]. High vWF levels may also predict the occurrence of cardiovascular disease [10,32] and of diabetic neuropahty [33]. Whether endothelial dysfunction (other than increased vWF levels) occurs in (N)IDDM patients with *normal urinary albumin excretion* (and if so, at what stage) is controversial [14,26,29-31,34-40]. It is also unclear whether the prognostic value of vWF [10,19,32,33,41] is due to its specific functions, i.e. enhancement of platelet adhesion and factor VIII availability, or to the fact that it tends to parallel other types of endothelial dysfunction [13,26].

4. WHAT CAUSES ELEVATED vWF LEVELS AND ENDOTHELIAL DYSFUNCTION IN DIABETES?

Insulin-dependent diabetes mellitus

Poor glycaemic control is associated with high vWF levels and endothelial dysfunction [13,16,40], but the relation is relatively weak. This is consistent with current thinking on the pathogenesis of nephropathy, which postulates that hyperglycaemia is necessary but not sufficient to cause severe microangiopathy [1].

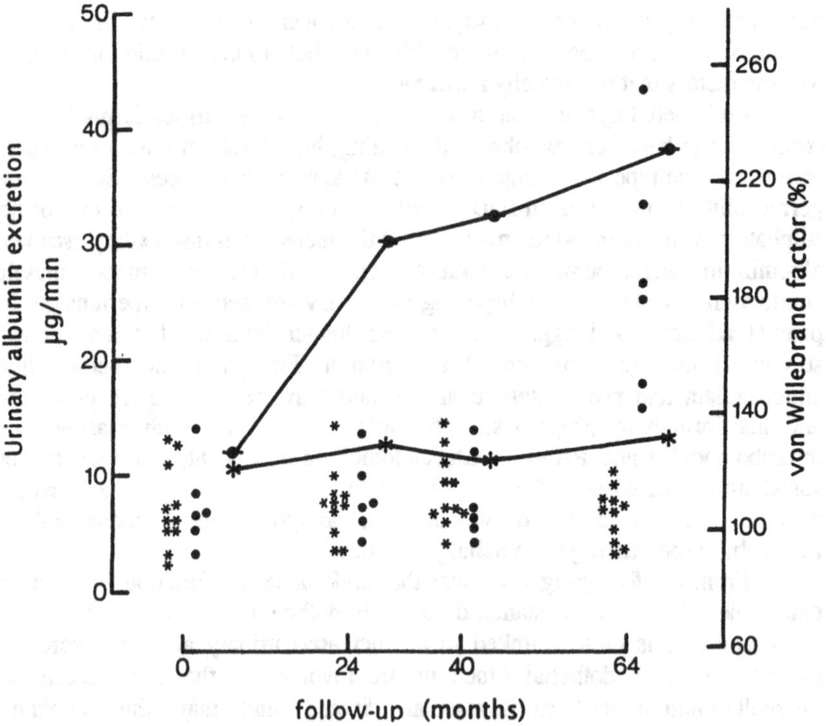

Figure 21-1 Time course of urinary albumin excretion (UAE; reference < 15 μg/min) and plasma von Willebrand factor level (vWF; reference range 50-150%) in insulin-dependent diabetes mellitus. All patients had normal UAE at the start of the follow-up (t=0). UAE remained normal in 11 patients (*); in six patients (•), microalbuminuria was present at the final follow-up (t=64). The figure shows the individual values of UAE (* and •) and the medians of the vWF levels (*-*) and (•-•). The figure illustrates that high vWF levels, indicating endothelial dysfunction, are present in patients in whom microalbuminuria develops. The increase in vWF (present at t=24) precedes the development of microalbuminuria (at t=24). Reproduced with permission [19].

Elevated levels of vWF have been shown to be related to increases in growth hormone, fibrin generation, and blood pressure; endothelial dysfunction, in turn, may enhance fibrin formation and increase peripheral vascular resistance, thus creating the potential for vicious cycles of increasing vascular damage (see ref. 26 for a more detailed discussion). Except for hypertension , the importance of these factors in the initiation and progression of diabetic complications has not been definitely established [1,13,14].

Non-insulin-dependent diabetes mellitus

In NIDDM, the causes of high vWF levels, or of other types of endothelial dysfunction, have not been elucidated. The most likely candidates are hyperglycaemia, hyperinsulinaemia, hypertension and dyslipidaemia, i.e. the chief components of the insulin resistance syndrome [12].

Although glucose is clearly toxic to cultured human endothelial cells [42], the relationship between measures of hyperglycaemia and cardiovascular disease incidence in NIDDM is not particularly strong [8-11,32], nor is the relationship with vWF [10]. Possible explanations include unknown protective factors in human endothelium *in vivo* or an overriding influence of other components of the insulin resistance syndrome. Moreover, it may be the *interplay* among the components of the insulin resistance syndrome which may prove crucial.

The effects of hyperinsulinaemia on endothelial function have not yet been extensively studied. Endothelial cells do have insulin receptors; insulin can increase endothelial production of endothelin [43], a potent vasoconstrictor and mitogen. Plasma levels of endothelin have been reported to be elevated in NIDDM [44]. Hyperinsulinaemia may, in addition, increase plasma levels of PAI-1, which inhibits fibrinolysis and facilitates the persistence of fibrin, which can damage the endothelium [34]. Recent data indicate that hyperinsulinaemia is also related to high vWF levels [45]. On the other hand, insulin is a vasodilator, at least partly through increasing nitric oxide synthesis or action [46]. In addition, insulin infusion in healthy volunteers is associated with a *decrease* in plasma endothelin levels [47, and unpublished observations].

Similarly, data on the relationship between hypertension or dyslipidaemia and endothelial dysfunction in NIDDM are scarce. In our cohort study, blood pressure and lipid levels were not strongly related to vWF levels [10]. Lipid levels did not predict the development of increases in urinary albumin excretion either [10,48]; rather, serum HDL-cholesterol levels seem to decrease *after* microalbuminuria develops [10,48]. Microalbuminuria may be associated with a slightly increased blood pressure [7,10,49], but whether this is the cause of microalbuminuria or the consequence of the processes underlying the development of microalbuminuria (e.g. endothelial dysfunction) is not clear. It is also unclear whether *progression* (as opposed to *development*) of microalbuminuria is principally related to generalised endothelial dysfunction or to local renal mechanisms [50].

It is becoming increasingly clear that insulin resistance and endothelial dysfunction – by whatever measure – are linked [26,45,46,51-53]. In general however, the relationship between the insulin resistance syndrome and endothelial dysfunction appears extremely complex in that endothelial dysfunction may not only be the *result* of the insulin resistance syndrome, but may in addition *cause or contribute* to insulin resistance (through loss of insulin-mediated, endothelium-dependent vasodilation [46], through impaired capillary recruitment [51,52] and through delaying transendothelial insulin transport [53]), blood pressure elevation (through loss of endothelium-dependent vasodilatation), and – at least theoretically – dyslipidaemia (through loss of endothelium-bound lipoprotein lipase activity).

To add even more complexity to this issue, recent studies have indicated that increased adipose tissue and muscle expression of tumour necrosis factor-α (TNF-α) in human obesity may induce insulin resistance [54]. TNF-α can induce the synthesis of other cytokines and alter endothelial function. Thus adipose tissue-derived cytokines may conceivably provide yet another link between insulin resistance and endothelial dysfunction [51,55].

5. vWF: USE IN CLINICAL RESEARCH AND PRACTICE

The data reviewed strongly suggest that plasma vWF level may be useful as an estimate of endothelial injury in diabetes, similar to its proposed use in vasculitis [13].

The development of microalbuminuria was accompanied by an increase in vWF from (median) 121 to 203% in IDDM [16], and from 116 to 219% in NIDDM [10]. The baseline level of and the change in vWF were strongly related to the development of microalbuminuria in NIDDM and explained 60% of its variance [10]. An increase in vWF level may precede and predict the development of microalbuminuria both in IDDM [19] and in NIDDM [10].

As reviewed above, microalbuminuria *in general* clusters with hypertension, severe retinopathy and atherosclerotic cardiovascular disease in both IDDM and NIDDM. There is some recent evidence, however, for heterogeneity among these relationships and for a role of vWF in distinguishing microalbuminuria with vs microalbuminuria without a tendency for severe extrarenal disease. The EURODIAB IDDM Complications Study found, in a Europe-wide study of over 3000 IDDM patients, that the albumin excretion rate correlated significantly with both systolic blood pressure and the plasma vWF concentration, but only in subjects with diabetic retinopathy. Around half of the patients with microalbuminuria had no clinical evidence of retinopathy, and in this group there was no association of increasing albumin excretion with either blood pressure or endothelial dysfunction [56,57]. In NIDDM, there is some evidence – although by no means undisputed – that both dipstick-positive proteinuria [58] and microalbuminuria [59] are morphologicaly heterogeneous. Fioretto et al. have recently shown that endothelial dysfunction, as estimated by plasma vWF, was present only in those microalbuminuric patients who, on renal biopsy, had either typical diabetic glomerulopathy or atypical patterns of injury but not in those with (near-) normal histology [59,60]. In our prospective study in NIDDM, microalbuminuria was associated with an increased risk of new cardiovascular events *only* when endothelial dysfunction was present [10]. Thus, both in IDDM and, perhaps even more so, in NIDDM, the interrelationships among microalbuminuria, endothelial dysfunction, renal histology and diabetic retinopathy appear somewhat more heterogeneous than previously thought.

Several problems remain, however. First, the normal range of vWF, from 50-150%, is quite wide, suggesting that changes in vWF may be a more sensitive marker than a single value. Second, the intra-person day-to-day variability of vWF levels may be as high as 20%, although this can be reduced to about 10% by carefully standardising the blood sampling procedure [13].

6. CONCLUSION

Endothelial dysfunction is present from the earliest increase in urinary albumin excretion in diabetes, and may in fact precede it. Endothelial dysfunction may explain why microalbuminuria appears to be a marker of a high risk of (extrarenal) cardiovascular disease in diabetes. Elevated and/or increasing plasma vWF levels reflect endothelial injury and dysfunction. The vWF plasma level may serve as a useful marker for the state of the vascular endothelium in trials aiming to prevent or delay progression of cardiovascular and renal disease in diabetes.

REFERENCES

1. Deckert T, Feldt-RasmussenB, Borch-Johnsen K, Jensen T, Kofoed-Enevoldsen A. Albuminuria reflects widespread vascular damage. The Steno hypothesis. Diabetologia 1989; 32:219-226
2. Parving HH, Hommel E, Mathiesen ER, et al. Prevalence of microalbuminuria, arterial hypertension, retinopathy and neuropathy in patients with insulin-dependent diabetes. BMJ 1988; 296:156-160.
3. Krolewski AS, Kosinski EJ, Warram JH, et al. Magnitude and determinants of coronary disease in juvenile onset insulin-dependent diabetes mellitus. Am J Cardiol 1987; 59:750-755.
4. Deckert T, Yokoyama H, Mathiesen E, et al. Cohort study of predictive value of urinary albumin excretion for atherosclerotic vascular disease in patients with insulin dependent diabetes. BMJ 1996; 312:871-874.
5. Dinneen SF, Gerstein HC. The association of microalbuminuria and mortality in non-insulin-dependent diabetes mellitus. A systematic overview of the literature. Arch Intern Med 1997; 157:1413-1418.
6. Nelson RG, Pettitt DJ, Carraher MJ, Baird HR, Knowler WC. Effect of proteinuria on mortality in non-insulin dependent diabetes mellitus. Diabetes 1988; 37:1499-1504.
7. Gall MA, Rossing P, Skott P, et al. Prevalence of micro- and macroalbuminuria, arterial hypertension, retinopathy and large vessel disease in European Type 2 (non-insulin-dependent) diabetic patients. Diabetologia 1991; 34:655-661.
8. Damsgaard EM, Froland A, Jorgensen OD, Mogensen CE. Eight-nine year mortality in known non-insulin-dependent diabetes and controls. A prospective study. Kidney Int. 1992; 41:731-735.
9. Mattock MB, Morrish NJ, Viberti GC, Keen H, Fitzgerald AP, Jackson G. Prospective study of microalbuminuria as predictor of mortalitity in non-insulin-dependent diabetes mellitus. Diabetes 1992; 41: 736-741.
10. Stehouwer CDA, Nauta JJP, Zeldenrust GC, Hackeng WHL, Donker AJM, den Ottolander GJH. Albuminuria, cardiovascular disease, and endothelial dysfunction in non-insulin-dependent diabetes mellitus. Lancet 1992; 340:319-323.
11. Gall M-A, Borch-Johnsen K, Hougaard P, Nielsen FS, Parving H-H. Albuminuria and poor glycemic control predict mortality in non-insulin-dependent diabetes mellitus. Diabetes 1995; 44:1301-1309.
12. DeFronzo RA, Ferranini E. Insulin resistance: A multifaced syndrome responsible for NIDDM, obesity, hypertension, dyslipidemia, and atheroslerotic cardiovascular disease. Diabetes Care 1991;14:173-194.
13. Stehouwer CDA, Donker AJM. Urinary albumin excretion and cardiovascular disease risk in diabetes mellitus: Is endothelial dysfunction the missing link? J Nephrol 1993; 6:72-92.

14. Stehouwer CDA, Schaper NC. The pathogenesis of vascular complications of diabetes mellitus: One voice or many? Eur J Clin Invest 1996; 26:535-543.
15. Jensen T. Increased plasma level of von Willebrand factor in type 1 (insulin-dependent) diabetic patients with incipient nephropathy. BMJ 1989; 298:27-28.
16. Stehouwer CDA, Stroes ESG, Hackeng WHL, Mulder PGH, den Ottolander GJH. von Willebrand factor and development of diabetic nephropathy in insulin-dependent diabetes mellitus. Diabetes 1991; 40:971-976 [erratum,Diabetes 1991; 40:1746].
17. Schmitz A, Ingerslev J. Haemostatic measures in Type 2 diabetic patients with microalbuminuria Diabetic Med 1990; 7:521-525.
18. Collier A, Rumley A, Rumley AG, et al. Free radical activity and hemostatic factors in NIDDM patients with and without microalbuminuria. Diabetes 1992;41:909-913.
19. Stehouwer CDA, Fischer HRA, van Kuijk AWR, Polak BCP, Donker AJM. Endothelial dysfunction precedes develoment of microalbuminuria in insulin-dependent diabetes mellitus. Diabetes 1995; 44:561-564.
20. Chen JW, Gall M-A, Deckert M, Jensen JS, Parving H-H. Increased serum concentration of von Willebrand factor in non-insulin-dependent diabetic patients with and without diabetic nephropathy. BMJ 1995; 311:1405-1406.
21. Stehouwer CDA, Zellenrath P, Polak BCP, et al. von Willebrand factor and early diabetic retinopathy: No evidence for a relationship in patients with Type 1 (insulin-dependent) diabetes mellitus and normal urinary albumin excretion. Diabetologia 1992; 35:555-559.
22. Meyer D, Girma JP. von Willebrand factor: Structure and function. Thromb Haemost 1993; 70:111-118.
23. Wagner DD. The Weibel-Palade body: The storage granule for von Willebrand factor and P-selectin. Thromb Haemost 1993; 70:105-110.
24. Collier A, Leach JP, McLellan A, Jardine A, Morton JJ, Small M. Plasma endothelinlike immunoreactivity levels in insulin-dependent mellitus patients with microalbuminuria. Diabetes Care 1992; 15:1038-1040.
25. Elliot TG, Cockcroft JR, Groop PH, Viberti GC, Ritter JM. Inbition of nitric oxide synthesis in forearm vasculature of insulin-dependent diabetic patients: blunted vasoconstriction in patients with microalbuminuria. Clin Sci 1993; 83:687-693
26. Stehouwer CDA, Lambert J, Donker AJM, van Hinsbergh VWM. Endothelial dysfunction and pathogenesis of diabetic angiopathy. Cardiovasc Res 1997; 34: 55-68.
27. Ross R. The pathogenesis of atherosclerosis: A perspective for the 1990s. Nature 1993; 362:801-809.
28. Diamond JR, Karnovsky MJ. Focal and segmental glomerulosclerosis: analogies to atherosclerosis. Kidney Int 1988; 33: 917-924.
29. McVeigh GE, Brennan GM, Johnston GD, et al. Impaired endothelium-dependent and independent vasodilation in patients with type 2 (non-insulin-dependent) diabetes mellitus. Diabetologia 1992; 35: 771-776.
30. Ting HH, Timini FK, Boles KS, Creager SJ, Ganz P, Creager MA. Vitamin C improves endothelium-dependent vasodilation in patients with non-insulin dependent diabetes mellitus. J Clin Invest 1996; 97:22-28.
31. Goodfellow J, Ramsey MW, Luddington LA, et al. Endothelium and inelastic arteries: an early marker of vascular dysfunction in non-insulin-dependent diabetes. BMJ 1996; 312:744-745.
32. Strandl E, Balletshofer B, Dahl B, et al. Predictors of 10-year macrovascular and overall mortality in patients with NIDDM: The Munich General Practitioner Project. Diabetologia 1996; 39: 1540-1545.
33. Plater ME, Ford I, Dent MT, Preston FE, Ward JE. Elevated von Willebrand factor antigen predicts deterioration in diabetic periperal nerve function. Diabetologia 1996; 39:336-343.
34. Juhan-Vague I, Vague P. "Hyperinsulinemia and its effects of coagulation and fibrinolysis in cardiovascular diseasae". In *Atherosclerotic Cardiovascular Disease, Hemostasis and Endothelial Function*. Francis RB, ed. New York: Marcel Dekker, 1992; pp 141-182.
35. Calver A, Collier J, Vallance P. Inhibition and stimulation of nitric oxide synthesis in the human forearm arterial bed of patients with insulin-dependent diabetes. J Clin Invest 1992; 90:2548-2554.
36. Smits P, Kapma J, Jacobs MC, Lutterman J, Thien T. Endothelium-dependent vascular relaxation in patients with type 1 diabetes. Diabetes 1993; 42: 148-153.

37. Smulders RA, Stehouwer CDA, Olthof GC, et al. Plasma endothelin levels and vascular effects of intravenous L-arginine infusion in subjects with uncomplicated insulin-dependent diabetes mellitus. Clin Sci. 1994; 87:37-43.
38. Kool MJF, Lambert J, Stehouwer CDA, Hoeks APG, Struijker Boudier HAJ, van Bortel LMAB. Vessel wall properties of large arteries in uncomplicated insulin-dependent diabetes mellitus. Diabetes Care 1995; 18: 618-624.
39. Lambert J, Aarsen M, Donker AJM, Stehouwer CDA. Endothelium-dependent and –independent vasodilation of large arteries in normoalbuminuric insulin-dependent diabetes mellitus. Arterioscl Thromb Vasc Biol 1996; 16: 705-711.
40. Lehmann ED, Riley WA, Clarkson P, Gosling RG. Non-invasive assessment of cardiovascular disease in diabetes mellitus. Lancet 1997; 350 (suppl I):14-19.
41. Thompson SG, Kienast J, Pyke SD, Haverkate F, van de Loo JC. Hemostatic factors and the risk of myocardial infarction or sudden death in patients with angina pectoris. N Engl J Med 1995; 332:635-641.
42. Lorenzi M. Glucose toxicity in the vascular complications of diabetes; the cellular perspective. Diabetes Metab Rev 1992; 8: 85-103.
43. Hattori Y, Kasai K, Nakamura T, Emoto T, Shimodi SI. Effect of glucose and insulin on immuno-reactive endothelin-1 release from cultured porcine aortic endothelial cells. Metabolism 1991; 40:165-169.
44. Takahashi K, Ghatei MA, Lam HC, O'Halloran DJ, Bloom SR. Elevated plasma endothelin in patients with diabetes mellitus. Diabetologia 1990; 33:306-310.
45. Conlan MG, Folsom AR, Finch A, et al. Associations of factor VIII and von Willebrand factor with age, race, sex and risk factors for atherosclerosis. The Atherosclerosis Risk in Communities (ARIC) Study. Thromb Haemost 1993; 70:380-385.
46. Baron AD. The coupling of glucose metabolism and perfusion in human skeletal muscle. The potential role of endothelium-derived nitric oxide. Diabetes 1996; 45: Suppl. 1: S105-S109.
47. Polderman KH, Stehouwer CDA, van Kamp GJ, Gooren LJG. Effects of insulin infusion on endothelium-derived vasoactive substances. Diabetologia 1996; 39: 1284-1292.
48. Niskanen L, Uusitupa M, Sarlund H, et al. Microalbuminuria predicts the development of serum lipoprotein abnormalities favouring atherogenesis in newly diagnosed type 2 (non-insulin-dependent) diabetic patients. Diabetologia 1990; 33:237-243.
49. Haffner SM, Morales PA, Gruber MK, Hazuda HP, Stern MP. Cardiovascular risk factors in non-insulin-dependent diabetic subjects with microalbuminuria. Arteriosclerosis Thromb 1993; 13:205-210.
50. Smulders YM, Rakic M, Stehouwer CDA, Weijers RNM, Slaats EH, Silberbusch J. Determinants of progression of microalbuminuria in patients with NIDDM. Diabetes Care 1997; 20:999-1005.
51. Serné EH, Stehouwer CDA, ter Maaten JC, et al. Insulin resistance and hypertension: Role for microcirculation? Diabetologia 1997; 40 (suppl. 1): A246 (abstract).
52. Rattigan S, Clark MG, Barrett EJ. Hemodynamic actions of insulin in rat skeletal muscle. Evidence for capillary recruitment. Diabetes 1997; 46: 1381-1388.
53. Castillo C, Bogardus C, Bergman R, et al. Interstitial insulin concentrations determine glucose uptake rates but not insulin resistance in lean and obese men. J Clin Invest 1994; 93: 10-16.
54. Hotamisligil GS, Peraldi P, Budavari A, Ellis R, White MF, Spiegelman BM. IRS-1 mediated inhibition of insulin receptor tyrosine kinase activity in TNF-α and obesity-induced insulin resistance. Science 1996; 271: 665-668.
55. Yudkin JS, Stehouwer CDA, Emeis JJ, Coppack SW. Insulin resistance syndrome and endothelial damage – role of adipose tissue derived pro-inflammatory cytokines. Diabetologia 1997; 40 (suppl.1): A305 (abstract).
56. Stephenson JM, Fuller JH, Viberti G-C, Sjolie A-K, Navalesi R, the EURODIAB IDDM Complications Study Group. Blood pressure, retinopathy and urinary albumin excretion in IDDM: The EURODIAB IDDM Complications Study. Diabetologia 1995; 38:599-603.
57. Greaves M, Malia RG, Goodfellow K, et al. Fibrinogen and von Willebrand factor in IDDM: relationships to lipid vascular risk factors, blood pressure, glycaemic control and urinary albumin excretion rate: the EURODIAB IDDM complications study. Diabetologia 1997; 40:698-705.
58. Parving HH, Gall MA, Skott P, et al. Prevalence and causes of albuminuria in non-insulin-dependent diabetic patients. Kidney Int 1992; 41:758-762.

59. Fioretto P, Mauer M, Brocco E et al. Patterns of renal injury in NIDDM patients with microalbuminuria. Diabetologia 1996; 39:1569-1576.
60. Fioretto P, Stehouwer CDA, Mauer M, et al. Heterogeneous nature of microalbuminuria in NIDDM: Studies of endothelial function and renal structure. Diabetologia 1998 41:233-236.

22. SMOKING AND DIABETIC NEPHROPATHY

Peter T. Sawicki
Medizinische Klinik und Poliklinik, Klinik f. Stoffwechselkrankheiten und Ernährung, Düsseldorf, Germany

In 1978, Christiansen reported that cigarette smoking is a risk factor for the development of diabetic nephropathy [1]. He found a significantly higher prevalence of persistent proteinuria among patients who were or had been cigarette smokers. In a later study by Telmer et al. [2], the earlier findings were confirmed in a greater number and better characterised group of Type 1 diabetic patients. In 668 patients, the prevalence of diabetic nephropathy was significantly higher among heavy smokers (more than 10 cigarettes per day for more than 1 year) than among other patients, that is 19% vs. 12%. In addition, a higher frequency of clinical nephropathy was found with increasing cigarette consumption. Among patients who smoked a maximum of 10 cigarettes per day, about 13% had clinical diabetic nephropathy, whereas it was more than 25% among those patients who smoked 30 cigarettes per day. An association between smoking and nephropathy was also observed by Nordén and Nyberg [3]. They compared smoking habits in 47 matched pairs of Type 1 diabetic patients with and without nephropathy. Patients with nephropathy had a significantly higher smoking index than their controls. There were also more current smokers, more heavy smokers, and fewer individuals who had never smoked in the nephropathy group than in the control group. With respect to retinopathy, study results had been controversial [4]. It is of note, that in these early studies glycosylated haemoglobin values had not been included into the analyses as a possible confounding factor.

In a later cross-sectional case-control study the association between current cigarette smoking, macroproteinuria, and retinopathy, including glycosylated haemoglobin values has been re-examined [5]. Out of a cohort of 1254 Type 1 diabetic patients, 90 female and 102 male cigarette-smoking patients with a duration of diabetes of at least 6 years were pair-matched with non-smoking patients with respect to sex, duration of diabetes, and age. The percentages of patients with macroproteinuria or proliferative retinopathy were significantly higher in smokers than in non-smokers, although the difference with respect to proliferative retinopathy was significant only for women. On the other hand, glycosylated haemoglobin values and the percentages of patients with hypertension were comparable between smokers and non-smokers. After an average duration of diabetes of 14 years, macroproteinuria was found in 19% of the smoking and 8% of the non-smoking patients, whereas the percentages of patients with normal proteinuria or without retinopathy were comparable between the two groups. Since ex-smokers had been included in the non-smokers patient groups, the associations between smoking and nephropathy might have been underestimated. The main results of this latter study were supported by an observation by Stegmayr and Lithner [6] who found that 21 of 22 uraemic Type 1 diabetic patients were tobacco users, whereas this was the case in only 10 out of 22 well-matched non-uraemic patients selected from their diabetes outpatient clinic. An association between proteinuria and smoking has also been found among Type 1 diabetic patients who survived for 40 years or more [7].

Recent prospective studies support the concept that cigarette smoking is a relevant factor in the clinical course of diabetic nephropathy [8-17]. In a clinic-based study Chase et al. [10] evaluated the association of smoking and progression of albuminuria (borderline and abnormal, over 7.6 µg/min) in young insulin-dependent adults aged about 20 years with a diabetes duration of about 11 years and a rather low prevalence and mild degrees of nephropathy (only 3% were considered to be hypertensive). Over a follow-up period of 2 to 3.5 years the progression of albuminuria and of retinopathy was greater in smokers. Albuminuria decreased significantly when subjects ceased smoking. Smoking remained a significant factor in the logistic regression model for albuminuria when controlled for possible confounding factors, such as glycohaemoglobin levels; the odds ratio of developing a significant increase of albuminuria was 2.2 times higher for smokers.

Other studies have been confirmatory [11,12,15]. In a four-year prospective study the factors predicting albuminuria were evaluated in 172 normotensive, insulin-dependent diabetic patients without overt nephropathy [11]. Initial urinary albumin excretion and glycosylated haemoglobin were the major predictors of the level of albuminuria after four years, whereas weaker associations were found with a history of hospital admission, smoking and treatment of blood pressure. In another observational study including a cohort of 148 non-microalbuminuric, non-hypertensive insulin-dependent diabetic patients followed for four years, poor glucose control, an early rise of arterial pressure and smoking were implicated in the development of persistent microalbuminuria [15]. Ekberg et al. [9,12] reported an association between glomerular hyperfiltration and smoking in insulin-treated patients. The prevalence of hyperfiltration in smokers was 41% compared to 18% in non-smokers.

Although these data strongly suggest an association of smoking with the development and/or progression of diabetic renal damage, other explanations are possible. Thus, it could be, that smoking influences renal tubule and permeability functions independent of any specific effects on clinical propensity to nephropathy and renal insufficiency. Alternatively, smoking may not be directly related to nephropathy at all; the smoking status may merely be an indicator for particular patterns of health behaviour that are due to affect renal function detrimentally.

Some clarification of this question comes from a study by Sawicki et al. [17]. In a prospective investigation possible factors associated with the progression of diabetic nephropathy over a period of one year have been evaluated. The study

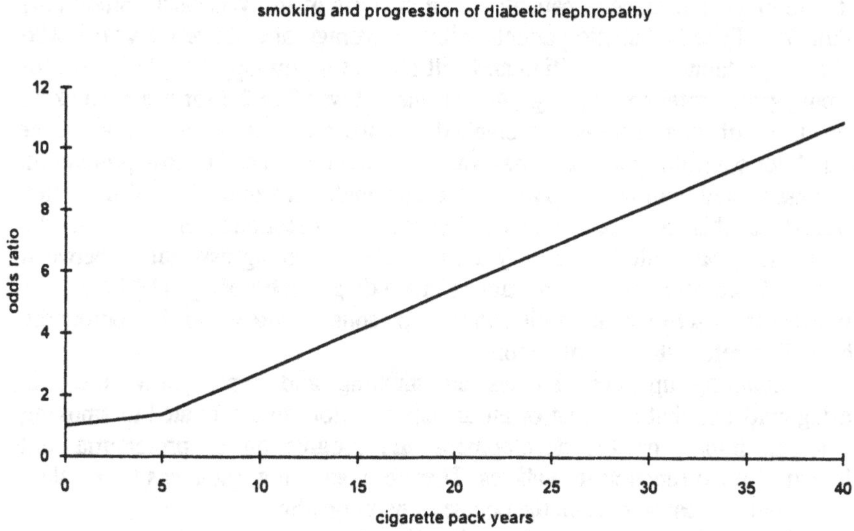

Figure 22-1 Results from logistic regression analysis [17]. Estimated odds ratios for progression of diabetic nephropahty and number of cigarette pack years.

included 92 Type 1 diabetic patients with long duration of diabetes, hypertension and diabetic nephropathy. All patients were under intensified insulin and antihypertensive therapy. Consequently, these patients had well controlled blood glucose and blood pressure values throughout the observation period. A progression of renal disease was defined according to the stage of nephropathy as an increase in proteinuria or serum creatinine or a decrease in glomerular filtration rate. Progression of nephropathy was found in 53% of smokers as compared to 11% of non-smokers and 33% of ex-smokers. The adjusted odds ratio for progression of nephropathy between smokers (including ex-smokers) and never-smokers was 6.7. It was concluded that smoking represents an important factor associated with progression of diabetic nephropathy in patients who are intensively treated for hypertension. There was a dose dependent increase of risk for progression of nephropathy with the number of smoked cigarettes, figure 22-1.

Further support for a direct role of smoking on the progression of nephropathy comes from observations derived from patients with lupus nephritis [13]. In a retrospective cohort study an inception cohort of 160 adults with lupus nephritis were followed-up for a median of 6.4 years. Hypertension and smoking status at the onset of nephritis were strongly and independently associated with differences in the time to development of end-stage renal disease. The median time to end-stage renal disease was 145 months among smokers and it was longer than 273 months among non-smokers. These effects persisted in multivariable analyses adjusted for differences among patients in age, gender, socio-economic status, renal histology, and immunosuppressive treatment.

Associations between smoking and progression of proteinuria have also been found in Type 2 diabetic patients. In an analysis of the Wisconsin Study [14] including 794 Type 2 diabetic patients with an average age above 60 years, who were free of proteinuria at recruition and still alive at follow-up, the relative risk of developing gross proteinuria during a 4-year interval was 2 to 2.5 for heavy smokers (highest level of total pack-years smoked) compared to those who had never smoked. After controlling for other risk variables, the incidence of gross proteinuria was also associated with higher glycosylated haemoglobin values. It is of note, that in contrast to this prospective study, several cross-sectional analyses of the Wisconsin study had failed to identify a consistent and strong association between smoking and diabetic late complications, including nephropathy [18,19,20]. A possible reason is selective mortality, that is, persons who developed nephropathy may have died before their examination.

Summing up these studies on smoking and nephropathy, there is increasing evidence that smoking or an unknown factor closely related to smoking has a strong impact on the development and progression of proteinuria and impairment of renal function in diabetes. Therefore, smoking status has to be taken into account in clinical studies on the course of nephropathy.

The mechanisms by which smoking increases albuminuria/proteinuria and promotes nephropathy are unknown. Interestingly, abnormality on urine analysis, including proteinuria, has also been found to be more common in male and female smokers in a population-based study, but the reasons for this finding remained unclear [21].

Smoking a cigarette induces acute haemodynamic and metabolic changes mediated through adrenergic mechanisms. The smoking associated sympathetic discharge is physiologically reflected by a transient rise of pulse rate and blood pressure [22]. In addition to sympathetic stimulation, smoking a cigarette is followed by transient increases of plasma cortisol, ACTH, and aldosterone levels in hypertensive subjects [23]. Despite these complex acute haemodynamic and hormonal effects, in epidemiological studies smoking has not been found to increase the risk of hypertension [24]. However, recent studies have revealed that by continuous monitoring of blood pressure heavy smoking is associated with sustained and substantial increases in blood pressure during the day [25,26]. The blood pressure increasing effect of smoking is short-lived, i.e. it lasts for about half an hour and can therefore be missed during the blood pressure measurement in the clinic. We have studied 10 normotensive controls and 15 hypertensive patients with diabetic nephropathy (5 with and 10 without autonomic neuropathy) during a non-smoking and a smoking day of one cigarette every 30 minutes for eight hours [27]. During smoking systolic blood pressure increased 12 mmHg in normals and by 8 mmHg in patients with diabetic nephropathy and without autonomic neuropathy but did not change significantly in patients with autonomic neuropathy. No significant changes in diastolic blood pressure occurred. Mean proteinuria increased only in diabetic nephropathic patients without autonomic neuropathy by 21 mg $mmol^{-1}$.

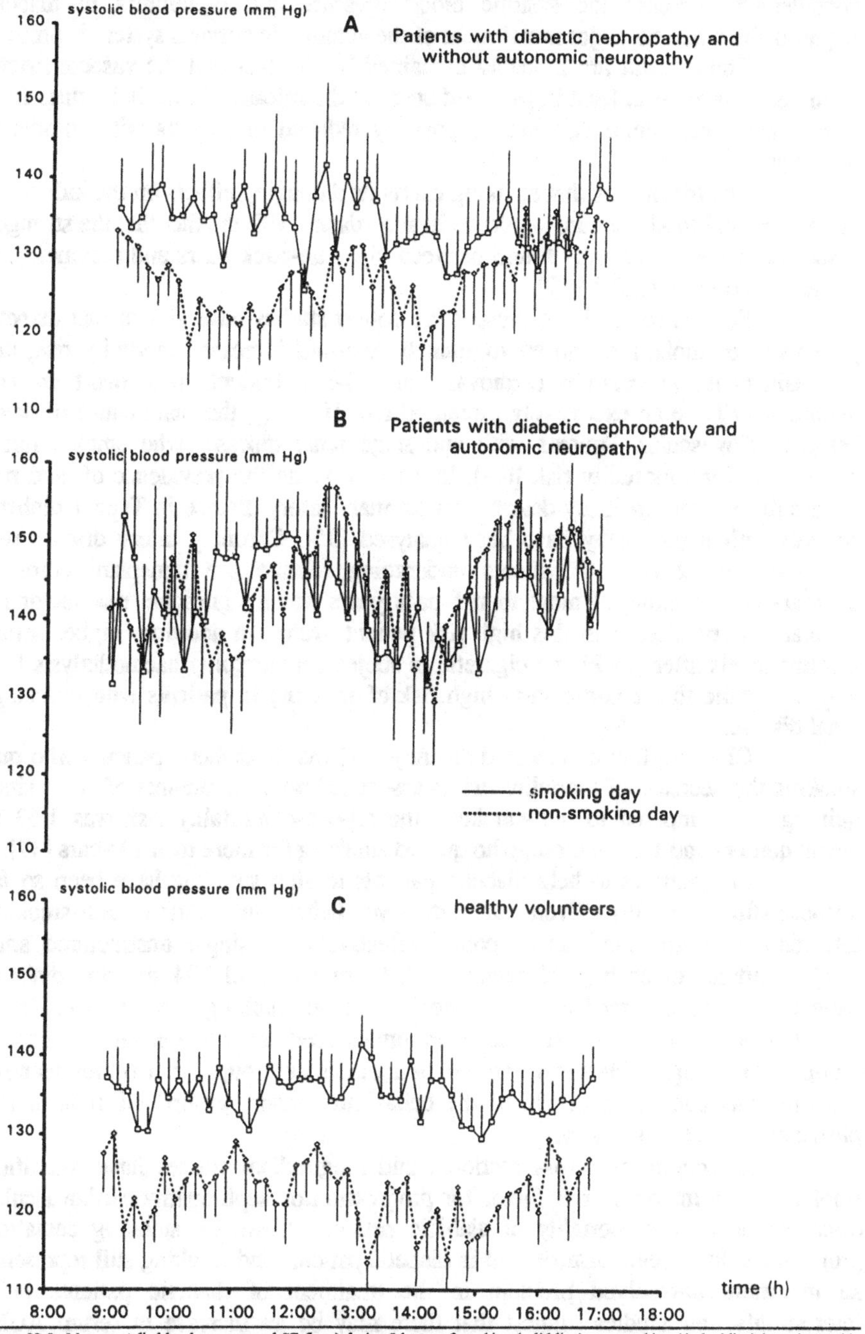

Figure 22-2. Mean systolic blood pressure and SE (bars) during 8 hours of smoking (solid line) non-smoking (dashed line) in patients with diabetic nephropathy and without automatic neuropathy (A), patients with diabetic nephropathy and autonomatic neuropahty (B) and healty volunteers (C). From: Sawicki et al.: Effects of smoking on blood pressure and proteinuria in patients with diabetic nephropathy. J Intern Med 1996; 239; 345-352. Copyrignt, Blackwell Science Ltd.

These results indicate that smoking two cigarettes per hour is sufficient to considerably increase the systolic blood pressure and proteinuria in diabetic nephropathy when no major impairment of the autonomic nervous system is present.

These result are probably explained by the fact that the vasoconstrictor action of nicotine is at least in part mediated via the release of catecholamines from sympathetic nerve endings, which is possibly reduced in patients with autonomic neuropathy.

The hypothesis that smoking exerts its damaging effects on the kidney via an increase in blood pressure would be in accordance with the fact that the strongest associations are consistently found between cigarette-pack years and parameters of kidney function [1,2,6,8,14,17].

Several recent large prospective cohort studies have shown that diabetic patients who smoke have an approximately two-fold increased mortality risk, and the main cause of death is cardiovascular [28-34]. Patients with overt diabetic nephropathy have an excessively increased risk of dying, the main cause of death being cardiovascular. Patients with end stage renal disease, who smoke, run a particularly high mortality risk [6,8]. In a recent study the prevalence of, and risk factors for, angiographically determined coronary artery disease in Type 1 diabetic patients with nephropathy have been analysed [35]. Coronary artery disease was diagnosed in 52 of 110 patients undergoing routine pre transplant coronary angiography. Smoking of more than 5 pack-years was a significant risk factor for coronary artery disease in this high risk patient group. In addition, higher serum nicotine levels after smoking a cigarette in subjects undergoing haemodialysis [36] may contribute to the particularly high risk of smoking in patients with end stage renal disease.

Chaturvedi et al. reported recently [37] that in diabetic patients who quit smoking the decrease of mortality risk is associated with the number of years since quitting. As compared to non-smokers, the all-cause mortality risk was 1.53 in recent quitters and 1.25 in those, who quitted smoking for more than 10 years [37].

Programmes to help diabetic patients to stop smoking have been so far unsuccessful [4,38,39]. Even an extensive behaviour therapy anti-smoking intervention programme was as poorly effective as a single unstructured anti-smoking advice given by a physician [40]: Form a total of 794 smoking diabetic patients only 11% agreed to participate in a »stop smoking programme«. These patients who wanted to stop smoking were randomised either to a behaviour therapy group or to a single »physicians anti-smoking advice« group. After 6 months non-smoking was confirmed in 5% of the behaviour therapy group and 16% of the physicians advice group only.

In conclusion, cross sectional and longitudinal studies have identified smoking as an important risk factor for progression of nephropathy cardiovascular diseases and overall mortality in diabetic patients. However, smoking cessation programmes have been unsuccessful in diabetic patients and smoking still represents an important unresolved problem in the treatment of diabetic patients [41]. Interestingly new studies suggest that there may be an increase in serum AGE-products in patients who smoke [42]. The general problems regarding smoking dependence and quitting have recently been discussed [43-47].

REFERENCES

1. Christiansen JS. Cigarette smoking and prevalence of microangiopathy in juvenile-onset insulin-dependent diabetes mellitus. Diabetes Care 1978; 1: 146-149.
2. Telmer S, Christiansen JS, Andersen AR, Nerup J, Deckert T. Smoking habits and prevalence of clinical diabetic microangiopathy in insulin-dependent diabetics. Acta Med Scand 1984; 215: 63-68.
3. Nordén G, Nyberg G. Smoking and diabetic nephropathy. Acta Med Scand 1984; 215: 257-261.
4. Mühlhauser I. Smoking and diabetes. Diabetic Med 1990; 7: 10-15.
5. Mühlhauser I, Sawicki P, Berger M. Cigarette-smoking as a risk factor for macroproteinuria and proliferative retinopathy in Type 1 (insulin-dependent) diabetes. Diabetologia 1986; 29: 500-502.
6. Stegmayr B, Lithner F. Tobacco and end stage diabetic nephropathy. BMJ 1987; 295: 581-582.
7. Borch-Johnsen K, Nissen H, Henriksen E, Kreiner S, Salling N, Deckert T, Nerup J. The natural history of insulin-dependent diabetes mellitus in Denmark: 1. Long-term survival with and without late diabetic complications. Diabetic Med 1987; 4: 201-210.
8. Stegmayr BG. A study of patients with diabetes mellitus (type 1) and end-stage renal failure: tobacco usage may increase risk of nephropathy and death. J Intern Med 1990; 228: 121-124.
9. Ekberg G, Grefberg N, Larsson LO, Vaara I. Cigarette smoking and glomerular filtration rate in insulin-treated diabetics without manifest nephropathy. J Intern Med 1990; 228: 211-217.
10. Chase HP, Garg SK, Marshall G, Berg CL, Harris S, Jackson WE, Hamman RE. Cigarette smoking increases the risk of albuminuria among subjects with Type 1 diabetes. JAMA 1991; 265: 614-617.
11. Watts GF, Harris R, Shaw KM. The determinants of early nephropathy in insulin-dependent diabetes mellitus: a prospective study based on the urinary excretion of albumin. Q J Med 1991; 79 (288): 365-378.
12. Ekberg G, Grefberg N, Larsson LO. Cigarette smoking and urinary albumin excretion in insulin-treated diabetics without manifest nephropathy. J Intern Med 1991; 230: 435-442.
13. Ward MM, Studenski S. Clinical prognostic factors in lupus nephritis. The importance of hypertension and smoking. Arch Intern Med 1992; 152: 2082-2088.
14. Klein R, Klein BEK, Moss SE. Incidence of gross proteinuria in older-onset diabetes. A population-based perspective. Diabetes 1993; 42: 381-389.
15. Microalbuminuria Collaborative Study Group, United Kingdom. Risk factors for development of microalbuminuria in insulin dependent diabetic patients: a cohort study. BMJ 1993; 306: 1235-1239.
16. Mühlhauser I, Verhasselt R, Sawicki PT, Berger M. Leukocyte count, proteinuria and smoking in type 1 diabetes mellitus. Acta Diabetol 1993; 30: 105-107.
17. Sawicki PT, Didjurgeit U, Mühlhauser I, Bender R, Heinemann L, Berger M. Smoking is associated with progression of diabetic nephropathy. Diabetes Care 1994; 17: 126-131.
18. Klein R, Klein BEK, Davis MD. Is cigarette smoking associated with diabetic retinopathy? Am J Epidemiol 1983; 118: 228-238.
19. Klein R, Klein BEK, Moss S, DeMets DL. Proteinuria in diabetes. Arch Intern Med 1988; 148: 181-186.
20. Klein R, Klein BEK, Linton KLP, Moss SE. Microalbuminuria in a population-based study of diabetes. Arch Intern Med 1992; 152: 153-158.
21. Dales LG, Friedman GD, Siegelaub AB, Seltzer CC, Ury HK. Cigarette smoking habits and urine characteristics. Nephron 1978; 20: 163-170.
22. Cryer PE, Haymond MW, Santiago JV, Shah SD. Norepinephrine and epinephrine release and adrenergic mediation of smoking-associated hemodynamic and metabolic events. N Engl J Med 1976; 295: 573-577.
23. Baer L, Radichevich I. Cigarette smoking in hypertensive patients-blood pressure and endocrine responses. Am J Med 1985; 78: 564-568.
24. Green MS, Jucha E, Luz Y. Blood pressure in smokers and non-smokers: epidemiologic findings. Am Heart J 1986; 111: 932-940.
25. Mann SJ, James GD, Wang RS, Pickering TG. Elevation of ambulatory systolic blood pressure in hypertensive smokers. A case control study. JAMA 1991; 265: 2226-2228.

26. Groppelli A, Giorgi DMA, Omboni S, Parati G, Mancia G. Persistent blood pressure increase induced by heavy smoking. J Hypertens 1992; 10: 495-499.
27. Sawicki PT, Mühlhaser I, Bender R, Pethke W, Heinemann L, Berger M. Effects of smoking on blood pressure and proteinuria in patients with diabetic nephropathy. J Intern Med 1996: 239: 345-352.
28. Klein R, Moss SE, Klein BEK, DeMets DL. Relation of ocular and systemic factors to survival in diabetes. Arch Intern Med 1989; 149: 266-272.
29. Moy CS, LaPorte RE, Dorman JS, Songer TJ, Orchard TJ, Kuller LH, Becker DJ, Drash AL. Insulin-dependent diabetes mellitus mortality. The risk of cigarette smoking. Circulation 1990; 82: 37-43.
30. Rosengren A, Welin L, Tsipogianni A, Wilhelmsen L. Impact of cardiovascular risk factors on coronary heart disease and mortality among middle aged diabetic men: a general population study. BMJ 1989; 299: 1127-1131.
31. Morrish NJ, Stevens LK, Head J, Fuller JH, Jarrett RJ, Keen H. A prospective study of mortality among middle-aged diabetic patients (the London cohort of the WHO multinational study of vascular disease in diabetics) II: associated risk factors. Diabetologia 1990; 33: 542-548.
32. Ford ES, DeStefano F. Risk factors for mortality from all causes and from coronary heart disease among persons with diabetes. Findings from the National Health and Nutrition Examination Survey I. Epidemiological follow-up study. Am J Epidemiol 1991; 133: 1220-1230.
33. Manson JE, Colditz GA, Stampfer MJ, Willett WC, Krolewski AS, Rosner B, Arky RA, Speizer FE, Hennekens CH. A prospective study of maturity-onset diabetes mellitus and risk of coronary heart disease and stroke in women. Arch Intern Med 1991; 151: 1141-1147.
34. Stamler J, Vaccaro O, Neaton JD, Wentworth D. Diabetes, other risk factors, and 12-yr. cardiovascular mortality for men screened in the multiple risk factor intervention trial. Diabetes Care 1993; 16: 434-444.
35. Manske CL, Wilson RF, Wang Y, Thomas W. Prevalence of, and risk factors for, angiographically determined coronary artery disease in Type 1 diabetic patients with nephropathy. Arch Intern Med 1992; 152: 2450-2455.
36. Perry RJ, Griffiths W, Dextraze P, Solomon RJ, Trebbin WM. Elevated nicotine levels in patients undergoing hemodialysis. A role in cardiovascular mortality and morbidity? Am J Med 1984; 76: 241-246.
37. Chaturvedi N, Stevens L, Fuller. The World Health Organisation Multinational Study Group. Which features of smoking determine mortality risk in former cigarette smokers with diabetes? Diabetes Care 1997; 20:1266-1272.
38. Ardron M, MacFarlane IA, Robinson C, van Heyningen C, Calverley PMA. Anti-smoking advice for young diabetic smokers: is it a waste of breath? Diabetic Med 1988; 5: 667-670.
39. Fowler PM, Hoskins PL, McGill M, Dutton SP, Yue DK, Turtle JR. Anti-smoking programme for diabetic patients: the agony and the ecstasy. Diabetic Med 1989; 6: 698-702.
40. Sawicki PT, Didjurgeit U, Mühlhauser I, Berger M. Behaviour therapy versus doctor's anti-smoking advice in diabetic patients. J Intern Med 1993; 234: 407-409.
41. Mühlhauser I, Bender R, Bott U, Jorgens V, Grusser M, Wagener W, Overmann H, Berger M. Cigarette-smoking and progression of retinopathy and nephropathy in type-1 diabetes. Diabetic Med 1996; 13: 536-543.
42. Baumgartl H-J, Standl E, Vlassara H, Bucala R. Increase in serum ages ("advanced glycosylation end-products") in IDDM patients who smoke (Abstract). Diabetologia 1996; 39: Suppl. 1: A291.
43. Fortmannn SP. Smoking: No time for complacency. Cardiovasc Risk Factors 1996; 6: 123-125.
44. Joossens L. Trends in uptake and quitting smoking in Europe. Cardiovasc Risk Factors 1996; 6: 126-129.
45. Kunze M. Epidemiology of nicotine dependence and general aspectss of smoking cessation. Cardiovasc Risk Factors 1996; 6: 130-134.
46. Fagerström KO, Säwe U. The pathophysiology of nicotine dependence: treatment options and the cardiovascular safety of nicotine. Cardiovasc Risk Factors 1996; 6: 135-143.
47. Wilhelmsen L. Benefits of quitting smoking for cardiac disease. Cardiovasc Risk Factors 1996; 6: 144-147.
48. Hansen HP, Rossing K, Jacobsen P, Jensen BR, Parving H-H. The acute effect of smoking on systemic hemodynamics, kidney and endothelian functions in insulin-dependent diabetic patients with microalbuminuria. Scand J Clin Lab Invest 1996; 56: 393-399.

23. LIGHT MICROSCOPY OF DIABETIC GLOMERULOPATHY: THE CLASSIC LESIONS

Steen Olsen
Department of Pathology, Aarhus Kommunehospital, Aarhus, Denmark

The history of our knowledge of the light microscopy of diabetic glomerulopathy began with the famous paper by Kimmelstiel and Wilson in 1936 [1]. With some justification, it can be said that it has been completed by the careful analysis of large series by Thomsen 1965 [2] and Ditscherlein 1969 [3], the first mentioned taking advantage of the introduction of percutaneous renal biopsies.

Histologic lesions of the renal glomerulus in diabetics were not totally unknown when Kimmelstiel and Wilson reported their findings, but the exact relationship of these alterations to the diabetic state was unclear. Kimmelstiel and Wilson were the first investigators to draw attention to the characteristic »intercapillary«, nodular thickening of mesangial regions and its association with a clinical syndrome consisting of severe proteinuria, edema, hypertension, and eventually a decrease in renal function.

The histology of diabetic glomerulopathy described here rests upon the cornerstones mentioned above as well as on other important contributions published by several authors, among them Allen [4], Bell [5-7], Fahr [8], Spühler and Zollinger [9], Muirhead et al. [10], and Randerath [11]. The juxtaglomerular arterioles will be included in the discussion due to their close functional and anatomic connection with the glomerulus.

1. THE DIFFUSE LESION

This consists of a uniform widening of the mesangial regions (figure 23-1). It is particularly well exhibited in sections stained by periodic acid-Schiff (PAS) or by silver methenamine that display structures often described as finger-like radiations from the glomerular hilum.

2. THE NODULAR LESION

As the volume of the mesangial matrix increases, some mesangial regions become more prominent than others and may take on a globular shape (figure 23-2). The mesangial nodule is thus created by a gradual increase of the diffuse lesion and the distinction between them is arbitrary. Several nodules may be present in each glomerulus, but usually only a few of the mesangial regions are affected in this way.

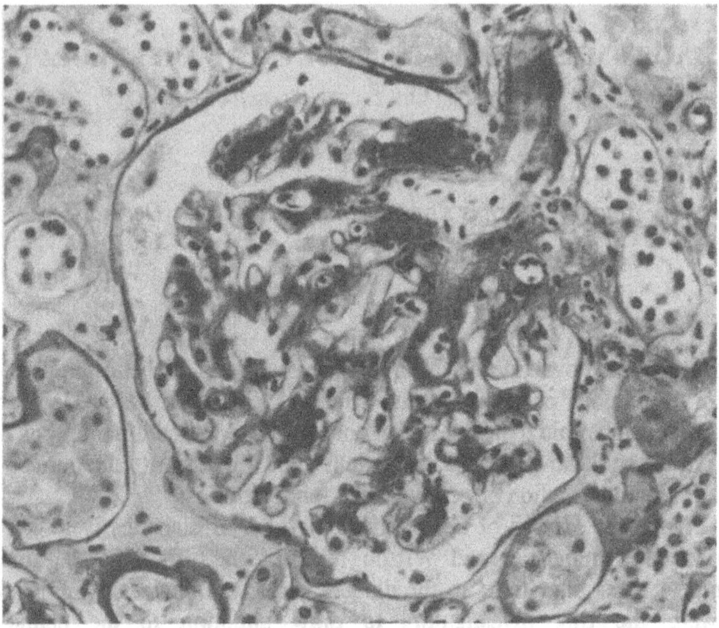

Figure 23-1 Diabetic glomerulosclerosis, diffuse type. There is slight increase of PAS-positive material in all mesangial regions, radiating from the vascular pole (*upper right*). PAS-hamematoxylin.

The nodules are distributed in a horseshoe-shaped area corresponding to the peripheral mesangium [12]. The other mesangial regions present the diffuse lesion. Small nodules contain evenly distributed mesangial cells, but, in medium-sized or large nodules, the central areas are almost always acellular. The periphery of the nodule contains one or a few layers of mesangial cells. Around the nodule, a ring of capillaries is present and they may be dilated. It has been suggested that the formation of the nodule is preceded by focal mesangiolysis [13,14].

3. THE FIBRINOID CAP

Insudative lesions consists of deposits of plasma proteins and lipids within renal arterioles (arteriolar hyalinosis), glomerular capillaries (fibrinoid or fibrin cap) and Bowman's capsule (capsular drop). The fibrin cap [8,9,15-17] is situated in the peripheral capillary wall and has a crescentic shape (figure 23-3).

If the basement membrane is stained by silver methenamine, the cap appears to be situated between this and the endothelium. Its structure is homogeneous although small vacuoles may be seen in which lipids can be demonstrated in frozen sections stained by oil-red.

4. THE CAPSULAR DROP

This lesion [1,3] is situated on the inner side of the capsule of Bowman. It sometimes looks like a drop (figure 23-4), but it may also be more extended, as a slender, fusiform deposit. Its outer border is formed by the capsule of Bowman; its inner projects toward the urinary space.

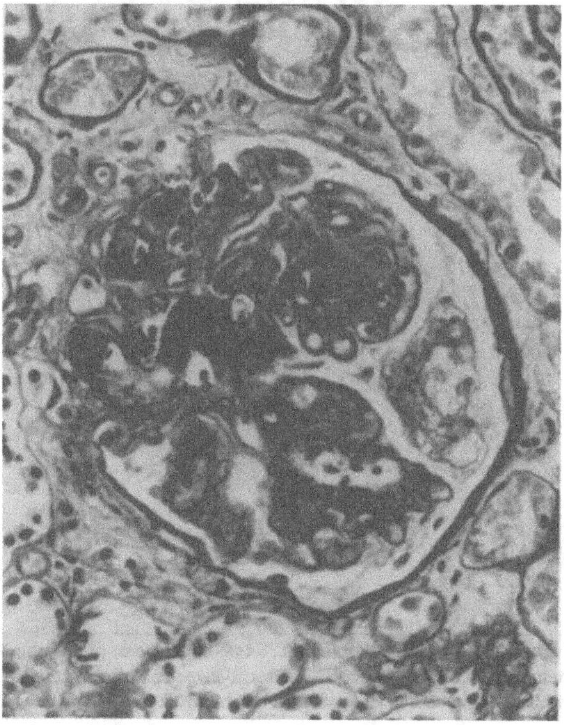

Figure 23-2 Diabetic glomerulschlerosis. The diffuse component is more marked than in figure 23-1 and a nodule has been formed from a particulary voluminous mesangial region. PAS-haematoxylin.

5. ARTERIOLAR HYALINOSIS

In the early stage of arteriolar hyalinosis (or hyaline arteriolosclerosis), small drops of strongly eosinophilic material accumulate in the wall of the juxtaglomerular arterioles. They may be situated in the intima or in the media. They gradually increase in size and eventually involve the whole arteriolar wall, which then appears as a strongly thickened, homogeneous structure. Arteriolar hyalinosis in diabetes involves the afferent arteriole as well as the efferent arteriole (figure 23-5).

6. STAINING CHARACTERISTICS AND HISTOCHEMISTRY

Histochemical studies have been published by several authors [10,17,18]. The most important results are presented in table 23-1. The fibrinoid cap, capsular drop, and arteriolar hyalinosis are identical in staining characteristics, which is why some authors have included them in one group.

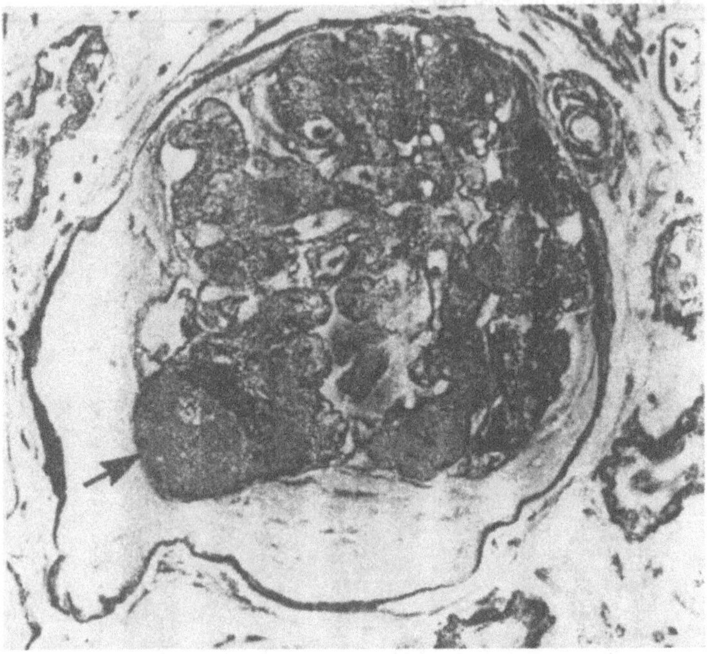

Figure 23-3 Fibrinoid cap in diabetic glomerulosclerosis. Totally obsolescent glomerulus with several fibrinoid caps, one of them indicated by an arrow. The crescent-shaped pale area to the left is subcapsular, fibrotic tissue. The PAS-positive glomerular basement membranes from a solid, retracted tuft. PAS-haematoxylin.

Reports on immunofluorescence data are not unanimous. Some investigators have found immunoglobulin G (IgG), in a finely linear pattern along the capillary walls [19,20]. We found [21] that the reaction was weak and only present in some cases.

The nodules were negative. Exudative lesions are positive for fibrinogen, C3, β-lipoprotein, and (weakly) for IgG [21]. Some authors have reported the presence of insulin and/or antiinsulin, detectable by immunfluorescence, but we as well as Westberg and Michael [20] could not demonstrate these proteins. The different results may partly be due to technical differences and partly to subjective interpretations.

7. DEVELOPMENT OF THE LESIONS BY TIME

The most powerful determinant for the appearance and development of glomerular and vascular lesions in diabetes is duration of the diabetic state [2]. Diffuse glomerulopathy can be demonstrated by ultrastructural morphometry after a few years of diabetes [22], but is usually not distinct light-microscopically until 5-10 years after the onset of the disease. Nodular glomerulosclerosis demands at least 15 years of diabetes to develop. The nodules tend to disappear with marked glomerular

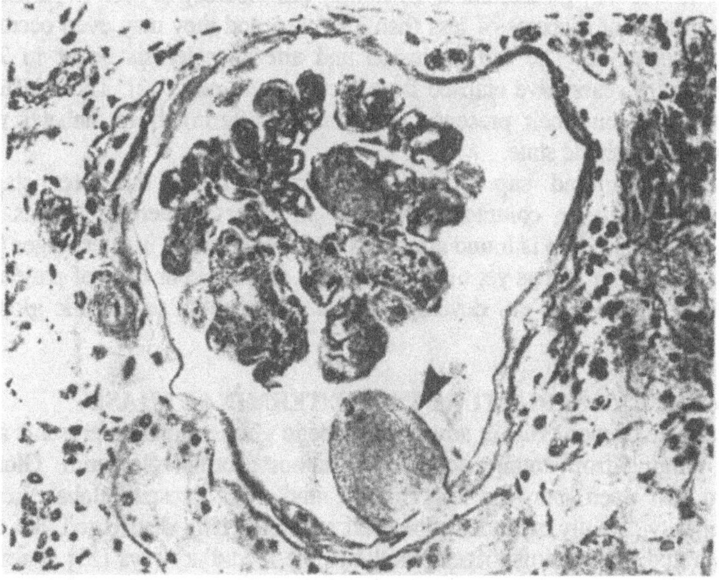

Figure 23-4 Capsular drop in diabetic glomeruloschlerosis. A large, drop-shaped deposit (*arrow*). PAS-haematoxylin.

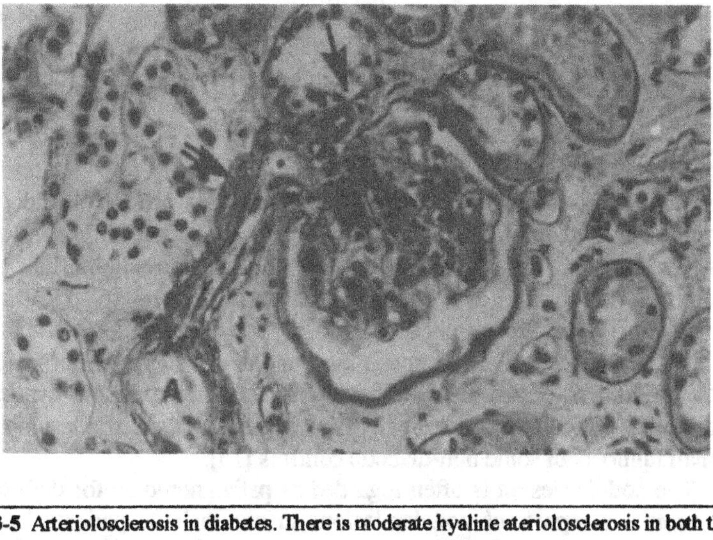

Figure 23-5 Arteriolosclerosis in diabetes. There is moderate hyaline ateriolosclerosis in both the afferent (*double arrow*) and the efferent (*arrow*) arterioles. A, interlobular artery. PAS-haematoxylin.

obsolescence. Whereas the precise onset of the diabetic disease is known in insulin dependent diabetes (IDDM) this is not the case with non-insulin dependent diabetes

(NIDDM) in which the disease may have been present several years before diagnosis. This is why glomerular nodules may occasionally be seen in patients with a *known* duration of diabetes of less than 15 years, and they may even occur at the time diagnosis made. The diffuse lesion and arteriolosclerosis occur in 20% of patients before 5 years have elapsed from the apparent onset [2]. These lesions are nonspecific, and thus their presence in a patient suffering from diabetes may be unrelated to the diabetic state.

The fibrinoid cap occurs most frequently in the later stages of glomerulopathy, but, in contradistinction to all other glomerular lesions in this disease, the capsular drop is found almost as often in earlier as in later stages [2].

A peculiar and as yet unexplained fact is that about 60% of patients with long-standing diabetes do *not* develop clinical nephropathy or diabetic glomerular changes.

8. GLOMERULAR STRUCTURE IN THE TERMINAL PHASE

The appearance of glomeruli in advanced diabetic glomerulopathy presents a broad spectrum ranging from totally occluded to almost normal glomeruli. Glomeruli, which are still open, may be hypertrophic and often present global mesangial hypercellularity. Totally occluded glomeruli are not evenly distributed, but tend to be concentrated in radiating stripes parallel to the medullary rays [23]. There is no difference in the severity of glomerular involvement between deep and superficial cortical zones. The total number of glomeruli decreases with progression of the diabetic nephropathy, at least in IDDM [24].

It is important to realize that this terminal pattern is not exclusively due to glomerular alterations specific for diabetes. Ischemic scarring and focal glomerular sclerosis occur and may indicate that causes other than progression of diabetic glomerular lesion may be partially responsible for the development of renal failure, such as vascular constriction with glomerular ischemia and lesions due to hyperfunction of remaining glomeruli.

9. SPECIFICITY OF THE LESIONS

The diffuse lesion is completely nonspecific and may be present in older people without diabetes. The combination of arteriolosclerosis and the diffuse lesion often occurs in hypertension, but involvement of both the afferent arteriole and the efferent arteriole is regarded as a strong indication of diabetes [6,25,26] although even this combination is not entirely specific [15].

All insudative lesions are much more numerous and/or larger in diabetics than in controls but they are not specific. Even capsular drops and hyalinosis of efferent arterioles which have traditionally been regarded as specific lesions may be seen in small numbers in some non-diabetic controls [15].

The nodular lesion is often regarded as pathognomonic for diabetes. It is true that numerous reports of nodular lesions in non-diabetic patients have been published [for a list, see ref. 3]. Most of these reports can be criticized, however, either because of doubt as to absence of diabetes or to lack of application of precise criteria for the morphologic diagnosis. There are, however, well documented cases on record with typical nodular glomerulopathy without diabetes [27,28].

Table 23-1 Staining characteristics of diabetic glomerular lesions

Stain	Diffuse	Nodular	Exudative[a]
Haematoxylineosin	+red	+red	++red
V. Gieson-Hansen	+red	+red	++yellow
Masson-trichrome	++blue	++blue	+++red
Phosphotungstic acid-haematoxylin	0	0	+++deep blue
PAS after diastase	++	++	+++
Silver-methenamine	++black	+/- black fibrils in pale matrix	0
Alcian-blue	+	0	0
Congo red, other amyloid stains	0	0	0
Neutral fat	0	(+) occasionally	+ fat vacuoles

[a]Exudative lesions are fibrinoid caps, capsular drops, and arteriolar hyalinosis

Although the *typical* nodular lesion is very strongly associated with diabetes, there exist nevertheless other conditions in which glomerular nodules may occur. Since these may present diagnostic difficulties, they will be briefly mentioned here. For a detailed report and illustrations, the reader is referred to an earlier publication [29].

In renal *amyloidosis*, abnormal homogeneous substance is deposited in the peripheral as well as mesangial parts of the glomerular capillary walls. In rare cases, the deposits may take on the shape of typical diabetic nodules with an acellular center. They can be correctly classified by the use of amyloid stains and by demonstration of typical fibrils on electron microscopy.

Some types of advanced *glomerulonephritis* (mesangial proliferative, membrano-proliferative) have a histology that resembles nodular glomerulosclerosis. In glomerulonephritis, however, there is a distinct hypercellularity and the central, acellular area that is so characteristic for diabetes is not present. Nodules in glomerulonephritis involve all mesangial areas and are of almost equal size. Immunodeposits are usually present, but are faint or absent in diabetes.

Glomerular nodules may also be present in various *dysproteinemias* (e.g. multiple myeloma and heavy-chain disease [30-35].

The clinical picture may often solve the diagnostic problem, but the occurrence of glomerular nodules in these diseases should be a reminder to the pathologist not to postulate the presence of diabetes on the prima facie detection of nodular structures in the glomeruli.

10. OTHER RENAL DISEASES IN DIABETES MELLITUS

Many reports have been published of *glomerulonephritis* occurring in patients with diabetic renal disease and this combination has been thought to be more frequent than could be explained by mere coincidence [34,35]. Autopsy studies have - on the other hand - shown that complicating glomerular disease is rare and probably not exceeding prevalence in the general population [36]. Glomerulonephritis complicating IDDM seems to be comparatively rare [37,38], probably around 2-3% in unselected cases with proteinuria and duration of diabetes of more than 10 years. Recently it has been reported that glomerulonephritis may be more common in NIDDM [for literature see ref. 39]. Published data are, however, conflicting. The rates of glomerulonephritis vary between 0 and 69% and those of other complicating renal diseases between 0 and 20%. Geographical differences and variable criteria for histopathological diagnosis may have been partly responsible, but the main cause of the diverging results are probably selection of patients for study. Most of the investigations are based upon patients referred to a nephrologic department and in some reports is was explicitly stated that the biopsies were made due to presence of symptoms and signs considered to be caused by other diseases than diabetes. It is clear that this will favour inclusion of patients with complicating renal disease. Pinel et al. [40], on the other hand, in their investigation of patients with NIDDM have excluded all patients with clinical renal disease other than the presence of micro- or macroalbuminuria. In this particular study no complicating renal disease was found at all.

Investigating a consecutive series of renal biopsies from 53 patients with NIDDM and microalbuminuria, Brocco et al. did not find any with complicating glomerulonephritis [41].

None of the studies published until now permit the conclusion that complicating glomerulonephritis in NIDDM is more frequent than in the general population.

Other complicating diseases. Atheroma emboli may be found in the intrarenal vessels as a complication to diabetic macroangiopathy (atherosclerosis in the aorta and renal arteries). Papillary necrosis is also a well known complication. Other renal diseases occurring in the same age as NIDDM such as amyloidosis and myeloma are probably unrelated to the diabetic state.

It is well established that long term diabetic nephropathy is associated with marked *interstitial fibrosis, tubular atrophy* and *mononuclear cell infiltration.* Formerly these changes were interpreted as evidence of complicating chronic pyelonephritis [3]. Since they were shown to be correlated to the renal microvascular alterations characteristic for long term diabetes, it was later on suggested that they were due to chronic ischemia [42,43]. Lane et al [44] found in IDDM that mesangial volume fraction, severity of arteriolar hyalinosis, percentage of globally sclerosed glomeruli, and interstitial volume fraction for total renal cortex were significantly correlated and all four structural parameters correlated with glomerular filtration rate and urinary albumin excretion. Stepwise multiple regression analysis suggested, however, that they are partially independent. Gambara et al [45] described a special subgroup of patients with diabetic renal disease in which the severe interstitial changes were not clearly correlated with glomerular or vascular lesions. Similar observations were reported by another group of investigations who analysed patients with microalbuminuria [41] and described three patterns of renal morphology. One had normal structure, another had typical diabetic glomerular changes and a third group had absent or mild glomerular changes together with disproportionately severe tubulointerstitial changes and/or arteriolar hyalinosis. Conceivably such changes may not be due to ischemia but to the diabetic metabolic abnormality, like diabetic glomerulopathy although with other pathogenesis.

REFERENCES

1. Kimmelstiel P, Wilson C. Intercapillary lesions in the glomeruli of the kidney. Am J Pathol 1936; 12: 83-105.
2. Thomsen AC. *The Kidney in Diabetes Mellitus* (thesis). Copenhagen: Munksgaard, 1965.
3. Ditscherlein G. *Nierenveränderungen bei Diabetikern*. Jená: G. Fischer, 1969.
4. Allen AC. So-called intercapillary glomerulosclerosis: a lesion associated with diabetes mellitus. Arch Pathol Lab Med 1941; 32: 33-51.
5. Bell ET. Renal lesions in diabetes mellitus. Am J Pathol 1942; 18: 744-745.
6. Bell ET. Renal vascular disease in diabetes mellitus. Diabetes 1953; 2: 376-389.
7. Bell ET. *Diabetes Mellitus: A Clinical and Pathological Study of 2529 Cases.* Springfield IL: Thomas, 1960.
8. Fahr T. Über Glomerulosklerose. Virschows Arch (Pathol Anat) 1942; 309: 16-33.
9. Spühler O, Zollinger HU. Die diab. Glomerulosklerose. Dtsch Arch Klin Med 1943; 190: 321-379.
10. Muirhead EE, Montgomery POB, Booth E. The glomerular lesions of diabetes mellitus: cellular hyaline and acellular hyaline lesions of »intercapillary glomerulosclerosis« as depicted by histochemical studies. Arch Intern Med 1956; 98: 146-161.
11. Randerath E. Zur Frage der intercapillären (diabetischen) Glomerulosklerose. Virchows Arch (Pathol Anat) 1953; 323: 483-523.
12. Sandison A, Newbold KM, Howie AJ. Evidence for unique distribution of Kimmelstiel-Wilson nodules in glomeruli. Diabetes 1992; 41: 952-955.
13. Stout LC, Kumar S, Whorton EB. Focal mesangiolysis and the pathogenesis of the Kimmelstiel-Wilson nodule. Hum Pathol 1993; 24: 77-89.
14. Yafumi S, Hiroshi K, Shin-Ichi T, Mitsuhiro Y, Hitoshi Y, Yoshitaka K, Nobu H. Mesangiolysis in diabetic glomeruli: Its role in the formation of nodular lesions. Kidney Int 1988; 34: 389-396.
15. Stout LC, Kumar S, Whorton EB. Insudative lesions - their pathogenesis and association with glomerular obsolescence in diabetes: A dynamic hypothesis based on single views of advancing human diabetic nephropathy. Hum Pathol 1994; 25: 1213-1227.
16. Barrie HJ, Aszkanazy CL, Smith GW. More glomerular changes in diabetics. Can Med Assoc J 1952; 66: 428-431.
17. Koss LG. Hyaline material with staining reaction of fibrinoid in renal lesions in diabetes mellitus. Arch Pathol Lab Med 1952; 54: 528-547.
18. Rinehart JF, Farquhar MG, Jung HC, Abul-Haj SK. The normal glomerulus and its basic reactions in disease. Am J Pathol 1953; 29: 21-31.
19. Gallo GR. Elution studies in kidneys with linear deposition of immunoglobulin in glomeruli. Am J Pathol 1970; 61: 377-394.
20. Westberg NG, Michael AF. Immunohistopathology of diabetic glomerulosclerosis. Diabetes 1972; 21: 163-174.
21. Frøkjær Thomsen O. Studies of diabetic glomerulosclerosis using an immunofluorescent technique. Acta Pathol Microbiol Scand (A) 1972; 80: 193-200.
22. Østerby R, Gundersen HJG, Nyberg G, Aurell M. Advanced diabetic glomerulopathy. Quantitative structural characterization of nonoccluded glomeruli. Diabe 1987; 36: 612-619.
23. Hørlyck A, Gundersen HJG, Østerby R. The cortical distribution pattern of diabetic glomerulopathy. Diabetologia 1986; 29: 146-150.
24. Bendtsen TF, Nyengaard JR. The number of glomeruli in Type 1 (insulin-dependent) and Type 2 (non-insulin dependent) diabetic patients. Diabetologia 1992; 35: 844-850.
25. Allen AC. *The Kidney: Medical and Surgical Diseases*, 2nd ed. London: Churchill, 1962; pp 38.
26. Heptinstall RH. *Pathology of the Kidney*, 3rd ed. Boston: Little, Brown and Company, 1983; Ch. 26.
27. Da-Silva EC, Saldanha LB, Pestalozzi MS, Del-Bueno IJ, Barros RT, Marcondes M, Nussenzveig I. Nodular diabetic glomerulosclerosis without diabetes mellitus. Nephron 1992; 62: 289-291.

28. Kanwar YS, Garces J, Molitch ME. Occurrence of intercapillary nodular glomerulosclerosis in the absence of glucose intolerance. Am J Kidney Dis 1990; 15: 281-283.
29. Olsen TS. Mesangial thickening and nodular glomerular sclerosis in diabetes mellitus and other diseases. Acta Pathol Microbiol Scand (A) 1972; 80: 203-216.
30. Sølling K, Askjær S-A. Multiple myeloma with urinary excretion of heavy chain components of IgG and nodular glomerulosclerosis. Acta Med Scand 1973; 194: 23-30.
31. Gallo GR, Feiner HD, Katz LA, Feldman GM, Correa EB, Chuba JV Buxbaum JN. Nodular glomerulopathy associated with nonamyloidotic kappa light chain deposits and excess immunoglobulin light chain synthesis. Am J Pathol 1980; 99: 621-644.
32. Sølling K, Sølling J, Jacobsen NO, Frøkjær Thomsen O. Nonsecretory myeloma associated with nodular glomerulosclerosis. Acta Med Scand 1980; 207: 137-143.
33. Schubert GE, Adam A. Glomerular nodules and long-spacing collagen in kidneys of patients with multiple myeloma. J Clin Pathol 1974; 27: 800-805.
34. Wehner H, Bohle A. The structure of the glomerular capillary basement membrane in diabetes mellitus with and without nephrotic syndrome. Virchows Arch (Pathol Anat) 1974; 364: 303-309.
35. Yum M, Maxwell DR, Hamburger R, Kleit SA. Primary glomerulonephritis complicating diabetic nephropathy. Hum Pathol 1984; 15: 921-927.
36. Waldherr R, Ilkenhans C, Ritz E. How frequent is glomerulonephritis in diabetes mellitus type II ? Clin Nephrol 1992; 37: 271-273.
37. Mauer SM, Steffes MW, Ellis EN, Sutherland DER, Brown DM, Goetz FC. Structural-functional relationships in diabetic nephropathy. J Clin Invest 1984; 74: 1143-1155.
38. Richards N, Greaves I, Lee S, Howie A, Adu D, Michael J. Increased prevalence of renal biopsy findings other than diabetic glomerulopathy in type II diabetes mellitus. Nephrol Dial Transplant 1992; 7: 397-399.
39. Olsen S, Mogensen CE. How often is type II diabetes mellitus complicated with non-diabetic renal disease? A material of renal biopsies and an analysis of the literature. Diabetologia 1996; 39: 1638-1645.
40. Pinel NBF, Bilous R, Corticelli P, Halimi S, Cordonnier D. *Renal Biopsies in 30 Micro- and Macroalbuminuric Non-Insulin Dependent (NIDDM) Patients: Heterogeneity of Renal Lesions.* Heidelberg: European Diabetic Nephropathy Study Group, 1995.
41. Brocco E, Fioretto P, Mauer M, Saller A, Carraro A, Frigato C, Chiesura-Corona M, Bianchi L, Baggio B, Maioll M, Abaterusso C, Velussi M, Sambatoro M, Virgili F, Ossi E, Nosadini R. Renal structure and function in non-insulin dependent diabetic patients with microalbuminuria. Kidney Int. 1997; 52: Suppl. 63: S40-S44.
42 Bohle A, Wehrmann M, Bogenschütz B, Müller CA. The pathogenesis of chronic renal failure in diabetic nephropathy. Path Res Pract 1991; 187: 251-259.
43. Bader R, Bader H, Grund KE, Mackensen-Hahn S, Christ H, Bohle A. Structure and function of the kidney in diabetic glomerulosclerosis. Correlations between morphological and functional parameters. Path Res Pract 1980; 167: 204-216.
44. Lane PH, Steffes M, Fioretto P, Mayer SM. Renal interstitial expansion in insulin-dependent diabetes mellitus. Kidney Int 1993; 43: 661-667.
45. Gambara V, Remuzzi G, Bertani T. Heterogenous nature of renal lesions in type II diabetes. J Am Soc Nephrol 1993; 3: 1458-1466.

24. RENAL ULTRASTRUCTURAL CHANGES IN MICROALBUMINURIC IDDM-PATIENTS

Hans-Jacob Bangstad, Susanne Rudberg and Ruth Østerby
Department of Pediatrics, Aker Diabetes Research Centre, Aker University Hospital, Oslo, Norway, Department of Woman and Child Health, Pediatric Unit, Karolinska Institute, Stockholm, Sweden and Laboratory for Electron Microscopy, Aarhus Kommunehospital, Aarhus, Denmark

Associations between early stages of diabetic nephropathy and structural changes is far from clarified. Some reports present rather marked changes in patients in the preclinical stage whereas others found very moderate changes in the early stage of nephropathy. Hence the issue is still a challenge to further studies. This chapter concentrates on the renal morphological changes in patients with insulin dependent diabetes mellitus (IDDM) and early nephropathy and the influence of blood glucose control on these structural changes.

1. METHODS AND STRUCTURES IN QUESTION

The increased thickness of the glomerular basement membrane (BM) and the mesangial expansion with accumulation of matrix are the most characteristic changes in diabetic glomerulopathy [1]. The methodology involved in the measurement of BM thickness is described in detail elsewhere [2]. The relative increase of mesangium and of mesangial matrix is expressed as volume fractions, e.g. mesangium per glomerulus, matrix per mesangium or per glomerulus. The volume fractions are relative measures, estimating the composition of glomeruli and mesangial regions. These parameters are the quantitative expressions of the characteristic appearance of diabetic glomerulopathy. The matrix star volume (3-5) is an estimate of the confluence and/or convexity and size of the individual branches of the matrix. Another estimate, the matrix "thickness", corresponds to the arbitrary thickness of the matrix if transposed to form an even layer on the urinary surface of the mesangial region [4,5]. An overall expression of the glomerulopathy is the structural index (BMT/10 + matix/glomerular volume fraction in % + matrix star volume). Of decisive importance for obtaining reliable data describing the earliest stages is a sufficient and unbiased sampling. In order to reduce the imprecision in the estimates of the mesangial volume fraction, a method with complete cross-sections at 3 levels per glomerulus has been advocated [6]. With respect to the arteriolar changes the matrix/media volume fraction of the afferent and the efferent arterioles were studied according to the methods recently described [7].

2. PATIENTS WITH MICROALBUMINURIA VS. HEALTHY CONTROLS

We have studied two series of kidney biopsies from 38 normotensive young IDDM patients as baseline data for prospective studies [8,9]. Most of the diabetic patients had AER in the low range with median of 31 µg/min (range 15-194). Their mean age was 19 years (14-29) and diabetes duration 11 years (6-18). The microalbuminuric (MA) patients showed a clear increment in BM thickness with a mean of 586 nm (95% confidence interval 553-619 nm) versus 350 nm (315-384) in the non-diabetic control group. All of the MA patients had BM thickness above the normal range. The average BM thickening during the years with diabetes was approximately 21 nm per year. This approximation was based on the assumption that the patients had a BM thickness at onset of diabetes corresponding to the mean BMT of the control group, i.e. 350 nm. A significant parallel matrix expansion in the microalbuminuric patients vs. the normal controls was observed. Matrix/glomerular volume fraction was 0.12 (0.11-0.13) vs. 0.09 (0.08-0.10) and matrix star volume 28 μm^3 (26-31) vs. 14 μm^3 (11-17) in the two groups respectively [10].

Fioretto et al. presented structural data (BMT and mesangial/glomerular volume fraction) in 33 patients with AER above 15 µg per minute. Both parameters were increased compared with those in controls and correlated with AER. Matrix parameters were not investigated. Observations different from those in our series were very high figures for mesangial volume fraction also in the low range of microalbuminuria. Furthermore, several patients had decreased creatinine clearance and hypertension [11].

It is hardly surprising that it is possible with sensitive methods to show morphological changes in IDDM-patients with clinical indications of renal impairment (microalbuminuria), when compared to healthy controls, but the extent of the changes should be emphasized.

3. MICROALBUMINURIA VS. NORMOALBUMINURIA

In the 60ies several reports indicated that morphological changes were present at the onset of IDDM. Later studies clearly showed that the glomeruli are normal at that time [12] and the impact of that observation was supported by studies of identical twins discordant for IDDM [13]. In a clinical setting the transition from normo- to microalbuminuria is of utmost importance. Walker et al. compared two groups of IDDM patients [4], one with normoalbuminuria (n=9, AER <20 µg/min) and one with microalbuminuria (n=6). Even though the number of patients was low, a significant increment in BM thickness, mesangial/glomerular volume fraction and also the matrix parameters was found in patients with MA compared to those with NA. The patients in the normoalbuminuric (NA) group were slightly younger and had a shorter duration of diabetes than the MA-group, although the differences were not statistically significant. The group of patients with microalbuminuria was very heterogeneous with a wide range in diabetes duration. Since the biopsies in that study and the biopsies in our microalbuminuric patients were analysed at the same laboratory, and as clinical data were rather similar in the two studies, we compared the normo- and microalbuminuric groups and thus with a greater number of patients (n=17) we confirmed Walker's principal findings. These results differ from those presented by Fioretto et al. [11], who found no difference between patients with normo- and low-grade microalbuminuria (< 32 μg/min). Further, their observations in the normoalbuminuric group are remarkable as increased BMT and mesangial volume fraction are demonstrated. The latter parameter (with a mean of 0.30) is in fact markedly higher than that observed in our microalbuminuric group (0.21) and expresses advanced glomerulopathy. The high prevalence of hypertension (15%) in the normoalbuminuric patients does not seem to fully explain the discrepancies between the studies.

Another recent American study reported analogous findings in children and adolescents with diabetes duration between five and twelve years [14]. In that study a high frequency of BM-thickening and increased mesangial volume fraction was found in more than fifty percent of the patients, most of whom (48/59) had normal AER. However, since concurrent analysis of valid control cases was not performed and details of morphometry are not given, this percentage should be taken with great reserve. Yet, the two reports stating occurrence of advanced lesions in cases with normal AER lead to the question whether European and American populations are really that different, or whether patient selection or quantitative methodology are part of the explanation of discrepancies.

4. EXTRA-GLOMERULAR CHANGES

In advanced stages of nephropathy several structural compartments in the kidney display distinct abnormalities. The hyalinosis of efferent and afferent arterioles was described a long time ago. Increase in the interstitial tissue has in fact been incriminated as the major determinant of the late fall in renal function [15]. Some information on these structures during earlier phases of nephropathy has been obtained in recent years.

Semiquantitative studies of the hyalinosis of arterioles have dealt with a very broad clinical range. The results showed that the score of arteriolar lesions correlated with the severity of glomerulopathy and interstitial expansion and also with renal function [16]. Clearly in this composite picture with affection of all compartments it is not possible to determine which is the most important in terms of the further progression of nephropathy, in particular since abnormalities in one compartment may be very closely and causally related to that in others.

In a quantitative ultrastructural study the composition of arteriolar walls was estimated in NA and MA IDDM patients and in controls [7]. All of the patients had clinical blood pressure within the normal range. Increased matrix was found in afferent and efferent arterioles in the MA patients, showing that matrix abnormalities have developed in this location at the earliest stage of nephropathy.

Quantitative data are now available in the baseline biopsies described above [10]. A significant difference in the matrix/media volume fraction was found between the microalbuminuric patients and the controls both regarding the afferent (0.44 ± 0.06 vs 0.33 ± 0.07, $p < 10^{-4}$) and the efferent arterioles (0.55 ± 0.10 vs 0.45 ± 0.10, $p = 10^{-2}$). The matrix/media volume fraction of the afferent arterioles was highly correlated to the glomerular parameters (BMT, r=0.44, mesangial/glomerular volume fraction, r=0.69 and matrix/glomerular volume fraction, r=0.70) whereas the positive correlation of the efferent arteriole did not reach statistical significance.

Interstitial expansion is a companion of advanced glomerulopathy and vasculopathy. The interstitium expressed as fraction of cortical space has been shown to correlate with AER and creatinine clearance, as well as with glomerular and arteriolar changes, considering a wide range of functional impairment [16]. We estimated the interstitial volume fraction in the MA patients with low grade albuminuria, and found that it was increased compared to controls already in this early phase [5,17]. A positive correlation with the degree of glomerulopathy was found, indicating parallel or maybe even interactive processes. In addition, an association between interstitial changes and a decline in GFR in the early stage of microalbuminuria was shown [17].

5. GLOMERULOPATHY AND BLOOD GLUCOSE CONTROL

The impact of long term hyperglycaemia on the development of structural changes has been demonstrated in several studies of experimental diabetes (18-23). Previous studies in diabetic patients have dealt with the conditions in transplanted kidneys. In one prospective 5-years' study renal transplant recipients were allocated to maximized or standard control [24]. A beneficial effect of maximized control was observed, since the increment in mesangial matrix volume fraction was less than in the standard treated group, whereas the differences between the two groups in BM thickening and mesangial volume fraction failed to reach statistical significance. A few studies have dealt with patients who received kidney as well as pancreas transplants. Although the results are not absolutely lucid the various series do indicate some beneficial effect in terms of preventing early changes [25,26] if complete normalisation is obtained, or preventing the further progression of moderately expressed glomerulopathy [27].

In our own series we studied the relationship between structural changes and preceding blood glucose control. The estimated yearly increment of BMT and matrix volume fraction from onset of diabetes correlated with mean HbA_{1c} from the year preceding the study, which probably reflects the long term blood glucose control [5]. Recently a study in adolescents confirmed this by finding that 5-year mean HbA1c in addition to diabetes duration and GFR, was a variable with an independent influence on the glomerulopathy index [9].

One of the prospective studies has been concluded after 2 and a half years period (8). The patients were randomized to either intensive insulin treatment by continuous subcutaneous insulin infusion (CSII) or conventional treatment (CT,- mostly multiple injections). It should be noticed that the mean HbA_{1c}-values in the two groups were rather high, and that the difference between the groups was modest, although significant, 8.7% and 9.9% respectively (normal range 4.3-6.1%). The AER was for most of the patients in the low microalbuminuric range throughout the study. In fact, 38 % of the patients had AER <15 µg/min at the end of the study and thus by definition had no longer microalbuminuria. The main finding of the study was that in the CSII-group none of the matrix-parameters increased, whereas they all increased (not significantly for matrix/glomerular volume fraction and matrix-thickness) in the CT-group. The BM thickness increased in both groups,- but the increment during the study period was significantly larger in the CT-group [140 nm

(50-230) vs. 56 nm (27-86)]. The association between blood glucose control and structure was confirmed when all the patients were considered together. A strong correlation was found between mean HbA_{1c} during the study and increase in BM thickness and matrix/glomerular volume fraction (figure 24-1). We thus showed that

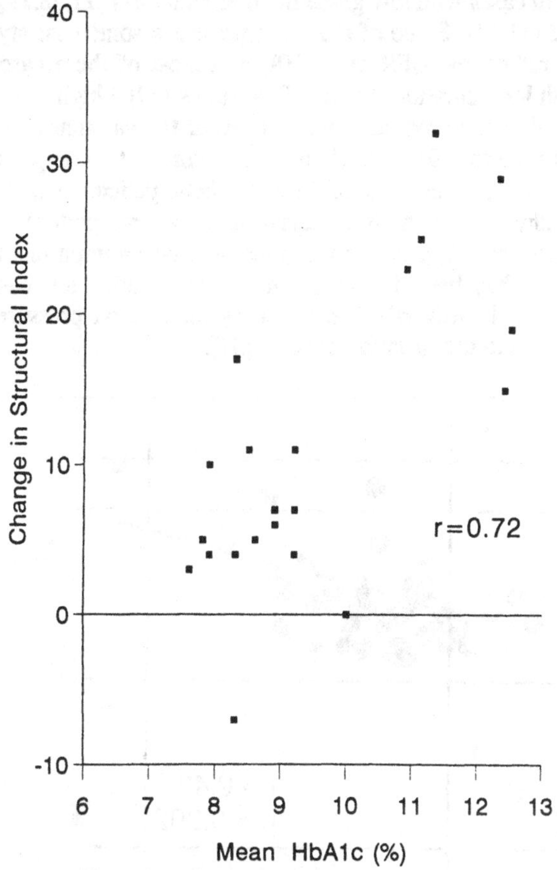

Figure 24-1. Results of a prospective study showing change in structural index (basement membrane thickness/10 + matrix volume fraction of the glomerulus,%) vs. mean HbA_{1c} during 26-34 months in 21 IDDM-patients with microalbuminuria. Reference no. 8.

the progression of morphological changes in the glomerulus can be identified within a short period of only 2-3 years. Furthermore, we observed that reduced mean blood glucose levels clearly retarded the progression of morphological changes in the glomeruli. However, the glycated haemoglobin level achieved in the CSII-treated group (8.7%) was not sufficient to stop the progression of morphological changes.

6. GLOMERULAR STRUCTURE VERSUS ALBUMIN EXCRETION AND SYSTEMIC BLOOD PRESSURE

AER is an important parameter of kidney function in the early stages of nephropathy. In the combined group of NA and MA-patients Walker et al. [4] found a significant correlation between AER and the severity of glomerular lesions. Also within groups of MA-patients correlation between AER and structural parameters are observed [8,10,11]. However, it is not a very close correlation (figure 24-2) and in conflict with this general observation are the reports mentioned above of rather advanced glomerulopathy in cases with low grade microalbuminuria [11,28,29], and even in normoalbuminuria [11,14]. Some of the cases present a somewhat atypical picture with concurrently rather low GFR and AER, and most of these cases are female IDDM-patients with long duration. In one of the series [29] a high frequency of totally occluded glomeruli was found, and enlargement of the vascular pole area in the open glomeruli was marked [30]. This change may represent a compensation to falling GFR and might influence the level of AER. Diabetic patients with a slow development of nephropathy may exhibit a deviating structural pattern where changes of arterioles and arteries (diabetic microangiopathy) play an important role.

One of our series has been followed for six years after the baseline biopsy. It was revealed that primarily BMT, but also systolic blood pressure and mean 6-yearHbA_{1c} contributed to the variation of AER [31].

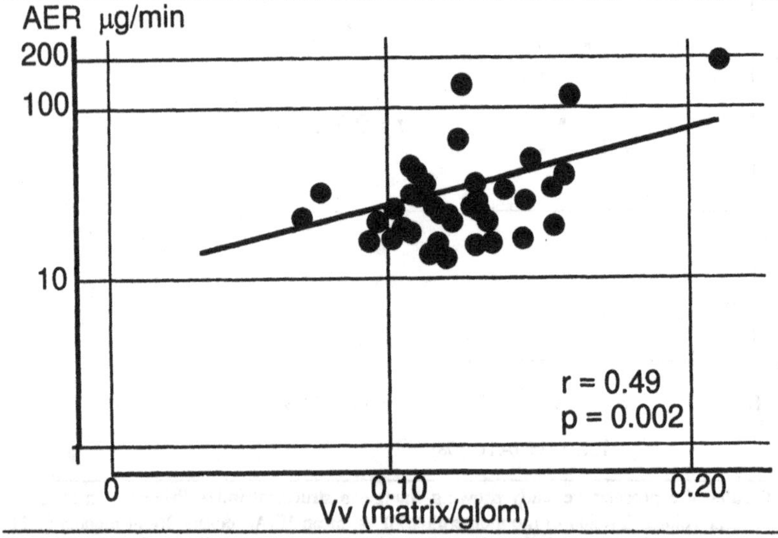

Figure 24-2. Urinary albumin excretion rate vs. mesangial matrix volume fraction, V_V(matrix/glom) in baseline biopsies from 38 young, normotensive IDDM patients with microalbuminuria. Reference no. [10].

It is still unclear whether the elevation of blood pressure observed in diabetic nephropathy precedes, develops in parallel with or follows the initial increment of AER [32,33]. In our prospective study none of the patients had arterial hypertension (>150/90 mmHg), but 24 hours ambulatory blood pressure was not measured [8]. No associations between blood pressure (BP) and glomerular parameters were found, neither at baseline nor at follow-up, but all patients had BP within a fairly narrow range. Similarly, in the study by Rudberg et al [9] 5-year mean systolic and diastolic blood pressure preceding the renal biopsy in the transitional stage from normo- to microalbuminuria, did not predict the degree of diabetic glomerulopathy changes. This might indicate that BP has little impact on the initiation of structural lesions. But as mentioned above, systolic blood pressure at baseline of the prospective study correlated with the level of AER 6 years later. Also, Chavers et al. reported on a group of MA-patients with AER in the medium range (65 μg/min) with elevated BP (and/or reduced GFR) and found that they had more advanced structural changes than MA-patients with normal BP and GFR [34].

7. MECHANISMS OF ALBUMINURIA

The urinary excretion of negatively charged proteins, e.g. albumin, is restricted by the negatively charged basement membrane. In the aforementioned prospective study [8] the charge selectivity index (clearances of IgG/IgG_4) was not associated with BM thickness at the beginning of the study. However, a striking correlation was found between the increase of BM thickness and the loss of charge selectivity during the study [35]. This may imply that the increase in BM thickness takes place concomitant with qualitative changes (e.g. loss of negative charge).

It is not known which substances that are responsible for the early thickening of BM and matrix expansion in diabetes. In the BM collagen IV predominates quantitatively, while laminin and heparan-sulphate proteoglycan probably play an important role as well. The mesangial matrix contains in addition collagen V, fibronectin, and chondroitin/dermatan sulphate proteoglycans [36]. Short-term experimental studies show that hyperglycaemia induces increased production of most of the aforementioned proteins [37-39], increased levels of the proteins' respective mRNA [40,41], increased matrix synthesis [42], and reduced amount of heparan-sulphate proteoglycan [43,44]. Furthermore, hyperglycaemia leads to accumulation of advanced glycated end products of proteins (AGE). These glycated proteins do contribute to the formation of pathological tissue deposits (45). In our study [8] the level of AGEs at the start of the study was related to the changes in structural parameters during the study period [46].

Even if we have demonstrated a close linkage between long term hyperglycaemia and change in structural parameters, and also an association between renal function and glomerulopathy in the early stages of nephropathy, we still lack the deeper insight into the mechanisms behind the increment in albumin leakage.

The increase in BM thickness in itself is unlikely to be responsible for the increased albumin excretion rate, but qualitative changes, e.g. reduced negative charge and/or presence of large pores, which develop concomitantly with the increase in thickness, may be decisive. An interesting observation in advanced glomerulopathy [47] and occasionally also in the early stage in microalbuminuric patients [1] is capillary loops with extremely thin and fluffy BM, contrasting markedly the other capillaries in the biopsies. They may be an expression of a compensatory glomerular growth, setting in at this early stage, and could represent the "large pores". The BM-thickening develops in parallel with matrix expansion. Matrix changes, quantitative and qualitative, may interfere with the function of the mesangial cells [48]. One immediate consequence of the matrix expansion is that the distance between mesangial cells increases. This may impair the cell to cell interaction. Mesangial cell function plays a role in many aspects of glomerular physiology [49].

Altogether, the present data indicate that the increased loss of albumin across the glomerular filtration barrier is a sign associated with early structural lesions of diabetic glomerulopathy.

REFERENCES

1. Østerby R (1993) Renal pathology in diabetes mellitus. Curr Opin Nephrol Hypertens 2:475-483
2. Hirose K, Østerby R, Nozawa M, Gundersen HJ (1982) Development of glomerular lesions in experimental long-term diabetes in the rat. Kidney Int 21:889-895
3. Gundersen HJ, Bendtsen TF, Korbo L, et al (1988) Some new, simple and efficient stereological methods and their use in pathological research and diagnosis. APMIS 96:379-394
4. Walker JD, Close CF, Jones SL, et al (1992) Glomerular structure in type-1 (insulin-dependent) diabetic patients with normo- and microalbuminuria. Kidney Int 41:741-748
5. Bangstad H-J, Østerby R, Dahl-Jørgensen K, et al (1993) Early glomerulopathy is present in young, type 1 (insulin-dependent) diabetic patients with microalbuminuria. Diabetologia 36:523-529
6. Østerby, R. Research methodologies related to renal complications: structural changes. In: *Research Methodologies in Human Diabetes, vol.2. Diabetes Forum Series V, Part II*, edited by Mogensen, C.E. and Standl, E. Berlin,New York: Walter de Gruyter & Co., 1995, p. 289-309.
7. Østerby R, Bangstad H-J, Nyberg G, Walker JD, Viberti GC (1995) A quantitative ultrastructural study of juxtaglomerular arterioles in IDDM patients with micro- and normoalbuminuria. Diabetologia 38:1320-1327
8. Bangstad H-J, Østerby R, Dahl-Jørgensen K, Berg KJ, Hartmann K, Hanssen KF (1994) Improvement of blood glucose control retards the progression of morphological changes in early diabetic nephropathy. Diabetologia 37:483-490
9. Rudberg S, Østerby R, Dahlquist G, Nyberg G, Persson B (1997) Predictors of renal morphological changes in the early stage of microalbuminuria in adolescents with IDDM. Diabetes Care 20:265-271
10. Østerby R, Bangstad H-J, Rudberg S (1998) Structural changes in microalbuminuria. Effect of intervention. Nephrol Dial Transplant, in press.
11. Fioretto P, Steffes MW, Mauer SM (1994) Glomerular structure in nonproteinuric IDDM patients with various levels of albuminuria. Diabetes 43:1358-1364
12. Østerby R (1974) Early phases in the development of diabetic glomerulopathy. Acta Med Scand Suppl 574:3-82
13. Steffes MW, Sutherland DE, Goetz FC, Rich SS, Mauer SM (1985) Studies of kidney and muscle biopsy specimens from identical twins discordant for type I diabetes mellitus. N Engl J Med 312:1282-1287
14. Ellis EN, Warady BA, Wood EG, et al (1997) Renal structural-functional relationship in early diabetes mellitus. Pediatr Nephrol 11:584-591
15. Ziyadeh FN, Goldfarb S (1991) The renal tubulointerstitium in diabetes mellitus. Kidney Int 39:464-475
16. Lane PH, Steffes MW, Fioretto P, Mauer SM (1993) Renal interstitial expansion in insulin-dependent diabetes mellitus. Kidney Int 43:661-667
17. Rudberg S, Østerby R (1997) Decreasing glomerular filtration rate - an indicator of more advanced diabetic glomerulopathy in the early course of microalbuminuria in IDDM adolescents? Nephrol Dial Transplant 12:1282-1283
18. Mauer SM, Brown DM, Matas AJ, Steffes MW (1978) Effects of pancreatic islet transplantation on the increased urinary albumin excretion rates in intact and uninephrectomized rats with diabetes mellitus. Diabetes 27:959-964
19. Rasch R (1979) Prevention of diabetic glomerulopathy in streptozotocin diabetic rats by insulin treatment. Diabetologia 16:319-324
20. Rasch R (1979) Prevention of diabetic glomerulopathy in streptozotocin diabetic rats by insulin treatment. The mesangial regions. Diabetologia 17:243-248

21. Steffes MW, Brown DM, Basgen JM, Mauer SM (1980) Amelioration of mesangial volume and surface alterations following islet transplantation in diabetic rats. Diabetes 29:509-515
22. Orloff MJ, Yamanaka N, Greenleaf GE, Huang YT, Huang DG, Leng XS (1986) Reversal of mesangial enlargement in rats with long-standing diabetes by whole pancreas transplantation. Diabetes 35:347-354
23. Kern TS, Engerman RL (1987) Kidney morphology in experimental hyperglycemia. Diabetes 36:244-249
24. Barbosa J, Steffes MW, Sutherland DE, Connett JE, Rao KV, Mauer SM (1994) Effect of glycemic control on early diabetic renal lesions. A 5-year randomized controlled clinical trial of insulin-dependent diabetic kidney transplant recipients. JAMA 272:600-606
25. Wilczek HE, Jaremko G, Tyden G, Groth CG (1995) Evolution of diabetic nephropathy in kidney grafts. Evidence that a simultaneously transplanted pancreas exerts a protective effect. Transplantation 59:51-57
26. Nyberg G, Holdaas H, Brekke IB, et al (1996) Glomerular ultrastructure in kidneys transplanted simultaneously with a segmental pancreas to patients with type 1 diabetes. Nephrol Dial Transplant 11:1029-1033
27. Bilous RW, Mauer SM, Sutherland DE, Najarian JS, Goetz FC, Steffes MW (1989) The effects of pancreas transplantation on the glomerular structure of renal allografts in patients with insulin-dependent diabetes. N Engl J Med 321:80-85
28. Lane PH, Steffes MW, Mauer SM (1992) Glomerular structure in IDDM women with low glomerular filtration rate and normal urinary albumin excretion. Diabetes 41:581-586
29. Østerby R, Schmitz A, Nyberg G, Asplund J (1998) Renal structural changes in insulin dependent diabetic patients with albuminuria. Comparison of cases with onset of albuminuria after short or long duration. APMIS in press
30. Østerby R, Asplund J, Bangstad H-J, et al (1997) Glomerular volume and the glomerular vascular pole area in patients with insulin-dependent diabetes mellitus. Virch Arch 431:351-357
31. Bangstad H-J, Østerby R, Hartmann A, Berg TJ, Dahl-Jørgensen K, Hanssen KF (1997) Renal morphological changes predict urinary albumin excretion rate 6 years later in patients with IDDM and microalbuminuria. Diabetologia 40:2085
32. Mogensen CE, Hansen KW, Østerby R, Damsgaard EM (1992) Blood pressure elevation versus abnormal albuminuria in the genesis and prediction of renal disease in diabetes. Diabetes Care 15:1192-1204
33. Poulsen PL, Hansen KW, Mogensen CE (1994) Ambulatory blood pressure in the transition from normo- to microalbuminuria. A longitudinal study in IDDM patients. Diabetes 43:1248-1253
34. Chavers BM, Bilous RW, Ellis EN, Steffes MW, Mauer SM (1989) Glomerular lesions and urinary albumin excretion in type I diabetes without overt proteinuria. N Engl J Med 320:966-970
35. Bangstad HJ, Kofoed-Enevoldsen A, Dahl-Jørgensen K, Hanssen KF (1992) Glomerular charge selectivity and the influence of improved blood glucose control in type 1 (insulin-dependent) diabetic patients with microalbuminuria. Diabetologia 35:1165-1169
36. Silbiger S, Crowley S, Shan Z, Brownlee M, Satriano J, Schlondorff D (1993) Nonenzymatic glycation of mesangial matrix and prolonged exposure of mesangial matrix to elevated glucose reduces collagen synthesis and proteoglycan charge. Kidney Int 43:853-864
37. Brownlee M, Spiro RG (1979) Glomerular basement membrane metabolism in the diabetic rat. In vivo studies. Diabetes 28:121-125
38. Roy S, Sala R, Cagliero E, Lorenzi M (1990) Overexpression of fibronectin induced by diabetes or high glucose: phenomenon with a memory. Proc Natl Acad Sci U S A 87:404-408
39. Cagliero E, Roth T, Roy S, Lorenzi M (1991) Characteristics and mechanisms of high-glucose-induced overexpression of basement membrane components in cultured human endothelial cells. Diabetes 40:102-110
40. Poulsom R, Kurkinen M, Prockop DJ, Boot Handford RP (1988) Increased steady-state levels of laminin B1 mRNA in kidneys of long-term streptozotocin-diabetic rats. No effect of an aldose reductase inhibitor. J Biol Chem 263:10072-10076
41. Ledbetter S, Copeland EJ, Noonan D, Vogeli G, Hassell JR (1990) Altered steady-state mRNA levels of basement membrane proteins in diabetic mouse kidneys and thromboxane synthase inhibition. Diabetes 39:196-203

42. Ayo SH, Radnik RA, Garoni JA, Glass WF, Kreisberg JI (1990) High glucose causes an increase in extracellular matrix proteins in cultured mesangial cells. Am J Pathol 136:1339-1348
43. Shimomura H, Spiro RG (1987) Studies on macromolecular components of human glomerular basement membrane and alterations in diabetes. Decreased levels of heparan sulfate proteoglycan and laminin. Diabetes 36:374-381
44. Olgemoller B, Schwaabe S, Gerbitz KD, Schleicher ED (1992) Elevated glucose decreases the content of a basement membrane associated heparan sulphate proteoglycan in proliferating cultured porcine mesangial cells. Diabetologia 35:183-186
45. Brownlee M, Vlassara H, Cerami A (1984) Nonenzymatic glycosylation and the pathogenesis of diabetic complications. Ann Intern Med 101:527-537
46. Berg TJ, Bangstad HJ, Torjesen PA, Østerby R, Bucala R, Hanssen KF (1997) Advanced glycation end products in serum predict changes in the kidney morphology of patients with insulin-dependent diabetes mellitus. Metabolism 46:661-665
47. Østerby R, Nyberg G (1987) New vessel formation in the renal corpuscles in advanced diabetic glomerulopathy. J Diabet Complications 1:122-127
48. Kashgarian M, Sterzel RB (1992) The pathobiology of the mesangium. Kidney Int 41:524-529
49. Hawkins NJ, Wakefield D, Charlesworth JA (1990) The role of mesangial cells in glomerular pathology. Pathology 22:24-32

25. RENAL STRUCTURE IN NON INSULIN DEPENDENT DIABETIC PATIENTS WITH MICROALBUMINURIA

Paola Fioretto, Michael Mauer and Romano Nosadini.
Department of Internal Medicine and Center of the National Research Council for the Study of Aging, University of Padova, Italy;
Department of Pediatrics, University of Minnesota, Minneapolis, MN, USA;
Department of Internal Medicine, University of Sassari, Italy.

RENAL STRUCTURAL CHANGES IN DIABETIC NEPHROPATHY

Although far more than 50 % of diabetic patients receiving renal replacement therapy have type 2 diabetes [1-5], the renal pathology and natural history of diabetic nephropathy (DN) in type 2 diabetes has been studied much less intensly than in type 1 diabetes and thus many important questions remain unclear. The clinical manifestations of DN, proteinuria, declining GFR and increasing blood pressure, are similar in type 1 and type 2 diabetes [6-7], as they are in many other renal diseases; nevertheless whether these clinical features are the consequences of similar underlying renal lesions is not entirely known. In type 1 diabetes it is generally accepted that glomerulopathy represents the most important structural change, leading to progressive renal function loss [8-13]; concomitantly and roughly proportionally to the degree of glomerulopathy, the arterioles, tubules and interstitium also undergo structural changes, including hyalinosis of the arteriolar wall, thickening and reduplication of tubular basement membranes, tubular atrophy and interstitial expansion and fibrosis [8-14]. These lesions become progressive and severe only when glomerulopathy is far advanced. Quantitative morphometric studies have demonstrated that the lesion most closely related to the decline in renal function in type 1 diabetes is mesangial expansion, caused predominantly by mesangial matrix accumulation [12, 15]. We have also recently observed, in sequential renal biopsies of type 1 diabetic patients performed 5 years apart, that the only structural change associated with increasing albuminuria was mesangial expansion [13]; GBM width, interstitial expansion and the number of globally sclerosed glomeruli did not change over 5 years in this group of patients, several of whom were studied while in transition from normal to microalbuminuria or from microalbuminuria to overt nephropathy. Thus in type 1 diabetes severe arteriolar, tubular and interstitial lesions are rare unless advanced diabetic glomerulopathy is present.

When overt nephropathy develops in patients with type 1 diabetes of at least 10 years duration, advanced diabetic glomerulopathy is almost always present, while non-diabetic renal diseases are rare in such patients (Mauer, unpublished data). In proteinuric type 2 diabetic patients, on the contrary, the prevalence of non diabetic renal lesions has been reported to be high (approximately 30%). Parving et al reported that 23% of type 2 diabetic patients with proteinuria had non-diabetic glomerulopathies, which these authors classified as minimal lesion nephropathy, mesangio-proliferative glomerulonephritis (GN) and sequelae of GN [16]. Heterogeneity in renal lesions has also been reported by Gambara et al, who found that only 37 % of proteinuric type 2 diabetic patients had typical changes of DN [17]. Khan et al observed the presence of non diabetic renal disease in 42% of 153 type 2 patients with overt nephropathy [18]; the occurrence of non diabetic renal diseases was much lower (12%) in the series of 33 proteinuric patients studied by Olsen and Mogensen [19]. In all these studies, with the exception of the study of Parving, however, patients were referred to the nephrologist and kidney biopsies were performed for clinical indications; thus many of these renal biopsies were presumably performed bacause the patient's clinical course was considered to be atypical for diabetic nephropathy. Therefore, these studies may not describe the usual type 2 patients with diabetic nephropathy, but those with an unusual clinical course; also the different results may reflect differences in the criteria for kidney biopsy. A large autopsy study on type 2 diabetic patients did not confirm a high incidence of non-diabetic renal diseases [20]. Thus the available data on renal structure in type 2 diabetic patients with proteinuria are contradictory.

Quantitative morphometric studies in type 2 diabetes are scarce; in Japanese type 2 patients with a wide range of renal function, morphometric measures of diabetic glomerulopathy showed correlations to renal functional paramethers similar to those observed in type 1 diabetes [21]. However, more recent studies suggest a high incidence of normal glomerular structure among microalbuminuric and proteinuric Japanese type 2 diabetic patients [22]. In caucasian type 2 diabetic patients diabetic glomerulopathy has been estimated by Østerby et al. in a proteinuric group [23]; in this study all the morphometric glomerular paramethers were on average abnormal, however some patients had glomerular structure within the normal range. In type 1 diabetic patients with overt nephropathy, on the other hand, glomerular structure was always severely altered [12, 23 and Fioretto and Mauer, unpublished data]. We have recently studied a group of non-proteinuric caucasian type 2 diabetic patients, and found that, although diabetic glomerular structural parameters were more altered on average in patients with microalbuminuria, several patients despite persistent microalbuminuria had normal glomerular structure [24]; also compared to patients with type 1 diabetes and comparable renal function, diabetic glomerulopathy was less in patients with type 2 diabetes.

MICROLABUMINURIA IN TYPE 2 DIABETES

Microalbuminuria (MA) antedates clinical proteinuria in both type 1 [25-27] and type 2 diabetes [28-29]; however the predictive value of MA is quite different in type 1 and type 2 diabetes in that only approximately 20% of type 2 patients with MA progress to overt nephropathy over a decade of follow-up in contrast to over 80% of type 1 patients [29]. In fact MA in type 2 diabetes is a better predictor of cardiovascular mortality than of end stage renal disease [28, 30-31]. The low predictive value of MA for overt proteinuria in type 2 diabetes may in part be accounted for by the high mortality from cardiovascular disease, which can interrupt the progression to clinical nephropathy. However, other explanations are tenable, including the possibility that MA in type 2 diabetes, at least in a subset of patients, may not be associated with the same underlying abnormalities which are so common in patients with type 1 diabetes and MA. Nonetheless, to date there is no full explanation to the clinical observation that only a subgroup of type 2 diabetic patients with MA progresses to overt nephropathy, while in the majority renal function remains stable. It can be hypothesized that MA in type 2 patients may be either consequent to diabetic glomerulopathy, as in type 1 diabetes, and progress to overt nephropathy, or be due to other renal lesions or reflect altered vascular permeability due to regional or generalized endothelial dysfunction [7, 32]. The structural basis for MA in type 1 diabetes has been studied by us and others and it is now established that when albuminuria exceeds 30 μg/min diabetic glomerulopathy, with thickening of the glomerular basement membrane and mesangial expansion is usually well established [33]. Only one study to date evaluated renal structure in MA type 2 diabetics [34]; surprisingly these authors, who described diagnostic heterogeneity in proteinuric type 2 diabetic patients [17], reported that all 16 MA type 2 diabetic patients had classic diabetic glomerulopathy.

For these reasons we have undertaken the study of renal function and structure in MA type 2 diabetic patients in order to describe the renal structural concomitants of this functional disturbance and to test the above mentioned hypotheses. The light microscopy results of this study have been recently reported [35-36] and are summarized here.

RENAL STRUCTURE IN MICROALBUMINURIC TYPE 2 DIABETIC PATIENTS

Study design and patient population

In recent years we have been inviting patients with type 2 diabetes to participate to an ongoing multicentered study of renal structural-functional relationships. Patients are admitted to the University of Padova for research evaluation of renal structure and function; kidney biopsy in this study is never performed for clinically indicated diagnostic purposes. All type 2 diabetic patients willing to participate are accepted regardless of renal function, unless serum creatinine exceeds 2.0 mg/dl or unless clinical controindication to renal biopsy is present. Patients are defined as MA when albumin excretion rate (AER) is ≤20 μg/min but ≤200 μg/min in at least two of three consecutive sterile 24 hour urine collections. To date light microscopic slides from 53 MA patients have been evaluated (35,36). Thirty-five of the 53 patients (all caucasians) were males. Age was 58±8 years (Mean±1SD), known diabetes duration was 11±7 years and HbA1c was 8.3±1.8% (normal range: 4.1-6.1 %). Glomerular filtration rate (GFR), determined by the plasma clearance of [51] Cr-EDTA (37), was 99±28 ml/min/1.73 m^2 (normal range in a group of 19 age and sex matched normal controls: 85-135) and AER was 61 (20-199) μg/min (median, range) (normal values: 5 (0-14)). Blood pressure (BP) was measured at least 10 times in supine position and patients were defined hypertensive when BP values exceed 140/85 mm Hg [38], or when on antihypertensive therapy regardless of BP levels. Using these criteria all but 9 patients were receiving antihypertensive therapy, and the majority of them were on ACE-inhibors. Overall, according to the criteria described above, 78% of these patients were hypertensive.

Renal structure

Percutaneous kidney biopsies were performed in all patients, and renal tissue immediately fixed and embedded for light, electron and immunofluorescence microscopy studies [39]. For comparison kidney biopsies were obtained from 36 (17 M/19F) kidney donors at the time of renal transplantation, at the University of Minnesota; these controls were matched for age with the diabetic patients (age: 55.7±7 years, range: 45-69).

Light microscopy. The initial reading of the biopsy material made apparent the inadequacy of existing descriptive systems, which had largely been based on observations of research biopsies in type 1 diabetes. In fact all type 1 patients with at least 10 years of diabetes duration and overt nephropathy that we have reviewed have obvious diabetic glomerulopathy and diabetic glomerulopathy is also usually quite advanced in MA type 1 patients. In this series, however, many type 2 patients with MA did not have glomerulopathy, or they had mild mesangial expansion by light microscopy; in fact the majority of the MA type 2 patients had normal or near normal glomerular structure, with or without tubulo-interstitial and arteriolar changes.

Thus we proposed a new classification system which included 3 major groups:

Category C I) Normal or near normal renal structure. These patients (15 M/7F, 41%) had biopsies which were normal or showed mild mesangial expansion, tubulo-interstitial changes or arteriolar hyalinosis (Figure 25-1A).
Category C II) Typical diabetic nephropathology. These patients (9M/5F, 26%) had established diabetic lesions with an approximately balanced severity of glomerular, tubulo-interstitial and arteriolar changes. This picture is typical of that seen in type 1 diabetic patients with obvious light microscopic DN changes (Figure 25-1B).

Category C III) Atypical patterns of renal injury. These patients (11M/6F, 33%) had relatively mild diabetic glomerular changes considering the disproportionately severe renal structural changes including:

(a) Tubular atrophy, tubular basement membrane thickening and reduplication and interstitial fibrosis (tubulo-interstitial lesions) (Figure 25-1C).

(b) Advanced glomerular arteriolar hyalinosis commonly associated with atherosclerosis of larger vessels (Figure 25-1D).

(c) Global glomerular sclerosis.

In C III group these patterns were present in all possible combinations (Figures 25-25-1C and 25-1D); however important tubulo-interstitial changes were observed in all but 1 patient, who had very severe arteriolar hyalinosis lesions; these tubulo-interstitial lesions were often associated with arteriolar changes and in some patients with global glomerulosclerosis.

In the age matched control group, 3/36 subjects had important tubulo-interstitial changes. Several normal controls had mild arteriolar hyalinosis lesions; 6 controls had more advanced arteriolar lesions scores, sometimes comparable to those observed in patients in categories II and III.

In this series of 53 patients we did not find cases of any definable non diabetic renal disease. The difference between our findings and those in previous reports in proteinuric type 2 patients (see above) may be explained by the study design, in that patients in the present study had kidney biopsies performed on the basis of a research protocol as opposed to biopsies performed for clinical indications based upon atypical course.

Clinical features in relation to patterns of lesions

Age was similar in the three groups; known duration of type 2 diabetes was different among groups, with group CII and CIII patients having longer duration than CI patients [14±6 and 13±8 yrs vs 7±3, $p<0.05$ for both]. HbA1c levels were significantly different among groups with CII patients having the highest HbA1c values. Body mass index (BMI) was also different among groups (ANOVA, $p<0.02$); BMI was only mildly increased in CII patients (26±4) and was significanty higher in CI (30±4) and CIII patients (29±3) compared to CII (t-tests, $p<0.05$ for both). AER levels were similar in the three groups (median: 56, 58 and 69 µg/min respectively); GFR was lower in CII patients (86±37 ml/min/1.73 m^2) than in CI (109±19) and CIII patients (96±20, $p<0.05$ for both). Systolic and diastolic blood pressure values were similar in the three groups as was the prevalence of hypertension (84% in CI, 73% in CII and 79% in CIII).

Diabetic retinopathy was present in all C II patients, background in 6 and proliferative in 8. None of the patients in C I and C III had proliferative retinopathy, while background diabetic retinopathy was observed in 9 of C I and 6 of C III patients. Thus, all C II patients had diabetic retinopathy and all patients with proliferative retinopathy had "typical" DN.

From the clinical features in the three groups we hypothesize that the "atypical" patterns of renal injury observed in many of our patients are probably

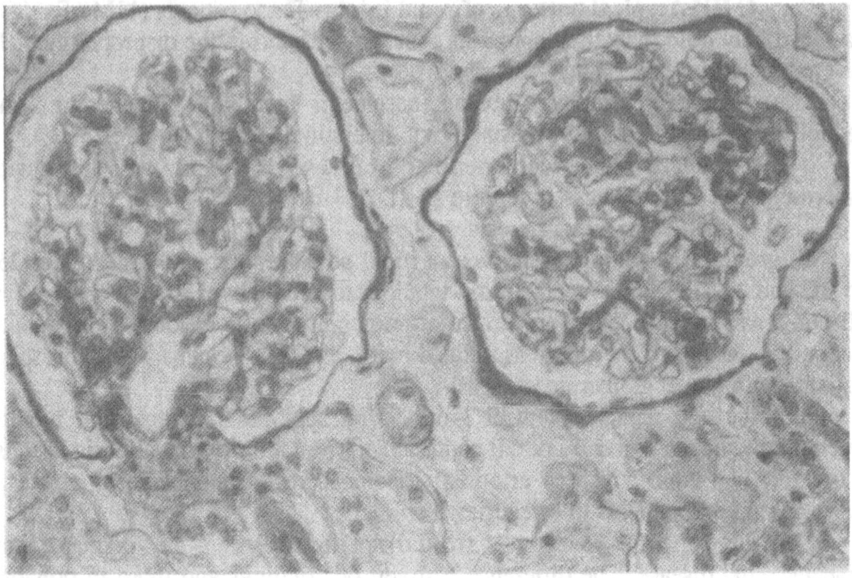

Figure 25-1A Glomeruli from a patient in category C I. Glomerular structure is near normal with minimal mesangial expansioin (PAS)

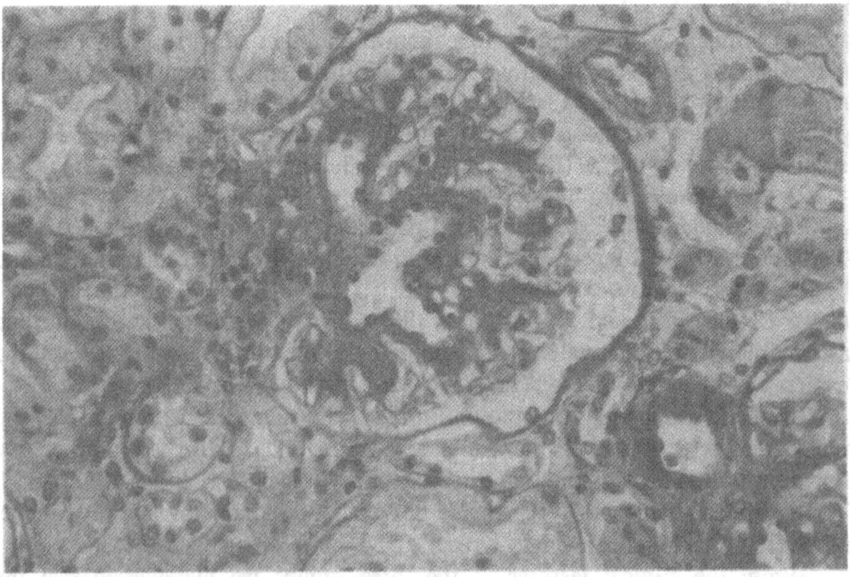

Figure 25-1B Glomerulus from a patient in category C II, with well established diabetic nephropathy. Diffuse mesangial expansion, moderate ateriolar hyalinosis, and mild interstitial fibrosis are present (PAS).

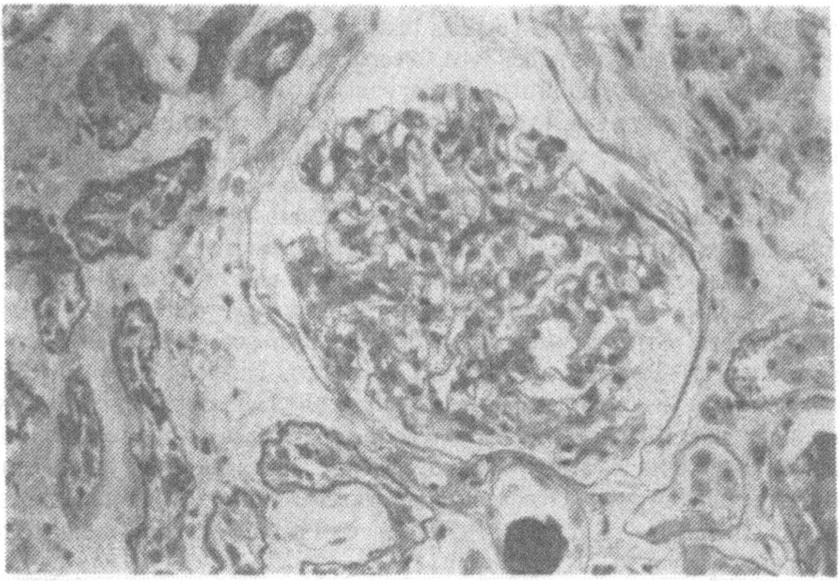

Figure 25-1C Glomerulus from a patient in category C III (a), with near normal glomerular structure and TBM thickening, tubular atrophy and severe interstitial fibrosis (PAS).

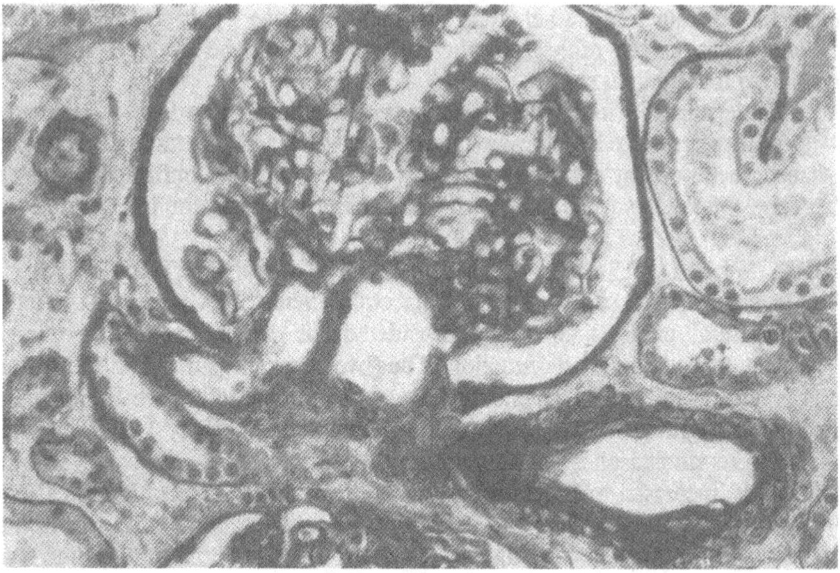

Figure 25-1D Glomerulus from a patient in category C III (b), with mild mesangial expansion and severe arteriolar hyalinosis, affecting both afferent and efferent glomerular arterioles (PAS).

related to hyperglycemia. This suggests that hyperglycemia may cause different patterns of renal injury in older type 2 compared to younger type 1 diabetic patients. The tubulo-interstitial and vascular changes could also be related to aging, atherosclerosis and systemic hypertension. However, hypertension was present in almost all patients in all 3 structural categories, and "per se" cannot account for the different lesions observed in category III. Further, mean age was similar in category II and III patients (60 years), despite the different patterns of renal injury in the two groups, and our observations in a large number of age-matched normal controls argue that aging, per se, is not sufficient to explain most of the renal structural changes observed in C III patients. Thus it can be hypothesized that the heterogeneity in renal structure might reflect the heterogeneous nature of type 2 diabetes "per se". Patients with "typical" DN lesions had long known diabetes duration, worse metabolic control and they all had diabetic retinopathy; interestingly their BMI only slightly exceeded normal values, as opposed to clearly increased BMI values in category I and III patients. This suggests that the different underlying pathophysiologic mechanisms responsible for type 2 diabetes in these groups of patients may also underlie different renal pathophysiologic mechanisms or responses.

A remarkably high number of MA type 2 patients (41%) had normal or near normal renal structure (C I). They tended to be younger and to have shorter diabetes duration than patients with renal lesions (categories II and III). Although we do not have an explanation for the abnormal AER in these patients, it is possible that MA in this subset is a clinical manifestation of generalized endothelial dysfunction rather than of renal damage "per se". The clinical predictive significance of MA in these patients would be of great interest to elucidate in longitudinal studies.

These must obviously be considered to be preliminary data. In particular, category III patients are hypothesized to represent alternative pathologic expression of diabetic nephropathy and this new observation needs to be confirmed in this and other series of patients from a variety of racial, ethnic and cultural backgrounds.

ENDOTHELIAL FUNCTION IN RELATION TO RENAL STRUCTURE

Since in a substantial subset of type 2 diabetic patients MA is not associated to renal structural changes, we have considered the possibility that it may be consequent to endothelial dysfunction. Thus we have measured von Willebrand factor (vWF) plasma levels, an endothelial-derived protein indicative of endothelial function, in a group of MA patients undergoing kidney biopsy [40]. Thirty-two patients were studied and, contrary to our hypothesis, vWF plasma levels were significantly increased only in patients with renal structural abnormalities (both allocated in category II-typical and category III-atypical patterns) and was normal in patients with normal renal structure (Category I) [40]. The results of this study do not provide an explanation for MA in patients without renal injury, and the nature of MA in there patients remains unknown. vWF plasma levels, however, represent only one measure of endothelial function, and further physiologic studies are necessary. Nevertheless, from these studies on vWF and renal structure we suggest that there are two types of MA in type 2 diabetes: one associated with increased vWF plasma levels, established renal structural lesions and frequently diabetic retinopathy, and the other characterized by normal vWF plasma levels, normal renal structure and absent or mild diabetic retinopathy. Whether these two types of MA have a different prognostic impact in terms of end stage renal disease and cardiovascular events deserves longitudinal studies.

CONCLUSIONS

These preliminary results, far from clarifying the mechanisms responsible for MA in type 2 diabetic patients, clearly demonstrate the complexity and the problematic nature of this renal functional abnormality in these patients. They also encourage and stimulate further investigation and new directions of research. Thus, to better understand the pathophysiologic mechanisms responsible for MA in type 2 diabetes we are currently studying markers of endothelial function. These studies will clarify the relationships between endothelial function and renal lesions in type 2 diabetic patients with MA.

Also, given the subset of MA patients with disproportionaly severe tubulo-interstitial lesions, a better understanding of tubular function and vascular injury needs to be developed in these patients [36].

Finally, longitudinal detailed renal structural and functional studies of these patients are crucial to the understanding of the clinical implications of these complex processes.

REFERENCES

1. Cordonnier DJ, Zmirou D, Benhamou PY, Halimi S, Ledoux F, Guiserix J. Epidemiology, development and treatment of end-stage renal failure in type 2 diabetes. The case of mainland France and of overseas French territories. Diabetologia 1993; 36: 1109-1112.
2. Stephen SGW, Gillaspry JA, Clyne D, Mejia A, Pollok VE. Racial differences in the incidence of end stage renal disease in type 1 and type 2 diabetes mellitus. Am J Kidney Dis 1990; 15: 562-567.
3. Ritz E, Nowack R, Fliser D, et al. Type II diabetes mellitus: is the renal risk adequately appreciated? Nephrol Dial Transplant 1991; 6: 679-682.
4. Catalano C, Postorino M, Kelly PJ. Diabetes mellitus and renal replacement therapy in Italy: prevalence, main characteristic and complications. Nephrol Dial Transplant 1990; 5: 788-796.
5. Mauer M, Mogensen CE, Friedman E. Diabetic Nephropathy. In: Schrier RW, Gottschalk CW (eds). Diseases of the kidne, 6th edn. Little Brown& Co. 1996, Vol 3, pp 2019-2062.
6. Mogensen CE, Shmitz A, Christiensen CK. Comparative renal pathophysyology relevant to IDDM and NIDDM patients. Diabetes Metab Rev 1988; 4: 453.
7. Shmitz A. Nephropathy in non-insulin dependent diabetes mellitus and perspectives for intervention. Diab Nutr Metab 1995; 7: 135-148.
8. Mauer SM, Steffes MW, Brown DM. The kidney in diabetes. Am J Med 1981; 70: 603-612.
9. Fioretto P, Mogensen CE, Mauer SM. Diabetic nephropathy. In: Pediatric nephroplogy, ed by Holliday MA, Barratt TM, Avner ED, New York, Williams and Wilkins, 1994; 576-585.
10. Lane PH, Steffes MW, Fioretto P, Mauer SM. Renal interstitial expansion in insulin-dependent diabetes mellitus. Kidney Int 1993; 43: 661-67.
11. Gellman DD, Pirani CL, Soothill JF, Muehrcke RC, Maduros W, Kark RM. Structure and funtion in diabetic nephropathy: the importance of diffuse glomerulosclerosis. Diabetes 1959; 8: 251-256.
12. Mauer SM, Steffes MW, Ellis EN, Sutherland DER, Brown DM, Goetz FC. Structural functional relationships in diabetic nephropathy. J Clin Invest 1984; 74: 1143-55.
13. Fioretto P, Steffes MW, Sutherland DER, Mauer M. Sequential renal biopsies in IDDM patients: structural factors associated with clinical progression. Kidney Int 1995; 48:1929-1935 .

14. Brito P, Fioretto P, Drummund K, Kim Y, Steffes MW, Basgen JM, Mauer M. Proximal tubular basement membrane width in insulin-dependent diabetes mellitus. Kidney Int, 1998; 53:754-762.
15. Steffes MW, Bilous RW, Sutherland DER, Mauer SM. Cell and matrix components in the glomerular mesangium in type I diabetes. Diabetes 1992; 41: 679-84.
16. Parving H-H, Gall M-A, Skøtt P, Jørgensen HE, Løkkegaard H, Jørgensen F, Nielsen B, Larsen S. Prevalence and causes of albuminuria in non-insulin-dependent diabetic patients. Kidney Int 1992; 41: 758-762.
17. Gambara V, Mecca G, Remuzzi G, Bertani T. Heterogeneous nature of renal lesions in type II diabetes. JASN 1993; 3: 1458-1466.
18. Kahn S, Seghal V, Appel GB, D'Agati V. Correlates of diabetic and non-diabetic renal disease in NIDDM. JASN 1995; 6: 451 (Abs).
19. Olsen S, Mogensen CE. Non-diabetic renal disease in NIDDM proteinuric patients may be rare in biopsies from clinical practice. Diabetologia 1996, 39: 1638-1645.
20. Waldherr R, Ilkenhans C, Ritz E. How frequent is glomerulonephritis in diabetes mellitus type II? Clinical Nephrology 1992; 37: 271-273.
21. Hayashi H, Karasawa R, Inn H et al. An electron microscopic study of glomeruli in Japanese patients with non-insulin dependent diabetes mellitus. Kidney Int 1992; 41: 749-757.
22. Moiya T, Moriya R, Yajima Y, Steffes MW, Mauer M. Urinary albumin excretion is a weaker predictor of diabetic nephropathy lesions in Japanese NIDDM patients than in Caucasian IDDM patients. JASN, 1997, 8: 116A (abs).
23. Østerby R, Gall MA, Schmitz A, Nielsen FS, Nyberg G, Parving HH. Glomerular structure and function in proteinuric type 2 (non insulin dependent) diabetic patients. Diabetologia 1993; 36: 1064-1070.
24. Fioretto P, Mauer M, Velussi M, Carraro A, Muollo B, Brocco E, Baggio B, Crepaldi G, Nosadini R. Ultrastructural measures of glomerular extracellular matrix accumulation in non-proteinuric type 2 diabetic patients. JASN 1996, 7:1356 (abs).
25. Viberti GC, Hill RD, Jarrett RJ, Argyropoulos A, Mahmud U, Keen H. Microalbuminuria as a predictor of clinical nephropathy in insulin-dependent diabetes mellitus. Lancet 1982 i: 1430-32.
26. Parving H-H, Oxenbøll B, Svensen PAA, Christiansen JS, Andersen AR. Early detection of patients at risk of developing diabetic nephropathy: a longitudinal study of urinary albumin excretion. Acta Endocrinol Copenh 1982; 7, 100: 550-52.
27. Mogensen CE, Christensen CK. Predicting diabetic nephropathy in insulin-dependent diabetic patients. N Engl J Med 1986; 331: 89-93.
28. Mogensen CE. Microalbuminuria predicts clinical proteinuria and early mortality in maturity-onset diabetes. N Engl J Med 1984; 310: 356-360.
29. Mogensen CE. Microalbuminuria as a predictor of clinical diabetic nephropathy. Kidney International 1987; 31: 673-689.
30. Schmitz A, Vaeth M. Microalbuminuria: a major risk factor in type 2 diabetes. A 10 year follow-up study of 503 patients. Diab Med 1988; 5: 126-134.
31. Jarrett RJ, Viberi GC, Argyropoulos A, Hill RD, Mahmud U, Murrells TJ. Microalbuminuria predicts mortality in non-insulin-dependent diabetes. Diab Med 1984; 1: 17-19.
32. Stehouwer CDA, Nauta JJP, Zeldenrust GC, Hackeng WHL, Donker AJM, den Ottolander GJH (1992). Urinary albumin excretion, cardiovascular disease, and endothelial dysfunction in non-insulin dependent diabetes mellitus. Lancet 1992; 340: 319-323.
33. Fioretto P, Steffes MW, Mauer M. Glomerular structure in non proteinuric IDDM patients with various levels of albuminuria. Diabetes 1994; 43: 1358-1364.
34. Ruggenenti P, Mosconi L, Bianchi L, Cortesi L, Campana M, Pagani G, Mecca G, Remuzzi G. Long-term treatment with either Enalapril or Nitrendipine stabilizes albuminuria and increases glomerular filtration rate in non-insulin-dependent diabetic patients. Am J Kidney Dis 1994; 24: 753-761.
35. Fioretto P, Mauer M, Brocco E, Velussi M, Frigato F, Muollo B, Sambataro M, Abaterusso C, Baggio B, Crepaldi G, Nosadini R. Patterns of renal injury in type 2 (non insulin dependent) diabetic patients with microalbuminuria. Diabetologia, 1996, 39: 1569-1576.
36. Brocco E, Fioretto P, Mauer M, Saller A, Carraro A, Frigato F, Chiesura-Corona M, et al. Renal structure and function in non-insulin dependent diabetic patients with microalbuminuria. Kidney Int., 1997; 52, suppl. 63:40-44.
37. Sambataro M, Thomaseth K, Pacini G, et al. Plasma clearance of 51 Cr-EDTA provides a precise and convenient technique for measurement of glomerular filtration rate in diabetic humans. JASN 1996; 7: 118-127.

38. The Fifth Report of the Joint National Committee on Detection, Evaluation, and Treatment of High Blood Pressure. Arch Int Med 1993; 153: 154.
39. Ellis EN, Basgen JM, Mauer SM, Steffes MW. Kidney biopsy technique an evaluation. In Methods in Diabetes Research, Volume II Clinical Methods. Clarke WL, Larner J, Pohl SL, Eds. New York, John Wiley & Sons, 1986; 633-47.
40. Fioretto P, Stehouwer CDA, Mauer M, Chiesura-Corona M, Brocco E, Carraro A, Bortoloso E, van Hinsberg V, Crepaldi G, Nosadini R. Heterogeneous nature of microalbuminuria in NIDDM: studies of endothelial function and renal structure. Diabetologia, 1998; 41:233-236.

26. SODIUM-HYDROGEN ANTIPORT, CELL FUNCTION AND SUSCEPTIBILITY TO DIABETIC NEPHROPATHY

Roberto Trevisan And Giancarlo Viberti

Department of Clinical and Experimental Medicine, University of Padua, Padua, Italy and Division of Medicine, Guy's and St Thomas's Medical and Dental School, London, United Kingdom

The annual incidence of diabetic nephropathy rises rapidly over the first 15-20 years of diabetes, but declines sharply afterward for longer disease duration [1]. This pattern of risk indicates that only a subset of diabetic patients are susceptible to renal damage and, indeed, clinical renal disease cumulatively develops in approximately 30% of insulin-dependent diabetic (IDDM) patients [2] and between 15 and 60% of non-insulin-dependent diabetic (NIDDM) patients, depending on their ethnic origin[3]. Familiar clustering of diabetic nephropathy has been shown both in IDDM [4] and NIDDM patients [5]. These findings are consistent with the possibility that genetic factors may explain the liability to or protection from renal disease of diabetic patients.

Recent reports suggest that raised blood pressure levels play an important role not only in the progression of renal complications, but also in the initiation of the multistage process leading to end-stage renal failure. Two prospective studies have shown that the patients who progress to microalbuminuria have either raised or rising blood pressure before microalbuminuria becomes persistent [6,7]. Raised blood pressure [8] and an increased frequence of cardiovascular disease [9] are also more prevalent in parents of diabetic patients with nephropathy. Taken together, these findings indicate that a familial predisposition to hypertension and cardiovascular disease may be an important determinant of susceptibility to renal disease and its cardiovascular complications in diabetes.

In accord with these observations, studies of sodium-lithium countertransport activity, an intermediate phenotype of essential hypertension and its vascular complications [10,11], have shown significant elevation in the rate of this cation transport system in IDDM [12,13] and NIDDM patients [14] with proteinuria or microalbuminuria and hypertension. Diabetic patients with high sodium-lithium countertransport activity display a clustering of metabolic and haemodynamic risk factors for renal and cardiovascular complications well before the development of overt renal disease [15]. The activity of sodium-lithium countertransport also shows significant familial aggregation [16].

These results have raised growing interest in the search for intermediate phenotypes significantly associated with diabetic nephropathy, poorly influenced by environment, stable with age, easy to quantify and possibly dependent upon a single major gene effect. Such intermediate phenotypes can be useful for early diagnosis and would help clarify the molecular mechanisms leading to diabetic nephropathy.

BASIC PROPERTIES OF THE Na^+/H^+ ANTIPORT

Sodium/lithium countertransport however is not operating in vivo and, therefore, the pathophysiological implication of this abnormality remains uncertain. Sodium-lithium countertransport has similarities of operation with the ubiquitous physiological Na^+/H^+ antiport [17].

Na^+/H^+ antiport is a membrane transport system found in all eukaryotic cells. Under normal physiological conditions, Na^+/H^+ antiport employs the sodium concentration gradient from extracellular to intracellular fluid to drive protons out of the cells in exchange for an influx of sodium ions. This transport is activated cooperatively by an increase in the cytosolic proton concentration through a proton regulatory site [18]. Molecular biology studies have revealed the presence of at least five different isoforms of Na^+/H^+ antiport. The first isoform, referrred to as NHE1, ubiquitously expressed in most cell types, is sensitive to amiloride and activated by growth factors. The human cDNA coding for this protein has been cloned and the gene is located on the short arm of chromosome 1. It encodes a protein of 815 aminoacids with two distinct domains [19]. The N-terminal domain contains 10-12 transmembrane segments, while the C-terminus is largely cytoplasmic. The second isoforms (NHE2) is expressed on the apical membrane of polarized epithelia and it is involved in the transcellular transport of Na, Cl and bicarbonate. The structure and the functional implications of the other isoforms require further investigations.

Na^+/H^+ antiport is involved in three major cellular events: 1) intracellular pH regulation, 2) cell volume control and 3) stimulus-response coupling and cell proliferation. At kidney level, this transport system plays an important role in Na reabsorption [18].

Many studies have shown that the Na^+/H^+ antiporter is activated in response to growth factors and various cell activating agents such as hormones, chemotactic peptides and phorbol esters. The sequence of intracellular events triggered by growth factors binding to their membrane receptors is as yet not fully understood. The trophic action of these compounds appears in part to be dependent on the elevation of intracellular free calcium and the activation of phospholipase C that mediates the formation of inositol triphosphate and diacylglycerol which, in turn, activates protein kinase C. The effect on the Na^+/H^+

antiport is triggered by an increase of the affinity of the antiporter protein for H^+ at the internal H^+ regulatory site [18]. A phosphorilation step is required for this activation of Na^+/H^+ antiport.

Na^+/H^+ ANTIPORT ACTIVITY IN DIABETIC NEPHROPATHY

An increased leukocyte Na^+/H^+ antiport activity has been reported in IDDM patients with nephropathy [20] as well as in patients with essential hypertension [21]. IDDM patients with microalbuminuria and raised blood presssure have also higher red blood cell Na^+/H^+ antiport activity [22]. In all these cases the increased activity was due to a raised maximal velocity of the antiport. These observations are consistent with the view that arterial hypertension or the predisposition to it are important components in the pathogenensis of diabetic nephropathy.

In all these studies, however, measurements were performed soon after blood sampling and a potential effect of the disturbed metabolic milieu of the diabetes state on the transporter activity, therefore, could not be excluded. These studies could not establish whether the higher activity of this cell-membrane transport system was an intrinsic abnormality of these cells.

Skin fibroblasts and Epstein-Barr-immortalized lymphoblasts offer a useful approach that allows dissection of the primary (possibly genetic) abnormalities from those that may be secondary to the diabetic milieu, since these cells, once removed, can be cultured for several passages under well defined metabolic conditions. In serially passaged skin fibroblasts we have demonstrated, by determining amiloride-sensitive ^{22}Na uptake, a significantly greater Na^+/H^+ antiport activity in IDDM patients with overt nephropathy than in long-term IDDM patients without nephropathy, whose activity was similar to that of a non-diabetic control group [23]. A kinetic analysis of Na^+/H^+ exchange revealed that the raised activity was caused by an increased maximal velocity (V_{max}) for extracellular Na^+. The external Na^+ concentration that yields 50% of the V_{max} (Km) was similar in the three groups. This abnormality was associated to a higher intracellular pH in exponentially growing cultures of fibroblasts of patients with nephropathy.

These results were confirmed by other studies, where Na^+/H^+ antiport activity and intracellular pH were determined by a different technique that used the pH-sensitive dye, BCECF [24, 25]. Growing fibroblasts from IDDM patients with nephropathy were more alkaline compared to both normoalbuminuric IDDM patients or normal controls. This was associated with a raised Na^+/H^+ antiport activity. This abnormal phenotype is also conserved in Epstein-Barr-immortalised lymphoblasts of IDDM patients with nephropathy [26]. In this cellular model, the kinetic analysis of Na^+/H^+ antiport activity demonstrated that maximal velocity was increased and that Hill coefficient was reduced when compared with cells from normoalbuminuric IDDM patients and nondiabetic control subjects. Both in fibroblasts and in immortalised lymphoblasts by means of specific polyclonal antisera to the carboxyl terminus of NHE-1, it was shown that the elvated maximal velocity of Na^+/H^+ exchange was not caused by an increased NHE-1 density, which was similar in IDDM patients with and without nephropathy, but by an increased turnover rate per site [26,27]. The persistence of these abnormalities in long-term cultured cells from insulin-dependent diabetic patients with nephropathy are consistent with an intrinsic overactivity of the Na^+/H^+ antiport and with an increased responsiveness to the action of growth factors. The importance of genetic factors was confirmed by the close association of maximal velocities of antiport activities found in long-term cultured skin fibroblasts of IDDM sibling pairs [28].

The similarity between the kinetic abnormalities of Na^+/H^+ antiport described in cells from IDDM patients with nephropathy and those reported in cells from patients with essential hypertension supports the contention that an inherited predisposition to essential hypertension may be implicated in increasing the risk of diabetic nephropathy. It is of note that a similar increased maximal velocity of Na^+/H^+ antiport without differences in Km have also been described in NIDDM patients with microalbuminuria and/or hypertension [29].

The abnormalities of Na^+/H^+ antiport activity do not seem to reflect modifications in Na^+/H^+ antiport gene(s). Linkage analysis has yielded no evidence for NHE-1 as a candidate gene in hypertension, and the possibility that the increased maximal velocity could be caused by an increased gene expression was excluded both in patients with essential hypertension and in IDDM patients with nephropathy.

It is more likely that alterations in some of the regulatory pathways of the Na^+/H^+ exchange are important for its overactivity in diabetic nephropathy. Although inhibition of protein kinase C in lymphocytes of IDDM patients with albuminuria normalizes the elevated activity of the antiporter [30], a recent report was unable to observe an increased net phosphorylation of NHE-1 in immortalized lymphoblasts from IDDM patients with nephropathy [31]. Therefore additional post-translational mechanisms for activation of NHE-1 has to be involved.

More insight into the relationship between the disturbed milieu of diabetes and the Na^+/H^+ antiport activity has come from a study by Williams et al. in which incubation of vascular smooth muscle cells in high glucose increased Na^+/H^+ antiport activity [32]. Davies et al. [33] demonstrated that elevated glucose concentrations significantly increased Na^+/H^+ antiport activity and turnover number only in immortalized lymphoblasts from IDDM patients with nephropathy. Thus high glucose levels appear to exaggerate the differences in Na^+/H^+ antiport activity that are already present between cells from patients with and without nephropathy during euglycaemic conditions.

CELL FUNCTION IN DIABETIC NEPHROPATHY

Increased Na^+/H^+ antiport activity has been found to be associated with enhanced smooth muscle cell [34], skin fibroblast [35] and lymphoblasts [36] proliferation in response to growth factors in essential hypertension. In hypertensive patients a significant correlation between Na^+/H^+ antiport activity in lymphocytes and left ventricular hypertrophy has also been described [37].

In fibroblasts of insulin-dependent diabetic patients with nephropathy, an enhanced DNA synthesis and abnormalities in DNA cell cycle and in the cell life span have been reported [23, 25, 38]. This abnormality suggests a difference in the ability of these cells to enter the synthetic S phase after mitogen stimulation. The positive correlation found between Na^+/H^+ antiport activity and DNA synthesis [23] indicates that the antiport may be involved in this altered cell function. Similar results were also found in immortalized lymphoblasts from IDDM patients with nephropathy, which demonstrated an increased cell proliferation rate that was further magnified by the incubation of cells in high glucose concentration [33]. Whether the enhanced activity of Na^+/H^+ antiport reflects the appropriate response to an abnormal growth tendency or constitutes a primary permissive factor leading to cell function disturbances remains to be clarified. However recent data suggest that raised Na^+/H^+ antiport activity is secondary rather than primary to disturbances in cell growth in that the inhibition of Na^+/H^+ antiport by ethyl-isopropylamiloride did not prevent the increased DNA synthesis in cells from diabetic patients with nephropathy [25].

Na^+/H^+ antiport can be activated by extracellular matrix molecules, such as fibronectin [39], and any interaction between extracellular matrix production and Na^+/H^+ antiport is of particular importance in view of the relevance of excessive matrix deposition to the sclerotic process of diabetic nephropathy. We have found that long-term cultured fibroblasts derived from IDDM patients with nephropathy exhibit an increased total collagen synthesis compared with that of patients without nephropathy and normal controls [40]. Moreover, high glucose concentrations increased collagen synthesis in cells from all subjects, exaggerating the difference already present in normal glucose concentration between cells from IDDM patients with nephropathy and those from patients without nephropathy and normal subjects.

The persistence of all these abnormalities in ion transport and cell function despite serial passaging of cells in identical media in vitro indicates a likely genetic control of these intermediate phenotypes.

This body of data supports the view that the reason for an increased susceptibility to diabetic nephropathy resides in the host cell response to diabetes-induced dysregulation of a number of growth factors and vasoactive compounds whose expression and circulating or tissue levels are increased. Therefore increased concentrations of growth factors and plasma glucose may exert a more profound effect in that subset of diabetic patients characterized by an intrinsic overactivity of Na^+/H^+ antiport activity or prediposed to overreact to any hypertrophic or hyperplastic stimulus. The connection between enahnced sodium-hydrogen antiport activity and diabetic glomerulosclerosis remains speculative, but it could be mediated by increased tubular sodium reabsorption as well as hypertrophic/hyperplastic processes of mesangial and smooth muscle cells in the vessel wall, combined with excessive matrix deposition.

The recent advances in molecular biology should better clarify the relation between Na^+/H^+ antiport activity, cell growth and extracellular matrix production and, in particular, elucidate the interaction between diabetes and those cells functions regulated by Na^+/H^+ antiport activity. The knowledge of the cellular and molecular mechanisms responsible for those abnormalities may lead to effective primary prevention strategies.

REFERENCES

1. Krolewski AS, Warram JH, Rand LI, Kahn CR. Epidemiologic approach to the etiology of type 1 diabetes mellitus and its complications. N Engl J Med 1987; 317:1390-1398.
2. Andersen AR, Christiansen JS, Andersen JK, Kreiner S, Deckert T. Diabetic nephropathy in type 1 (insulin-dependent) diabetes: an epidemiological study. Diabetologia 1983; 25: 496-501.
3. Viberti GC, Walker JD, Pinto J. Diabetic Nephropathy. In : International Textbook of diabetes mellitus. Alberti KGMM, DeFronzo RA, Keen H, Zimmet P. eds. John Wiley & Sons Ltd. 1992; vol 2: 1267-1328.
4. Seaquist ER, Goetz FC, Rich S, Barbosa J. Familial clustering of diabetic kidney disease. Evidence for genetic susceptibility to diabetic nephropathy. N Engl J Med 1989; 320: 1161-5.
5. Petitt DJ, Saad MF, Bennett PH, Nelson RG, Knowler WC. Familial predisposition to renal disease in two generations of PIma Indians with Type 2 (non-insulin-dependent) diabetes mellitus. Diabetologia 1990; 33: 438-43.
6. Microalbuminuria Collaborative Study group. Risk factors for development of microalbuminuria in insulin-dependent diabetic patients: a cohort study. Br Med J1993; 306: 1235-9.
7. Poulsen PL, Hansen KW, Mogensen CE. Ambulatory blood pressure in the transition from normo- to microalbuminuria; a longitudinal study in IDDM patients. Diabetologia 1993; 36 (Suppl. 1) A214.
8. Viberti GC, Keen H, Wiseman MJ. Raised blood pressure in parents of proteinuric insulin-dependent diabetic patients. Br Med J 1987; 295: 575-577.
9. Earle K, Walker J, Hill C, Viberti GC. Familial clustering of cardiovascular disease in patients with insulin dependent diabetes and nephropathy. N Engl J Med 1992; 326: 673-677.
10. Williams RR, Hunt SC, Kuida H, Smith JB, Ash KO. Sodium-lithium countertransport in erythrocytes of hypertension prone families in Utah. Am J Epidemiol 1983; 118: 338-44.
11. Morgan DB, Steward AD, Davidson C. Relations between erythrocyte lithium efflux, blood pressure and family history of hypertension And cardiovascular disease. Studies in a factory workforce and hypertension clinic. J Hypertens 1986; 4: 609-615.
12. Mangili R, Bending JJ, Scott G, Li LK, Gupta A, Viberti GC. Increased sodium-lithium countertransport activity in red cells of patients with insulin-dependent diabetes and nephropathy. N Engl J Med 1988; 318: 146-150.
13. Jones SL, Trevisan R, Tariq T, Semplicini A, Mattoch M, Walker JD, Nosadini R, Viberti GC. Increased sodium-lithium countertransport activity in insulin-dependent diabetic patients with microalbuminuria. Hypertension 1990; 15: 570-575.
14. Morocutti A, Barzon I, Solini A, Sambataro M, Cipollina MR, Velussi M, Duner E, Muollo B, Crepaldi G, Nosadini R. Poor metabolic control and predisposition to hypertension, rather than hypertension itself, are risk factors for nephropathy in type 2 diabetes. Acta Diabetol 1992; 29: 123-129.
15. Trevisan R, Nosadini R, Fioretto P, Semplicini A, Donadon v, Doria A, Nicolosi G, Zanuttini D, Cipollina MR, Lusiani L, Avogaro A, Crepaldi G, Viberti GC. Clustering of risk factors in hypertensive insulin-dependent diabetics with high sodium-lithium countertransport. Kidney Int 1992; 41: 855-861.
16. Walker JD, Tariq T, Viberti GC. Sodium-lithium countertransport activity in red cells of patients with insulin-dependent diabetes and nephropathy and their parents. Br Med J 1990; 301: 635-8.
17. Canessa M, Morgan K, Semplicini A. Genetic differences in lithium- sodium exchange and regulation of the sodium-hydrogen exchanger in essential hypertension. J Cardiovasc Pharmacol 1988; 12 (Suppl. 3): S92-S98).
18. Seifter JL, Aronson PS. Properties and physiological roles of the plasma membrane sodium-hydrogen exchanger. J Clin Invest 1986; 78: 859-864.

19. Sardet C, Franchi A, Pouyssegur J: Molecular cloning, primary structure, and expression of the human growth factor-activatable sodium-hydrogen antiporter. Cell1989; 56: 271-280

20. Ng LL, Simmons D, Frighi V, Garrido MC, Bomford J, Hockaday TDR. Leucocyte Na^+/H^+ antiport activity in type 1(insulin-dependent) diabetic patients with nephropathy. Diabetologia 1990; 33: 371-77.

21. Ng LL, Dudley C, Bomford J, Hawley D. Leucocyte intracellular pH and Na^+/H^+ antiport activity in human hypertension. J Hypertens 1989; 7: 471-475.

22. Semplicini A, Mozzato MG, Samà B, Nosadini R, Fioretto P, Trevisan R, Pessina A, Crepaldi G, Dal Palù D. Sodium-hydrogen and lithium-sodium exchange in red cells of normotensive and hypertensive patients with insulin-dependent diabetes mellitus. Am J Hypertens 1989; 2: 174-77.

23. Trevisan R, Li LK, Messent J, Tariq T, Earle KA, Walker JD, Viberti GC. Na/H antiport activity and cell growth in cultured skin fibroblasts of IDDM patients with nephropathy. Diabetes 1992; 41: 1239-46.

24. Davies JE, Ng LL, Kofoed-Enevoldsen A, Li LK, Earle A, Trevisan R, Viberti GC. Intracellular pH and Na^+/H^+ antiport activity of cultured skin fibroblasts from diabetics. Kidney Int 1992; 42: 1184-1190.

25 Lurbe A, Fioretto P, Mauer M, LaPointe MS, Battle D. Growth phenotype of cultured skin fibroblasts from IDDM patients with and without nephropathy and overactivity of the Na/H antiporter. Kidney Int 1996; 50: 1684-1693.

26. Ng LL, Davies JE, Siczkowski M, Sweeney FP, Quinn PA, Krolewski B, Krolewski AS. Abnormal sodium-hydrogen antiporter phenotype and turnover of immortalized lymphoblasts from type 1 diabetic patients with nephropathy. J Clin Invest 1994; 93: 2750-57.

27. Siczkowski M, Davies JE, Sweeney FP, Kofoed-Enevoldsen A, Ng LL. Na/H exchanger isoform-1 abundance in skin fibroblasts of type 1 diabetic patients with nephropathy. Metabolism 1995; 44: 791-795.

28. Trevisan R, Fioretto P, Mauer SM, Duner E, Cipollina MR, Trevisan M, Barbosa J, Nosadini R. Concordance for sodium-hydrogen antiport activity in insulin-dependent diabetic sibling pairs. Diabetologia 1995; 38 (Suppl. 1): A230.

29. Trevisan R, Cipollina MR, Duner E, Trevisan M, Nosadini R. Abnormal sodium hydrogen antiport activity in cultured fibroblasts from non-insulin-dependent diabetic patients with hypertension and microalbuminuria. Diabetologia 1996; 39: 717-724.

30. Ng LL, Simmons D, Frighi V, Garrido MC, Bomford J. effect of protein kinase C modulators on the leucocyte sodium-hydrogen antiport in type 1 diabetic subjects with albuminuria. Diabetologia 1990; 33: 278-84.

31. Sweeney FP, Siczkowski M, Davies JE, Quinn PA, McDonald J, Krolewski B, Krolewski AS, Ng LL. Phosphorylation and activity of Na^+/H^+ exchanger isoform 1 of immortalized lymphoblasts in diabetic nephropathy. Diabetes 1995; 44:1180-85.

32. Williams B, Howard RL. Glucose-induced changes in Na/H antiport activity and gene expression in cultured vascular smooth muscle cells: role of protein kinase C. J Clin Invest 1994; 93: 2623-31.

33. Davies JE, Siczkowski M, Sweeney FP, Quinn PA, Krolewski B, Krolewski AJ, Ng LL. Glucose-induced changes in turnover of Na^+/H^+ exchanger of immortalized lymphoblasts from type 1 diabetic patients with nephropathy. Diabetes 1995; 44: 382-88.

34. Berk BC, Vallega G, Muslin AJ, Gordon HM, Canessa M, Alexander RW. Spontaneously hypertensive rat vascular muscle cells in culture exhibit increased growth and Na/H exchange. J Clin Invest 1989; 83: 822-29.

35. Guicheney P, Wauquier I, Paquet JL, Meyer P. Enhanced response to growth factors and to angiotensin II of spontaneously hypertensive rat skin fibroblasts in culture. J Hypertens 1991; 9 (Suppl. 1): 23-28.

36. Rosskopt D, Fromter E, Siffert W. Hypertensive sodium-proton exchanger phenotype persists in immortalized lymphoblasts from essential hypertensive patients. J Clin Invest 1993; 92: 2553-59.

37. Strazzullo P, De Simone G, Celentano A, Iacone R, Ragone E, Pagano E, Tammaro P, Canessa M. Sodiul-hydrogen echange and cardiac hypertrophy in patients with primary hypertension. J Hypertens 1991; 9 (Suppl. 6): S306-S307.

38. Morocutti A, Earle KA, Sethi M, Piras G, Pal K, Richards D, Rodeman P, Viberti GC. Premature sensescence of skin fibroblasts from insulin-dependent diabetic patients with kidney disease. Kidney Int 1996; 50: 250-256.

39. Schwartz MA, Lechene C, Ingber DE. Insoluble fibronectin activates the Na^+/H^+ antiporter by clustering and immobilizing integrin , independent of cell shape. Proc Natl Acad Sci (USA) 1991; 88: 7849-7853.

40. Trevisan R, Yip J, Sarika L, Li LK, Viberti GC. Enhanced collagen synthesis in cultured skin fibroblasts from insulin-dependent diabetic patients with nephropathy. J Am Soc Nephrol 1997 ; 8 : 1133-1139.

27. ADVANCED GLYCATION END-PRODUCTS AND DIABETIC RENAL DISEASE

Mark E Cooper MB BS PhD FRACP
Associate Professor, Department of Medicine, University of Melbourne, Austin & Repatriation Medical Centre (Repatriation Campus), West Heidelberg Australia

George Jerums MB BS MD FRACP
Director of Endocrinology, Endocrine Unit, Austin & Repatriation Medical Centre (Austin Campus), Heidelberg Australia

Since there is chronic hyperglycaemia in diabetes, there is an acceleration of the Maillard or browning reaction [1]. This is a spontaneous reaction between glucose and proteins, lipids or nucleic acids, particularly on long-lived proteins such as the collagens [1]. There is a sequence of biochemical reactions, many of which are still poorly defined, leading to the formation of a range of advanced glycation end-products [AGEs], some of which are fluorescent. These modified long-lived tissue proteins are formed as a result not only of glycation but also oxidative processes and many of these AGEs are now considered glycoxidation products [2]. Over the last decade, an increasing number of AGEs have been identified [3]. However, the identity of the AGEs linked to diabetic complications and in particular to renal disease has not been clearly determined.

Initial studies involved assessment of AGEs by measuring their specific fluorescence in tissue homogenates. It was clearly shown that these fluorescent AGEs were increased in the aorta from diabetic rats [4]. Further studies were performed in diabetic animals and confirmed increased AGEs in the diabetic kidney [5, 6] and retina [7], sites of diabetic microvascular disease. In clinical studies, Monnier et al were able to demonstrate increased AGE levels with age, diabetic patients having an even further increase in AGE levels, as assessed by specific fluorescence [8]. In addition, levels of collagen-linked fluorescence from human skin increased with the severity of retinopathy, suggesting that there is a link between the severity of complications and cumulative exposure to hyperglycaemia [8]. However, in that study, the trend for collagen-linked fluorescence to be linked with levels of proteinuria did not reach statistical significance.

More recently, other techniques have been developed to assay AGEs.

Mogensen, C.E. (ed.), THE KIDNEY AND HYPERTENSION IN DIABETES MELLITUS.

Non-fluorescent AGEs such as carboxymethylysine (CML) have been assayed and a relationship between this AGE and diabetic complications has been shown [9]. Using a radioreceptor assay, Makita et al have reported increased AGE levels in diabetic patients, particularly in the setting of renal impairment [10]. Various antibodies to AGEs have now been developed and using a immunohistochemical techniques, increased AGE levels have been reported in both human and experimental diabetes [11, 12]. Our own group using a radioimmunoassay has detected increased AGE levels in the diabetic kidney [12] and using immunohistochemistry we have localised this increase in AGE levels to the glomerulus [13]. Beisswenger et al have used an ELISA technique to detect AGEs in serum and noted increased AGE levels in diabetic patients with complications including retinopathy and nephropathy [14].

AGE RECEPTORS

Over the last few years, a number of AGE binding sites have been identified. The first binding site to be cloned has been termed RAGE and was initially identified in endothelial cells [15]. Our own group has recently detected RAGE in various other sites including the kidney, retina, nerve and blood vessels, sites of diabetes associated vascular injury [13]. Further studies have suggested that RAGE has a central role in the development of vascular disease in diabetes by influencing various pathological processes including expression of adhesion molecules involved in mononuclear cell recruitment and hyperpermeability [16, 17]. Vlassara's group has cloned at least 3 different proteins which bind to AGEs [18]. The role of these proteins remains an area of intensive investigation and it has been postulated that they may mediate a range of functions including clearance of AGEs and activation of intracellular messengers such as protein kinase C [18]. These AGE-binding sites have been identified in cultured mesangial cells [18]. Other proteins such as lysozyme can also bind AGEs [19] but the significance of these ligand-receptor interactions has still not been fully delineated. It is still uncertain whether these AGE-binding proteins act primarily to clear AGEs which would be viewed as a beneficial effect or whether they are mainly involved in activating a range of pathological processes which lead to diabetic complications.

AGES AND CYTOKINES

In vitro AGEs have been shown to activate a range of cytokines which may be relevant to diabetic complications. In the non-diabetic mouse, *in vivo* injection of *in vitro* prepared AGEs has been shown to not only lead to increased gene expression of TGFß and type IV collagen in the kidney [20] but also to lead to histological changes with some resemblance to diabetic nephropathy [21]. These changes included mesangial expansion and glomerulosclerosis. Recently, our group has shown that activation of gene expression of the prosclerotic cytokine, TGFß1 is closely linked to AGE accumulation in blood vessels [22]. Furthermore, the inhibitor of advanced glycation, aminoguanidine, prevented diabetes associated overexpression of TGFß1 and type IV collagen in these blood vessels [22]. Recently, AGEs have been shown *in vitro* to activate vascular endothelial growth factor (VEGF) [23], a cytokine implicated in diabetes associated retinal neovascularisation and increased vascular permeability [24]. It is not yet known if these effects also occur in the kidney, a major site of VEGF production.

AGES, RECEPTORS AND CYTOKINES

It is likely that AGEs lead to diabetic complications via both receptor and receptor-independent pathways. It is postulated that AGEs activate a range of cytokines which mediate important pathological processes involved in tissue remodelling including cell adhesion, extracellular matrix accumulation, vascular permeability and cell proliferation (Fig. 27-1). This involves cytokines such as the anti-adhesin, SPARC [25], adhesins such as VCAM-1 [16], the prosclerotic cytokine, TGFß1 [22], vascular endothelial growth factor [23] and PDGF, a cytokine which promotes cell proliferation [26].

INHIBITORS OF ADVANCED GLYCATION

Pharmacological inhibitors of AGE-dependent pathways have been developed. Aminoguanidine is a hydrazine derivative which prevents AGE formation [4]. This effect has been attributed to its ability to bind to reactive dicarbonyl and aldehyde products of early glycation and glycoxidation such as 3-deoxyglucosone [2]. Aminoguanidine has been shown in experimental models of diabetes to not only reduce tissue AGE levels but also to retard the development of neuropathy, retinopathy and nephropathy [6, 7, 27]. Our own studies in the streptozotocin diabetic rat have shown that aminoguanidine, administered for 32 weeks from the induction of diabetes, retarded the development of albuminuria and mesangial expansion [6]. Aminoguanidine therapy also prevented diabetes-related increases in fluorescent AGEs.

Subsequent studies in our laboratory have explored whether aminoguanidine is more effective when administered early or late in the evolution of experimental diabetic nephropathy. Four groups of diabetic rats were studied over 32 weeks, one receiving no therapy, the second receiving aminoguanidine throughout, the third receiving aminoguanidine for the first 16 weeks only and the fourth receiving aminoguanidine for the last 16 weeks [12]. Untreated diabetic rats showed an exponential increase in albuminuria over the 8 month study period whereas rats treated with aminoguanidine showed decreased levels of albuminuria, in proportion to the duration of treatment. This study confirmed that *in vivo* generation of AGEs in the kidney is time dependent and closely linked to the development of experimental diabetic nephropathy.

New, more potent inhibitors of advanced glycation have been developed recently. Two of these, ALT462 and ALT486, are approximately 5 and 20 times respectively, more potent than aminoguanidine in their ability to inhibit fluorescence generated on reaction of lysozyme with ribose and both are approximately 20 times as potent as aminoguanidine in preventing diabetes-related decreases in rat tail collagen solubility *in vivo* [28]. Of particular interest is the thiazolium compound, phenacylthiazolium bromide (PTB) which reacts with and cleaves covalent, AGE-derived protein cross-links. Daily intraperitoneal injections of PTB in streptozotocin diabetic rats have been shown to ameliorate AGE cross-links in rat tail collagen over 32 weeks and to halve IgG binding to red blood cell surfaces over 4 weeks [29]. If

PTB or related compounds can be shown to have similar effects in large arteries, retina or kidney, this would provide a conceptual basis for the reversal of AGE-mediated tissue damage, which till now has been regarded as irreversible.

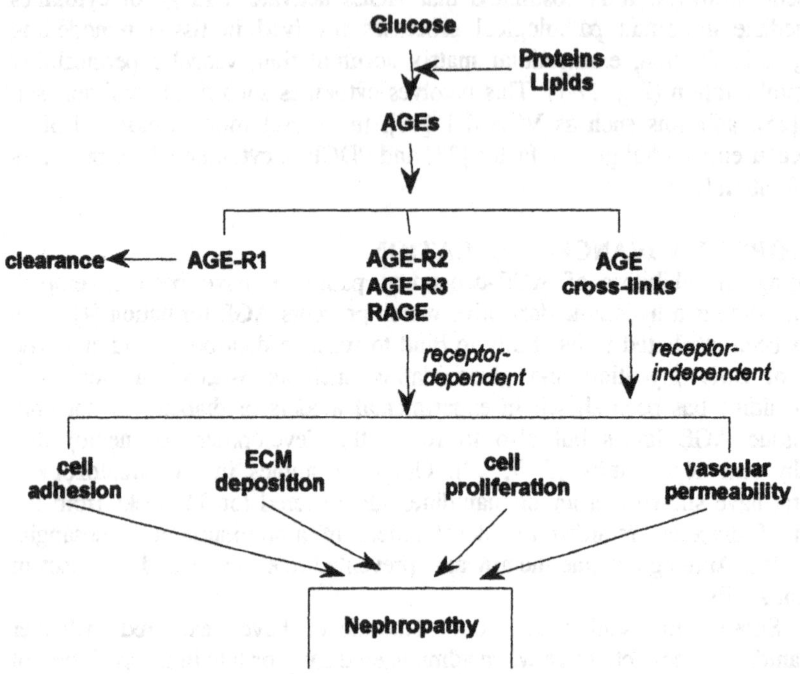

Figure 27-1.

CLINICAL STUDIES

Makita et al. have shown that the highest levels of AGEs are observed in patients with end-stage renal disease, in the absence or presence of diabetes [10]. Furthermore, aminoguanidine, as outlined previously, has been shown in experimental studies to attenuate the development of diabetic nephropathy. Therefore, a range of clinical studies are in progress focussing on the role of aminoguanidine in end-stage renal disease and in diabetic patients with nephropathy, either with overt renal disease or microalbuminuria [30]. Two separate studies known as Action 1 and Action 2 have completed the randomisation phase and involve evaluation of the effects of aminoguanidine in type I and type II diabetic patients with overt proteinuria and impaired renal function [31]. The results of these clinical trials as well as planned studies with newer inhibitors of advanced glycation are awaited with interest. It is clearly evident that the findings of these studies will have direct relevance to the management of diabetic patients with renal disease. Furthermore, these agents have the potential to influence other diabetic vascular complications.

REFERENCES

1. Brownlee M. Lilly Lecture 1993. Glycation and diabetic complications. Diabetes 1994; 43: 836-41.
2. Fu MX, Wells-Knecht KJ, Blackledge JA, Lyons TJ, Thorpe SR, Baynes JW. Glycation, glycoxidation, and cross-linking of collagen by glucose. Kinetics, mechanisms, and inhibition of late stages of the Maillard reaction. Diabetes 1994; 43: 676-683.
3. Wells-Knecht KJ, Brinkmann E, Wells-Knecht MC, Litchfield JE, Ahmed MU, Reddy S, Zyzak DV, Thorpe SR, Baynes JW. New biomarkers of maillard reaction damage to proteins. Nephrol Dial Transplantation 1996; 11 (Suppl 5): 41-47.
4. Brownlee M, Vlassara H, Kooney A, Ulrich P, Cerami A. Aminoguanidine prevents diabetes-induced arterial wall protein cross-linking. Science 1986; 232: 1629-1632.
5. Nicholls K, Mandel T. Advanced glycosylation end products in experimental murine diabetic nephropathy: effect of islet grafting and of aminoguanidine. Lab Invest 1989; 60: 486-489.
6. Soulis-Liparota T, Cooper M, Papazoglou D, Clarke B, Jerums G. Retardation by aminoguanidine of development of albuminuria, mesangial expansion, and tissue fluorescence in streptozocin-induced diabetic rat. Diabetes 1991; 40: 1328-34.
7. Hammes H, Martin S, Federlin K, Geisen K, Brownlee M. Aminoguanidine treatment inhibits the development of experimental diabetic retinopathy. Proc Natl Acad Sci USA 1991; 88: 11555-11558.
8. Monnier V, Vishwanath V, Frank K, Elmets G, Dauchot P, Kohn R. Relation between complications of type I diabetes mellitus and collagen-linked fluorescence. N Engl J Med 1986; 314: 403-408.
9. Dyer DG, Dunn JA, Thorpe SR, Bailie KE, Lyons TJ, McCance DR, Baynes JW. Accumulation of Maillard reaction products in skin collagen in diabetes and aging. J Clin Invest 1993; 91: 2463-9.
10. Makita Z, Radoff S, Rayfield EJ, Yang Z, Skolnik E, Delaney V, Friedman EA, Cerami A, Vlassara H. Advanced glycosylation end products in patients with diabetic nephropathy. N Engl J Med 1991; 325: 836-842.
11. Makita Z, Bucala R, Rayfield EJ, Friedman EA, Kaufman AM, Korbet SM, Barth RH, Winston JA, Fuh H, Manogue KR, et al. Reactive glycosylation endproducts in diabetic uraemia and treatment of renal failure. Lancet 1994; 343: 1519-22.
12. Soulis T, Cooper M, Vranes D, Bucala R, Jerums G. The effects of aminoguanidine in preventing experimental diabetic nephropathy are related to duration of treatment. Kidney Int 1996; 50: 627-634.
13. Soulis T, Thallas V, Youssef S, Gilbert RE, McWilliam B, Murray-McIntosh RP, Cooper ME. Advanced glycation end products and the receptor for advanced glycated end products co-localise in organs susceptible to diabetic microvascular injury: immunohistochemical studies. Diabetologia 1997; 40: 619-628.
14. Beisswenger PJ, Makita Z, Curphey TJ, Moore LL, Jean S, Brinck Johnsen T, Bucala R, Vlassara H. Formation of immunochemical advanced glycosylation end products precedes and correlates with early manifestations of renal and retinal disease in diabetes. Diabetes 1995; 44: 824-9.
15. Schmidt A, Vianna M, Gerlach M, Brett J, Ryan J, Kao C, Esposito H, Hegarty W, Hurley W, Clauss M, Wang F, Pan Y, Tsang T, Stern D. Isolation and characterisation of two binding proteins for advanced glycation end products from bovine lung which are present on the endothelial cell surface. J Biol Chem 1992; 267: 14987-14997.
16. Schmidt AM, Hori O, Chen JX, Li JF, Crandall J, Zhang J, Cao R, Yan SD, Brett J, Stern D. Advanced glycation endproducts interacting with their endothelial receptor induce expression of vascular cell adhesion molecule-1(VCAM-1) in cultured human endothelial cells and in mice. A potential mechanism for the accelerated vasculopathy of diabetes. J Clin Invest 1995; 96: 1395-1403
17. Wautier JL, Zoukourian C, Chappey O, Wautier MP, Guillausseau PJ, Cao R, Hori O, Stern D, Schmidt AM. Receptor-mediated endothelial cell dysfunction in diabetic vasculopathy. Soluble receptor for advanced glycation end products blocks hyperpermeability in diabetic rats. J Clin Invest 1996; 97: 238-243.

18. Li Y, Mitsuhashi T, Wojciechowicz D, Shimizu N, Li J, Stitt A, He C, Banerjee D, Vlassara H. Molecular identity and distribution of advanced glycation endproducts receptors: Relationship of p60 to OST-48 and p90 to 80K-H membrane proteins. Proc Natl Acad Sci USA 1996; 93: 11047-11052.
19. Li YM, Tan AX, Vlassara H. Antibacterial activity of lysozyme and lactoferrin is inhibited by binding of advanced glycation-modified proteins to a conserved motif. Nature Medicine 1995; 1: 1057-1061.
20. Yang CW, Vlassara H, Peten EP, He CJ, Striker GE, Striker LJ. Advanced glycation end products up-regulate gene expression found in diabetic glomerular disease. Proc Natl Acad Sci USA 1994; 91: 9436-9440.
21. Vlassara H, Striker LJ, Teichberg S, Fuh H, Li YM, Steffes M. Advanced glycation end products induce glomerular sclerosis and albuminuria in normal rats. Proc Natl Acad Sci USA 1994; 91: 11704-11708.
22. Rumble JR, Cooper ME, Soulis T, Cox A, Wu L, Youssef S, Jasik M, Jerums G, Gilbert R. Vascular hypertrophy in experimental diabetes: role of advanced glycation end products. J Clin Invest 1997; 99: 1016-1027.
23. Yamagishi S, Yonekura H, Yamamoto Y, Katsuno K, Sato F, Mita I, Ooka H, Satozawa N, Kawakami T, Nomura M, Yamamoto H. Advanced glycation end products-driven angiogenesis in vitro. J Biol Chem 1997; 272: 8723-8730.
24. Ferrara N, Davissmyth T, Ferrara N, Yuan F, Chen Y, Dellian M, Safabakhsh N, Ferrara N, Jain RK. The biology of vascular endothelial growth factor. Endocrine Reviews 1997; 18: 4-25.
25. Gilbert RE, McNally PG, Cox A, Dziadek M, Rumble J, Cooper ME, Jerums G. SPARC Gene Expression is Reduced in Early Diabetes Related Kidney Growth. Kidney Int 1995; 48: 1216-1225.
26. Isaka Y, Fujiwara Y, Ueda N, Kaneda Y, Kamada T, Imai E. Glomerulosclerosis induced by in vivo transfection of transforming growth factor-beta or platelet-derived growth factor gene into the rat kidney. J Clin Invest 1993; 92: 2597-601.
27. Kihara M, Schmelzer JD, Poduslo JF, Curran GL, Nickander KK, Low PA. Aminoguanidine effects on nerve blood flow, vascular permeability, electrophysiology, and oxygen free radicals. Proc Natl Acad Sci USA 1991; 88: 6107-11.
28. Kochakian M, Manjula B, Egan J. Chronic dosing with aminoguanidine and novel advanced glycosylation end product formation inhibitors ameliorates cross-linking of tail tendon collagen in streptozotocin-induced diabetic rats. Diabetes 1996; 45: 1694-1700.
29. Vasan S, Zhang X, Zhang X, Kapurniotu A, Bernhagen J, Teichberg S, Basgen J, Wagle D, Shih D, Terlecky I, Bucala R, Cerami A, Egan J, Urlich P. An agent cleaving glucose-derived protein cross-links in vitro and in vivo. Nature 1996; 382: 275-278.
30. Bucala R, Vlassara H. Advanced glycosylation end products in diabetic renal and vascular disease. Am J Kidney Dis 1995; 26: 875-88.
31. Wuerth J-P, Bain R, Mecca T, Park G, Cartwright K, Pimagedine Investigator Group. Baseline data from the Pimagedine Action trials. Diabetologia 1997; 40 (Suppl 1): A548.

28. PROTEIN KINASE C IN DIABETIC RENAL INVOLVEMENT, THE PERSPECTIVE OF ITS INHIBITION

Daisuke Koya
Third Department of Medicine, Shiga University of Medical Science, Seta, Otsu Shiga 520-21, Japan

George L. King
Research Division, Joslin Diabetes Center, Department of Medicine, Brigham and Women's Hospital and Harvard Medical School, Boston, MA 02215, USA

The Diabetes Control and Complication Trial recently reported that the strict maintenance of euglycemia by intensive insulin treatment can prevent the development and progression of diabetic nephropathy [1], suggesting the adverse effects of hyperglycemia on metabolic pathways are main cause of chronic complications in diabetes such as kidney disease. The importance of hyperglycemia in the development of diabetic nephropathy is supported by the results of Heilig et al. who have found that the overexpression of glucose transporter 1 (GLUT1) into glomerular mesangial cells enhanced the production of extracellular matrix components which can contribute mesangial expansion and finally glomerulosclerosis, even in normal glucose levels [2]. Multiple biochemical mechanisms have been proposed to explain the adverse effects of hyperglycemia. Activation of diacylglycerol (DAG) -protein kinase C (PKC) pathway [3,4], enhanced polyol pathway related with myo-inositol depletion [5], altered redox state [6], overproduction of advanced glycation products [7], and enhanced growth factor and cytokine production [8.9] have all been proposed as potential cellular mechanisms by which hyperglycemia induces the chronic diabetic complications.

In this article, evidence regarding the activation of DAG-PKC pathway will be briefly reviewed. The possibility that changes in PKC activities could be causing diabetic vascular complications has been discussed frequently due to the finding that PKC activation can increase vascular permeability, extracellular matrix synthesis, contractility, leukocyte attachment, cell growth, and angiogenesis [10,11,12]. All of these vascular functions have been reported to be abnormal in diabetic state. When the DAG level and PKC activities were first quantitated, we and Craven et al. showed that elevating 5 to 20 mM of glucose increased both DAG and PKC levels in vascular cells or tissue including renal glomeruli, retina, and aorta

[13,14,15,16]. Recently, possible activation of DAG-PKC have also been reported in the liver and skeletal muscle of insulin resistant diabetic animals, suggesting that the activation of DAG-PKC signal transduction pathway by hyperglycemia may also induce insulin resistance in those tissues.

It is not surprising that the activation of PKC could affect such a wide range of tissues since PKC is a family of serine and threonine kinases which act as intracellular signal transduction system for many cytokines and hormones [10,11]. Different PKC isoforms are also one of the major downstream targets for lipid signaling molecules and can be classified according to their structure differences. Conventional PKCs (a, b1, b2, g) are sensitive to both Ca++ and DAG whereas new PKCs (d, e, h, q, m) are sensitive to DAG but insensitive to Ca++ due to the loss of C1 region. Atypical PKCs (z, l) may also sensitive to other phospholipids such as the products of phosphatidylinositol-3-kinase.

The sources of cellular DAG are multiple with the majority derived from the hydrolysis of polyphosphoinositides or phophatidylcholine by phospholipase C or D, respectively [10,11,12]. The mechanism by which PKC is activated by diabetes and by hyperglycemia appears to be related to increase in de novo synthesis of DAG through glycolytic pathway [13,14].

We and others have found the activation of DAG-PKC pathway in glomeruli of diabetic rats and cultured mesangial cells exposed to high concentrations of glucose [13,15,17]. Multiple PKC isoforms are activated in each vascular tissues of diabetic animal models. Among them PKC b isoforms appear to be most consistently increased. We have reported that PKC a and b1 exhibited a greater increase in membranous fractions of diabetic glomeruli and mesangial cells exposed to elevated glucose levels using immunoblotting study [17], whereas PKC b2 was reported to be preferentially activated in aorta and heart of diabetic rats [16]. Interestingly, Kikkawa et al. have reported that PKC z as well as PKC a was activated in rat glomerular mesangial cells exposed to high concentrations of glucose [8], although the mechanism for PKC z activation, which is independent on DAG, is unclear.

Functionally, the activation of DAG-PKC pathway have been correlated with many vascular changes in enzymatic activities, gene expressions, contractility, extracellular matrix synthesis, and cell growth and differentiation. To determine those vascular or renal dysfunctions which are due to specifically the activation of PKC b isoform, we have designed a specific inhibitor to PKC b isoform (LY333531) and studied its effect on glomerular cells or tissues from diabetic animals. The specificity of PKC b inhibitor LY333531 was evaluated by in vitro study to examine the PKC isoform-induced phosphorylation of myelin basic protein. LY333531 inhibited PKC b1 and b2 with a half-maximal inhibitory constant (IC50) of 4.5 and 5.9 nM, respectively, whereas the IC50 was 250 nM or greater for other PKC isoforms [15]. Furthermore, its specificity was confirmed in vivo study to examine the phosphorylation of PKC a and b1, which has been shown to correspond to PKC isoform specific activation, in isolated glomeruli from control and streptozotocin-induced diabetic rats with or without LY333531 (10 mg/kg body wt/day) [17]. Diabetes enhanced phosphorylation of both PKC a and b1 by 60 and 60%, respectively. PKC b specific inhibitor LY333531 prevented the increase in phosphorylation of PKC b1 but not PKC a, suggesting the specific PKC b isoform inhibition of LY333531 even in vivo [16].

The effect of PKC b isoform inhibitor LY333531 on renal hemodynamics were examined first. These functional parameters included glomerular filtration rates (GFR) and urinary albumin excretion rates (UAE). Treatment with LY333531 orally at the start of diabetes normalized GFR and glomerular PKC activity in a dose-dependent manner [15]. Treatment with also ameliorated the increase in urinary albumin excretion rate in diabetic rats 12 wks after the onset of diabetes [15], suggesting that PKC b activation may cause the early hemodynamic and histological abnormalities which have been implicated to be responsible for glomerular injury leading to the progression of diabetic nephropathy. One possible mechanisms to explain renal hyperfiltration is the increase in vasodilatory prostanoids such as prostaglandin (PG) E2 and PGI2 which have been noted in the kidney of diabetic patients and animals with glomerular hyperfiltration [19,20]. We have reported that the possible overproduction of glomerular PGE2 in the glomeruli of diabetic rats could be due to an enhanced synthesis of arachidonic acid via the activation of cytosolic phospholipase A2 (cPLA2) by PKC since specific inhibitor of PKC b isoform was able to decrease PGE and arachidonic acid release by hyperglycemia [17]. Haneda et al. have found that the increase in mitogen-activated protein kinase (MAPK) activity, which was dependent on diabetes-induced activation of PKC pathway, was able to enhance cPLA2 activity, resulting in increase in arachidonic acid release in glomerular mesangial cells exposed to elevated glucose levels [21]. Williams et al. have also reported similar findings showing that PKC activation by glucose increased PGE2 production through cPLA2 and it was normalized in the presence of PKC inhibitors such as H-7 or staurosporine in glomerular mesangial cells [22]. Those results strongly support that diabetes-induced hyperfiltration could be due to an overproduction of vasodilatory prostanoids through the activation of cPLA2 which was due to the activation of PKC-MAPK pathway.

Another important biochemical change induced by DAG-PKC activation is the inhibition of Na+-K+ ATPase , an integral component of the sodium pump, which is involved in the maintenance of cellular integrity and functions such as contractility, growth, and differentiation [23]. Its inhibition has been well established in the vascular and neural tissues of diabetic patients and diabetic experimental animals [5]. However, the mechanisms by which hyperglycemia can inhibit Na+-K+ ATPase is still unclear especially regarding the role of PKC. We have found that PKC activation induced by diabetes or hyperglycemia can lead to the inhibition of Na+-K+ ATPase and PKC b inhibitor prevented the decrease of Na+-K+ATPase induced by hyperglycemia, suggesting the importance of PKC b activation in the development of mesangial or glomerular dysfunctions which are due to the inhibition of Na+-K+ ATPase activity in diabetes [17].

One of the most important glomerular pathological changes in diabetic nephropathy is structural alterations including glomerular hypertrophy, basement membrane thickening, and mesangial expansion due to accumulation of extracellular matrix components such as collagen and fibronectin [24]. A close relation is also found between mesangial expansion and the declining surface area available for glomerularfiltration. Thus, the mechanisms responsible for mesangial expansion are closely related to the formation of nodular glomerulosclerosis, resulting in end stage diabetic nephropathy.

Although multiple mechanisms are probably involved in causing mesangial expansion, many studies have recently focused on the role of transforming growth factor b (TGF-b), a multifunctional cytokine, in the regulation of extracellular matrix production in diabetic nephropathy [8,9]. TGF-b can stimulate the production of extracellular matrix such as type IV collagen, fibronectin and laminin in cultured mesangial cells and epithelial cells [25,26]. Increase in gene and protein expressions of TGF-b were found in glomeruli from diabetic animal models as well as human diabetics [27,28,29], suggesting that overexpression of TGF-b might be responsible for the development of mesangial expansion in diabetic nephropathy. This hypothesis was strengthen by the fact that inhibition of TGF-b activity with neutralizing antibody attenuates the increase in mRNA expressions of type IV collagen and fibronectin in renal cortex and glomeruli of diabetic animal models [30.31]. Since PKC is well known stimulator for synthesis of type IV collagen and fibronectin [32], it has been postulated that PKC activation might be involved in the enhancement of TGF-b expression in diabetes. To substantiate this hypothesis, we have examined the effect of PKC b inhibitor LY333531 on the gene expressions of TGF-b1, type IV collagen, and fibronectin in glomeruli of control and diabetic rats [17]. In the glomeruli of diabetic rats, the expression of TGF-b1 mRNA was significantly increased compared to control rats [17]. Treatment with LY333531 abrogated the enhanced glomerular expression of TGF-b mRNA in diabetic rats [17]. LY333531 also prevented mRNA overexpression of extracellular matrix components such as type IV collagen and fibronectin in the glomeruli of diabetic rats, again supporting the importance of PKC b activation and TGF-b expression in causing extracellular matrix overproduction.

In summary, a great deal of evidence have accumulated to indicate a pivotal role of PKC b activation in causing many of the pathophysiological abnormalities associated with the development and progression of diabetic nephropathy. The ability of PKC b specific inhibitor LY333531 to prevent diabetes-induced glomerular hyperfiltration, increase in albuminuria, inhibition of Na+-K+ ATPase, and glomerular overexpression of TGF-b and extracellular matrix components suggested that PKC b activation induced by diabetes lies in intracellular signaling pathway leading to these abnormalities. The availability of PKC b inhibitor LY333531 provided an important insight into the molecular pathogenesis of diabetic nephropathy and clinical studies using PKC b inhibitor LY333531 which are ongoing will determine the therapeutic usefulness of PKC b inhibition in diabetic nephropathy and other diabetic complications.

ACKNOWLEDGEMENTS

This work was supported by a grant NIH EY05110 provided by National Institutes of Health.

REFERENCES

1. The Diabetes Control and Complications trial Research Group: The effecttof intensive treatment of diabetes on the development and progression of long-term complications in insulin-dependent diabetes mellitus. N Engl J Med 329:977-986, 1993
2. Heilig CW, Concepcion LA, Riser BL, Freytag SO, Zhu M, Cortes P: Overexpression of glucose transporters in rat mesangial cells cultured in a normal glucose milieu mimics the diabetic phenotype. J Clin Invest 96:1802-1814, 1995
3. King GL, Ishii H, Koya D: Diabetic vascular dysfunctions: A model of excessive activation of protein kinase C. Kidney Int 52:S77-S85, 1997
4. DeRubertis FR, Craven PA: Activation of protein kinase C in glomerular cells in diabetes. Mechanisms and potential link to the pathogenesis of diabetic glomerulopathy. Diabetes 43: 1-8, 1994
5. Greene D, Lattimer SA, Sima AAF: Sorbitol, phosphoinositides and sodium-potassium-ATPase in the pathogenesis of diabetic complications. N Engl J Med 316: 599-606, 1987
6. Williamson JR, Chang K, Frangos M, Hasan KS, Ido Y, Kawamura T, Nyengaard JR, Van den Enden M, Kilo C, Tilton RG: Hyperglycemic pseudohypoxia and diabetic complications. Diabetes 42: 801-813, 1993
7. Brownlee M, Cerami A, Vlassara H: Advanced glycosylation end products in tissue and the biochemical basis of diabetic complications N Engl J Med 318: 1315-1321, 1988
8. Sharama K, Ziyadeh FN: Hyperglycemia and diabetic kidney disease. Mechanisms and potential link to the pathogenesis of diabetic glomerulopathy. Diabetes 43: 1-8, 1994
9. Mogyorosi A, Ziyadeh FN: Update on pathogenesis, markers and management of diabetic nephropathy. Curr Opin Nephrol Hyperten 5:243-253, 1996
10. Nishizuka Y: Intracellular signaling by hydrolysis of phospholipids and activation of protein kinase C. Science 258: 607-614, 1992
11. Nishizuka Y: Protein kinase C and lipid signaling for sustained cellular responses. FASEB J 9:484-496, 1995
12. Liscovitch M, Cantley LC: Lipid second messengers. Cell 77:329-334, 1994
13. Craven PA, Davidson CM, DeRubertis FR: Increase in diacylglycerol mass in isolated glomeruli by glucose from de novo synthesis of glycerolipids. Diabetes 39:667-674, 1990
14. Inoguchi T, Pu X, Kunisaki M, Higashi S, Feener EP, King GL: Insulin's effect on protein kinase C and diacylglycerol induced by diabetes and glucose in vascular tissue. Am J Physiol 267: E369-E379, 1994
15. Ishii H., Jirousek MR, Koya D, Takagi C, Xia P, Clermont A, Bursell S-E, Kern TS, Ballas LM, Heath WF, Stramm LE, Feener EP, King GL: Amelioration of vascular dysfunctions in diabetic rats by an oral PKC b inhibitor. Science, 272: 728-731, 1996
16. Inoguchi T, Battan R, Handler E, Sportsman JR, Heath WF, King GL: Preferential elevation of protein kinase C bII and diacylglycerol levels in the aorta and heart of diabetic rats: differential reversibility to glycemic control by islet cell transplantation. Proc Natl Acad Sci USA 89: 11059-11063, 1992
17. Koya D, Jirousek MR, Lin Y-W, Ishii H, Kuboki K, King GL: Characterization of PKC b isoform activation on the gene expression of transforming growth factor b, extracellular matrix components, and prostanoids in the glomeruli of diabetic rats. J Clin Invest, 100:115-126, 1997
18. Kikkawa R, Haneda M, Uzu T , Koya D, Sugimoto T, Shigeta Y:Translocation of protein kinase C a and z in rat glomerular mesangial cells cultured under high glucose conditions. Diabetologia 37: 838-841, 1994
19. Craven PA, Caines MA, DeRubertis FR: Sequential alterations in glomerular prostaglandin and thromboxane synthesis in diabetic rats:relationship to the hyperfiltration of early diabetes. Metabolism 36:95-103, 1987
20. Perico N, Benigni A, Gabanelli M, Piccinelli A, Rog M, Riva CD, Remuzzi G: Atrial natriuretic peptide and prostacyclin synergistically mediate hyperfiltration and hyperfusion of diabetic rats. Diabetes 41:533-538

21. Haneda M, Araki S-I, Togawa M, Sugimoto T, Isono M, Kikkawa R: Mitogen-activated protein kinase cascade is activated in glomeruli of diabetic rats and glomerular mesangial cells cultured under high glucose conditions. Diabetes 46: 847-853, 1997
22. Williams B, Schreier RW: Glucose-induced protein kinase C activity regulates arachidonic acid release and eicosanoid production by cultured glomerular mesangial cells. J Clin Invest 92: 2889-2896, 1993
23. Vasilets LA, Schwarz W: Structure-function relationships of cation binding in Na+/K+-ATPase. Biochim Biophys Acta 1154:201-222, 1993
24. Ziyadeh FN: The extracellular matrix in diabetic nephropathy. Am J Kidney Dis 22:736-744, 1993
25. MacKay K, Striker LJ, Stauffer JW, Agodoa LY, Striker GE: Transforming growth factor b. Murine glomerular receptors and responses of isolated glomerular cells. J Clin Invest 83:1160-1167, 1989
26. Nakamura T, Miller D, Ruoslahti E, Border WA: Production of extracellular matrix by glomerular epithelial cells is regulated by transforming growth factor-b1 Kidney Int 41:1213-1221, 1992
27. Yamamoto T, Nakamura T, Noble NA, Ruoslahti E, Border WA: Expression of transforming growth factor b is elevated in human and experimental diabetic nephropathy. Proc Natl Acad Sci USA 90:1814-1818, 1993
28. Nakamura T, Fukui M, Ebihara I, Osada S, Nagaoka I, Tomino Y, Koide H: mRNA expression of growth factors in glomeruli from diabetic rats. Diabetes 42:450-456, 1993
29. Sharma K, Ziyadeh FN: Renal hypertrophy is associated with upregulation of TGF-b1 gene expression in diabetic BB rat and NOD mouse. Am J Physiol 267:F1094-F1101, 1994
30. Ziyadeh FN, Sharma K, Ericksen M, Wolf G: Stimulation of collagen gene and protein synthesis in murine mesangial cells by high glucose is mediated by autocrine activation of transforming growth factor-b. J Clin Invest 93:536-542, 1994
31. Sharma K, Jin Y, Gua J, Ziyadeh FN: Neutralization of TGF-b by anti-TGF-b antibody attenuates kidney hypertrophy and the enhanced extracellular matrix gene expression in STZ-induced diabetic mice. Diabetes 45:522-530, 1996
32. Fumo P, Kuncio GS, Ziyadeh FN: PKC and high glucose stimulates collagen a1(IV) transcriptional activity in a reporter mesangial cell line. Am J Physiol 267: F632-F638, 1994

29. BIOCHEMICAL ASPECTS OF DIABETIC NEPHROPATHY

Erwin D. Schleicher
Department of Medicine IV, University of Tübingen, Germany

The dominant histological feature of diabetic nephropathy is the thickening of the glomerular basement membrane and expansion of the mesangial matrix [1-3]. The changes correlate strongly with the clinical onset of proteinuria, hypertension and kidney failure. Although more than 50 years have elapsed since Kimmelstiel and Wilson [4] described in diabetic glomeruli the distinctive periodic acid-schiff (PAS)-reactive nodular deposits, progress in elucidating the pathobiochemistry has been slow. Recent investigations with electron microscopic, immunochemical and biochemical methods have led to an improved understanding of the structure-function relationship of the glomerular filtration unit in normal and pathological conditions [5].

MOLECULAR STRUCTURE AND FUNCTION OF GLOMERULAR EXTRACELLULAR MATRIX

The extracellular matrix of the glomerulus consists of the basement membrane interposed between endothelial and epithelial cells and the closely adjoining extracellular matrix surrounding the mesangial cells. The structural and functional properties of the matrix components are summarized in table 29-1. The basement membrane representing the size and charge selective area of the filtration unit is composed of a filamentous network of collagen type IV fibrils. Immunohistochemical studies revealed that the collagen IV chains are inhomogenously distributed within the glomerulus. The $\alpha 1,\alpha 2$-chains are primarily detected in the mesangial matrix whereas the $\alpha 3,\alpha 4$-chains are exclusively found in the glomerular basement membrane [6]. The basement membranes also contain a proteoglycan which consists of three heparan sulfate side chains covalently attached to the protein core [10,11]. It has been convincingly shown that the negatively charged heparan sulfate chains form the anionic barrier of the glomerular filtration unit [5,12,13]. A detailed review of this heparan sulfate proteoglycan (HSPG) and its changes in diabetes is given in the following chapter. The traces of fibronectin found in normal glomerular matrices are probably derived from plasma since the tissue specific fibronectin A+ which contains the extra domain A is not detected in normal glomeruli [14]. The mesangial matrix, although developmentally and morphologically distinct from the glomerular basement membrane, contains essentially the same components but in different distributions.

Several functions of the matrix components can now be explained by features of these components on the molecular level. Specific cell-matrix adhesion molecules which are intercalated in the cellular plasma membrane recognize well-defined amino acid sequences found in collagen, laminin and fibronectin [9,15]. Furthermore, these adhesion molecules (integrins) which are in contact with the cytoskcleton influence cell migration and cell proliferation. Changes in matrix composition may therefore alter cellular adhesion, migration and proliferation and thus influencing repair processes [15]. The finding that HSPG by virtue of its side chains specifically binds polypeptide growth factors like basic fibroblast growth factor (bFGF) or transforming growth factor ß (TGF-ß) is important in this context. It has been suggested that the matrix-bound growth factors may act as a reservoir for vascular repair mechanisms [16]. The anti-proliferative role of heparan sulfate on mesangial cells underlines the possible importance of this the proteoglycan in glomerular matrix [17].

Table 29-1. Structure and function of the major components of the glomerular basement membrane and mesangial matrix

Component	Structure	Function
Collagen type IV	Triplehelix with non-helical segments; 5 different chains with approximately 1700 amino acids are known [6,9] Chains are unequally distributed in the glomerular matrix [6]	Mechanical scaffold; Size selective filter; Binding to cell adhesion molecules
Collagen type VI	3 different chains [8]	Formation of microfibrils
Laminin	3 different poly-peptide chains MW 800 KD [9]	Cell adhesion Integrin binding
Heparan sulfate proteoglycan (HSPG)	Coreprotein MW 470 KD [7,10] 3 heparan sulfate side chains	Integrin binding Charge selective filter Antiproliferative Binding of humoral factors

STRUCTURAL AND FUNCTIONAL GLOMERULAR ALTERATIONS IN DIABETES

The first major change after the onset of diabetes is the increased volume of the whole kidney [18] and the glomeruli [19]. These hypertrophical glomeruli have normal structural composition. After a few years the amount of glomerular matrix material is increased [1,3]. Biochemical determinations indicate an increased amount of collagen in the glomerular extracellular matrices [20]. More recently, an increase in collagen type VI in the glomerular matrix of diabetic patients has been documented [21]. On the basis of immunochemical measurement, it has become evident that the HSPG content of glomerular matrix is lower in diabetic patients [22] consistent with previous chemical analyses of the heparan sulfate chains [23,24]. These immunochemical measurements, although yielding reliable quantitative values, were performed with preparations of glomerular matrices which contain firstly, both the basement membrane and the mesangial matrix and secondly a mixture of glomeruli which may be affected to a variable degree. Therefore, immunohistochemical studies have been performed to distinguish the changes within the different compartments of the glomerulus and between the individual glomeruli.

These immunohistochemical studies, summarized in table 23-2, indicate that in diabetic kidneys with slight lesions only a minor increase in all basement membrane components was found except for HSPG. More pronounced diffuse glomerulo-sclerosis showed a further increase in basement membrane components, especially collagen IV α1,α2-chains in the expanded mesangial matrix. However, HSPG which was entirely absent from the enlarged matrix could only be observed in the periphery of the glomeruli. The staining of collagen IV α3,α4-chain showed a similar distribution as found for HSPG however, with intense staining of the thickened glomerular basement membrane [6]. To this stage of nephropathy the accumulation of excess matrix material can be attributed to quantitative changes of the components present in normal glomeruli. In contrast, pronounced nodular lesions exhibited a strong decrease of collagen IV α1,α2-chains, laminin, and HSPG which were only detectable in the periphery of the noduli. Staining sequential sections with collagen VI antiserum or PAS revealed coincidence of both stainings indicating that the noduli consist mostly of collagen type VI [8]. Peripheral areas of these noduli were also positive for collagen III which was not detected in earlier lesions. It appears that in diffuse glomerulosclerosis an increase in normal matrix components occurs while the nodular glomerulosclerosis is characterized by qualitative changes (table 29-2). Morphological and structural changes occurring in the interstitium, tubuli or glomerular arterioles are a concomitant of diabetic nephropathy [1].

The likelihood that increased matrix content occurring in diffuse glomerulo-sclerosis is the consequence of increased synthesis coupled with decreased degradation is supported by in vivo and in vitro studies of collagen metabolism in glomeruli obtained from diabetic animals [20,25,26]. An increased synthesis was unequivocally demonstrated by extracellular matrix gene expression. Fukui et al. [27] showed increased steady state mRNA levels of the collagen IV α1-chain, laminin B1 and B2 and fibronectin while the collagen I α1-chain was unchanged in the kidneys of diabetic rats after one month of diabetes. The message for HSPG was decreased after induction of diabetes and increased steadily afterwards. The changes in mRNA levels which preceded the glomerular matrix expansion could be prevented by normalisation of blood glucose by insulin treatment. Recent *in situ* hybridization studies revealed that mRNA transcript levels of α_1(IV) collagen are increased more than twofold in glomerular and proximal tubular cells in long-term (12 months) diabetic rats [28]. In the glomerulum, mainly mesangial cells showed enhanced α_1(IV) collagen expression. The α_1(IV) collagen deposition in the mesangial matrix was similarly increased. Chronic treatment with a modified heparin preparation completely prevented the increased α_1(IV) collagen deposition and expression and the overt albuminuria in diabetic rats. Taken together, these results indicate that the increased synthesis of collagen IV, laminin and fibronectin is the biochemical correlate of the expansion of the mesangial matrix and the thickening of glomerular basement membrane observed histologically. The occurrence of decreased degradation of matrix components has also been documented [26].

Table 29-2. Changes of glomerular matrix composition in different stages of diabetic glomerulosclerosis (GS)*

	diffuse GS		nodular GS	
	GBM	mesangium	GBM	mesangium
laminin	↑	↑	↑	↓
collagen IV				
α1,α2-chain	↑	↑	↑	↓
α3,α4-chain	↑	-	↑	↑
HSPG	↓→	↓	↓	-
fibronectin A+	-	n.d.	-	↑
collagen III	-	-1)	-	↑2)
collagen VI	↓	↑3)	↓	↑↑

↑ = increased; ↓ = decreased; → = unchanged; - = not detectable; *see also [6-8]; n.d. = not determined; 1)traces in late diffuse GS; 2)only peripheral; 3)focally

Extensive studies have shown that the changes in glomerular ultrastructure are closely associated with renal function [2,3]. Comparing the immunohistochemical findings with clinical data Nerlich et al. [7] found that the increase in the glomerular matrix components was consistently associated with impaired renal filter function. Late stage nodular glomerulosclerosis associated with decrease of all basement membrane components and increase in collagen III and VI coincided with severe renal insufficiency. In all cases, even in early diffuse glomerulosclerosis, HSPG was decreased.

INVOLVEMENT OF GROWTH FACTORS IN THE DEVELOPMENT OF DIABETIC NEPHROPATHY

The morphological changes occurring in diabetic micro- and macroangiopathy have led to the idea that growth hormone or other growth factors may play an active role in mediating these alterations [29]. In a recent study with experimental animals Nakamura et al. [30] demonstrated the gene expression of different growth factors including TGF-ß, bFGF and platelet derived growth factor in glomeruli of diabetic rats within 4 weeks after induction of diabetes. The gene expression was relatively specific since other growth factors like IGF-I were unchanged. Insulin treatment partially ameliorated the induction of growth factors. In a related study Yamamoto et al. [14] report that in glomeruli of diabetic rats there is a slow, progressive increase in the expression of TGF-ß mRNA and TGF-ß protein. A more recent report showed that the induction of glomerular TGF-β_1 synthesis is significant after 14 days of diabetes indicating that the increased TGF-β_1 production is an early event in diabetes [31]. A key action of TGF-ß is the induction of extracellular matrix production and specific matrix proteins, known to be induced by TGF-ß, were increased in diabetic rat glomeruli. Corresponding changes were found in patients with diabetic nephropathy, whereas glomeruli from normal subjects or individuals with other glomerular diseases were essentially negative. These findings suggest that TGF-ß plays a pivotal role in the glomerular matrix expansion that occurs in diabetic nephropathy. A causal relationship between TGF-ß expression and matrix accumulation in the acute model of glomerular nephritis was proven by preventing matrix accumulation with TGF-ß antiserum [32,33]. Furthermore, addition of oligonucleotides antisense to TFG-β_1 attenuated the high glucose-induced matrix production indicating that hyperglycemia induces TFG-β_1 synthesis in mesangial cells [34].

BIOCHEMICAL PATHWAYS INVOLVED IN THE PATHOGENESIS OF DIABETIC GLOMERULOPATHY

The biochemical mechanisms leading to the quantitative and finally qualitative alterations of the glomerular matrix and to the induction of growth factors are not well understood. Epidemiological studies indicate that the development of diabetic nephropathy is linked to hyperglycaemia [35,36]. Three pathobiochemical pathways are favoured in the current discussion:

The first possibility involves the direct action of elevated glucose on the cells. Ayo and coworkers reported that prolonged exposure to high glucose concentration leads to an increase in collagen IV, laminin and fibronectin synthesis on the protein and mRNA level in mesangial cells [37]. Furthermore, mesangial cells exposed to elevated glucose synthesize less HSPG [38]. The HSPG biochemistry in diabetes is discussed in detail in the suceeding chapter. Studies with epithelial, endothelial and mesangial cells revealed that all three cell types of the glomerulus produce more collagen type IV when exposed to elevated glucose levels [39]. In recent studies the effect of periodic changes in glucose concentration on mesangial matrix production was examined. Mesangial cells cultured in daily changed high (25 mM) and low (5 mM) glucose concentrations produced more collagen III and IV than cell cultured continuously in low or high glucose medium. The data indicate the deleterious effects of fluctuating glucose levels on the development of diabetic glomerulosclerosis [40]. A recent approach using mesangial cells with overexpressed glucose transporter provides a more direct evidence for the involvement of glucose in matrix production [41]. Mesangial cells transduced with the human glucose transporter 1 gene had an increased glucose uptake (5-fold) and net utilization (43-fold) and exerted enhanced synthesis of matrix components when cultured in <u>normal</u> glucose concentration. Thus increased cellular glucose flux enhances matrix production in mesangial cells. These in vitro experiments suggest that hyperglycaemia rather than hyperinsulinaemia or hyperosmolarity is the cause of enhanced matrix synthesis [37,39]. Recent in vitro studies suggest how elevated glucose concentrations may exert their effects on cellular metabolism. High glucose levels induce the transcription and secretion of TGF-ß in mesangial cells [42] and elevate cellular transcripts of TGF-α and bFGF in vascular muscle cells [43]. Several reports provide evidence for the involvement of glucose-induced activation of protein kinase C in the elevated synthesis of matrix components [44,46]. PKC activation may be also involved in the elevation of lipooxygenase products [35] which may lead to increased matrix production [47]. Application of an PKC inhibitor (preferentially inhibiting the β-isoform) ameliorated the glomerular filtration rate, albumin excretion rate, and retinal circulation in diabetic rats in a dose-responsive manner, in parallel with its inhibition of PKC activities [48]. (see also preceeding chapter).

The second pathomechanism linking elevated glucose levels with diabetic nephropathy may be the non-enzymatic glycosylation (glycation) of matrix proteins which are freely accessible to glucose. The extent of glycation is dependent on proteins' half lives and the mean glucose level of the patient during the life time of the respective protein [49,50]. The amount of glycation in these tissues seemed to be related to the extent and severity of the patients' late complications [50]. More recent approaches suggest that the development of diabetic late complications may be linked to the formation of advanced glucosylation end-products (AGE-products) [51]. The AGE-products result from the slow decomposition of glycated proteins. With time highly reactive products are formed which may yield new modifications on the same or the neighbouring protein. These AGE-products lead to synthesis and secretion of cytokines like tumour necrosis factor, interleukin-1 and IGF-1 when bound to a specific AGE-receptor identified on macrophages [52]. AGE-products also act on mesangial cells via platelet derived growth factor causing the cells to synthesize increased amounts of collagen IV, laminin and HSPG [53] while prolonged exposure to glycated matrices reduced collagen synthesis and proteoglycan charge [54]. Recently, pentosidine a well defined AGE-product has been implicated in the pathogenesis of diabetic nephropathy [55]. To prevent the formation of AGEs and possibly diabetic microangiopathy e.g. nephropathy the AGE inhibitor aminoguanidine has been suggested to have beneficial effects [56].

The third pathochemical mechanism involves intracellular formation of sorbitol from glucose catalysed by aldose reductase [57]. Chronic hyperglycaemia leads to sorbitol accumulation in a variety of tissues like peripheral neurons, lense and renal tubuli [58]. The initial hypothesis that sorbitol accumulation causes tissue damage is unlikely to operate in kidney [36]. The inositol depletion theory suggested by Greene and coworkers explains tissue damages as impairment of myo-inositol uptake leading to a decrease of phosphatidyl-inositides in the cell membrane [57]. Although the cellular inositol uptakes is competitively inhibited by D-glucose [59] and non-competitively inhibited by hyperosmolar intracellular sorbitol [60], recent studies show that cells may counterregulate inositol depletion [45,61]. Thus, it is not generally agreed that the increase in intracellular sorbitol is the cause of the

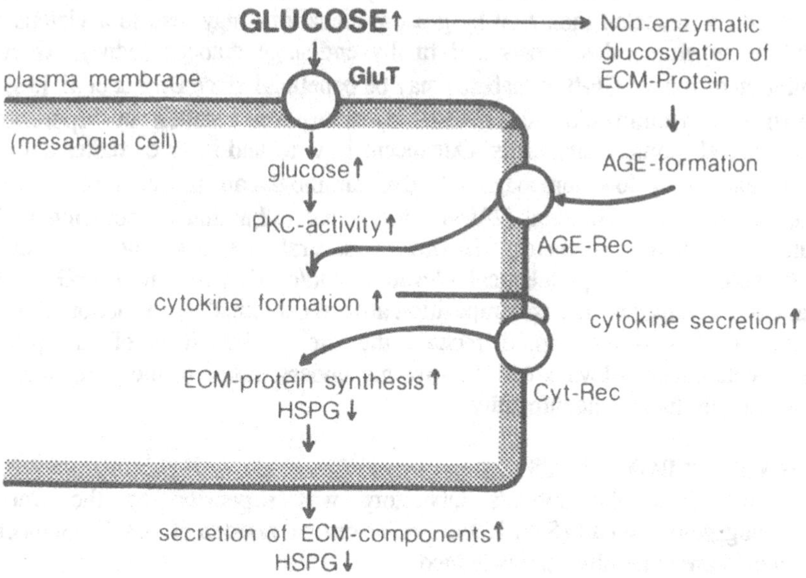

Fig. 29-1 Sequence of molecular mechanisms possibly involved in the alterations of glomerular matrix proteins in diabetes. Two possibilities are shown by which elevated glucose may alter cellular metabolism and the metabolism of glomerular extracellular matrix components. AGE-Rec and Cyt-Rec indicate the receptors for AGE-products and cytokines, respectively. ECM = extracellular matrix; AGE = advanced glucosylation end products; PKC = protein kinase C; GluT = glucose transporter.

impaired function of the affected tissues in diabetes. Furthermore, after treatment of diabetic rats for six months with the aldose reductase inhibitor tolrestat only a slight reduction in the urinary albumin excretion rate was observed indicating that other mechanism are operating in diabetic nephropathy.

CONCLUSIONS

The morphological observations of an expanded matrix in diabetic glomeruli are now supported by the immunohistochemical findings showing an increased deposition of normally occurring matrix components. The biochemical findings suggest that increased glucose concentrations stimulate the synthesis of the matrix components like fibronectin, laminin and collagen IV either by direct action or via formation of AGE products (figure 29-1). The increased matrix synthesis is probably mediated by cytokines. In particular, glucose-induced TGF-ß expression would explain the progressive accumulation of matrix material in diabetic patients with chronic hyperglycaemia since TGF-ß is unique among the cytokines in (i) stimulating the synthesis of matrix, (ii) inhibiting matrix degradation and (iii) inhibiting mesangial proliferation. The latter property of TGF-ß is consistent with the absence of mesangial cell proliferation in diabetic glomerulopathy. The in vitro and in vivo results indicate that diabetes induces a wound repair-like mechanism in glomeruli. A failure to turn off TGF-ß production due to a defect in TFG-ß regulation or repeated induction by glucose elevations may lead to a vicious cycle resulting in glomerulosclerosis and finally end-stage diabetic kidney. Therefore, inhibition of renal TGF-β in diabetes may be beneficial since Border et al. [32] have shown that neutralization of TFG-β_1 by antiserum resulted in suppresion of experimental glomerulonephritis. Our recent in vitro and in vivo studies show that application of a low anticoagulant glycosaminoglycan prevents renal TFG-β_1 induction [63] and structural [28] and functional (albuminuria) occuring in long-term experimental diabetes. However, several characteristics of diabetic nephropathy like the paradoxical elevation and/or decrease in HSPG, and the qualitative changes in matrix composition are not explained by the action of TGF-ß. Further studies which should include the use of inhibitors of the proposed pathobiochemical pathways will improve our understanding of the pathobiochemistry leading to diabetic nephropathy.

ACKNOWLEDGEMENTS

The work from the author's laboratory was supported by the Deutsche Forschungsgemeinschaft (Schl 239/6-2). The critical notions of Drs. K. Gempel and J. Guretzki are gratefully acknowledged.

REFERENCES

1. Mauer SM, Ellis E, Bilous RW, Steffes MW. »The pathology of diabetic nephropathy.« In *Complications of Diabetes Mellitus*, Draznin B, Melmed S, LeRoith D, eds. New York: Alan R Liss Inc., 1989; pp 95-101.
2. Mauer SM, Steffes MW, Ellis EN, Sutherland DER, Brown DM, Goetz FC. Structural-functional relationships in diabetic nephropathy. J Clin Invest 1984; 74: 1143-1155.
3. Østerby R, Gall MA, Schmitz A, Nielsen FS, Nyberg G, Parving H-H. Glomerular structure and function in proteinuric type 2 (non-insulin-dependent) diabetic patients. Diabetologia 1993; 36: 1064-1070.
4. Kimmelstiel P, Wilson C. Intercapillary lesions in the glomeruli of the kidney. Am J Pathol 1936; 12: 83-89.
5. Farquhar MG. »The glomerular basement membrane: A selective macromolecular filter.« In *Cell Biology of Extracellular Matrix*, Hay E, ed. New York, London: Plenum Press, 1981; pp 335-378.
6. Kim Y, Kleppel M, Butkowski R, Mauer M, Wieslander J, Michael A. Differential expression of basement membrane collagen chains in diabetic nephropathy. Am J Pathol 1991; 138: 413-420.
7. Nerlich A, Schleicher E. Immunohistochemical localization of extracellular matrix components in human diabetic glomerular lesions. Am J Pathol 1991; 139: 889-899.
8. Schleicher ED, Nerlich A, Sauer U, Wiest I, Specks U, Timpl R. Immunhistochemische Untersuchungen zur Verteilung Kollagen Typ VI bei diabetischer Nephropathie (abstract). Diabetes und Stoffwechsel 1993; 2: 185.
9. Timpl R. Structure and biological activity of basement membrane proteins. Eur J Biochem 1989; 180: 487-503.
10. Kallunki P, Tryggvason K. human basement membrane heparan sulfate proteoglycan core protein: A 467-kD protein containing multiple domains resembling elements of the low density lipoprotein receptor, laminin, neural cell adhesion molecules, and epidermal growth factor. J Cell Biol 1992; 116: 559-571.
11. Schleicher ED, Wagner EM, Olgemöller B, Nerlich AG, Gerbitz KD. Characterization and localization of basement membrane-associated heparan sulphate proteoglycan in human tissues. Lab Invest 1989; 61: 323-332.

12. Stow JL, Sawada H, Farquhar MG. Basement membrane heparan sulfate proteoglycans are concentrated in the laminae rarae and in podocytes of the rat renal glomerulus. Proc Natl Acad Sci USA 1985; 82: 3296-3300.
13. van den Born J, van den Heuvel PWJ, Bakker MAH, Veerkamp JH, Assmann KJM, Berden JHM. A monoclonal antibody against GBM heparan sulfate induces an acute selective proteinuria in rats. Kidney Int 1992; 41: 115-123.
14. Yamamoto T, Nakamura T, Noble NA, Ruoslahti E, Border WA. Expression of transforming growth factor ß is elevated in human and experimental diabetic nephropa-thy. Proc Natl Acad Sci USA 1993; 90: 1814-1818.
15. Ruoslahti E. »Extracellular matrix in the regulation of cellular functions.« In *Cell to Cell Interaction*, Burger MM, Sordat B, Zinkernagel RM, eds. Basel: Karger, 1990; pp 88-98.
16. d'Amore PA. Modes of FGF release in vivo and in vitro Cancer and Metastasis Reviews 1990; 9: 227-238.
17. Wright TC, Casellot JJ, Diamond JR, Karnovsky MJ. »Regulation of cellular proliferation by heparin and heparan sulfate.« In *Heparin*, Lane DA, Lindahl U, eds. London: Edward Arnold, 1989; pp 295-316.
18. Steffes MW, Østerby R, Chavers B, Mauer, MS. Mesangial expansion as a central mechanism for loss of kidney function in diabetic patients. Diabetes 1989; 38: 1077-1081.
19. Østerby R, Gundersen HJG. Glomerular size and structure in diabetes mellitus: early abnormalities. Diabetologia 1975; 11: 225-259.
20. Spiro RG. »Pathogenesis of diabetic glomerulopathy: a biochemical view.« In *The Kidney and Hypertension in Diabetes Mellitus*, Mogensen CE, ed. Boston: Martinus Nijhoff Publishing, 1988; pp 117-130.
21. Mohan PS, Carter WG, Spiro RG. Occurrence of type VI collagen in extracellular matrix of renal glomeruli and its increase in diabetes. Diabetes 1990; 39: 31-37.
22. Shimomura H, Spiro RG. Studies on macromolecular components of human glomerular basement membrane and alterations in diabetes: decreased levels of heparan sulfate proteogly-can. Diabetes 1987; 36: 374-381.
23. Parthasarathy N, Spiro RG. Effect of diabetes on the glycosaminoglycan component of the human glomerular basement membrane. Diabetes 1982; 31: 738-741.
24. Schleicher E, Wieland OH. Changes of human glomerular basement membrane in diabetes mellitus. Eur J Clin Chem Clin Biochem 1984; 22: 223-227.
25. Haneda M, Kikkawa R, Horide N, Togawa M, Koya D, Kajiwara N, Ooshima A, Shigeta Y. Glucose enhances type IV collagen production in cultured rat glomerular mesangial cells. Diabetologia 1991; 34: 198-200.
26. Schaefer RM, Paczek L, Huang S, Teschner M, Schaefer L, Heidland A. Role of glomerular proteinases in the evolution of glomerulosclerosis. Eur J Clin Chem Clin Biochem 1992; 30: 641-646.
27. Fukui M, Nakamura T, Ebihara I, Shirato I, Tomino Y, Koide H. ECM gene expression and its modulation by insulin in diabetic rats. Diabetes 1992; 41: 1520-1527.
28. Ceol M, Nerlich A, Baggio B, Anglani A, Sauer U, Schleicher E, Gambaro G. Increased glomerular α_1 (IV) collagen expression and deposition in long-term diabetic rats in prevented by chronic glycosminoglycan treatment. Lab Invest 1996; 74; 484-495.
29. Flyvbjerg A. Growth factors and diabetic complications. Diabetic Med 1990; 7: 387-390.
30. Nakamura T, Fukui M, Ebihara I, Osada S, Nakaoka I, Tomino Y, Koide H. mRNA Expression of growth factors in glomeruli from diabetic rats. Diabetes 1993; 42: 450-456.
31. Park IS, Kiyomoto H, Abboud SL, Abboud HE. Expression of transforming growth factor-beta and type IV collagen in early streptozotocin-induced diabetes. Diabetes 1997; 46: 473-480.
32. Border WA, Okuda S, Languino LR, Sporn MB, Ruoslahti E. Suppression of experimental glomerulonephritis by antiserum against transforming growth factor beta 1. Nature 1990; 346: 371-374.
33. Sharma K, Ziyadeh FN. Perspectives in diabetes.Hyperglycemia and diabetic kidney disease. The case for transforming growth factor-β as a key mediator. Diabetes 1995; 44: 1139-1146.
34. Kolm V, Sauer U, Olgemöller B, Schleicher ED. High glucose-induced TGF-beta 1 regulates mesangial production of heparan sulfate proteoglycan.Am J Physiol 1996; 270 : F812-21.
35. Kern TS, Engerman TL. Arrest of glomerulopathy in diabetic dogs by improved diabetic control. Diabetologia 1990; 21: 178-183.

36. Larkins RG, Dunlop ME. The link between hyperglycaemia and diabetic nephropathy. Diabetologia 1992; 35: 499-504.
37. Ayo SH, Radnik RA, Glass IIWF, Garoni JA, Rampt ER, Appling DR, Kreisberg JI. Increased extracellular matrix synthesis and mRNA in mesangial cells grown in high-glucose medium. Am J Physiol 1990; 260: F185-F191.
38. Olgemöller B, Schwaabe S, Gerbitz KD, Schleicher ED. Elevated glucose decreases the content of a basement membrane associated proteoglycan in proliferating mesangial cells. Diabetologia 1992; 35: 183-186.
39. Danne T, Spiro MJ, Spiro RG. Effect of high glucose on type IV collagen production by cultured glomerular epithelial, endothelial, and mesangial cells. Diabetes 1993; 42: 170-177.
40. Takeuchi A, Throckmorton DC, Brogden AP, Yoshizawa N, Rasmussen H, Kashgarian M. Periodic high extracellular glucose enhances production of collagens III and IV by mesangial cells. Am Physiol Soc 1995; 268: F13-F19.
41. Heilig CW, Concepcion LA, Riser BL, Freytag SO, Zhu M, Cortes P. Overexpression of glucose transporters in rat mesangial cells cultured in a normal glucose milieu mimics the diabetic phenotype. J Clin Invest 1995; 96: 1802-1814.
42. Wolf G, Sharma K, Chen Y, Ericksen M, Ziyadeh FN. High glucose-induced proliferation in mesangial cells is reserved by autocrine TGF-ß. Kidney Int 1992; 42: 647-656.
43. McClain DA, Paterson AJ, Roos MD, Wei X, Kudlow JE. Glucose and glucosamine regulate growth factor gene expression in vascular smooth muscle cells. Proc Natl Acad Sci USA 1992; 89: 8150-8154.
44. Ayo SH, Radnik R, Garoni JA, Troyer DA, Kreisberg JA. High glucose increases diacylglycerol mass and activates protein kinase C in mesangial cells. Am J Physiol 1991; 261: F571-F577.
45. Guzman NJ, Crews FT. Regulation of inositol transport by glucose and protein kinase C in mesangial cells. Kidney Int 1992; 42: 33-40.
46. Craven PA, DeRubertis FR. Protein kinase C is activated in glomeruli from streptozotocin diabetic rats. Possible mediation by glucose. J Clin Invest 1989; 83: 1667-1675.
47. Ledbetter SR, Copeland EJ, Noonan D, Vogeli G, Hassel JR. Altered steady-state in mRNA levels of basement membrane proteins in diabetic mouse kidneys and thromboxane synthase inhibition. Diabetes 1990; 39: 196-203.
48. Ishii H, Jirousek MR, Koya D, Takagi C, Xia P, Clermont A, Bursell SE, Kern TS, Ballas LM, Heath WF, Stramm LE, Feener EP, King GL. Amelioration of vascular dysfuntions in diabetic rats by an oral PKC beta inhibitor. Science 1996; 272: 728-731.
49. Brownlee M, Cerami A, Vlassara H. Advanced glucosylation end products in tissue and the biochemical basis of diabetic complications. N Engl J Med 1988; 318: 1315-1321.
50 Vogt BW, Schleicher ED, Wieland OH. ε-Aminolysine bound glucose in human tissues obtained at autopsy: increase in diabetes mellitus. Diabetes 1982; 31: 1123-1127.
51. Ledl F, Schleicher E. New aspects of the Maillard reaction in foods and in the human body. Angew Chem Intern Ed Engl 1990; 29: 565-594.
52. Vlassara H, Brownlee M, Cerami A. Noval macrophage receptor for glucose-modified proteins is distinct from previously described scavenger receptors. J Exp Med 1986; 164: 1301-1309.
53. Doi T, Vlassara H, Kirstein M, Yamada Y, Striker GE, Striker LJ. Receptor-specific increase in extracellular matrix production in mouse mesangial cells by advanced glycosylation end products is mediated via platelet-derived growth factor. Proc Natl Acad Sci USA 1992; 89: 2873-2877.
54. Silbiger S, Crowley S, Shan Z, Brownlee M, Satriano J, Schlöndorff D. Nonenzymatic glycation of mesangial matrix and prolonged exposure of mesangial matrix to elevated glucose reduces collagen synthesis and proteoglycan charge. Kidney Int 1993; 43: 853-864.
55. Sell DR, Carlson EC, Monnier VM. Differential effects of type 2 (non-insulin-dependent) diabetes mellitus on pentosidine formation in skin and glomerular basement membrane. Diabetologia 1993; 36: 936-941.
56. Soulis T, Cooper ME, Sastra S, Thallas V, Panagiotopoulos S, Bjerrum O, Jerums G. Relative contributions of advanced glycation and nitric oxide synthase inhibition to aminioguanidine-mediated renoprotection in diabetic rats. Diabetologia 1997; 40: 1141-1151.
57. Greene D. The pathogenesis and its prevention of diabetic neuropathy and nephropathy. Metabolism 1988; 37: suppl. 1: 25-29.

58. Schmolke M, Schleicher E, Guder WG. Renal sorbitol, myo-inositol and glycerophosphorylcholine in streptozotocin-diabetic rats. Eur J Clin Chem Clin Biochem 1992; 30: 607-614.
59. Olgemöller B, Schwaabe S, Schleicher ED, Gerbitz KD. Competitive inhibition by glucose of myo-inositol incorporation into cultured porcine mesangial cells. Biophys Biochem Acta 1990; 1052: 47-52.
60. Li W, Chan LS, Khatami M, Rockey JH: Non-competitive inhibition of myo-inositol transport in cultured bovine retinal capillary pericytes by glucose and reversal by sorbinil. Biochim Biophys Acta 1986; 857: 198-208.
61. Olgemöller B, Schleicher E, Schwaabe S, Gerbitz KD. Upregulation of myo-inositol transport compensates for competitive inhibition by glucose. Diabetes 1993; 42: 1119-1125.
62. Mc Caleb ML, Mc Kean ML, Hohman TC, Laver N, Robinson WG. Intervention with aldose reductase inhibitor, tolrestat, in renal and retinal lesions of streptozotocin diabetic rats. Diabetologia 1991; 34: 659-701.
63. Schleicher E, Ceol M, Sauer U, Nerlich A, Baggio B, Anglani F, Gambaro G. TGF-β1 renal overexpression in long-term diabetic rats and in high glucose mesangial cell cultures: Inhibition by heparin (Abstract). Diabetologia 1996; 39: Suppl. 1: A43.

30. THE STENO HYPOTHESIS AND GLOMERULAR BASEMENT MEMBRANE BIOCHEMISTRY IN DIABETIC NEPHROPATHY

Allan Kofoed-Enevoldsen
Department of Endocrinology, Herlev Hospital, University of Copenhagen, Herlev, Denmark

INTRODUCTION

So far, at the biochemical level, the pathogenesis of diabetic nephropathy is unresolved. Not surprisingly perhaps since even our understanding of the biochemical fundaments of normal glomerular function remains incomplete. In addition, when exploring the pathogenesis of diabetic nephropathy, we are likely to witness the composite course of succeeding stages, each of which may have its own pathogenetic trait.

The Steno hypothesis [1] suggests that impairment of heparan sulphate metabolism is a key-event in the development of diabetic nephropathy, and identifies impaired heparin sulphate metabolism as the link between diabetic nephropathy and the associated generalized cardiovascular disease. It may seem risky to postulate a single mechanism as a key feature in the pathogenesis of diabetic nephropathy, having recognised the possible complexity of the disease process. On the other hand however, the need to forward specific hypotheses is augmented by our current stage of incomplete knowledge, the alternative being to go on »fishing trips« with the risk of getting the net plugged with trivial catch.

LOSS OF CHARGE SELECTIVITY AND THE DEVELOPMENT OF ALBUMINURIA

Urinary protein excretion is normal from the onset of diabetes, except during episodes of poor metabolic control. After some years, the urinary excretion of albumin and other large plasma proteins eventually start to increase. With reservation to the expected effect of more aggressive metabolic and blood pressure control, ultimately 30 to 40% of all IDDM patients will progress to clinical diabetic nephropathy. The cumulative incidence of microalbuminuria (30-300 mg/24 h) is not known, but the overall prevalence seems to be around 20% [2].

Reduced glomerular charge selectivity may serve as the pathophysiological fundament of the initial rise in urinary albumin excretion. Glomerular charge selectivity is effective for proteins of a wide size range, e.g. from 61 Å ferritin molecules to 30 Å horse radish peroxidases [3]. It has been calculated that a 30%

decrease in the glomerular filtration barrier charge (from 150 to 100 meq/l) may cause a 25-fold increase in the fractional clearance of albumin [4]. In comparison, a doubling of the effective pore radius may not cause more than a 5-fold increase in the fractional albumin clearance [4]. Glomerular charge-selectivity can not be quantitated directly in man, but may be estimated from measurements of the relative clearance of differently charged, similarly sized endogenous proteins.

The first indication of reduced glomerular charge-selectivity in microalbuminuric IDDM patients was published by Viberti et al. [5] and succeeding studies have confirmed this finding [6]. In the later study, patients with urinary albumin excretion in the range 30-100 mg/24 h had a 50% reduction in the total-IgG:IgG_4 selectivity index compared both to normoalbuminuric patients and to healthy control subjects. As strict metabolic control may retard the progression of microalbuminuria, Bangstad et al. studied the effect of intensified insulin treatment on the total-IgG:IgG_4 selectivity index in microalbuminuric IDDM patients and saw a significant normalization of total-IgG:IgG_4 selectivity index within a few months [7]. Although in our study [6] no accompanying impairment of glomerular size selectivity using dextran clearance during the early stages of diabetic nephropathy could be demonstrated, formation of a subtle non-size-selective glomerular shunt - as suggested in advanced diabetic nephropathy [8,9] - may however still explain the observed changes in the proposed charge sensitive indices [10].

In conclusion, current data are in accordance with an initial impairment of glomerular charge selectivity as responsible for the development of microalbuminuria.

THE GLOMERULAR BASEMENT MEMBRANE

The structural domain responsible for glomerular charge selectivity includes the glomerular basement membrane [3]. Anionic sites present in the glomerular basement membrane may be of crucial importance for maintenance of charge selectivity. Heparitinase treatment removes 80-100% of the anionic sites from the lamina rara externa, indicating that within the lamina rara externa these sites are predominantly composed of heparan sulphate glycosaminoglycan [11]. In addition removal of glomerular basement membrane heparan sulphate glycosaminoglycan by heparinase treatment induces increased permeability for albumin [12]. Van Den Born et al. [13] demonstrated that a rapid loss of charge-selectivity and onset of proteinuria can be induced in rats by injecting a monoclonal antibody directed towards the heparan sulphate glycosaminoglycan chain whereas antibodies directed towards the heparan sulphate core protein or other glomerular basement membrane components had no effect. Thus loss of glomerular basement membrane anionic sites, i.e. heparan sulphate glycosaminoglycan, may lead to loss of charge selectivity and development of albuminuria [14,15].

Quantitative measurement of glomerular basement membrane heparan sulphate in IDDM patients with microalbuminuria [11] disclosed a 30-40% reduction in number of heparinase digestible anionic sites in the glomerular basement membrane lamina rare externa in IDDM patients with urinary albumin excretion above 200 mg/24 h. No reduction in the number of sites was however found in 3 patients with urinary albumin excretion in the range from 30 to

100 mg/24 h compared to 5 patients with normal urinary albumin excretion. Shimomura & Spiro [16] and Parthasarathy & Spiro [17] found a 70% decrease in glomerular basement membrane heparan sulphate core protein and a 40% decrease in glomerular basement membrane heparan sulphate glycosaminoglycan content in patients with »histological evidence of varying degrees of diabetic glomerulopathy«. Semiquantitative immunohistochemical measurements have indicated a reduction in HS core protein in the glomerular basement membrane of patients with advanced diabetic nephropathy [18]. In contrast two studies found normal immunohistochemical staining of HS core protein while segmental or absent staining was observed with an antibody directed against the heparan sulphate glycosaminoglycan chain in IDDM patients with diabetic nephropathy [14,19]. Thus in man, demonstration of significant changes in basement membrane HS content is restricted to advanced diabetic nephropathy.

Animal experiments provide diverging results regarding the impact of poorly controlled diabetes on glomerular basement membrane heparan sulphate. A 50% decreased de novo synthesis of overall glomerular heparan sulphate in isolated glomeruli from diabetic rats was found by Reddi et al. [20] whereas Klein et al. [21] found no significant change. Incorporation of newly synthesized heparan sulphate into the glomerular basement membrane was reduced 30-60% in two studies [21] [22]. In vivo labelling of newly synthesized glomerular basement membrane heparan sulphate has suggested either a decrease [23] or no change [21,24]. Steady-state glomerular basement membrane heparan sulphate content per glomeruli has been measured in three studies, showing either a 60% decrease [25] or no significant change [26,27]. Sulphation of heparan sulphate was 50% decreased in one study [27] and not significantly changed in two [24,26].
Fukui et al. [28] reported a specific 50% decrease in glomerular heparan sulphate core protein (HSPG2) mRNA expression after 4 weeks of diabetes duration. In our STZ- and spontaneously diabetic rats, no significant reduction in kidney cortex HSPG2 mRNA was seen after 4 weeks of diabetes when comparing animals in poor and good metabolic control [29]. Thus, although animal studies offer a variety of results, the all round trend for heparan sulphate is either »unchanged« or »reduced«. It is not possible to pin-point one single pathobiochemical mechanism.

A state of "dyscoordinated matrix remodeling " may result from diabetes, as diabetes may be associated with a decrease in the ratio between the biosynthesis heparan sulphate and the rate of biosynthesis of several other extracellular matrix components. In the isolated perfused rat kidney, reactive oxygen species produced a 10 to 20-fold decrease in heparan sulphate core protein synthesis and glomerular basement membrane ^{35}S incorporation, whereas collagen IV and laminin were only slightly affected [30]. In cultured porcine mesangial cells high glucose induced a 10 to 50% decrease in basement membrane heparan sulphate core protein, whereas the content of fibronectin remained unchanged [31]. In contrast, Doi et al. [32] found a general increment in mRNA for both collagen IV, laminin *and* heparan sulphate core protein in mouse mesangial cells exposed to advanced glycosylation end-product-modified albumin. Several studies have found a stimulatory effect of high glucose on collagen IV synthesis rate and mRNA expression in vitro in rat mesangial cells, human umbilical vein endothelial cells, and mouse proximal tubular cells [33,34,55], a tendency markedly contrasting to the findings of impaired rather than stimulated heparan sulphate synthesis as discussed above. Thus a reduction in basement membrane heparan sulphate may result from a *dys*coordinated regulation of the synthesis of basement membrane components.

The mechanisms by which diabetes influences glomerular extracellur matrix metabolism are possibly several. *Mechanical stress*, e.g. cyclic stretching of mesangial cells, induces VEPF (vascular endothelial factor) and TGF-b expression by mesangial and endothelial cells with concomitant alteration of matrix synthesis. *Metabolic factors* including polyol pathway activation and reactive nonenzymatic glycation products may through induction of protein kinase C activity induce TGF-β expression and other factors potentially influencing the regulation and balancing of extracellular matrix synthesis [15,35,36].

The summary above is primarily related to diabetes-induced changes in glomerular basement membrane heparan sulphate obtained in IDDM patients and models of type 1 diabetes mellitus. In defiance of a vast amount of studies reported, a definite description of the pathobiochemistry of diabetic nephropathy may not be for long time yet.

THE STENO HYPOTHESIS

The Steno hypothesis states that *»Decreased concentration of heparan sulphate in the extracellular matrix explains the simultaneous occurrence of albuminuria and premature atherosclerosis in IDDM. The decrease in heparan sulphate is caused by the combined effect of poor metabolic control and genetic factors, possibly mediated through inhibition of the glucosaminyl N-deacetylase«* [1]. Thus besides establishing a connection with albuminuria, decreased heparan sulphate concentration is suggested to be involved in the development of premature atherosclerosis among patients with diabetic nephropathy.

Endothelial cell surface and vascular smooth muscle cell basement membrane heparan sulphate express a variety of anti-atherogenic properties. These include increasing antithrombin III activity, interaction with lipoprotein lipase, maintenance of cellular adhesion, and regulation of cellular proliferation [37-39]. Extensive reviews of the background for hypothesising a role for heparan sulphate in the development of premature atherosclerosis can be found in [40] and [41].

The methodological difficulties in measuring the whole body vascular heparan sulphate are not less than those of quantitating glomerular basement membrane heparan sulphate. A suggested approach is measurement of the plasma concentration of prothrombin fragment 1+2 which may provide a close-up indirect estimate of the effective concentration of vascular heparan sulphate. The rationale is that a reduction in endothelial heparan sulphate content will reduce the antithrombin III mediated inhibition of coagulation factor-Xa in turn leading to the production of increased amounts of prothrombin fragment 1+2 by factor-Xa induced convertion of prothrombin to thrombin. The Steno hypothesis has postulated this mechanism to cause increased fibrin deposition and increasing the plasma concentration of von Willebrand factor. Indeed increased plasma concentration of prothrombin fragment 1+2 was reported in IDDM patients with microalbuminuria [42]. In contrast however, another study could not confirm this finding [43] although a positive correlation between prothrombin fragment 1+2 and transcapillary escape rate of albumin (known to be elevated in diabetic nephropathy) was found.

The mechanism behind the increased transcapillary escape rate of albumin in patients with microalbuminuria or clinical diabetic nephropathy, according to the Steno hypothesis, may be loss of subcutaneous capillary charge-selectivity much parallel to the hypothesized mechanism behind the development of increased urinary albumin excretion. Again studies specifically addressing this hypothesis provides diverging results. Estimating capillary charge selectivity from interstitial fluid concentrations of differently charged endogenous proteins we found no evidence of reduced charge selectivity in patients with nephropathy [44]. In contrast, Bent-Hansen et al. [45] - using exogenous tracers and possibly a more sensitive study design - have presented data to support the hypothesized reduction in general capillary charge selectivity.

The Steno hypothesis finally proposes that diabetes-induced impairment of heparan sulphate metabolism may be mediated by inhibition of the key enzyme glucosaminyl N-deacetylase. This enzyme plays a key role in the biosynthesis of heparan sulphate, since N-deacetylation is prerequisite to N-sulphation and further modifications of the newly synthesized glucosaminoglycan polymer. Prompted by the original demonstration by Kjellén et al. [46] of diabetes-induced reduction in hepatic heparan sulphate sulphation, several studies have demonstrated that experimental diabetes per se leads to inhibition of N-deacetylase activity [29,47-49]. The degree of inhibition correlates to blood glucose control reducing activity by 40-50% when blood glucose exceeds 15 mmol/l, and may be completely prevented by near-normalisation of blood glucose by intensified insulin treatment. An intriguing finding relating the role of inhibition of N-deacetylase to the development of diabetic nephropathy is the apparent correlation between glomerular N-deacetylase activity and urinary albumin excretion [29,49]. Finally our animal experiments have indicated that genetic factors seem to influence the vulnerability of the N-deacetylase towards diabetes-induced inhibition, as evident from studies including different rat strains [29,48,49]. Measurements of N-deacetylase activity in patients with diabetic nephropathy have been performed to in *in vitro* studies of fibroblast cell cultures and in white blood cells (neutrophil grannulocytes). In the latter study poor metabolic control was associated with reduced N-deacetylase activity [50]. No major constitutive reduction in N-deacetylase activity was found in cultured skin fibroblasts from IDDM patients with diabetic nephropathy [51]. However the possibility that activation of protein kinase A might be involved in the diabetes-induced N-deacetylase inhibition was suggested in this experiment. Insulin inhibits protein kinase A activity by decreasing its binding of cAMP [52] and insulin resistance is associated with a decrease in insulin-induced protein kinase A down-regulation [53]. Our study may, therefore, have identified a general pathway, i.e. protein kinase A activation, for down-regulation of N-deacetylase activity in diabetes. This mechanism could provide an explanation for the postulated association between the development of diabetic nephropathy and the presence of insulin resistance [54].

Ongoing studies directed at specific pharmacological intervention towards the impairment of heparan sulfate metabolism have provided encouring results. *In vitro*, heparin stimulates heparan sulfate biosynthesis and in experimental diabetes it has been shown to prevent the development of diabetes induced albuminuria and basement membrane thickening (*Gambaro et al 1992).* In IDDM patients with elevated urinary albumin excretion 1-3 months of low-dose heparin treatment lead to a significant decrease in albuminuria [55,56].

CONCLUSION

Since the publication of the first studies relating heparan sulphate to diabetic nephropathy a decade has passed during which the Steno hypothesis has found both support and neglect. As a working hypothesis, it remains a valuable guiding tool when exploring the pathogenesis of diabetic nephropathy.

However, improvement of methodological means for quantitative and qualitative measurements of cell surface and basement membrane heparan sulphate may be essential to allow for further significant progress in our understanding of the disease process.

REFERENCES

1. Deckert T, Feldt-Rasmussen B, Borch-Johnsen K, Jensen T, Kofoed-Enevoldsen A. Albuminuria reflects widespread vascular damage. Diabetologia 1989; 32: 219-26.
2. Mathiesen ER. Prevention of diabetic nephropathy: Microalbuminuria and perspectives for intervention in insulin-dependent diabetes. Dan Med Bull 1993; 40: 273-285.
3. Kanwar YS. Biophysiology of glomerular filtration and proteinuria. Lab Invest 1984; 51: 7-21.
4. Deen WM, Satvat B. Determinants of the glomerular filtration of proteins. Am J Physiol 1981; 241: F162-F170.
5. Viberti GC, Mackintosh D, Keen H. Determinants of the penetration of proteins through the glomerular barrier in IDDM. Diabetes 1983; 32: Suppl. 2: 92-95.
6. Deckert T, Kofoed-Enevoldsen A, Vidal P, Nørgaard K, Andreasen HB, Feldt-Rasmussen B. Size- and charge selectivity of glomerular filtration in IDDM patients with and without albuminuria. Diabetologia 1993; 36: 244-251.
7. Bangstad H-J, Kofoed-Enevoldsen A, Dahl-Jørgensen K, Hanssen KF. Glomerular charge selectivity and the influence of improved blood glucose control. Diabetologia 1992; 35: 1165-1169.
8. Myers BD, Winetz JA, Chui F, Michaels AS. Mechanisms of proteinuria in diabetic nephropathy - A study of glomerular barrier function. Kidney Int 1982; 21: 633-641.
9. Deen WM, Bridges CR, Brenner BM, Myers BD. Heterosporous model of glomerular size selectivity, application to normal and nephrotic humans. Am J Physiol 1985; 249: F374-F389.
10. Kofoed-Enevoldsen A. Heparan sulphate in the metabolism of diabetic nephropathy. Diabetes/Metabolism Reviews 1995; 11: 137-160.
11. Vernier RL, Steffes MW, Sisson-Ross S, Mauer SM. Heparan sulfate proteoglycan in the glomerular basement membrane in type 1 diabetes mellitus. Kidney Int 1992; 41: 1070-1080.
12. Rosenzweig LJ, Kanwar Y. Removal of sulfated (heparan sulfate) or nonsulfated (hyaluronic acid) glycosaminoglycans results in increased permeability of the glomerular basement membrane to ^{125}I-bovine serum albumin. Lab Invest 1982; 47: 177-184.
13. Van Den Born J, Van Den Heuvel LPWJ, Bakker MAH, Veerkamp JH, Assmann KJM, Berden JHM. A monoclonal antibody against GBM heparan sulfate induces an acute selective proteinuria in rats. Kidney Int 1992; 41: 115-123.
14. Tamsma JT, van den Born J, Bruijn JA, Assmann KJM, Weening JJ, Berden JHM, Wieslander J, Schrama E, Hermans J, Veerkamp JH, Lemkes HHPJ, van der Woude FJ. Expression of glomerular extracellular matrix components in human diabetic nephropathy – decrease of heparan sulphate in the glomerular basement membrane. Diabetologia 1994; 37: 313-320.

15. Riser BL, Cortes P, Zhao X, Bernstein J, Dumler F, Narins RG, Hassett CC, Sury-Sastry KS, Atherton J, Holcomb MA. Intraglomerular pressure and mesangial stretching stimulate extracellular matrix formation in the rat. J Clin Invest 1992; 90: 1932-1943.
16. Shimomura H, Spiro RG. Studies on macromolecular components of human glomerular basement membrane and alterations in diabetes. Diabetes 1987; 36: 374-381.
17. Parthasarathy N, Spiro RG. Effect of diabetes on the glycosaminoglycan component of the human glomerular basement membrane. Diabetes 1982; 31: 738-741.
18. Nerlich A, Schleicher E. Immunohistochemical localization of extracellular matrix components in human diabetic glomerular lesions. Am J Pathol 1991; 139: 889-899.
19. Van Den Born J, Van Den Heuvel LPWJ, Bakker MAH, Veerkamp JH, Assmann KJM, Weening JJ, Berden JHM. The distribution of GBM heparan sulfate proteoglycan core protein and side chains in human glomerular diseases by monoclonal antibodies. Kidney Int 1993; 43: 454-463.
20. Reddi AS, Ramamurthi R, Miller M, Dhuper S, Lasker N. Enalapril improves albuminuria by preventing glomerular loss of heparan sulfate in diabetic rats. Biochem Med Metab Biol 1991; 45: 119-131.
21. Klein DJ, Brown DM, Oegema TR. Glomerular proteoglycans in diabetes. Diabetes 1986; 35: 1130-1142.
22. Kanwar YS, Rosenzweig LJ, Linker A, Jakubowski ML. Decreased de novo synthesis of glomerular proteoglycans in diabetes. Proc Natl Acad Sci USA 1983; 80: 2272-2275.
23. Cohen MP, Surma ML. Effect of diabetes on in vivo metabolism of 35S-labelled glomerular basement membrane. Diabetes 1984; 33: 8-12.
24. Klein DJ, Oegema TR, Brown DM. Release of glomerular heparan-^{35}SO4 proteoglycan by heparin from glomeruli of streptozotocin-induced diabetic rats. Diabetes 1989; 38: 130-139.
25. Wu V-Y, Wilson B, Cohen MP. Disturbances in glomerular basement membrane glycosaminoglycans in experimental diabetes. Diabetes 1987; 36: 679-683.
26. Templeton DM. Retention of glomerular basement membrane proteoglycans accompanying loss of anionic site staining in experimental diabetes. Lab Invest 1989; 61: 202-211.
27. Cohen MP, Klepser H, Wu V-Y. Undersulfation of glomerular basement membrane heparan sulfate in experimental diabetes and lack of correction with aldose reductase inhibition. Diabetes 1988; 37: 1324-1327.
28. Fukui M, Nakamura T, Ebihara I, Shirato I, Tomino Y, Koide H. ECM gene expression and its modulation by insulin in diabetic rats. Diabetes 1992; 41: 1520-1527.
29. Kofoed-Enevoldsen A, Noonan D, Deckert T. Diabetes mellitus induced inhibition of glucosaminyl N-deacetylase - effect of short-term blood glucose control. Diabetologia 1993; 36: 310-315.
30. Kashihara N, Watanabe Y, Makino H, Wallner EI, Kanwar Y. Selective decreased de novo synthesis of glomerular proteoglycans under the influence of reactive oxygen species. Proc Natl Acad Sci USA 1992; 89: 6309-6313.
31. Olgemöller B, Schwaabe S, Gerbitz KD, Schleicher ED. Elevated glucose decreases the content of a basement membrane associated heparan sulphate proteoglycan in proliferating cultured porcine mesangial cells. Diabetologia 1992; 35: 183-186.
32. Doi T, Vlassara H, Kirstein M, Yamada Y, Striker GE, Striker LJ. Receptor-specific increase in extracellular matrix production in mouse mesangial cells by advanced glysosylation end products is mediated via platelet-derived growth factor. Proc Natl Acad Sci USA 1992; 89: 2873-2877.
33. Cagliero E, Roth T, Roy S, Lorenzi M. Characteristics and mechanisms of high-glucose-induced overexpression of basement membrane components in cultures human endothelial cells. Diabetes 1991; 40: 102-110.
34. Ziyadeh FN, Snipes ER, Watanabe M, Alvarez RJ, Goldfarb S, Haverty TP. High glucose induces cell hypertrophy and stimulates collagen gene transcription in proximal tubule. Am J Physiol 1990; 259: F704-F714.
35. Shankland SJ, Scholey JW. Expression of transforming growth factor-ß1 during diabetic renal hypertrophy. Kidney Int 1994; 46: 430-442.
36. Border WA, Noble NA, Yamamoto T, Harper JR, Yamaguchi Y, Pierschbacher MD, Ruoslahti. Natural inhibitor of transforming growth factor-ß protects against scarring in experimental kidney disease. Nature 1992; 360:361-364.

37. Mulder M, Lombardi P, Jansen H, van Berkel TJC, Frants RR, Havekes LM. Heparan sulphate proteoglycans are involved in the lipoprotein lipase-mediated enhancement of the cellular binding of very low density and low density lipoproteins. Biochem Biophys Res Commun 1992; 185: 582-587.
38. Sudhalter J, Folkman J, Svahn CM, Bergendal K, D'Amore PA. Importance of size, sulfatation and anticoagulant activity in the potentiation of acidic fibroblast growth factor by heparin. J Biol Chem 1989; 264: 6892-6897.
39. Turnbull JE, Fernig DG, Ke Y, Wilkinson MC, Gallagher JT. Identification of the basic fibroblast growth factor binding sequence in fibroblast heparan sulfate. J Biol Chem 1992; 267: 10337-10341.
40. Deckert T, Jensen T, Feldt-Rasmussen B, Kofoed-Enevoldsen A, Borch-Johnsen K, Stender S. Albuminuria a risk marker of atherosclerosis in insulin dependent diabetes mellitus. Cardiovasc Risk Factors 1991; 1: 347-360.
41. Deckert T, Kofoed-Enevoldsen A, Nørgaard K, Borch-Johnsen K, Feldt-Rasmussen B, Jensen T. Microalbuminuria - implications for micro and macrovascular disease. Diabetes Care 1992; 15: 1181-1191.
42. Gruden G, Cavallo-Perin P, Bazzan M, Stella S, Bruno A, Pagano G. Haemostatic alterations in microalbuminuric insulin-dependent diabetic patients (Abstract). Diabetologia 1993; 36: Suppl. 1: A215.
43. Myrup B, Rossing P, Jensen T, Gram J, Kluft C, Jespersen J. Prothrombin fragment 1+2, a marker of thrombin formation, is related to transcapillary escape rate of albumin in insulin-dependent diabetic patients (Abstract). Diabetologia 1993; 36: Suppl. 1: A71.
44. Kofoed-Enevoldsen A, Bent-Hansen L, Deckert T. Transcapillary filtration of plasma protein in long-term type 1 (insulin-dependent) diabetic patients. Scand J Clin Lab Invest 1992; 52: 591-597.
45. Bent-Hansen L, Feldt-Rasmussen B, Kverneland A, Deckert T. Plasma disappearance of glycated and non-glycated albumin in type 1 (insulin-dependent) diabetes mellitus - evidence for charge dependent alterations of the plasma to lymph pathway. Diabetologia 1993; 36: 361-363.
46. Kjellén L, Bielefeld D, Höök M. Reduced sulfatation of liver heparan sulfate in experimentally diabetic rats. Diabetes 1983; 32: 337-342.
47. Unger E, Pettersson I, Eriksson UJ, Lindahl U, Kjellén L. Decreased activity of the heparan sulfate modifying enzyme glucosaminyl N-deacatylase in hepatocytes from streptozotocin-diabetic rats. J Biol Chem 1991; 266: 8671-8674.
48. Kofoed-Enevoldsen A, Eriksson UJ. Inhibition of N-acetylheparosan deacetylase in diabetic rats. Diabetes 1991; 40: 1449-1452.
49. Kofoed-Enevoldsen A. Inhibition of glomerular glucosaminyl N-deacetylase in diabetic rats. Kidney Int 1992; 41: 763-767.
50. Kofoed-Enevoldsen A, Kotinis A, Deckert T. Poor metabolic control decreases n-deacetylase activity type-1 diabetic-patients (Abstract). Diabetologia 1994; 37: Suppl. 1: A3.
51. Kofoed-Enevoldsen A, Petersen JS, Deckert T. Glucosaminyl N-deacetylase in cultured fibroblasts - comparison of patients with and without diabetic nephropathy, and identification of a possible mechanism for diabetes-induced N-deacetylase inhibition. Diabetologia 1993; 36: 536-540.
52. Walkenbach RJ, Hazen R, Larner J. Reversible inhibition of cyclic AMP-dependent protein kinase by insulin. Mol Cell Biochem 1978; 19: 31-41.
53. Kida Y, Nyomba BL, Bogardus C, Mott DM. Defective insulin response of cyclic adenosine monophosphate-dependent protein kinase in insulin resistant humans. J Clin Invest 1991; 87: 673-679.
54. Trevisan R, Nosadini R, Fioretto P, Semplicini A, Donadon V, Doria A et al. Clustering of risk factors in hypertensive insulin-dependent diabetics with high sodium-lithium countertransport. Kidney Int 1992; 41: 855-861.
55. Myrup B, Hansen PM, Jensen T, Kofoed-Enevoldsen A, Feldt-Rasmussen B, Gram J, Kluft C, Jespersen J, Deckert T. Effect of low-dose heparin on urinary albumin excretion in insulin-dependent diabetes mellitus. Lancet 1995; 345: 421-422.
56. Tamsma JT, van der Woude FJ, Lemkes HH. Effect of sulphated glycosaminoglycans on albuminuria in patients with overt diabetic (type 1) nephropathy Nephrol Dial Transplant 1996; 11(1): 182-185.

31. VOLUME HOMEOSTASIS AND BLOOD PRESSURE IN DIABETIC STATES

James A. O'Hare, MD, FRCPI, MRCP
Diabetes Unit, Limerick Regional General Hospital, Limerick, Ireland

J. Barry Ferriss MD, FRCPI, FRCP
Department of Medicine, University Hospital, Cork, Ireland.

SUMMARY

Extra-cellular sodium and fluid volume expansion as measured using the isotopic technique of Total Exchangeable Sodium measurements is commonly seen in patients with both IDDM and NIDDM. The exact cause is not known but plausible factors include increased capillary permeability and subtle renal alterations in sodium handling. Intravascular volume is not expanded.

In IDDM patients with nephropathy and hypertension Total Exchangeable Sodium is further increased and positively related to Blood Pressure. By contrast Total Exchangeable Sodium is not clearly expanded in NIDDM patients with hypertension ab initio and is not related to blood pressure. In IDDM patients free of complications the renin-angiotensin-aldosterone system behaves normally. In nephropathy angiotensin 11 may be playing a role in hypertension in some patients. In NIDDM patients without nephropathy plasma renin is suppressed in both normotensive and hypertensives.

1. METABOLIC CONTROL INFLUENCES VOLUME HOMEOSTASIS.

Arterial pressure is maintained by the complex interaction of body fluid volumes and a host of local, neural and endocrine regulators [1]. Ketoacidosis and hyperosmolar non-ketotic coma are characterised by profound dehydration and sodium depletion deficits. In less severe states of poor metabolic control there an be mild stimulation of the renin angiotensin-aldosterone system in humans. With improvements in metabolic control there is an increase in plasma volume and of total exchangeable sodium (an isotopic measurement of metabolically active sodium) to above normal with subsequent down-regulation of the renin-angiotensin system [2]. By contrast studies in streptozotocin induced diabetes in rats are associated with paradoxical increase in fluid volumes, suppression of renin and stimulation of atrial natriuretic factor [3]. While these unexpected trends have not

Mogensen, C.E. (ed.), THE KIDNEY AND HYPERTENSION IN DIABETES MELLITUS.

been seen in most human studies, higher plasma atrial natriuretic peptide (ANP) and lower plasma renin activity (PRA) were found in poorly controlled diabetics in one report [4].

2. SODIUM RETENTION OCCURS IN NORMOTENSIVE DIABETICS.

Exchangeable sodium is frequently elevated in both IDDM and NIDDM normotensive diabetic patients without overt nephropathy [5,6,7]. Total body sodium measured by neutron activation analysis is also increased [8]. Extracellular volume is expanded [7,9] to a similar degree in IDDM patients with both elevated and normal glomerular filtration rates [9].

Sodium retention in the absence of elevated blood pressure might be explained by cardiac impairment, by altered vascular reactivity, or by a change in Starling's forces in the microcirculation. Significant myocardial dysfunction is unusual in insulin-dependant diabetics in good metabolic control [10]. Vascular reactivity to infused norepinephrine [5] and angiotensin II [11] is enhanced in diabetics without complications, findings which do not favour decreased vascular reactivity as a cause of sodium retention. Increased microvascular permeability to albumin [12,13] and fluid [14] have been demonstrated especially in patients with microvascular complications. The transcapillary escape rate of albumin is positively related to 24-h urinary albumin excretion and to exchangeable sodium in normotensive diabetics [15].

Sodium retention may result from a primary renal defect. Normotensive IDDM patients without clinically overt renal disease have impaired ability to excrete a water load [9] and have adiminished natriuresis in response to underwater immersion [16]. This impaired natriuresis occurs despite an increase in creatinine clearance and in filtered sodium, indicating enhanced tubular sodium reabsorption [9].

Physiological or elevated levels of insulin may stimulate sodium retention in the renal tubule [17,18] although infusions of insulin at physiological concentrations do not impair the natriuretic response to immersion in normal subjects [19]. Marked hyperinsulinaemia reduces urinary sodium excretion even in subjects and animals who are insulin resistant in respect of glucose metabolism [18,20]. However despite sodium retention insulin does not raise blood pressure acutely in diabetics [21]. Thus it is possible that the hyperinsulinaemia that occurs episodically in IDDM and that is seen in some patients with NIDDM contributes to sodium retention. Proximal tubular absorption of sodium may be amplified in the presence of hyperglycaemia [22 , 23].

Plasma Angiotensin 11 (24) and plasma aldosterone concentrations are generally normal or reduced (24) in metabolically well controlled patients. By contrast basal ANP concentrations are slightly elevated in IDDM [9] and NIDDM [26]. In IDDM patients the ANP response both to saline loading [9] and to water immersion [16] are normal. However the natriuretic response to a saline load remained impaired during ANP infusion [27] demonstrating the presence of impaired renal responsiveness to ANP. Nevertheless renal blood flow responsiveness to short term infusions of ANP was preserved in diabetics with established chronic renal failure [28].

It is possible that blood pressure is sodium dependent in such patients, albeit in the normal range. In contrast to normal subjects, normotensive diabetics without overt nephropathy show a weak positive association between systolic blood pressure and exchangeable sodium [29]. Exchangeable sodium in these patients also correlates with 24-h urinary albumin excretion [15] and sodium retention is a possible explanation for the small blood pressure rise often seen in patients with incipient nephropathy [7].

Blood volume appears to be normal in normotensive diabetics without long-term complications [5,6]. A small increase in blood volume may result in a substantial increase in blood pressure [30] however, and current techniques may not detect subtle changes.

Despite the presence of sodium retention, PRA is generally normal in IDDM patients without complications [25, 29-31]. In contrast PRA is suppressed in normotensive NIDDM compared with similar-aged control subjects [34], findings consistent with functional suppression by increased extracellular sodium.

3. HYPERTENSION IN NON-INSULIN DEPENDENT DIABETICS

Up to 50% of patients with NIDDM may have hypertension [35]. It is often present at the time diabetes is detected [36]. There are likely to be a variety of causes, including factors co-associating through insulin resistance [37], nephropathy from diabetes and other causes of hypertension.

We measured exchangeable sodium and PRA in hypertensive non-insulin dependent diabetic patients without overt nephropathy[34]. The findings were compared with those in control subjects, normotensive diabetics and patients with essential hypertension of similar age. Urinary albumin excretion was similar in normotensive and hypertensive diabetics and in patients with essential hypertension. It is unlikely that hypertension could be attributed to nephropathy in diabetic patients and was present at diagnosis of diabetes in most. Exchangeable sodium was similar in control subjects and in essential hypertension, as previously described [38]. Exchangeable sodium was elevated in normotensive non-insulin dependent patients, but was not clearly elevated in hypertensive diabetic subjects. A similar pattern has been described in non-nephropathic hypertensive diabetics when total body sodium was measured by neutron activation analysis [8]. Exchangeable sodium and blood pressure were not related in either hypertensive group [34]. On the other hand PRA was suppressed in both normotensive and hypertensive diabetic patients. Intravascular volume tended to be lower in both non-diabetic and diabetic hypertensives, compared with their control groups.

Thus, as in essential hypertension, the hypertensive NIDDM patient without nephropathy is not characterised by volume expansion, and PRA is appropriately suppressed. The findings contrast with those in nephropathic hypertension discussed below.

4. DIABETIC NEPHROPATHY

Overt diabetic nephropathy is associated with marked fluid retention and a disturbance of variety of endocrine regulators of volume homeostasis.

Exchangeable sodium is further increased in nephropathic patients compared with patients with uncomplicated diabetes [6], and is positively related to blood pressure in incipient [7) and overt nephropathy [6]. The causes of sodium retention may be multiple. The transcapillary escape rate of albumin is usually elevated [12] and in more advanced cases hypoalbuminemia may be present. Some patients develop neuropathic oedema secondary to loss of autonomic nervous regulation of microvascular blood flow in the lower extremities [39], and myocardial failure may also contribute to fluid retention [40]. Intravascular volume is not increased [6]. This is not surprising however, in the light of other forms of renal disease with hypertension [41].

Early reports of PRA and plasma aldosterone in patients with advanced diabetic nephropathy described diminished responses to volume depletion [42,43]. In patients with less severe disease and receiving an unrestricted sodium intake, plasma levels of renin, angiotensin II and aldosterone may not be suppressed [6,24], although low plasma angiotensin II concentrations (7) and aldosterone (7) have been reported in IDDM patients with and without nephropathy despite normal renin values. Higher renin levels have also been described in diabetic nephropathy [44]. The sodium-renin product which reflects the combined influence of exchangeable sodium and plasma renin activity, is increased in patients with diabetic nephropathy, compared with diabetic patients without complications and non-diabetic controls [6].

While overt hyporeninaemiac hypoaldosteronism is relatively rare [24], an elevation of circulating inactive renin is common and appears to be a marker for microvascular complications [45]. It's functional significance if any, is unknown. It is however possible that inappropriately normal PRA levels in patients with nephropathy might be in part related to inadvertent activation of prorenin during renin measurement (25) reported in IDDM patients.

Plasma ANP concentrations are elevated in diabetic nephropathy showing a marked increase during water immersion but renal cyclic GMP responses are blunted suggesting renal resistance to ANP [46]. PRA has been reported to suppress during water immersion in normal subjects and in diabetic patients with normal albumin excretion or micro albuminuria [47] but not in diabetic nephropathy [46].

In other forms of chronic renal failure, raised blood pressure can be to be related to sodium retention and inappropriate activity of the renin-angiotensin system. Exchangeable sodium may be elevated, PRA inappropriately high and blood pressure is positively related to both exchangeable sodium and the sodium-renin product [48,49]. Similar mechanisms seem to operate in patients with diabetic nephropathy; exchangeable sodium is increased and is positively related to blood pressure, while PRA is not suppressed despite marked sodium retention. Nocturnal fluid retention may also contribute to the reduced nocturnal decline in blood pressure (50).

5. IMPLICATIONS FOR MANAGEMENT OF HYPERTENSION

Dietary salt intake has been related to blood pressure in the non-diabetic population however in the EURODIEB study this has not been found in IDDM patients regardless of whether they are taking antihypertensives (51).In NIDDM patients moderate sodium restriction seems to modestly lower blood pressure (52)

In view of the evidence that hypertension in nephropathy be may be at least partly maintained by sodium retention and inappropriate activity of the renin-angiotensin system, initial treatment with diuretic seems logical. Weidmann et al. [53] studied a mixed group of mildly hypertensive diabetic patients, with and without long-term complications including nephropathy. Chlorthalidone produced a fall in blood pressure and in exchangeable sodium, while exaggerated pressor responses to norepinephrine, and angiotensin II were restored to normal. Plasma renin and aldosterone rose briskly, perhaps blunting the antihypertensive effect. ACE inhibition produces a substantial natriuresis in diabetic patients [27] supporting the role of abnormal sodium-renin relationships in some patients with diabetic nephropathy. Furthermore renal responsiveness to plasma ANP was restored. Combination therapy is often necessary in nephropathy to optimise blood pressure control (54).

REFERENCES

1. Guyton AC. The body's approach to arterial pressure regulation. In: Circulatory Physiology III. Arterial pressure regulation. Philadelphia: WB Saunders. 1980; 1-9.
2. Ferriss JB, O'Hare JA, Kelleher CCM, Sullivan PA, Cole MN, Ross HF, O'Sullivan DJ. Diabetic control and the angiotensin system, catecholamines and blood pressure. Hypertension 1985; (supplement 11) 7:58-63.
3. Allen TJ, Cooper ME, O'Brien RC, Bach LA, Jackson B, Jerums G. Glomerular filtration rate in streptozocin-induced diabetic rats. Diabetes 1990; 39: 1182-90.
4. Bell GM, Bernstein RK, Laragh JH, Atlas SA, James GD, Pecker MS, Sealey JE. Increased plasma atrial natriuretic factor and reduced plasma renin in patients with poorly controlled diabetes mellitus. Clin Sci 1989; 77: 177-82.
5. Weidmann P, Beretta-Picolli C, Trost BN. Pressor factors and responsiveness in hypertension accompanying diabetes mellitus. Hypertension 1985;7: Suppl 11:33-42.
6. O'Hare JA, Ferriss JB, Brady D, Twomey B, O'Sullivan DJ. Exchangeable sodium and renin in hypertensive diabetic patients with and without nephropathy. Hypertension 1985; (Suppl 11) 7: 43-48.
7. Feldt-Rasmussen B, Mathiesen ER, Deckert T, et al. Central Role for sodium in the pathogenesis of blood pressure changes independent of angiotension, aldosterone, and catecholamines in type 1 (insulin-dependent) diabetes mellitus. Diabetologia 1987; 30: 610-17.
8. Brennan BL, Roginsky MS, Cohn S. Increased total body sodium as a mechanism for suppressed plasma renin activity in diabetes mellitus. Clin Res 1979; 27: 591a.
9. Fioretto P, Sambataro M, Cipollina MR et al. Role of atrial natriuretic peptide in the pathogenesis of sodium retention in ID with and without nephropathy.Diabetes 1992; 41: 936-945.
10. Fisher BM, Gillin G, Ong-Tone L, Dargie HJ, Frier BM. Cardiac Function and insulin-dependant diabetes: radionuclide ventriculopathy in young diabetics. Diabetic Med 1985; 2: 251-256.
11. Drury PL, Smith GM, Ferriss JB. Increased vasopressor responsiveness to angiotensin II in type 1 (insulin-dependent) diabetic patients without complications. Diabetologia 1984; 27: 174-179.
12. O'Hare JA, Ferriss JB, Twomey B, O'Sullivan DJ. Poor metabolic control, hypertension and microangiopathy independently increase the transcapillary escape rate of albumin in diabetics. Diabetologia 1983; 25: 260-263.
13. Norgaard K, Jensen T, Feld-Rasmussen B. Transcapillary escape rate of albumin in hypertensive patients with type 1 (insulin dependent) diabetes mellitus. Diabetologia 1993; 36: 57-61.
14. Jaap AJ, Shore AC, Gardside IB, Gamble J, Tooke JE. Increased microvascular fluid permeability in young type 1 (insulin dependent) diabetic patients. Diabetologia 1993; 36: 648-52.
15. O'Hare JA, Ferriss JB. Transcapillary escape rate of albumin and extracellular fluid volume in diabetes. Diabetologia 1985; 28: 937-938.

16. O'Hare JP, Anderson JV, Millar ND, Dalton N, Tymms DJ, Blood SR, Corral RJ. Hormonal responses to blood volume expansion in diabetic subjects with and without autonomic neuropathy. Clin Endocrinol (Oxf) 1989; 30: 571-9.
17. Skott P, Hother-Nielsen O, Bruun NE, et al. Effects of insulin on kidney function and sodium excretion in healthy subjects. Diabetologia 1989; 32: 694-99.
18. Finch D, Davis G, Bower J, Kirshner K. Effect of insulin, on renal sodium handling in hypertensive rats. Hypertension 1990; 15: 514-518.
19. Brible A, Corrall RJM, Mattocks J, O'Hare JP, Roland JM. Insulin and the renal response to volume expansion in man. J. Physiol 1985; 364:66.
20. Rocchini AP, Katch V, Kvesel D, et al. Insulin and renal sodium retention in obese adolescents. Hypertension 1989; 14: 367-74.
21. Norgaard K, Feld-Rasmussen B. Sodium retention and insulin treatment in insulin-dependent diabetes mellitus. Acta Diabetol 1994;14:367-374.
22. Ferrari P, Weidman P. Insulin, insulin sensitivity and hypertension. Hypertension 1990; 8: 491-500.
23. Nosadini R, Sambataro M, Thomaseth K, Pacini G, Cipollina MR, Brocco E, Solini A, Carraro A, Vellusi M, Frigato F, Crepaldi G. Role of hyperglycaemia and insulin resistance in determining sodium retention in non-insulin dependent diabetes mellitus. Kid Int 1993;17:261-269.
24. Ferriss JB, Sullivan PA, Gonggrijp H, Cole M, O'Sullivan DJ. Plasma angiotensin II and aldosterone in unselected diabetic patients. Clin Endocrinol 1982; 17: 261-269.
25. Cronin CC, Barry D, Crowley B, Ferriss JB. Reduced plasma aldosterone concentrations in randomly selected patients with insulin dependent diabetes mellitus. Diabetic Med 1995;12:809-15.
26. Lalau JD, Wesreel PF, Tenenbaum F, et al. Natriuretic and vasoactive hormones and glomerular hyperfiltration in hyperglycaemic type 2 diabetic patients: effect of insulin treatment. Nephron 1993; 63: 296-302.
27. Fioretto P, Muollo B, Faronato PF, Opocher G et al. Relationships amongst natriuresis, atrial natriuretic peptide and insulin in insulin-dependent diabetes. Kid Intern 1992; 41: 813-821.
28. Kumic BR, Weisberg LS, Cuttler IM, Kumic PB. Effects of atrial natriuretic peptide versus mannitol on renal blood flow during radiocontrast infusion in chornic renal failure. J Lab Clin Med 1990; 116: 27-36.
29. O'Hare JA, Ferriss JB, Twomey BM, Cole M, Brady D, O'Sullivan DJ. Blood pressure may be sodium dependent in diabetic patients without overt nephropathy.Ir J Med Sci 1985; 154: 455-460.
30. Coleman TG, Guyton AC. Hypertension caused by salt loading in the dog. Cir Res 1969; 25: 153-160.
31. Christlieb AR, Kaldany A, D'Elia JA. Plasma renin activity and hypertension in diabetes mellitus. Diabetes 1976; 25: 969-974.
32. Moss S, Oster JR, Perez GO, Katz FH, Vaamonde CA. Renin-aldosterone responsiveness in uncomplicated juvenile-type diabetes mellitus. Horm Res 1978; 9: 130-136.
33. Drury PL, Bodansky HJ, Oddie CJ, Edwards CRW. Factors in the control of plasma renin activity and concentration in type 1 (insulin-dependent) diabetes. Clin Endocrinol 1984; 20:607-618.
34. O'Hare JA, Ferriss JB, Twomey BM, Brady D, O'Sullivan DJ. Essential hypertension and hypertension in diabetic patients without nephropathy. J. Hypertension {Suppl 2} 1983: 1: 200-203.
35. Fuller JH: Epidemiology of hypertension associated with diabetes mellitus. Hypertension (Suppl II) 1985: 7: 3-7.
36. United Kingdom Prospective Diabetes Study. Prevalence of hypertension and hypotensive therapy in patients with newly diagnosed diabetes.Hypertension [Suppl II] 1985; 7: 8-13.
37. O'Hare JA. Insulin resistance and hypertension. Current Opinion in endocrinology and Diabetes 1994; 1:147-152.
38. Beretta-Piccoli C, Davies DL, Boddy K, Browne JJ, Cumming AMM, East BW, Fraser R, Lever AF, Padfield PL, Semple PF, Robertson JIA, Weidmann P, Williams ED. Relation of arterial pressur e with body sodium, body potassium and plasma potassium in essential hypertension.Clin Sci 1982; 63: 257-270.

39. Watkins PJ, Edmonds ME. Sympathetic nerve failure in diabetes. Diabetologia 1983; 25:73-77.
40. D'Elia JA, Weinrauch LA, Healy RW, Libertino JA, Bradley RF, Leyland OS. Myocardial dysfunction without coronary artery disease in diabetic renal failure. Am J Cardiol 1979; 43: 193-199.
41. Beretta-Piccoli C, Weidmann P, Chatel R, Reubi F. Hypertension associated with early stage kidney disease. Am J Med 1976; 61: 739-747.
42. Christlieb AR, Kaldany A, D'Elia JA, Williams GH. Aldosterone responsiveness in patients with diabetes mellitus. Diabetes 1978; 27: 732-727.
43. Tuck ML, Sambhi MP, Levin L. Hyporeninemic hypoaldosteronism in diabetes mellitus. Diabetes 1979; 28: 237-241.
44. O'Donnell MJ, Lawson N, Barnett MJ. Activity of the unstimulated renin-aldosterone system in type 1 diabetes patients with and without proteinuria. Diabetic Med 1989; 6: 422-425.
45. Leutscher JA, Kraemer FB, Wilson DM, Schwartz Hc, Bryer-Ash M. Increased plasma inactive renin in diabetes mellitus: a marker of microvascular complications. N Eng J Med 1985; 312: 1412-1417.
46. Lieberman JS, Parra L, Newton L, Scandling JD, Loon N, Myers BD. Atrial natriuretic peptide response to changing plasma volume in diabetic nephropathy. Diabetes 1991; 39: 893-901.
47. O'Hare JP, Anderson JV, Millar ND, Bloom SR, Corral RGM. The relationship of the renin-angiotensin-aldosterone system to atrial natriuretic peptide and the natriuresis of volume expansion in diabetics with and without proteinuria
Postgrad Med J 1988; 64 (Suppl 3): 35-38.
48. Dathan JRE, Johnson DB, Goodwin FJ. The relationship between body fluid comprtment volumes, renin activity and blood pressure in chronic renal failure.
Clin Sci Mol Med 1985; 45: 77-88.
49. Ferriss JB, O'Hare JA, Cole M, Kingston SM, Twomey BM, O'Sullivan DJ. Blood pressure in diabetic patients: relationships with exchangeable sodium and renin activity.
Diabetic nephropathy 1986; 5: 27-30.
50. Mulec H, Blohme G, Kullenberg K, Nyberg G, Bjork S. Latent overhydration and nocturnal hypertension in diabetic nephropathy. Diabetologia 1995;38:216-220.
51. Colhoun H, Stevens LK Collodo Messa F, Fuller J and the EURODIAB IDDM Complications study. The relationshop of sodium and potassium excretion in the EURODIAB IDDM Diabetologia 1997;40: Suppl. 1 A366
52. Dobson PM, Beevers M, Hallworth R, Webberley MJ, Fletcher RF, Taylor KG. Sodium restriction and blood pressure in hypertensive type II diabetics: randomised blind controlled and crossover studies of moderate sodium restriction and sodium supplementation. BMJ 1989; 298: 227-230.
53. Weidmann P, Beretta-Piccoli C, Keusch G, Gluck Z, Mujagic M, Grimm M, Merier A, Ziegler WH. Sodium-volume factor, Cardiovascular reactivity and hypotensive mechanism of diuretic therapy in mild hypertension associated with diabetes mellitus. Am J Med 1976; 67: 779-784.
54. Nielsen FS, Rossing P, Gall M Skott P, Smidt UM, Parving H-H. Impact of lisinopril and atenolol on kidney function in hypertensive subjects with diabetic nephropathy. Diabetes 1994;43:1108-1113

32. PATHOGENESIS OF DIABETIC GLOMERULOPATHY: THE ROLE OF GLOMERULAR HEMODYNAMIC FACTORS

Sharon Anderson, M.D.
Division of Nephrology and Hypertension, Oregon Health Sciences University, Portland, OR, U.S.A

INTRODUCTION

Glomerular hyperfiltration in insulin-dependent (Type 1) diabetes mellitus of short duration has been recognized for many years [1-3], with increments in renal plasma flow (RPF) and nephromegaly [3]. With the finding of early hyperfiltration, Stalder and Schmid proposed that these early functional changes may predispose the subsequent development of diabetic glomerulopathy [1]. Early support for the hypothesis that renal hyperperfusion and hyperfiltration contribute to diabetic glomerulopathy emanated from the finding of diabetic glomerulopathy only in the non-stenosed kidney in the setting of unilateral renal artery stenosis [4].

Although glomerular hyperperfusion and hyperfiltration have long been recognized in early Type 1 diabetes [1-3], similar studies have only recently been performed in the much larger patient population with non-insulin-dependent (Type 2) diabetes. Studies reveal a wide range of renal hemodynamics in this group, but provide clear evidence for elevations of GFR and RPF in significant proportions of patients of Caucasian, Native- and Afro-American origin [5-11].

It has been proposed that the glomerular hyperfunction of early Type 1 diabetes predicts the later development of overt nephropathy and diabetic glomerulopathy [12,13], while others have failed to document such a relationship [14-16]. The reasons for these disparate results are as yet unclear. Likewise, the role of the glomerular hyperfiltration observed in Type 2 diabetic patients in the subsequent development of nephropathy remains to be established in longitudinal studies. However, preliminary results indicate a reduction in GFR over the first 2 years after diagnosis, with the greatest changes in the younger patients with initial GFR values greater than 120 ml/min [17]. Despite the controversy in human diabetes concerning the significance of hyperfiltration in the subsequent development of overt nephropathy, extensive experimental data provides considerable insight into the importance of hemodynamic factors in the initiation and progression of diabetic glomerulopathy [18,19].

Mogensen, C.E. (ed.), THE KIDNEY AND HYPERTENSION IN DIABETES MELLITUS.

RENAL HEMODYNAMICS IN EXPERIMENTAL DIABETES MELLITUS

Several animal models with spontaneous or induced diabetes have been used to study the role of altered hemodynamics in the development of diabetic glomerulopathy [18-21]. As in Type 1 diabetic patients, diabetic rats tend to exhibit reduced values for whole kidney GFR during periods of severe uncontrolled hyperglycemia; single nephron (SN) GFR and plasma flow rates are also normal or reduced in animals in such catabolic states [21]. In the more clinically applicable model of moderate hyperglycemia, whole kidney GFR and SNGFR increase by about 40% as compared to normal rats [21-23]. Reductions in intrarenal vascular resistances result in elevation of the glomerular capillary plasma flow rate, Q_A. Despite normal blood pressure levels, transmission of systemic pressures to the glomerular capillaries is facilitated by proportionally greater reduction in afferent compared to efferent arteriolar resistances. Consequently, the glomerular capillary hydraulic pressure (P_{GC}) rises. Thus, the observed single nephron hyperfiltration results from both glomerular capillary hyperperfusion and hypertension [21-23]. In longterm studies, diabetic rats develop morphologic changes reminiscent of those in the diabetic human, including glomerular basement membrane thickening, renal and glomerular hypertrophy, mesangial matrix thickening and hyaline deposition, and ultimately glomerular sclerosis [22-27].

Evidence that these glomerular hemodynamic maladaptations contribute to the development and progression of diabetic glomerulopathy has been shown by studies involving maneuvers which aggravate or ameliorate glomerular hyperperfusion and hyperfiltration, without affecting metabolic control. Uninephrectomy, which increases SNGFR, Q_A and P_{GC} in normal rats, accelerates the development of albuminuria and glomerular sclerosis in diabetic rats [28]. Intensification of glomerular lesions is observed in the unclipped kidney of diabetic rats with two-kidney Goldblatt hypertension, while the clipped kidney is substantially protected from glomerular injury [29]. Diabetic renal injury is similarly amplified by augmentation of dietary protein content, which increases glomerular perfusion and filtration [22].

By contrast, dietary protein restriction, which reduces SNGFR, Q_A and P_{GC} in other models, has clarified the role of hemodynamic factors in diabetic glomerulopathy. In long-term diabetes, low protein diets limited SNGFR by reducing the elevated P_{GC} and Q_A, and virtually prevented albuminuria and glomerular injury. In contrast, diabetic rats fed a high protein diet exhibited glomerular capillary hyperfiltration, hyperperfusion and hypertension, and marked increases in albuminuria and glomerular morphologic injury [22]. As there were no differences in metabolic control between the various groups, this study provided clear evidence that amelioration of the maladaptive glomerular hemodynamic pattern could prevent diabetic renal disease could dramatically lower the risk of diabetic glomerulopathy.

MECHANISMS OF HYPERFILTRATION IN DIABETES

The pathogenesis of diabetic hyperfiltration is multifactorial. Defective autoregulation at the afferent arteriole is a major defect, which has been demonstrated both experimentally [30] and clinically [31]. Numerous mediators for this effect have been proposed (Table 32-1), and are briefly reviewed here.

Table 32-1. POTENTIAL MEDIATORS OF DIABETIC HYPERFILTRATION
Hyperglycemia/insulinopenia
Extracellular fluid volume expansion
Blunted tubulo-glomerular feedback
Advanced glycosylation end-products
Impaired afferent arteriolar voltage-gated calcium channels
Atrial natriuretic peptide
Endothelial-derived relaxing factor
Vasodilator prostaglandins
Increased kallikrein-kinin activity
Increased plasma ketone bodies, organic acids
Increased plasma glucagon levels
Increased plasma growth hormone levels
Increased insulin-like growth factor-1
Altered responsiveness to catecholamines/angiotensin II
Abnormalities in calcium metabolism
Abnormal myo-inositol metabolism
Tissue hypoxia/abnormalities in local vasoregulatory factors

The metabolic milieu may contribute: hyperglycemia and/or insulinopenia *per se* [20,32], together with augmented growth hormone and glucagon levels [33,34]. Reduction of plasma glucose with initial institution of therapy reduces GFR in both Type 1 and 2 diabetes [32,35]. In moderately hyperglycemic diabetic rats, normalization of blood glucose levels reverses hyperfiltration [36], and insulin infusion reduces P_{GC} [37]. By contrast, insulin infusion sufficient to produce hyperinsulinemia, with euglycemia, increases P_{GC} and hyperfiltration in normal rats [38]. Further, infusion of blood containing early glycosylation products reproduces glomerular hyperfiltration in normal rats [39].

Diabetes is also characterized by other physiologic changes with hemodynamic consequences, including elevation of plasma atrial natriuretic peptide levels [40]; possible augmentation of endothelium-derived relaxing factor activity [41,42]; reduced glomerular receptor sites for the vasoconstrictive Ang II and thromboxane [43,44]; altered vascular responsiveness to catecholamines and Ang II [45-47]; blunting of the tubulo-glomerular feedback mechanism [48,49]; and functional impairment of renal afferent arteriolar voltage-gated calcium channels [50]. Each of these may contribute; for example, blockade of atrial natriuretic peptide action with an antibody [40] or a specific receptor antagonist [51] blunts hyperfiltration in diabetic rats. Enhanced activity of vasodilator prostaglandins is another mechanism proposed as a mediator of diabetic hyperfiltration, as prostaglandin synthetase inhibition results in significant reductions in SNGFR, Q_A and P_{GC} [52]. Diabetes-related abnormalities of other vasodilator mechanisms have also been suggested, with findings of elevated urinary metabolites of the kallikrein-kinin system [53]. However, studies with kinin receptor antagonists have thus far proven inconsistent [54-56].

Increased activity of the polyol pathway and related disturbances in cellular myo-inositol metabolism have been implicated in the pathogenesis of several diabetic microangiopathic complications. Dietary myo-inositol supplementation and pharmacologic inhibition of aldose reductase sometimes [57] though not always [58] prevent renal hypertrophy, hyperfiltration and proteinuria in diabetic rats.

ROLE OF GLOMERULAR CAPILLARY HYPERTENSION

Of the glomerular hemodynamic determinants of hyperfiltration, the available evidence suggests that glomerular capillary hypertension plays the key role in progression of renal injury. Long-term protection against albuminuria and glomerular sclerosis was obtained in normotensive diabetic rats by angiotensin converting enzyme inhibitor (ACEI) therapy in doses which modestly lowered systemic blood pressure, but selectively normalized P_{GC}, without affecting the supranormal SNGFR and Q_A [23]. Studies in a variety of experimental models, including diabetes, have consistently shown that interventions which control glomerular capillary hypertension are associated with marked slowing of the development of structural injury [59].

Little is yet known of the exact mechanism(s) by which glomerular capillary hypertension eventuates in structural injury. Recently, innovative new techniques using a variety of *in vitro* systems have been developed to address this question. These studies postulate that glomerular hemodynamic factors modify the growth and activity of glomerular component cells, inducing the elaboration or expression of cytokines and other mediators which then stimulate mesangial matrix production and promote structural injury. For instance, increased shear stress on endothelial cells enhances activity of such mediators as endothelin [60], nitric oxide [61,62], transforming growth factor-ß [63], and several cellular adhesion molecules [64], and modulates release of platelet derived growth factor [65,66]. Altered hemodynamics also influence mesangial cells: it has been postulated that expansion of the glomerular capillaries, and stretching of the mesangium in response to hypertension, might translate high P_{GC} into increased mesangial matrix formation [67]. Evidence for this mechanism comes from observations in microperfused rat glomeruli, in which increased hydraulic pressure was associated with increased glomerular volume; and in cultured mesangial cells, where cyclic stretching resulted in enhanced synthesis of protein, total collagen, collagen IV, collagen I, laminin, fibronectin, and transforming growth factor-ß (TGF-ß)[67-69]. Of particular relevance to diabetes, the accumulation of extracellular matrix caused by any degree of mechanical strain is aggravated in a milieu of high glucose concentration [71]. Additionally, growing mesangial cells under pulsatile conditions has been reported to stimulate protein kinase C, calcium influx, and proto-oncogene expression [72], and Ang II receptor and angiotensinogen mRNA levels [73], as well as altered extracellular matrix protein processing enzymes [73,74]. Recently, it has been noted that mediators of oxidant stress are induced by shear stress in vascular smooth muscle cells [75], as well as mechanical stretch in proximal tubular cells [76]. More evidence comes from the recent finding that application of pressure (comparable to elevated glomerular pressures in vivo) enhances mesangial cell matrix synthesis in cultured cells [77]. Given these new techniques, the cellular mechanisms by which glomerular hypertension leads to structural injury are in process of being elucidated.

ANTIHYPERTENSIVE THERAPY IN EXPERIMENTAL DIABETES

Further support for the notion that glomerular capillary hypertension constitutes a central mechanism of glomerular injury in experimental diabetes comes from studies comparing differing antihypertensive agents [18]. Of the agents studied, ACEI have consistently limited injury parameters (albuminuria and glomerular sclerosis) in normotensive diabetic rats, uninephrectomized diabetic rats, and diabetes superimposed on genetic hypertension [23,78-83], as well as in diabetic dogs [84]. In studies where glomerular hemodynamics were measured, the protection afforded by ACEI was associated with reduction of P_{GC}, due to preferential reduction of efferent arteriolar tone.

By contrast, conflicting results have been reported for antihypertensive regimens which fail to control glomerular hypertension. Agents such as dihydropyridine calcium channel blockers,β-blockers and combinations of vasodilators and diuretics ("triple therapy") have not resulted in structural and functional protection in experimental diabetes with any consistency [78-84]. Failure to exert longterm control of glomerular hypertension has frequently been found to contribute to lack of protection with these alternate agents.

That the beneficial effects of ACEI are due in large part to limitation of Ang II formation has been confirmed in studies showing that the beneficial hemodynamic [85] and structural [86] effects can be reproduced with specific Ang II receptor antagonists. Ang II possesses a number of physiological actions. Limitation of several of these have been postulated to contribute to the protective effect of ACEI, including control of systemic and glomerular hypertension; decreased mesangial and tubular macromolecular and solute transfer; decreased proteinuria with improved glomerular permselectivity; and limitation of glomerular hypertrophy and microvascular growth. Although experimental diabetes is characterized by glomerular enlargement, longterm protection with ACEI has been observed without consistent limitation of glomerular size [78,79,81]. The proposed beneficial mechanisms of ACEI are, however, not mutually exclusive. Indeed, though less emphasized, the renin-angiotensin system is now thought to participate in pathogenesis of tubulointerstitial injury, as well as glomerular injury, in the setting of diabetes [87].As has been recently reviewed, hyperglycemia and the renin-angiotensin system may act synergistically to promote fibrosis in the diabetic kidney, by mechanisms beyond hemodynamic factors.Although the role of aggressive control of hypertension in the preservation of renal function in diabetic nephropathy is clear, clinical studies directly comparing different antihypertensive agents have remained somewhat controversial. Of note, however, are recent meta-analyses [88,89] and clinical trials [90] which have found a superior ability of ACEI to slow the pace of diabetic nephropathy, as compared to other antihypertensive agents. Elucidation of the complex mechanisms that contribute to diabetic hyperfiltration remains a challenge. Many genetic, metabolic and hemodynamic factors act in concert with the end result of glomerular obsolescence. The enormity of the clinical problem of nephropathy in this highly susceptible patient population behooves continued intense research into pathogenetic mechanisms, and approaches to specific therapy of patients at risk for renal disease.

REFERENCES

1. Stalder G, Schmid R. 1959. Severe functional disorders of glomerular capillaries and renal hemodynamics in treated diabetes mellitus during childhood. Ann Paediatr, 193:129-138.
2. Ditzel J, Junker K. 1972. Abnormal glomerular filtration rate, renal plasma flow and renal protein excretion in recent and short-term diabetes. Br Med J, 2:13-19.
3. Mogensen CE, Andersen MJF. 1973. Increased kidney size and glomerular filtration rate in early juvenile diabetes. Diabetes, 22:706-712.
4. Berkman J, Rifkin H. 1973. Unilateral nodular diabetic glomerulosclerosis (Kimmelstiel-Wilson). Metabolism, 22:715-722.

5. Vora J, Dolben J, Dean J, Williams JD, Owens DR, Peters JR. 1992. Renal hemodynamics in newly presenting non-insulin-dependent diabetics. Kidney Int, 41:829-835.
6. Myers BD, Nelson RG, Williams GW, et al. 1991. Glomerular function in Pima Indians with non-insulin-dependent diabetes mellitus of recent origin. J Clin Invest, 88:524-530.
7. Palmisano JJ, Lebovitz HE. 1989. Renal function in Black Americans with type II diabetes. J Diab Compl, 3:40-44.
8. Nelson RG, Bennett PH, Beck GJ, Tan M, Knowler WC, Mitch WE, Hirschman GH, Myers BD. 1996. Development and progression of renal disease in Pima Indians with non-insulin-dependent diabetes mellitus. New Engl J Med, 335:1636-1642.
9. Nowack R, Raum E, Blum W, Ritz E. 1992. Renal hemodynamics in recent-onset Type II diabetes. Am J Kidney Dis, 20:342-347
10. Ritz E, Stefanski A. 1996. Diabetic nephropathy in Type II diabetes. Am J Kidney Dis, 27:167-194.
11. Wirta O, Pasternack A, Laippala P, Turjanmaa V. 1996. Glomerular filtration rate and kidney size after six years disease duration in non-insulin-dependent diabetic subjects. Clin Nephrol, 45:10-71.
12. Mogensen CE. 1986. Early glomerular hyperfiltration in insulin-dependent diabetics and late nephropathy. Scand J Clin Lab Invest, 46:201-206.
13. Rudberg S, Persson B, Dahlquist G. 1992. Increased glomerular filtration rate as a predictor of diabetic nephropathy - an 8 year prospective study. Kidney Int, 41:822-828.
14 Lervang H-H, Jensen S, Borchner-Mortensen J, Ditzel J. 1988. Early glomerular hyperfiltration and the development of late nephropathy in type 1 (insulin-dependent) diabetes mellitus. Diabetologia, 31:723-729.
15. Yip JW, Jones SL, Wiseman M, Hill C, Viberti GC. 1996. Glomerular hyperfiltration in the prediction of nephropathy in IDDM. A 10-year followup study. Diabetes, 45:1729-1733.
16. Mogensen CE. 1994. Glomerular hyperfiltration in human diabetes. Diabetes Care, 17:770-775.
17. Vora JP, Peters JR, Williams JD. 1993. Evolution of renal hemodynamics in non-insulin-dependent diabetics (NIDDMs): a 2 year study. J Am Soc Nephrol, 4:310 (abstr).
18. Anderson S. 1992. Antihypertensive therapy in experimental diabetes. J Am Soc Nephrol, 3 (Suppl 1):S86-S90.
19. O'Donnell MP, Kasiske BL, Keane WF. 1986. Glomerular hemodynamics and structural alterations in experimental diabetes. FASEB J, 2:2339-2347.
20. Park SK, Meyer TW. 1995. The effect of hyperglycemia on glomerular function in obese Zucker rats. J Lab Clin Med, 125:501-507.
21. Hostetter TH, Troy JL, Brenner BM. 1981. Glomerular hemodynamics in experimental diabetes mellitus. Kidney Int, 19:410-415.
22. Zatz R, Meyer TW, Rennke HG, Brenner BM. 1985. Predominance of hemodynamic rather than metabolic factors in the pathogenesis of diabetic glomerulopathy. Proc Natl Acad Sci (USA), 82:5963-5967.
23. Zatz R, Dunn BR, Meyer TW, Anderson S, Rennke HG, Brenner BM. 1986. Prevention of diabetic glomerulopathy by pharmacological amelioration of glomerular capillary hypertension. J Clin Invest, 77:1925-1930.
24. Seyer-Hansen K. 1983. Renal hypertrophy in experimental diabetes mellitus. Kidney Int, 23:643-646.
25. Seyer-Hansen K, Hansen J, Gundersen HJG. 1980. Renal hypertrophy in experimental diabetes. A morphometric study. Diabetologia, 18:501-505.
26. Steffes MW, Brown DM, Basgen JM, Mauer SM. 1980. Amelioration of mesangial volume and surface alterations following islet transplantation in diabetic rats. Diabetes, 29:509-515.
27. Mauer SM, Michael AF, Fish AJ, Brown DM. 1972. Spontaneous immunoglobulin and complement deposition in glomeruli of diabetic rats. Lab Invest, 27:488-494.
28. O'Donnell MP, Kasiske BL, Daniels FX, Keane WF. 1986. Effect of nephron loss on glomerular hemodynamics and morphology in diabetic rats. Diabetes, 35:1011-1015.
29. Mauer SM, Steffes MW, Azar S, Sandberg SK, Brown DM. 1978. The effect of Goldblatt hypertension on development of the glomerular lesions of diabetes mellitus in the rat. Diabetes, 27:738-744.
30. Hayashi K, Epstein M, Loutzenhiser R, Forster H. 1992. Impaired myogenic responsiveness of the afferent arteriole in streptozotocin-induced diabetic rats: role of eicosanoid derangements. J Am Soc Nephrol, 2:1578-1586.
31. Christensen PK, Hansen HP, Parving H-H. 1997. Impaired autoregulation of GFR in hypertensive non-insulin dependent diabetic patients. Kidney Int, 52:1369-1374.
32. Christiansen JS, Gammelgaard J, Tronier B, Svendsen PA, Parving H-H. 1982. Kidney function and size in diabetics before and during initial insulin treatment. Kidney Int, 21:683-688.

33. Parving H-H, Christiansen JS, Noer I, Tronier B, Mogensen CE. 1980. The effect of glucagon infusion on kidney function in short-term insulin-dependent juvenile diabetics. Diabetologia, 19:350-354.
34. Christiansen JS, Gammelgaard J, Orskov H, Andersen AR, Telmer S, Parving H-H. 1980. Kidney function and size in normal subjects before and during growth hormone administration for one week. Eur J Clin Invest, 11:487-490.
35. Vora J, Dolben J, Williams JD, Peters JR, Owens DR. 1993. Impact of initial treatment on renal function in newly-diagnosed Type 2 (non-insulin-dependent) diabetes mellitus. Diabetologia, 36:734-740.
36. Stackhouse S, Miller PL, Park SK, Meyer TW. 1990. Reversal of glomerular hyperfiltration and renal hypertrophy by blood glucose normalization in diabetic rats. Diabetes, 39:989-995.
37. Scholey JW, Meyer TW. 1989. Control of glomerular hypertension by insulin administration in diabetic rats. J Clin Invest, 83:1384-1389.
38. Tucker BJ, Anderson CM, Thies RS, Collins RC, Blantz RC. 1992. Glomerular hemodynamic alterations during acute hyperinsulinemia in normal and diabetic rats. Kidney Int, 42:1160-1168.
39. Sabbatini M, Sansone G, Uccello F, Giliberti A, Conte G, Andreucci VE. 1992. Early glycosylation products induce glomerular hyperfiltration in normal rats. Kidney Int, 42:875-881.
40. Ortola FV, Ballermann BJ, Anderson S, Mendez RE, Brenner BM. 1987. Elevated plasma atrial natriuretic peptide levels in diabetic rats. J Clin Invest, 80:670-674.
41. Mattar AL, Fujihara CK, Ribeiro MO, DeNucci G, Zatz R. 1996. Renal effects of acute and chronic nitric oxide inhibition in experimental diabetes. Nephron, 74:136-143.
42. Komers R, Allen TJ, Cooper ME. 1994. Role of endothelium-derived nitric oxide in the pathogenesis of the renal hemodynamic changes of experimental diabetes. Diabetes, 43:1190-1197.
43. Ballermann BJ, Skorecki KL, Brenner BM. 1984. Reduced glomerular angiotensin II receptor density in early untreated diabetes mellitus in the rat. Am J Physiol, 247:F110-F116.
44. Wilkes BM, Kaplan R, Mento PF, Aynedjian H Macica CM, Schlondorff D, Bank N. 1992. Reduced glomerular thromboxane receptor sites and vasoconstrictor responses in diabetic rats. Kidney Int, 41:992-999.
45. Christlieb AR. 1974. Renin, angiotensin and norepinephrine in alloxan diabetes. Diabetes, 23:962-970.
46. Kennefick TM, Oyama TT, Thompson MM, Vora JP, Anderson S. 1996. Enhanced renal sensitivity to angiotensin actions in diabetes mellitus in the rat. Am J Physiol, 271:F595-F602.
47. Ohishi K, Okwueze MI, Vari RC, Carmines PK. 1994. Juxtamedullary microvascular dysfunction during the hyperfiltration stage of diabetes mellitus. Am J Physiol, 267:F99-F105.
48. Blantz RC, Peterson OW, Gushwa L, Tucker BJ. 1982. Effect of modest hyperglycemia on tubuloglomerular feedback activity. Kidney Int, 22 (Suppl 12):S206-S212.
49. Vallon V, Blantz RC, Thomson S. 1995. Homeostatic efficiency of tubuloglomerular feedback is reduced in established diabetes mellitus in rats. Am J Physiol, 269:F876-F883.
50. Carmines PK, Ohishi K, Ikenaga H. 1996. Functional impairment of renal afferent arteriolar voltage-gated calcium channels in rats with diabetes mellitus. J Clin Invest, 98:2564-2571.
51. Zhang PL, Mackenzie HS, Troy JL, Brenner BM. 1994. Effects of an atrial natriuretic peptide receptor antagonist on glomerular hyperfiltration in diabetic rats. J Am Soc Nephrol, 4:1564-1570.
52. Jensen PK, Steven K, Blaehr H, Christiansen JS, Parving H-H. 1986. Effects of indomethacin on glomerular hemodynamics in experimental diabetes. Kidney Int, 29:490-495.
53. Mayfield RK, Margolius HS, Levine JH, Wohltmann HJ, Loadholt CB, Colwell JA. 1984. Urinary kallikrein excretion in insulin-dependent diabetes mellitus and its relationship to glycemic control. J Clin Endocrinol Metab 59:278-286.
54. Jaffa AA, Rust PF, Mayfield RK. 1995. Kinin, a mediator of diabetes-induced glomerular hyperfiltration. Diabetes, 44:156-160.
55. Vora JP, Oyama TT, Thompson MM, Anderson S. 1997. Interactions of the kallikrein-kinin and renin-angiotensin systems in experimental diabetes. Diabetes, 46:107-112.
56. Komers R, Cooper ME. 1995. Acute renal hemodynamic effects of ACE inhibition in diabetic hyperfiltration: role of kinins. Am J Physiol, 268:F588-F594.
57. Goldfarb S, Ziyadeh FN, Kern EFO, Simmons DA. 1991. Effects of polyol-pathway inhibition and dietary *myo*-inositol on glomerular hemodynamic function in experimental diabetes mellitus in rats. Diabetes, 40:465-471.
58. Daniels BS, Hostetter TH. 1989. Aldose reductase inhibition and glomerular abnormalities in diabetic rats. Diabetes, 38:981-986.

59. Anderson S. 1993. Pharmacologic interventions in experimental animals. In Prevention of Progressive Chronic Renal Failure. El Nahas AM, Mallick NP, Anderson S, eds. Oxford: Oxford Univ. Press, 1993.
60. Kuchan MJ, Frangos JA. 1993. Shear stress regulates endothelin-1 release via protein kinase C and cGMP in cultured endothelial cells. Am J Physiol, 264:H150-H156.
61. Buga GM, Gold ME, Fukuto JM, Ignarro LJ. 1991. Shear stress-induced release of nitric oxide from endothelial cells grown on beads. Hypertension, 17:187-193.
62. Awolesi MA, Sessa WC, Sumpio BE. 1995. Cyclic strain upregulates nitric oxide synthesis in cultured bovine aortic endothelial cells. J Clin Invest, 96:1449-1454.
63. Ohno M, Cooke JC, Dzau VJ, Gibbons GH. 1995. Fluid shear stress induces endothelial transforming growth factor beta-1 transcription and production. Modulation by potassium-channel blockade. J Clin Invest, 95:1363-1369.
64. Nagel T, Resnick N, Atkinson WJ, Dewey CF, Jr, Gimbrone, MA, Jr. 1994. Shear stress selectively upregulates intercellular adhesion molecule-1 expression in cultured human vascular endothelial cells. J Clin Invest, 94:885-891.
65. Ott MJ, Olsen JL, Ballermann BJ .1995. Chronic *in vitro* flow promotes ultrastructural differentiation of endothelial cells. Endothelium 3:21-30.
66. Malek AM, Gibbons GH, Dzau VJ, Izumo S. 1993. Fluid shear stress differentially modulates expression of genes encoding basic fibroblast growth factor and platelet-derived growth factor B chain in vascular endothelium. J Clin Invest 92:2013-2021.
67. Riser BL, Cortes P, Zhao X, Bernstein J, Dumler F, Narins RG. 1992. Intraglomerular pressure and mesangial stretching stimulate extracellular matrix formation in the rat. J Clin Invest, 90:1932-1943.
68. Yasuda T, Becker B, Kondo S, et al. 1994. Mechanical stretch/relaxation increases type 1 angiotensin II receptor expression and angiotensinogen mRNA in cultured rat mesangial cells. J Am Soc Nephrol, 4:554, (abstr)
69. Harris RC, Haralson MA, Badr KF. 1992. Continuous stretch-relaxation in culture alters rat mesangial cell morphology, growth characteristics, and metabolic activity. Lab Invest, 66:548-554.
70. Riser BL, Cortes P, Heilig C, Grondin J, Ladson-Wofford S, Patterson D, Narins RG. Cyclic stretching force selectively up-regulates transforming growth factor-ß isoforms in cultured rat mesangial ells. Am J Pathol, 148:1915-1923.
71. Cortes P, Zhao X, Riser BL, Narins RG. 1997. Role of glomerular mechanical strain in the pathogenesis of diabetic nephropathy. Kidney Int, 51:57-68.
72. Homma T, Akai Y, Burns KD, Harris RC. 1992. Activation of S6 kinase by repeated cycles of stretching and relaxation in rat glomerular mesangial cells. J Biol Chem, 267:23129-23135.
73. Yasuda T, Kondo S, Homma T, Harris RC. 1994. Mechanisms for accumulation of extracellular matrix in rat mesangial cells in response to stretch/relaxation. J Am Soc Nephrol, 4:824 (abstr)
74. Harris RC, Akai Y, Yasuda T, Homma T. 1995. The role of physical forces in alterations of mesangial cell function. Kidney Int 45 (Suppl 45):S17, 1995
75. Wagner CT, Durante W, Christodoulide N, Hellums JD, Schafer AI. 1997. Hemodynamic forces induce the expression of heme oxygenase in cultured vascular smooth muscle cells. J Clin Invest, 100:589-596.
76. Ricardo SD, Ding G, Eufemio M, Diamond JR. 1997. Antioxidant expression in experimental hydronephrosis: role of mechanical stretch and growth factors. Am J Physiol, 272:F789-F798.
77. Mattana J, Singhal PC. 1995. Applied pressure modulates mesangial cell proliferation and matrix synthesis. Am J Hypertension, 8:1112-1120.
78. Anderson S, Rennke HG, Garcia DL, Brenner BM. 1989. Short and long term effects of antihypertensive therapy in the diabetic rat. Kidney Int, 36:526-532.
79. Anderson S, Rennke HG, Brenner BM. 1992. Nifedipine versus fosinopril in uninephrectomized diabetic rats. Kidney Int, 41:891-897.
80. Cooper ME, Rumble JR, Allen TJ, et al. 1992. Antihypertensive therapy and experimental diabetic nephropathy. Kidney Int, 41:898-903.
81. Fujihara C, Padilha RM, Zatz R. 1992. Glomerular abnormalities in long-term experimental diabetes. Diabetes, 41:286-293.
82. Geiger H, Bahner U, Vaaben W, et al. 1992. Effects of angiotensin-converting enzyme inhibition in diabetic rats with reduced renal function. J Lab Clin Med, 120:861-867.
83. O'Brien R, Cooper ME, Jerums G, Doyle AE. 1993. The effects of perindopril and triple therapy in a normotensive model of diabetic nephropathy. Diabetes, 42:604-609.

84. Brown SA, Walton CL, Crawford P, Bakris GL. 1993. Long-term effects of antihypertensive regimens on renal hemodynamics and proteinuria. Kidney Int, 43:1210-1218.

85. Anderson S, Jung FF, Ingelfinger JR. 1993. Renal renin-angiotensin system in diabetes: functional, immunohistochemical, and molecular biologic correlations. Am J Physiol, 265:F477-F486.

86. Remuzzi A, Perico N, Amuchastegui CS, Malanchini B, Mazerska M, Battaglia C, Bertani C, Remuzzi G. 1993. Short- and long-term effect of angiotensin II receptor blockade in rats with experimental diabetes. J Am Soc Nephrol, 4:40-49.

87. Wolf G, Ziyadeh N. 1997. The role of angiotensin II in diabetic nephropathy: emphasis on nonhemodynamic mechanisms. Am J Kidney Dis, 29:153-163.

88. Kasiske BL, Kalil RSN, Ma JZ, Liao M, Keane WF. 1993. Effect of antihypertensive therapy on the kidney in patients with diabetes: a meta-regression analysis. Ann Intern Med, 118:129-138.

89. Böhlen L, de Courten M, Weidmann P. 1994. Comparative study of the effect of ACE-inhibitors and other antihypertensive agents on proteinuria in diabetic patients. Am J Hypertension, 7:84S-92S.

90. Lewis EJ, Hunsicker LG, Bain RP, Rohde RD. 1993. The effect of angiotensin-converting-enzyme inhibition on diabetic nephropathy. New Engl J Med, 329:1456-1462.

33. THE ROLE OF GROWTH HORMONE, INSULIN-LIKE GROWTH FACTORS, EPIDERMAL GROWTH FACTOR AND TRANSFORMING GROWTH FACTOR β IN DIABETIC KIDNEY DISEASE: AN UPDATE

Allan Flyvbjerg, Charlotte Hill, Birgitte Nielsen, Henning Grønbæk,, Martin Bak, Thora Chistiansen, Ann Logan and Hans Ørskov
University of Aarhus, Aarhus Kommunehospital, Aarhus, Denmark
and Department of Medicine, University of Birmingham, Birmingham, UK
Medical Research Lab. M and ,Medical Department M (Diabetes and Endocrinology)

INTRODUCTION

Various growth factors have been proposed to be players in different areas of diabetes mellitus including a possible relationship to the characteristic changes in metabolism and development of complications. In particular, growth hormone (*GH*) and insulin-like growth factors (*IGFs*) system have a long and distinguished history with relation both to the diabetic metabolic aberration and the pathogenesis of diabetic angiopathy. The published evidence covering this area has recently been reviewed [1-3]. Further, substantial evidence has suggested that some growth factors (i.e. *GH* and *IGFs*, epidermal growth factor (*EGF*), transforming growth factor β (*TGF-β*), platelet derived growth factor (*PDGF*), tumor necrosis factor α (*TNF-α*) and fibroblastic growth factors (*FGFs*)) have conceivable effects on the development of renal complications in diabetes as reviewed in *The Kidney and Hypertension in Diabetes Mellitus, Second Edition, 1994* [4]. The present review is an update of the topic with emphasis on *three* of the above mentioned growth factor systems. The first part of the review presents an update for a definite role of the GH/IGF system in the pathogenesis of the renal changes in experimental diabetes with focus on the renoprotective effects of long-acting somatostatin analogues and GH-receptor antagonists. In the second and third part, an update of the literature is presented suggesting a causal role for EGF and TGF-β in the development of diabetic kidney disease.

GROWTH HORMONE (GH) AND INSULIN-LIKE GROWTH FACTORS (IGFS)

The GH/IGF system constitutes a complex system of peptides in the circulation, extracellular space and in most tissues. Essentially all members of the axis are present in the kidney and IGF-I mRNA and peptide have been demonstrated in collecting tubules and the thin limb of Henle's loop [5-7], specific IGF-I receptors have been demonstrated in glomeruli and tubules of the kidney [8,9] and, in addition, all six IGF binding proteins (IGFBPs) are present in the kidney [7,10-12]. Several of the components of the renal GH/IGF axis are increased in experimental diabetes and may be involved in early diabetic renal changes and possibly also in the development of long-term diabetic renal changes [for review see 13-15]. Thus, the *early* diabetic renal hypertrophy is preceded by a transient increase in kidney IGF-I content with a peak 24-48 hours after diabetes induction [16-18]. Further, IGF-I accumulation and renal hypertrophy are directly proportional to the blood glucose levels in rats [19]. The demonstrated increase in kidney IGF-I is not likely caused by local production, as IGF-I mRNA levels are unaltered during the phase of early kidney growth [18,20] or even decreased [21,22]. Changes in GH binding protein (GHBP), GH- and IGF-I receptor number and affinity have been investigated in early experimental diabetes and reported to be unchanged [14,23], however, in *long-term* diabetes a sustained increase in renal GHBP mRNA and IGF-I receptor mRNA is seen [14,20,22]. The possible role of IGFBPs in renal IGF-I accumulation and *early* renal growth has been examined in diabetic rats using Western ligand blotting [24]. Diabetes induction was followed by a transient local increase in a 30 kDa IGFBP species (containing IGFBP-1) in the kidney [24]. The transient increase in the IGFBPs occured in parallel with the transient increase in kidney IGF-I content and thus preceded the diabetic renal growth. In addition, an early and sustained increase in renal IGFBP-1 and IGFBP-5 mRNAs is seen in *long-term* diabetic rats with a diabetes duration for six months [7,14]. In conclusion, these experimental data indicate that GH, IGF-I, and IGFBPs are involved in the development of both early and late diabetic renal changes. Further, this knowledge has stimulated testing of existing drugs with specific action on the GH/IGF system and innovation in drug development with potential use in the treatment of diabetic nephropathy.

MANIPULATION OF THE ALTERED GH/IGF AXIS IN DIABETIC KIDNEY DISEASE

Long-acting somatostatin analogues

The initial idea that somatostatin and its long-acting analogues could be used in the treatment of subjects with diabetes mellitus is based on the expected benefit of suppressing elevated circulating GH levels in order to minimize their deleterious effects on diabetic metabolism and to inhibit or prevent development of long-term diabetic complications. The biological half-life of native somatostatin is too short to allow its use in clinical therapy and accordingly, long-acting somatostatin analogues (e.g. octreotide and lanreotide) have been developed and opened the possibility of performing experimental and clinical trials. In *short-term experimental diabetes* octreotide administration for seven days from diabetes onset completely inhibits the initial renal hypertrophy and the kidney IGF-I accumulation in rats [17]. Further, lanreotide in a dose similar to the octreotide dose given above has been demonstrated to inhibit renal glomerular growth as well [25]. When a lower octreotide dose is used a partial inhibition of the diabetes associated renal growth is seen, which may suggest a dose dependent effect of octreotide on renal IGF-I accumulation and diabetic renal growth [26]. Series of recent experiments has shown that early intervention with somatostatin analogues after diabetes onset seems crucial for achievement of full inhibitory effects on morphological changes. If initiation of octreotide treatment is postponed as short as 3 to 9 days after diabetes induction the early diabetic renal hypertrophy is only partly inhibited, indicating that early intervention with somatostatin analogues is important [27]. Similar results were observed in a study in which octreotide treatment was initiated for 3 weeks after a period of untreated diabetes for 3 or 6 months, as a tendency only towards a reduction in renal volume was observed [28]. The effects of somatostatin analogues on circulating and local IGFBPs in diabetes have only been examined sparsely. Lanreotide has been shown to inhibit the diabetes associated increase in serum 30 kDa IGFBP species (containing IGFBP-1) in rats and further to reduce serum IGFBP-3 [25]. In addition, octreotide inhibits the increased renal levels of IGFBP-1 mRNA levels in early experimental diabetes, with no effect on hepatic IGFBP-1 mRNA levels [29]. This is in contrast to the effect of octreotide on IGFBP-1 mRNA levels in non-diabetic rats, in which a dose dependent stimulatory effect of octreotide on hepatic IGFBP-1 mRNA is seen along with unchanged renal IGFBP-1 mRNA levels (30). Accordingly, it may be hypothesized that somatostatin analogues may prevent some of the classic early diabetic renal changes by inhibiting the renal IGF-I accumulation through mechanisms involving effects on renal IGFBPs. The effects of somatostatin analogue treatment on diabetic renal morphological and functional changes have also been examined in *long-term experimental diabetes*. Six months octreotide treatment from the day of diabetes induction is followed by significant reductions of increase in kidney weight, kidney IGF-I levels, and urinary albumin excretion (UAE) when compared to untreated diabetic rats [31]. In addition, diabetic rats treated for 5 weeks with octreotide from diabetes onset showed a reduction in renal glomerular growth [33]. However, when octreotide treatment for 14 weeks was initiated in unilaterally nephrectomized diabetic rats on the day of diabetes induction 3 days after the nephrectomy, no effect of octreotide treatment on renal hypertrophy, UAE or glomerular hyperfiltration was observed [33]. The lack of effect of octreotide treatment on renal hypertrophy in this situation may be due to the late intervention as IGF-I accumulation had already peaked in the remaining kidney following uninephrectomy [16]; or to the low octreotide dose used [16]. In studies by Igarashi et al. [34,35] octreotide treatment for 2-3 weeks was followed by diminished kidney hypertrophy and albuminuria in uninephrectomized-diabetic rats following an untreated diabetes period of 15 weeks. A recent study from our group aimed at examining the effect of 3 weeks treatment with octreotide and an angiotensin-converting enzyme (ACE)-inhibitor (captopril) either alone or in combination following 3 months of untreated diabetes [36]. Octreotide treatment alone and in combination with captopril induced a significant reduction in kidney weight compared to placebo treated diabetic animals [36]. Further, the combined treatment of octreotide and captopril was followed by a significant reduction in UAE compared to placebo treated diabetic rats giving evidence for a definite effect of the combined treatment with octreotide and captopril on manifest experimental diabetic renal changes [36].

Clinical studies of native somatostatin and its analogues and their possible effects on kidney function and hypertrophy have progressed since Vora et al. [37], using intravenous native somatostatin, observed an immediate reduction in urinary flow, renal plasma flow (RPF) and glomerular filtration rate (GFR) in control subjects and patients with insulin dependent diabetes mellitus (IDDM). Acute infusion (2 to 3 hours) of the somatostatin analogue, octreotide, to IDDM diabetic patients induced a reduction in RPF and GFR, and in addition plasma GH and glucagon decreased significantly [38]. However, in another study only a trend towards lowering GFR and no effect on serum GH was observed following octreotide infusion [39]. In more long-term studies octreotide administration for 12 weeks in eleven IDDM patients induced a significant decrease in the elevated GFR along with a reduction in total kidney volume. Three of the patients were reexamined 12 weeks after cessation of octreotide treatment, and their GFR had risen to the level at the start of the study [40]. No clinical studies have yet reported on the possible long-term effects of somatostatin analogues on UAE in IDDM patients.

GH-receptor antagonists

Recently, a series of highly specific antagonists of the GH action has been developed for the potential therapeutic use in various conditions, including diabetes mellitus. Initially it was shown that alteration of single amino acids in the third α-helix of bovine (b)GH (residues 109-126) results in a GH antagonist [41-43]. *In vitro* experiments showed that this new group of GH antagonists binds to the GH receptor with the same affinity as native GH, but *in vivo* a phenotypic dwarf animal characterized by low circulating IGF-I levels and a proportional body composition develops when the GH antagonist is expressed in transgenic mice [41-43]. Recent studies have reported renoprotective effects of two of these GH antagonists in long-term diabetic transgenic mice that express the GH antagonist (bGH-G119R or hGH-G120R) [44-46]. Compared with transgenic diabetic mice expressing wild-type bGH or bGH, the diabetic mice expressing GH antagonists showed lesser glomerular damage [44,45], no increase in total urine protein [44], no glomerular hypertrophy [46] and no increase in glomerular α1 type IV collagen mRNA levels [46]. The inhibitory effects of GH antagonists in transgenic mice were seen without alteration in glycemic control as similar levels in blood glucose, insulin and Hb_{A1c} were seen in the different diabetic animals expressing wild-type bGH, GH antagonists or bGH [44,45]. These studies support the hypothesis that GH (and IGFs) are involved in the pathogenesis of diabetic kidney disease in experimental diabetes. New studies including exogenous administration of GH antagonists to diabetic animals models are in progress to fully elucidate the usefulness of the GH antagonists as a potential therapeutic agent. No clinical studies have yet appeared on the effects of this new group of GH-receptor antagonists on metabolism and diabetic complications in diabetic patients.

EPIDERMAL GROWTH FACTOR (EGF)

The kidney is one of the main sites of EGF synthesis and recent studies have suggested that the kidney is also a target organ of EGF [47]. The presence of EGF receptors has been demonstrated in several segments of the nephron [48], and EGF administered *in vivo* systemically or directly into the renal artery increases urine flow and urinary sodium and potassium excretion [49]. The demonstration of acute effects of EGF on renal function
[50,51] opens some intriguing possibilities for a physiological role of EGF in the kidney. Although one study [47] reported reduced urinary EGF excretion after reduction of renal mass, others reported increased urinary EGF excretion [52], increased renal EGF synthesis and a transiently increased amount of immunoreactive EGF in distal kidney tubules after unilateral nephrectomy [53].

In *experimental diabetes* a possible role for EGF in the *early* renal enlargement has been proposed. In a study by Guh et al. [54] a pronounced elevation in diurnal urine EGF excretion was seen, while no significant change was observed in renal EGF within the first 7 days after induction of diabetes. These findings were confirmed in a recent study by Gilbert et al. [55] where unchanged levels of kidney and plasma EGF were reported, within the first week after induction of diabetes, along with a three fold increase in urinary EGF excretion. In addition, renal EGF mRNA as measured both by Northern blotting and in situ hybridization, was increased by 4-8 times [55]. These studies implicate that EGF may play a role as a renotropic factor in early experimental diabetes.

So far no studies have been published on changes in the renal EGF content or EGF excretion in *long-term experimental diabetes*. However, several cross-sectional clinical studies have studied the possible role of EGF in diabetic nephropathy by measuring the urinary excretion of EGF in IDDM patients with and without incipient/overt nephropathy [56-59] and in NIDDM patients with incipient nephropathy (60]. In general, reduced urinary excretion of EGF is found in patients with elevated UAE in comparison with non-diabetic controls [56,57]. A significant inverse correlation between urinary excretion of EGF and UAE was reported in two studies [56,57], while absent in one study [58]. A consistent finding is, however, that urinary excretion of EGF correlates positively with GFR [56,58] and creatinine clearance [59]. In a recent study in NIDDM patients with incipient diabetic nephropathy, the effect of an ACE-inhibitor (enalapril) and an calcium antagonist (nitrendipine) on UAE and urinary EGF excretion was examined [60]. Interestingly, enalapril significantly reduced UAE and increased urinary EGF excretion, while nitrendipine had no significant effect on any of these parameters [60]. These studies demonstrate that the urinary excretion of EGF diminished with increasing nephron impairment, and that renal tubular function, as judged by urinary EGF excretion, is reduced early in the development of diabetic kidney disease. The decrease in urinary

EGF excretion with decreasing renal function is not specific for the renal changes seen in diabetic patients as it is also seen in patients with various *non*-diabetic glomerulopathies [61].

TRANSFORMING GROWTH FACTOR β (TGF-β)

TGF-β is a prominent member of a family of cell regulatory proteins and is unique among growth factors in its broad effects on extracellular matrix. TGF-β is a 25 kDa polypeptide, synthesized as an inactive precursor protein which may bind to a 125 kDa TGF-β binding protein, and is proteolytically changed into its active form. The kidney is both producing TGF-β and a target of TGF-β action, as both mRNA TGF-β, the active protein, and TGF-β receptors have been demonstrated in all cell types of the glomerulus [62-64] and by proximal tubule renal cells [65,66]. *In vitro*, TGF-β has been shown to modulate extracellular matrix production and interestingly both glomerular mesangial and epithelial cells increase synthesis of extracellular matrix proteins including protoglycans, fibronectin, type IV collagen and laminin in response to TGF-β [67-69]. In addition, TGF-β inhibits the synthesis of collagenases and stimulates tissue production of metalloproteinase inhibitors [70-72]. Both these mechanisms could lead to a reduced degradation of ECM and possibly contribute to matrix accumulation.

Evidence has been published recently for TGF-β playing a role in different forms of kidney diseases characterized by changes in structure and ECM. In cultured glomerular cells obtained from immunologically induced glomerulonephritis, increased amounts of active TGF-β can be detected [73]. Furthermore, both the administration of an antibody raised against TGF-β [74] or decorin [75], a natural inhibitor of TGF-β, to glomerulonephritic rats suppresses glomerular matrix production and prevents matrix accumulation in injured glomeruli. In addition, there is evidence for TGF-β playing a role in the development of *diabetic nephropathy*. High glucose concentrations increase TGF-β1 mRNA levels in both cultured mesangial cells and proximal tubular cells in vitro [62-66]. Further, the elevated glucose levels in vitro stimulate TGF-β1 gene expression and bioactivity, cellular hypertrophy and collagen transcription in proximal tubules [65] in addition to increased mesangial production of heparan sulfate proteoglycan [76].

In addition to the in vitro experiments mentioned above interesting experiments have been published recently on changes in renal TGF-β in *early experimental diabetes* in vivo. In a study performed in STZ-diabetic rats, an increase in glomerular TGF-β mRNA was reported as early as 24 hours after the onset of hyperglycaemia [77]. The animals were followed for up to two weeks with a sustained rise for the whole period and a three-fold increase in glomerular TGF-β levels could be demonstrated by use of immunohistochemistry [77]. Intensive insulin treatment to normalize blood glucose levels attenuated the rise in glomerular TGF-β expression [77]. Increased renal levels of TGF-β mRNA in the early course of diabetes associated renal hypertrophy have also been described both in the non-obese diabetic (NOD) mouse [78,79] and the diabetic BB rat [78]. In addition, a sustained increase in glomerular TGF-β mRNA levels in *long-term STZ-diabetic rats* with a diabetes duration for up to 24 weeks has been described [62].

Two *clinical studies* have been published dealing with changes in the renal expression of the TGF-β system [80,81]. Initially increased TGF-β immunostaining was described in glomeruli obtained from diabetic subjects [80]. This observation was confirmed and further extended in a recent study, in which increased glomerular and tubulointerstitial levels of all three TGF-β isoforms were reported in diabetic nephropathy, but also in several other conditions characterized by accumulation of extracellular matrix (i.e. IgA nephropathy, focal and segmental glomerulosclerosis, crescentic glomerulonephritis and lupus nephritis) [81]. Further, a positive correlation between TGF-β, fibronectin and plasminogen activator inhibitor-1 levels in glomeruli and tubulointerstitium was reported [81]. These studies support the hypothesis
that glucose induced rise in renal TGF-β expression and peptide in the kidney may be responsible for some of the renal changes that precede the development of diabetic nephropathy.

MANIPULATION OF THE ALTERED TGF-β AXIS IN DIABETIC KIDNEY DISEASE

Neutralizing antibodies

Data supporting the hypothesis that the glucose induced rise in renal TGF-β expression and peptide may be responsible for some of the renal changes that follow the development of diabetic nephropathy, have been published in recent elegant studies using neutralizing
antibodies. *In vitro* the glucose mediated increase in type IV collagen synthesis in mesangial cells is dependent on the autocrine action of TGF-β1, as neutralizing antibodies to TGF-β attenuate the rise [82]. Further, in a recent study *in vivo*, administration of a neutralizing TGF-β1,2,3 antibody to STZ-diabetic mice for nine days attenuated the elevated renal TGF-β1 and TGF-β Type II receptor mRNA levels and reduced both the diabetes associated renal/glomerular growth and enhanced renal expression of collagen IV and fibronectin [83].

Angiotensin converting enzyme (ACE) inhibition

It has been suggested that activation of the renal TGF-β system in diabetes may be mediated, besides a direct stimulatory effect of hyperglycaemia *per se*, through activation of the renin-angiotensin system, because exposure of mesangial cells *in vitro* to angiotensin II stimulates the expression of TGF-β and extracellular matrix proteins [84]. Further a recent study examined the effect of an ACE-inhibitor (captopril) on high-glucose induced changes in the TGF-β system and growth in LLC-PK_1 cells, a porcine kidney cell line analogous to the proximal tubule cell [85]. In this cell system high glucose increased TGF-β1 mRNA, TGF-β Type receptor I and II protein expressions and cellular hypertrophy, while cellular mitogenesis was inhibited. Captopril dose-dependently decreased TGF-β Type receptor I and II protein expressions and cellular hypertrophy, increased cellular hyperplasia while TGF-β mRNA was unchanged [85]. In a recent *in vivo* study the effect of ACE-inhibition (ramipril) on the interstitial expression of TGF-β1 and matrix accumulation was examined in STZ-diabetic rats [86]. Using different techniques it was shown that the diabetes associated tubularinterstitial increase in TGF-β1 and collagen IV (both mRNA and protein) was prevented by ACE-inhibition. Further, a recent study from our group has aimed at examining the possible effect of ACE-inhibition on the intrarenal (i.e. in particular the glomerular) changes in all TGF-β isoforms (TGF-β 1,2,3) and TGF-β receptors (Type I, Type II, Type III) in experimental diabetes [87]. STZ-diabetic and non-diabetic rats were treated for two and four weeks with enalapril or placebo. Enalapril partially prevented the diabetes associated renal hypertrophy and fully the increase in 24h UAE. Further, enalapril treatment decreased the glomerular levels of TGF-β Type I and TGF-β Type III receptor isoforms to values below non-diabetic control level while treatment decreased the glomerular TGF-β Type II receptor level to almost undetectable levels. The glomerular expression of the TGF-β isoforms were not dramatically influenced by treatment. These findings suggest that the TGF-β axis operating through a complex intrarenal system, may be a significant mediator of the renal changes observed in experimental diabetes. Moreover, ACE-inhibition has pronounced inhibitory effects on the elevated levels of the TGF-β receptors required for intracellular signaling through this growth factor system. These findings suggest a possible new mechanism of action for ACE-inhibitors.

SUMMARY AND CONCLUSIONS

This review has collected recent facets of evidence for the significance of growth factors in the development of diabetic kidney disease. The knowledge we have today indicates that growth factors, through a complex system may be responsible for both *early* and *long-term* renal changes in experimental diabetes. Further insight into these processes may be useful in the future development of new antagonists for trial in the treatment of diabetic kidney disease.

ACKNOWLEDGEMENTS

The work was supported by the Danish Medical Research Council (#9700592), The Danish Kidney Foundation, the Ruth König Petersen Foundation, the Danish Diabetes Association, the Novo Foundation, the Nordic Insulin Foundation, the Aage Louis Petersen Foundation, the Institute of Experimental Clinical Research, University of Aarhus, Denmark and the Aarhus University-Novo Nordisk Center for Research in Growth and Regeneration (Danish Medical Research Council Grant #9600822).

REFERENCES

1. Flyvbjerg A, Frystyk J, Sillesen IB, Ørskov H. Growth hormone and insulin-like growth factor I in experimental and human diabetes. In: Alberti KGMM, Krall LP (Eds), Diabetes Annual/6, Elsevier Science Publishers B.V., Amsterdam 1991; pp. 562-590.
2. Growth hormone and insulin-like growth factor I in human and experimental diabetes. Flyvbjerg A, Ørskov H, Alberti KGMM (Eds), John Wiley & Sons, Chichester 1993; pp. 1-322.

3. International symposium on glucose metabolism and growth factors. Flyvbjerg A, Alberti KGMM, Froesch ER, De Meyts P, von zür Mühlen A, Ørskov H (Eds), Metabolism 1995; 44 [Suppl 4]: pp. 1-123.
4. Flyvbjerg A, Nielsen B, Skjærbæk C, Frystyk J, Grønbæk H, Ørskov H. Roles of growth factors in diabetic kidney disease. In: Mogensen CE (Ed), The Kidney and Hypertension in Diabetes Mellitus, 2nd Edition, Kluwer Academic Publishers, Boston, Dordrecht, London, 1994, pp. 233-243.
5. Bortz JD, Rotwein P, DeVol D, Bechtel PJ, Hansen VA, Hammerman MR. Focal expression of insulin-like growth factor I in rat kidney collecting duct. J Cell Biol 1988; 107: 811-819.
6. Flyvbjerg A, Marshall SM, Frystyk J, Rasch R, Bornfeldt KE, Arnqvist H, Jensen PK, Pallesen G, Ørskov H. Insulin-like growth factor I in initial renal hypertrophy in potassium-depleted rats. Am J Physiol 1992; 262: F1023-F1031.
7. Landau D, Chin E, Bondy C, Domene H, Roberts CT, Grønbæk H, Flyvbjerg A, LeRoith D. Expression of insulin-like growth factor binding proteins in the rat kidney: Effects of long-term diabetes. Endocrinology 1995; 136: 1835-1842.
8. Arnqvist HJ, Ballermann BJ, King GL. Receptors for and effects of insulin and IGF-I in rat glomerular mesangial cells. Am J Physiol 1988; 254: C411-C416.
9. Pillion DJ, Haskell JF, Meezan E . Distinct receptors for insulin-like growth factor I in rat renal glomeruli and tubules. Am J Physiol 1988; 255: E504-E512.
10. Chin E, Bondy C. Insulin-like growth factor system gene expression in the human kidney. J Clin Endocrinol Metab 1992; 75: 962-968.
11. Shimasaki S, Shimonaka M, Zhang HP, Ling N. Identification of five different insulin-like growth factor binding proteins (IGFBPs) from adult rat serum and molecular cloning of a novel IGFBP-5 in rat and human. J Biol Chem 1991; 266: 10646-10653.
12. Shimasaki S, Gao L, Shimonaka M, Ling N. Isolation and molecular cloning of insulin-like growth factor-binding protein-6. Mol Endocrinol 1991; 5: 938-948.
13. Flyvbjerg A. The growth hormone/insulin-like growth factor axis in the kidney: Aspects in relation to chronic renal failure. J Pediatr Endocrinol 1994; 7: 85-92.
14. Flyvbjerg A, Landau D, Domene H, Hernandez L, Grønbæk H, LeRoith D. The role of growth hormone, insulin-like growth factors (IGFs), and IGF-Binding proteins in experimental diabetic kidney disease. Metabolism 1995; 44: 67-71.
15. Flyvbjerg A. Role of growth hormone, insulin-like growth factors (IGFs) and IGF-binding proteins in the renal complications of diabetes. Kidney Int 1997; 52 [Suppl 60]: S12-S19.
16. Flyvbjerg A, Thorlacius-Ussing O, Næraa R, Ingerslev J, Ørskov H. Kidney tissue somatomedin C and initial renal growth in diabetic and uninephrectomized rats. Diabetologia 1988; 31: 310-314.
17. Flyvbjerg A, Frystyk J, Thorlacius-Ussing O, Ørskov H. Somatostatin analogue administration prevents increase in kidney somatomedin C and initial renal growth in diabetic and uninephrectomized rats. Diabetologia 1989; 32: 261-265.
18. Flyvbjerg A, Bornfeldt KE, Marshall SM, Arnqvist HJ, Ørskov H. Kidney IGF-I mRNA in initial renal hypertrophy in experimental diabetes in rats. Diabetologia 1990; 33: 334-338.
19. Flyvbjerg A, Ørskov H. Kidney tissue insulin-like growth factor I and initial renal growth in diabetic rats: relation to severity of diabetes. Acta Endocrinol (Copenh) 1990; 122: 374-378.
20. Werner H, Shen Orr Z, Stannard B, Burguera B, Roberts CT Jr, LeRoith D. Experimental diabetes increases insulin-like growth factor I and II receptor concentration and gene expression in kidney. Diabetes 1990; 39: 1490-1497.
21. Bornfeldt KE, Arnqvist HJ, Enberg B, Mathews LS, Norstedt G. Regulation of insulin-like growth factor-I and growth hormone receptor gene expression by diabetes and nutritional state in rat tissues. J Endocrinol 1989; 122: 651-656.
22. Weiss O, Anner H, Nephesh I, Alayoff A, Bursztyn M, Raz I. Insulin-like growth factor I (IGF-I) and IGF-I receptor gene expression in the kidney of chronically hypoinsulinemic rat and hyperinsulinemic rat. Metabolism 1995; 44: 982-986.
23. Marshall SM, Flyvbjerg A, Frystyk J, Korsgaard L, Ørskov H. Renal insulin-like growth factor I and growth hormone receptor binding in experimental diabetes and after unilateral nephrectomy in the rat. Diabetologia 1991; 34: 632-639.

24. Flyvbjerg A, Kessler U, Dorka B, Funk B, Ørskov H, Kiess W. Transient increase in renal insulin-like growth factor binding proteins during initial kidney hypertrophy in experimental diabetes in rats. Diabetologia 1992; 35: 589-593.
25. Grønbæk H, Nielsen B, Frystyk J, Flyvbjerg A, Ørskov H. Effect of lanreotide, a somatostatin analogue, on diabetic renal hypertrophy, kidney and serum IGF-I and IGF binding proteins. Exp Nephrol 1996; 4: 295-303.
26. Steer KA, Sochor M, Kunjara S, Doepfner W, McLean P. The effect of a somatostatin analogue (SMS 201-995) on the concentration of phosphoribosyl pyrophosphate and the activity of the pentose phosphate pathway in the early renal hypertrophy of experimental diabetes in the rat. Biochem Med Metab Biol 1988; 39: 226-233.
27. Grønbæk H, Nielsen B, Frystyk J, Ørskov H, Flyvbjerg A. Effect of octreotide on experimental diabetic renal and glomerular growth: Importance of early intervention. J Endocrinol 1995; 147: 95-102.
28. Grønbæk H, Nielsen B, Østerby R, Harris AG, Ørskov H, Flyvbjerg A. Effect of octreotide and insulin on manifest renal and glomerular hypertrophy and urinary albumin excretion in long-term experimental diabetes in rats. Diabetologia 1995; 38: 135-144.
29. Weiss O, Rubinger D, Nephesh I, Moshe R, Raz I. The influence of octreotide on the IGF system gene expression in the kidney of diabetic rats [Abstract]. Diabetologia 1995; 38: A206.
30. Flyvbjerg A, Schuller AGP, van Neck JW, Groffen C, Ørskov H, Drop SLS. Stimulation of hepatic insulin-like growth factor binding protein-1 and -3 gene expression by octreotide in rats. J Endocrinol 1995; 147: 545-551.
31. Flyvbjerg A, Marshall SM, Frystyk J, Hansen KW, Harris AG, Ørskov H. Octreotide administration in diabetic rats: effects on renal hypertrophy and urinary albumin excretion. Kidney Int 1992; 41: 805-812.
32. Iwasaki S. Octreotide suppresses the kidney weight and glomerular hypertrophy in diabetic rats. Nippon Jinzo Gakkai Shi 1993; 35: 247-255.
33. Muntzel M, Hannedouche T, Niesor R, Noel LH, Souberbielle JC, Lacour B, Drueke T. Long-term effects of a somatostatin analogue on renal haemodynamics and hypertrophy in diabetic rats. Clin Sci 1992; 83: 575-581.
34. Igarashi K, Ito S, Shibata A. Effect of a somatostatin analogue (SMS 201-995) on urinary albumin excretion in streptozotocin-induced diabetic rats. J Japan Diab Soc 1990; 33: 531-538.
35. Igarashi K, Nakazawa A, Tani N, Yamazaki M, Ito S, Shibata A. Effect of a somatostatin analogue (SMS 201-995) on renal function and excretion in diabetic rats. J Diab Compl 1991; 5: 181-183.
36. Grønbæk H, Vogel I, Lancranjan I, Flyvbjerg A, Ørskov H. Effect of octreotide, captopril, or insulin on manifest long-term experimental diabetic renal changes. Kidney Int 1998; in press.
37. Vora J, Owens DR, Luzio SD, Atiea J, Ryder R, Hayes TM. Renal response to intravenous somatostatin in insulin-dependent diabetic patients and normal subjects. J Clin Endocrinol Metab 1987; 64: 975-979.
38. Pedersen MM, Christensen SE, Christiansen JS, Pedersen EB, Mogensen CE, Ørskov H. Acute effects of a somatostatin analogue on kidney function in type 1 diabetic patients. Diab Med 1990; 7: 304-309.
39. Krempf M, Ranganathan S, Remy JP, Charbonnel B, Guillon J. Effect of a long acting somatostatin analogue (SMS 201-995) on high glomerular filtration rate in insulin dependent diabetic patients. Int J Clin Pharmacol Ther Toxicol 1990; 28: 309-311.
40. Serri O, Beauregard H, Brazeau P, Abribat T, Lambert J, Harris A, Vachon L. Somatostatin analogue, octreotide, reduces increased glomerular filtration rate and kidney size in insulin-dependent diabetes. JAMA 1991; 265: 888-892.
41. Chen WY, Wight DC, Wagner TE, Kopchick JJ. Expression of a mutated bovine growth hormone gene suppresses growth of transgenic mice. Proc Natl Acad Sci USA 1990; 87: 5061-5065.
42. Chen WY, Wight DC, Chen N-Y, Coleman TA, Wagner TE, Kopchick JJ. Mutations in the third α-helix of bovine growth hormone dramatically affect its intracellular distribution *in vitro* and growth enhancement in transgenic mice. J Biol Chem 1991; 266: 2252-2258.
43. Chen WY, White ME, Wagner TE, Kopchick JJ. Functional antagonism between endogenous mouse growth hormone (GH) and a GH analog results in dwarf transgenic mice. Endocrinology 1991; 129: 1402-1408.

44. Chen N-Y, Chen WY, Bellush L, Yang C-W, Striker LJ, Striker GE, Kopchick JJ. Effects of streptozotocin treatment in growth hormone (GH) and GH antagonist transgenic mice. Endocrinology 1995; 136: 660-667.
45. Chen N-Y, Chen WY, Kopchick JJ. A growth hormone antagonist protects mice against streptozotocin induced glomerulosclerosis even in the presence of elevated levels of glucose and glycated hemoglobin. Endocrinology 1996; 137: 5163-5165.
46. Liu Z-H, Striker LJ, Phillips C, Chen N-Y, Chen Y, Kopchick JJ, Striker GE. Growth hormone expression is required for the development of diabetic glomerulosclerosis in mice. Kidney Int 1995; 48 [Suppl 51]: S37-S38.
47. Olsen PS, Nexø E, Poulsen SS, Hansen HF, Kirkegaard P. Renal origin of rat urinary epidermal growth factor. Reg Pept 1984; 10: 37-45.
48. Gustavson B, Cowley G, Smith JA, Ozanne B. Cellular localization of human epidermal growth factor receptor. Cell Biol Int Rep 1984; 8: 649-658.
49. Scoggins BA, Butkus A, Coghlan JP, et al. In vivo cardiovascular, renal and endocrine effects of epidermal growth factor in sheep. In: Labrie F, Prouix L (Eds), Endocrinology, Elsevier Science Publishers B.V., Amsterdam 1984; pp. 573-576.
50. Stanton RC, Seifter JL. Epidermal growth factor rapidly activates the hexose monophosphate shunt in kidney cells. Am J Physiol 1988; 253: C267-C271.
51. Vehaskari VM, Hering-Smith KS, Moskowitz DW, Weirer ID, Hamm LL. Effect of epidermal growth factor on sodium transport in the cortical collecting tubules. Am J Physiol 1989; 256: F803-F809.
52. Jørgensen PE, Kamper A-L, Munck O, Strandgaard S, Nexø E. Urinary excretion of epidermal growth factor in living human kidney doners and their recipients. Eur J Clin Invest 1995; 25: 442-446.
53. Jennische E, Andersson G, Hansson HA. Epidermal growth factor is expressed by cells in the distal tubulus during postnephrectomy renal growth. Acta Physiol Scand 1987; 129: 449-450.
54. Guh JY, Lai YH, Shin SJ, Chuang LY, Tsai JH. Epidermal growth factor in renal hypertrophy in streptozotocin-diabetic rats. Nephron 1991; 59: 641-647.
55. Gilbert RE, Cox A, McNally PG, Wu LL, Dziadek M, Cooper ME, Jerums G. Increased epidermal growth factor in experimental diabetes related renal growth. Diabetologia 1997; 40: 778-785.
56. Mathiesen ER, Nexø E, Hommel E, Parving H-H. Reduced urinary excretion of epidermal growth factor in incipient and overt diabetic nephropathy. Diab Med 1989; 6: 121-126.
57. Dagogo-Jack S, Marshall SM, Kendall-Taylor P, Alberti KGMM. Urinary excretion of human epidermal growth factor in the various stages of diabetic nephropathy. Clin Endocrinol (Oxf) 1989; 31: 167-173.
58. ter Meulen CG, Bilo HJ, van Kamp GJ, Gans RO, Donker AJ. Urinary epidermal growth factor excretion is correlated to renal function loss per se and not to the degree of diabetic renal failure. Netherlands J Med 1994; 44: 12-17.
59. Lev-Ran A, Hwang DL, Miller JD, Josefsberg Z. Excretion of epidermal growth factor (EGF) in diabetes. Clin Chim Acta 1990; 192: 201-206.
60. Josefsberg Z, Ross SA, Lev-Ran A, Hwang DL. Effects of enalapril and nitrendipine on the excretion of epidermal growth factor and albumin in hypertensive NIDDM patients. Diab Care 1995; 15: 690-693.
61. Mattila AL, Pasternack A, Viinikka L, Perheentupa B. Subnormal concentrations of urinary epidermal growth factor in patients with kidney disease. J Clin Endocrinol Metab 1986; 62: 1180-1183.
62. Nakamura T, Fukui M, Ebihara E, Osada S, Nagaoka I, Tomino Y, Koide H. mRNA expression of growth factors in glomeruli from diabetic rats. Diabetes 1993; 42: 450-456.
63. Ziyadeh FN, Chen Y, Davila A, Goldfarb S. Self limited stimulation of mesangial cell growth in high glucose: autocrine activation of TGF-β reduces proliferation but increases mesangial matrix. Kidney Int 1992; 42: 647-656.
64. Choi ME, Eung-Gook K, Ballerman BJ. Rat mesangial cell hypertrophy in response to transforming growth factor β1. Kidney Int 1993; 44: 948-958.
65. Ziyadeh FN, Snipes ER, Watanabe M, Alvarey RJ, Goldfarb S, Haverty TP. High glucose induces cell hypertrophy and stimulates collagen gene transcription in proximal tubule. Am J Physiol 1990; 259: F704-F714.

66. Rocco MV, Chen Y, Goldfarb S, Ziyadeh FN. Elevated glucose stimulates TGF-β gene expression and bioactivity in proximal tubules. Kidney Int 1992; 41: 107-114.
67. Nakamura T, Miller D, Rouslahti E, Border WA. Production of extracellular matrix by glomerular epithelial cells is regulated by transforming growth factor β1. Kidney Int 1992; 41: 1213-1221.
68. Humes HD, Nakamura T, Cieslinski DA, Miller D, Emmons RV, Border WA. Role of protoglycans and cytoskeleton in the effects of TGF-β1 on renal proximal tubule cells. Kidney Int 1993; 43: 575-584.
69. Roberts AB, McCune BK, Sporn MB. TGF-β1: Regulation of extracellular matrix. Kidney Int 1992; 41: 557-559.
70. Davies M, Thomas GJ, Martin J, Lovett DH. The purification and characterisation of a glomerular basement membrane degrading neutral proteinase from the rat mesangial cells. Biochem J 1988; 251: 419-425.
71. Edwards DR, Murphy G, Reynolds JJ, Whitman SE, Docherty AJP, Angel P, Heath JK. Transforming growth factor beta modulates the expression of collagenase and metalloproteinase inhibitor [Abstract]. EMBO J 1987; 6: 1899.
72. Lovett DH, Marti HP, Martin J, Grond J, Kashfarian DH. Transforming growth factor β1 stimulates mesangial cell synthesis of the 72 kD type IV collagenase independent of TIMP-1 [Abstract]. J Am Soc Nephrol 1991; 1: 578.
73. Okuda S, Languino LR, Ruoslahti E, Border WA. Elevated expression of transforming growth factor-β and proteoglycan production in experimental glomerulonephritis. Possible role in expansion of the mesangial matrix. J Clin Invest 1990; 86: 453-462.
74. Border WA, Okuda S, Languino LR, Sporn MB, Ruoslahti E. Suppression of experimental glomerulonephritis by antiserum against transforming growth factor β1. Nature 1990; 346: 371-374.
75. Border WA, Noble NA, Yamamoto T, Harper JR, Yamaguchi Y, Pierschbacher MD, Ruoslahti E. Natural inhibitor of transforming growth factor-β protects against scarring in experimental kidney disease. Nature 1992; 360: 361-364.
76. Kolm V, Sauer U, Olgemoller B, Schleicher ED. High glucose-induced TGF-β1 regulates mesangial production of heparan sulphate proteoglycan. Am J Physiol 1996; 70: F812-F821.
77. Shankland SJ, Scholey JW. Expression of transforming grwoth factor β1 during diabetic renal hypertrophy. Kidney Int 1994; 46: 430-442.
78. Sharma K, Ziyadeh FN. Renal hypertrophy is associated with upregulation of TGF-β1 gene expression in diabetic BB rat and NOD mouse. Am J Physiol 1994; 67: F1094-F1101.
79. Pankewycz OG, Guan J-X, Kline Bolton W, Gomez A, Benedict JF. Renal TGF-β regulation in spontaneously diabetic NOD mice with correlations in mesangial cells. Kidney Int 1994; 46: 748-758.
80. Yamamoto T, Nakamura T, Noble NA, Ruoslahti E, Border WA. Expression of transforming growth factor is elevated in human and experimental diabetic glomerulopathy. Proc Natl Acad Sci USA 1993; 90: 1814-1818.
81. Yamamoto T, Noble NA, Cohen AH, Nast CC, Hishida A, Gold LI, Border WA. Expression of transforming growth factor-β isoforms in human glomerular diseases. Kidney Int 1996; 49: 461-469.
82. Ziyadeh FN, Sharma K, Ricksen N, Wolf G. Stimulation of collagen gene expression and protein synthesis in murine mesangial cells by high glucose is mediated by autocrine activation of transforming growth factor β. J Clin Invest 1994; 93: 536-542.
83. Sharma K, Jin Y, Guo J, Ziyadeh FN. Neutralization of TGF-β by anti-TGF-β antibody attenuates kidney hypertrophy and the enhanced extracellular matrix gene expression in STZ-induced diabetic mice. Diabetes 1996; 45: 522-530.
84. Kagami S, Border WA, Miller DE, Noble NA. Angiotensin II stimulates extracellular matrix protein synthesis through induction of transforming growth factor-β expression in rat glomerular mesangial cells. J Clin Invest 1994; 93: 2431-2437.
85. Guh JY, Yang ML, Yang YL, Chang CC, Chuang LY. Captopril reverses high-glucose-induced growth effects on LLC-PK_1 cells partly by decreasing transforming growth factor-β receptor protein expression. J Am Soc Nephrol 1996; 7: 1207-1215.

86. Gilbert RE, Cox A, Wu LL, Allen TJ, Hulthen L, Jerums G, Cooper ME. Expression of transforming growth factor β1 and type IV collagen in the renal tubulointerstitium in experimental diabetes: effects of angiotensin converting enzyme inhibition. Diabetes 1998; in press.
87. Hill C, Logan A, Grønbæk H, Sheppard MC, Flyvbjerg A. Effect of ACE-inhibition on the altered intrarenal TGF-β system in experimental diabetic nephropathy [Abstract]. Nephrol Dialysis Transpl 1998; in press.

34. TRANSFORMING GROWTH FACTOR-BETA AND OTHER CYTOKINES IN EXPERIMENTAL AND HUMAN DIABETIC NEPHROPATHY

Fuad N. Ziyadeh, Dong Cheol Han and Andras Mogyorosi
Penn Center for Molecular Studies of Kidney Diseases, Renal Electrolyte and Hypertension Division, Department of Medicine, University of Pennsylvania, Philadelphia, PA, USA

EFFECTS OF HIGH AMBIENT GLUCOSE IN RENAL CELL CULTURE

Increased renal extracellular matrix production in diabetes is most likely the result of increased synthesis and/or decreased degradation rates [1-3]. To model the effects of the diabetic milieu on the kidney, various renal cell lines have been investigated under high ambient glucose concentrations in tissue culture. High glucose stimulates proximal tubular cell hypertrophy [4] and modulates mesangial cell growth [5]. It also stimulates the production of connective tissue molecules such as fibronectin and collagens in proximal tubular cells and in glomerular mesangial, epithelial, and endothelial cells [4, 6-12]. It is noteworthy that periodically elevated glucose levels in rat mesangial cell culture increase collagen production to a greater extent than a sustained elevation in ambient glucose concentration [13]. This may closely mimic the fluctuations of blood glucose levels in vivo. The seminal factor for renal cell damage by high glucose is likely to be intracellular high glucose accumulation and metabolism rather than simply the extracellular, ambient hyperglycemia. Rat mesangial cells transfected with the human glucose transporter GLUT1 gene demonstrate stimulated mesangial matrix synthesis despite physiologic extracellular glucose concentration [14].

Other effects of high glucose on extracellular matrix metabolism in human glomerular mesangial and glomerular epithelial cells involve a significant decrease in heparan sulfate proteoglycan (HSPG) synthesis and alterations in the sulfation pattern [15, 16]. This may cause profound changes in charge- and size-permselectivity of the glomerular basement membrane (GBM) in vivo that are believed to contribute to diabetic proteinuria.

Mogensen, C.E. (ed.), THE KIDNEY AND HYPERTENSION IN DIABETES MELLITUS.

ACTIVATION OF THE TGF-β SYSTEM IN RENAL CELLS CULTURED IN HIGH GLUCOSE

Several studies have concluded that high glucose induces biochemical alterations that stimulate the production of transforming growth factor-β (TGF-β) and other intermediary growth factors [17-20]. There are three known mammalian isoforms of TGF-β (β1, β2, and β3) [21]. They share similar actions in vitro but not in vivo [22, 23]. This is in part a consequence of differences in developmental regulation and diverse tissue expression. TGF-β is secreted as latent complexes, and these in turn exist in soluble forms or bound to extracellular matrix constituents [24, 25]. The latent complex is composed of the mature TGF-β dimer and the latency-associated peptide (LAP) which are products of the same gene [26]. Activation of latent TGF-β in vivo is largely controlled by proteases (e.g., plasmin) to cleave the LAP from the bioactive TGF-β dimer [27]. In certain tissues including glomeruli, the latent complex exists in association with the product of another gene, the latent TGF-β binding protein (LTBP). In the kidney, tubular epithelial cells secrete the small latent complex (mature TGF-β1 + LAP), while glomerular parenchymal and arteriolar cells secrete the large latent complex (mature TGF-β1 + LAP + LTBP) [28]. This pattern of tissue expression in the kidney implies differences in functional regulation.

Virtually every cell type produces TGF-β and expresses receptors for it. The Type I and Type II TGF-β signaling receptors are unique because their cytoplasmic regions contain a serine/threonine kinase domain [29]. The Type I receptor contains the serine/glycine rich (GS) domain preceding the kinase domain. The Type III receptor (betaglycan) has a very short cytoplasmic domain without intrinsic signal transduction activity and functions mostly to enhance the affinity of TGF-β to the Type II receptor. The first step in signaling is the engagement of the ligand with the Type II receptor. The Type I receptor then binds the ligand-bound Type II receptor forming a heterotetrameric complex. Phosphorylation of the Type I receptor at its GS domain by the Type II receptor is a sine qua non event in TGF-β signaling [30]. Both serine-threonine kinase activities in the TGF-β receptor complex are required for the profibrotic and antiproliferative actions of TGF-β [29, 31]. It has also become clear recently that TGF-β receptors transduce their signals through novel intracellular proteins, the products of the *Mad* genes *(Mothers against decapentaplegic)* in drosophila and the related *Sma* genes in *C. elegans* which are members of the growing family of intracellular transducing molecules in the TGF-β/activins/BMP (Bone Morphogenetic Proteins) superfamily [32, 33]. According to the recent change in the nomenclature, the mammalian homologues of Mad and Sma molecules are now called Smad proteins. In humans, Smad2, Smad3 and Smad4 may function as downstream transducing molecules in the TGF-β receptor system [34]. On the other hand, Smad7 is capable of antagonizing TGF-β signaling by associating with the TGF-β receptor [35].

TGF-β promotes renal cell hypertrophy and stimulates the glomerular and tubular production of a host of extracellular matrix molecules [1]. In addition, TGF-β inhibits the breakdown of newly synthesized extracellular matrix by stimulating the production of protease inhibitors (e.g. plasminogen activator inhibitors) [36], and by decreasing the production of matrix-degrading proteases (collagenase and stromelysin). There is ample evidence that, at least in part, the prosclerotic and hypertrophic effects of high ambient glucose in cultures of glomerular mesangial [5, 9], glomerular epithelial [12], and proximal tubular cells [4, 37] are mediated by increased production and activation of TGF-β[5, 9, 38]. Furthermore, high glucose upregulates gene expression of TGF-β in human mesangial [39] and proximal tubular [40] cells. Additionally, high ambient glucose upregulates TGF-β receptor mRNAs and proteins in cultured murine mesangial and porcine LLC-PK1 tubular epithelial cells [41, 42]. Neutralizing anti-TGF-β antibodies reverse the downregulation of collagenase activity in rat mesangial cells grown in high glucose concentration [43]. TGF-β1 antisense oligonucleotides [11] as well as TGF-β neutralizing antibodies [5, 9, 12, 39] attenuate the increased synthesis of extracellular matrix as well as the inhibition of cell proliferation caused by high ambient glucose concentrations.

TGF-β IN EXPERIMENTAL DIABETIC KIDNEY DISEASE

Elevated renal TGF-β mRNA and protein levels have been found in various experimental animal models of insulin-dependent diabetes mellitus [44]. In streptozotocin (STZ)-diabetic rats the increased mRNA and protein levels of TGF-β1 and type IV collagen were demonstrated by in situ hybridization and immunohistochemistry within 7 days of diabetes [45]. Similarly, renal cortical TGF-β expression is upregulated early in the course of diabetes in other models of spontaneous type 1 diabetes mellitus, such as in the BB rat and the NOD mouse within a few days of the development of diabetes [46]. This event is coincident with the development of kidney hypertrophy [46]. The development of renal hypertrophy is likely linked to the increased expression of TGF-β1 and the Type II TGF-β receptor in the mouse kidney [47]. TGF-β was found to be upregulated not only in the early but also in later stages of the disease in spontaneous and STZ-induced diabetic animals [48-51]. Moreover, STZ-induced diabetes in rats results in decreased activity of glomerular cathepsin and metalloprotease, factors which contribute to accumulation of extracellular matrix molecules [52]. In concordance with this finding, ex vivo glomeruli from STZ-diabetic rats for up to 40 weeks of diabetes demonstrate persistently upregulated TGF-β1 mRNA and protein levels in association with a relentless increase in extracellular matrix components [53-56]. The role of hyperglycemia in the upregulation of renal TGF-β and extracellular matrix molecules can be demonstrated by the attenuation of the expression of these molecules in the kidney cortex [47] and the glomerulus [45] after high-dose insulin treatment.

The importance of the renal TGF-β system in diabetic kidney disease is demonstrated by the significant attenuation of glomerular and renal hypertrophy achieved by short-term treatment (9 days) of STZ-diabetic mice with neutralizing monoclonal antibodies against TGF-β [47]. It is interesting to note that in this model, the mRNA expression of TGF-β as well as the Type II TGF-β receptor in the renal cortex is increased as early as 3 days after the onset of diabetes, and this is associated with increased urinary levels of total (active plus latent) TGF-β [47]. The renal upregulation of the alpha1 chain of type IV collagen and fibronectin mRNAs is significantly attenuated by intraperitoneal treatment of the diabetic mice with anti-TGF-β antibodies [47]. Clearly, a long-term study with administration of anti-TGF-β antibodies into diabetic animals is needed to further delineate the putative importance of the renal TGF-β system in chronic manifestations of diabetic kidney disease such as glomerulosclerosis and tubulointerstitial fibrosis.

HUMAN DIABETIC KIDNEY DISEASE AND TGF-β

The renal TGF-β system has been demonstrated to be upregulated in studies examining ex vivo kidney tissue derived from patients with diabetic nephropathy. Immunostaining for the three isotypes of TGF-β is increased in both the glomeruli and the tubulointerstitium in patients with established diabetic kidney disease [53, 57, 58]. TGF-β immunostaining is also enhanced in other renal diseases characterized by progressive tubulointerstitial fibrosis, in association with increased staining of the extracellular matrix proteins tenascin and fibronectin whose production is also TGF-β-dependent [57]. In addition to immunostaining, renal biopsy specimens from patients with diabetic kidney disease also show markedly increased glomerular expression of TGF-β mRNA by reverse transcriptase/polymerase chain reaction [59]. The level of glomerular TGF-β mRNA expression correlates closely with the degree of hyperglycemia, as measured by glycated hemoglobin, and by the severity of the sclerosis index.

A recent study [60] was designed to determine if diabetic patients demonstrate enhanced renal production of TGF-β. Aortic, renal vein, and urinary levels of TGFβ were measured in 14 type 2 diabetic and 11 non-diabetic control patients undergoing elective coronary artery catheterization. Renal blood flow was measured in all patients to calculate net mass balance of TGF-β across the kidney vascular bed. Diabetic patients demonstrated net renal production of immunoreactive TGF-β1 whereas non-diabetic patients demonstrated net renal extraction of circulating TGF-β1. Urinary levels of immunoreactive TGF-β were also significantly increased in the diabetic patients compared with non-diabetic controls. However, the diabetic patients exhibited substantial net renal production of TGF-β which translates into higher TGF-β concentrations in the renal veins and in the urine. Judging from the results of this study it is highly likely that diabetes as a disease is associated with increased net renal production of TGFβ1. The details of this phenomenon and the exact contribution of the different renal cells to TGFβ1 production will need to be investigated in future studies.

OTHER CYTOKINES IN DIABETIC RENAL DISEASE

In vitro studies recently demonstrated the importance of other growth factors in diabetic renal disease. These include platelet-derived growth factor (PDGF), basic fibroblast growth factor (bFGF), prostanoids, insulin-like growth factor-1, and angiotensin II (AII), and vascular endothelial growth factor (reviewed in [20]). Some features of these mediators will be highlighted here.

PDGF: PDGF-B expression is upregulated in glomeruli from diabetic rats [61]. PDGF is implicated in the link between high glucose levels and the TGF-β pathway. Studies in human mesangial cells have found that antibodies to PDGF inhibit high glucose-induced stimulation of TGF-β1 mRNA [39]. A study in human proximal tubular cells found that high ambient glucose was a sufficient stimulus to increase TGF-β1 mRNA levels, but that PDGF was required to cause secretion and bioactivity of TGF-β protein [40]. Of interest is that expression of the PDGF-β receptor is increased in mesangial and other vascular cells (such as vascular smooth muscle and capillary endothelial cells) exposed to high ambient glucose [62]. PDGF may also play a role in mediating glycation-stimulated matrix production in mesangial cells [63]. Neutralizing anti-PDGF antibody reduces the expression of α1(IV) collagen mRNA which is induced by advanced glycation-end (AGE) products in cultured mouse mesangial cells [64].

Endothelins: Glomerular expression of endothelin-1 (ET-1) mRNA is increased in STZ-diabetic rats [65] and urinary level of ET-1 is elevated in the diabetic BB rat [65]. An endothelin receptor A antagonist, FR139317, when administered to STZ-diabetic rats, attenuates the glomerular hyperfiltration and urinary protein excretion, and decreases glomerular mRNA levels of collagens, laminins, tumor necrosis factor (TNF)-alpha, PDGF-B, TGF-β, and bFGF [66]. Endothelin levels are higher in type 2 diabetic patients than the general population [67]; levels in type 2 diabetic patients with retinopathy are even higher than those without retinopathy. Treatment with the ACE inhibitor captopril reduces ET-1 levels in such patients [68]. The mechanism of ET-1 stimulation in diabetes remains to be established but is likely due to multiple factors including AII.

AII: An important concept in diabetes research has been the elucidation that AII is not only a vasoconstrictor which is crucial in mediating intraglomerular hypertension but it also behaves as a growth factor that can mediate some of the hypertrophic and profibrotic changes that are characteristic of diabetic renal disease (reviewed in [18]). Tissue culture studies have demonstrated that AII stimulates TGF-β production in proximal tubular cells [69] and mesangial cells [70]. The renal protective effect of angiotensin converting enzyme inhibitors [71, 72] may perhaps be partly related to the blockade of AII-induced TGF-β production in renal cells [69, 70]. Furthermore, captopril reverses the high-glucose-induced growth effects on LLC-PK1 cells in culture, partly by decreasing TGF-β receptor protein expression [42].

Thromboxane: Studies in experimental animal models have demonstrated increased renal thromboxane expression [73] and urinary excretion of thromboxane B2 shortly after the onset of diabetes [74-76]. The source of increased thromboxane production may be the diabetic glomerulus [77] and/or infiltrating platelets [78], however the mechanism of stimulation of thromboxane production in diabetes is not known. Addition of thromboxane analogues to mesangial cells in culture results in stimulation of fibronectin production [79], which appears to be mediated by protein kinase C (PKC) activation [80]. Inhibitors of thromboxane synthesis and its receptor have been found to ameliorate diabetes-induced albuminuria [77, 81], mesangial matrix expansion [77], but may not prevent thickening of the GBM [77, 82].

It should be noted that exogenous prostaglandin E_2 (PGE_2) or drugs capable of increasing endogenous PGE_2 dose-dependently decrease the extracellular matrix proteins and their mRNAs as well as TGF-β gene expression in the culture of rat mesangial cells [83]. The net balance between the actions of vasoconstrictive and vasodilatory eicosanoids may determine whether TGF-β bioactivity is enhanced or diminished.

IGF-1: A role for insulin-like growth factor-1 (IGF-1) in diabetic hypertrophy has been suggested [84, 85]. Continuos, 12-week subcutaneous infusion of the somatostatin analogue octreotide, which antagonizes the effects of growth hormone and IGF-1, has been reported to reduce renal volume and glomerular hyperfiltration in 11 patients with normoalbuminuric normotensive type 1 diabetic patients [86]. Growth hormone may also play a role in mediating diabetic renal pathology. Transgenic mice overexpressing growth hormone have renal and glomerular hypertrophy with associated glomerulosclerosis similar to that of diabetic nephropathy [87]. There is likely an important interaction or "cross-talk" between various growth factors, such as TGF-β, IGF-1, and PDGF, that may promote diabetic renal pathology (reviewed in [17]).

MECHANISMS OF RENAL UPREGULATION OF THE TGF-β SYSTEM IN THE DIABETIC STATE IN RELATIONSHIP TO OTHER MEDIATORS

Under high ambient glucose conditions, there are several interrelated alterations/crosstalk amongst various growth factors and signal transduction pathways related to autocrine/paracrine or even endocrine mechanisms. In general, the effects of high glucose concentration on renal cells may arise as a consequence of increased flux of glucose metabolism through the polyol pathway [88], increased de novo synthesis of diacylglycerol (DAG) and subsequent activation of PKC [89, 90], or increased non-enzymatic glycation activity [91, 92].

The mechanism underlying high glucose induced upregulation of the TGF-β1 system is predominantly regulated at a transcriptional level [93]. The promoter of human TGF-β1 has multiple AP-1-like consensus sites which are responsive to phorbol-ester/PKC stimulation [94]. High ambient glucose increases DAG content and activates PKC in diabetic glomeruli and mesangial cells [75, 80, 89, 95]. Phorbol esters and DAG activate PKC by increasing PKC's membrane affinity [96]. Increased DAG activates PKC which may then lead to activation of the mitogen-activated protein (MAP) kinase cascade [97] and the subsequent increased production of the AP-1 transcription complex (Jun and Fos) [98]. The AP-1 binding sequence is essential for regulation of the promoter activity of many relevant genes including, for example, the alpha2 chain of collagen type I [99] and TGF-β itself [94]. The mRNA level of *c-fos* is increased transiently within 24 hours and *c-jun* expression is increased persistently for 7 days in glomeruli isolated from STZ-diabetic rats [100]. Importantly, Kim et al have demonstrated that TGF-β1 protein positively autoregulates the expression of TGF-β1 mRNA in an AP-1-dependent fashion [101]. This positive feed-back loop greatly exaggerates the profibrogenic potential of TGF-β1 in progressive kidney diseases such diabetic nephropathy. Recent studies in STZ-diabetic rats have demonstrated marked attenuation of glomerular overexpression of mRNAs encoding TGF-β1, collagen type IV and fibronectin following chronic treatment with a novel PKC-beta selective inhibitor [51].

The trigger of chronic stimulation of TGF-β may also be related to the presence of protein glycation in long-standing diabetes [102]. Administration of AGE-modified proteins to normal mice elevates the mRNA levels of TGF-β1, alpha1(IV) collagen, and laminin B1, effects which are reversible by concomitant aminoguanidine therapy [103]. Exposure to glycated LDL increases TGF-β1 and fibronectin mRNA levels in cultured murine mesangial cells; the increased fibronectin message is reversible with anti-TGF-β antibody treatment [104]. Mesangial cells have been demonstrated to have specific receptors for AGE, which may result in enhanced matrix and cytokine production [64, 105].

Vasoactive humoral factors such as AII (reviewed in [18]), endothelins, and altered prostaglandin metabolism have all been implicated in the pathogenesis of diabetic nephropathy, and all these factors may upregulate the TGF-β/TGF-β receptor system in the diabetic kidney (reviewed in [17, 19]). As reviewed above, endothelins may stimulate TGF-β production because endothelin receptor antagonists decrease the overexpression of glomerular TGF-β1 mRNA in diabetic rats [66]. Thromboxane has also been demonstrated to stimulate TGF-β production in mesangial cells [80]. AII is also capable of stimulating TGF-β production in proximal tubular and mesangial cell cultures [69, 70].

In addition to the metabolic factors listed above, hemodynamic and mechanical forces are also operative in the diabetic state. Cyclic stretching/relaxation of mesangial cells in culture, which closely mimics the increased glomerular pressure in vivo [106-108], has been demonstrated to be associated with increased synthesis of TGF-β and extracellular matrix molecules. Fluid shear stress increases TGF-β1 mRNA and the synthesis of the active form of TGF-β in cultured bovine aortic endothelial cells [109].

Concluding Remarks: The characteristic lesions of diabetic nephropathy such as renal hypertrophy, increased glomerular hypertension, and altered extracellular matrix metabolism may be intimately related to the effects of high ambient glucose on various growth factors and cytokines that are increased locally or in the circulation. Recent studies using cell culture techniques and experimental animal models have provided important insight into the pathogenetic mechanisms of diabetic nephropathy (Table 34-1). Much attention has been devoted to identifying the role of TGF-β as a possible mediator of kidney disease. The data we have reviewed strongly support the hypothesis that elevated production and/or activity of TGF-β in the kidney is an important mediator of diabetic renal hypertrophy and of extracellular matrix expansion in experimental as well as human diabetic nephropathy. Ongoing genetic studies linking cytokines and growth factors especially the TGF-β/TGF-β receptor system may further shed light on the predictability of diabetic nephropathy in the population at risk, and beyond current practices [110].

Table 34-1: Mediators of Diabetic Renal Disease:

I.	Genetic predisposition
II.	Intra-renal hemodynamic stress*
II.	Metabolic perturbations
	A. Non-enzymatic glycation of circulating or structural proteins
	Amadori-glucose adducts*
	Advanced glycosylation end-products ('AGE')*
	B. Activation of pathways of glucose metabolism
	Polyol pathway (increased sorbitol)
	Pentose phosphate shunt (increased UDP glucose)
	de novo synthesis of diacylglycerol and stimulation of protein kinase C*
	Disordered *myo*-inositol metabolism
	Altered cellular redox state (increased $NADPH/NADP^+$, $NADH/NAD^+$)
	Oxidant injury*
	C. Activation of intra-renal cytokines and growth factors
	transforming growth factor-β
	angiotensin II**
	endothelins**
	thromboxane**
	platelet-derived growth factor**
	insulin-like growth factor-1

* Factors known to activate transforming growth factor-β

** Factors known to activate both protein kinase C and transforming growth factor-β

ACKNOWLEDGMENTS

Supported in part by a fellowship grant from the Juvenile Diabetes Foundation International (A.M.), National Institutes of Health grants (DK-44513 and DK-45191 to F.N.Z., and training grant DK-07006), and the DCI-RED Fund. Dr. D. C. Han is visiting scholar at the University of Pennsylvania and is supported by the Hyonam Kidney Laboratory, Soon Chun Hyang University, Seoul, Korea.

REFERENCES:

1. Ziyadeh FN: The extracellular matrix in diabetic nephropathy. *Am J Kid Dis* 22:736-744, 1993.
2. Ziyadeh FN: Renal tubular basement membrane and collagen type IV in diabetes mellitus. *Kidney Int* 43:114-120, 1993.
3. Cohen MP, and Ziyadeh FN: Role of Amadori-modified nonenzymatically glycated serum proteins in the pathogenesis of diabetic nephropathy. *J Am Soc Nephrol* 7:1-8, 1996.
4. Ziyadeh FN, Snipes ER, Watanabe M, Alvarez RJ, Goldfarb S, and Haverty TP: High glucose induces cell hypertrophy and stimulates collagen gene transcription in proximal tubule. *Am J Physiol* 259:F704-F714, 1990.
5. Wolf G, Sharma K, Chen Y, Ericksen M, and Ziyadeh FN: High glucose-induced proliferation in mesangial cells is reversed by autocrine TGF-b. *Kidney Int* 42:647-656, 1992.
6. Ayo SH, Radnik R, Garoni JA, and Kreisberg J: High glucose increases diacylglycerol mass and activates protein kinases C in mesangial cell culture. *Am J Physiol* 261:F571-F577, 1991.
7. Ayo SH, Radnik RA, Glass II WF, Garoni JA, Rampt ER, Appling DR, and Kreisberg JI: Increased extracellular matrix synthesis and mRNA in mesangial cells grown in high-glucose medium. *Am J Physiol* 260:F185-F191, 1991.
8. Haneda M, Kikkawa R, Horide N, Togawa M, Koya D, Kajiwara N, Ooshima A, and Shigeta Y: Glucose enhances type IV collagen production in cultured rat glomerular mesangial cells. *Diabetologia* 34:491-499, 1991.

9. Ziyadeh FN, Sharma K, Ericksen M, and Wolf G: Stimulation of collagen gene expression and protein synthesis in murine mesangial cells by high glucose is mediated by activation of transforming growth factor-b. *J Clin Invest* 93:536-542, 1994.
10. Wakisaka M, Spiro MJ, and Spiro RG: Synthesis of type VI collagen in cultured glomerular cells and comparison of its regulation by glucose and other factors with that of type IV collagen. *Diabetes* 43:95-103, 1994.
11. Kolm V, Sauer U, Olgemoller B, and Schleicher ED: High glucose-induced TGF-b 1 regulates mesangial production of heparan sulfate proteoglycan. *Am. J. Physiol.* 270:F812-F821, 1996.
12. van Det NF, Verhagen NAM, Tamsma JT, Berden JHM, Bruijn JA, Daha MR, and van der Woulde FJ: Regulation of glomerular epithelial cell production of fibronectin and transforming growth factor-b by high glucose, not by angiotensin II. *Diabetes* 46:834-840, 1997.
13. Takeuchi A, Throckmorton DC, Brogden AP, Yoshizawa N, Rasmussen H, and Kashgarian M: Periodic high extracellular glucose enhances production of collagens III and IV by mesangial cells. *Am J Physiol* 268:F13-F19, 1995.
14. Heilig CW, Concepcion LA, Riser BL, and Freytag SO, Zhu M, Cortes P: Overexpression of glucose transporters in rat mesangial cells cultured in a normal glucose milieu mimics the diabetic phenotype. J Clin Invest 96: 1802-1814, 1995.
15. van Det NF, van den Born J, Tamsa JT, Verhagen NAM, Berden JHM, Brujin JA, Daha MR, and van der Woude FJ: Effects of high glucose on the production of heparan sulfate proteoglycan by mesangial and epithelial cells. *Kidney Int* 49:1079-1089, 1996.
16. Kasinath BS, Block JA, Singh AK, Terhune WC, Maldonado R, Davalath S, and Wanna L: Regulation of rat glomerular epithelial cell proteoglycans by high-medium glucose. *Arch of Biochem and Biophys* 309:149-159, 1994.
17. Sharma K, and Ziyadeh FN: Biochemical events and cytokine interactions linking glucose metabolism to the development of diabetic nephropathy. *Semin Nephrol* 17:80-92, 1997.
18. Wolf G, and Ziyadeh FN: The role of angiotensin II in diabetic nephropathy: Emphasis on nonhemodynamic mechanisms. *Am J Kidney Dis* 29:153-163, 1997.
19. Hoffman BB, and Ziyadeh FN: The role of growth factors in the development of diabetic nephropathy. *Curr Opin Endocrin Diabetes* 3:322-329, 1996.
20. Abboud HE: Growth factors and diabetic nephropathy:an overview. *Kidney Int* 52 (suppl 60):S3-6, 1997.
21. Roberts AB, McCune BK, and Sporn MB: TGF-b: Regulation of extracellular matrix. *Kidney Int* 41:557-559, 1992.
22. MacKay K, Kondiah P, Danielpour D, Austin HA, and Brown PD: Expression of transforming growth factor-b1 and b2 in rat glomeruli. *Kidney Int* 38:1095-1100, 1990.
23. Roberts AB, Kim S-J, Noma T, Glick AB, Lafyatis R, Lechleider R, Jaakowlew SB, Geiser A, O'Reilly MA, Danielpour D, and Sporn MB. 1991. Multiple forms of TGF-b: distinct promoters and differential expression. In *Clinical Applications of TGF-b*. M. B. Sporn and A. B. Roberts, eds. Ciba Foundation Symposium, Chichester, U.K. p. 7-28.
24. Miyazano K, and Heldin C-H, ed. *Latent forms of TGF-b: Molecular structure and mechanisms of activation*. Clinical Application of TGF-b., G. R. Bock and J. Marsh, eds. 1991, Wiley, Chichester, UK. p. 81-92.
25. Paralkar VM, Vukicevvic S, and Reddi AH: Transforming growth factor b type 1 binds to collagen IV of basement membrane matrix: implications for development. *Dev Biol* 143:303-308, 1991.
26. Wakefield LM, Winokur TS, Hollands RS, Christopherson K, Levinson AD, and Sporn MB: Recombinant latent transforming growth factor b1 has a longer half-life in rats than active transforming growth factor b1, and a different tissue distribution. *J Clin Invest* 86:1976-1984, 1990.
27. Flaumenhaft R, Abe M, Mignatti P, and Rifkin DB: Basic fibroblast growth factor-induced activation of latent transforming growth factor-b in endothelial cells: regulation of plasminogen activator activity. *J Cell Biol* 118:901-909, 1992.
28. Ando T, Okuda S, Tamaki K, Yoshitomi K, and Fujishima M: Localization of transforming growth factor-b and latent transforming growth factor-b binding protein in rat kidney. *Kidney Int* 47:733-739, 1995.
29. Massague J, Attisano L, and Wrana JL: The TGF-b family and its composite receptors. *Trends Cell Biol* 4:172-178, 1994.
30. Wrana JL, Attisano L, Wieser R, Ventura F, and Massague J: Mechanism of activation of the TGF-b receptor. *Nature* 370:341-347, 1994.

31. Wieser R, Attisano L, Wrana JL, and Massague J: Signaling activity of transforming growth factor b type II receptors lacking specific domains in the cytoplasmic region. *Mol Cell Biol* 7239-7247, 1993.
32. Sekelsky JJ, Newfeld SJ, Raftery LA, Chartoff EH, and Gelbart WM: Genetic characterization and cloning of mothers against dpp, a gene required for decapentaplegic function in Drosophila melanogaster. *Genetics* 139:1347-1358, 1995.
33. Liu F, Hata A, Baker JC, Doody J, Carcamo J, Harland RM, and Massague J: A human Mad protein acting as a BMP-regulated transcriptional activator. *Nature* 381:620-623, 1996.
34. Zhang Y, Feng X, We R, and Derynck R: Receptor-associated Mad homologues synergize as effectors of the TGF-b response. *Nature* 383:168-172, 1996.
35. Hayashi H, Abdollah S, Qiu Y, Cai J, Xu Y, Grinnell BW, Richardson MA, Topper JN, Gimbrone MA, Wrana JL, and Falb D: The MAD-related protein Smad7 associates with the TGF-b receptor and functions as an antagonist of TGF-b signaling. *Cell* 89:1165-1173, 1997.
36. Laiho M, Saksela O, Andreasen PA, and Keski-Oja J: Enhanced production and extracellular deposition of the endothelial-type plasminogen activator inhibitor in cultured human lung fibroblasts by transforming growth factor-beta. *J Cell Biol* 103:2403-2410, 1986.
37. Ziyadeh FN, Simmons DA, Snipes ER, and Goldfarb S: Effect of *myo*-inositol on cell proliferation and collagen transcription and secretion in proximal tubule cells cultured in elevated glucose. *J Am Soc Nephrol* 1:1220-1229, 1991.
38. Rocco M, Chen Y, Goldfarb S, and Ziyadeh FN: Elevated glucose stimulates TGF-b gene expression and bioactivity in proximal tubule. *Kidney Int.* 41:107-114, 1992.
39. Di Paolo S, Gesualdo L, Ranieri E, Grandaliano G, and Schena FP: High glucose concentration induces the overexpression of transforming growth factor-b through the activation of a platelet-derived growth factor loop in human mesangial cells. *Am J Path* 149:2095-2106, 1996
40. Phillips AO, Steadman R, Topley N, and Williams JD: Elevated D-glucose concentrations modulate TGF-beta 1 synthesis by human cultured renal proximal tubular cells. The permissive role of platelet-derived growth factor. *Am J Pathol* 147:362-374, 1995.
41. Mogyorosi A, Hoffman BB, Guo J, Jin Y, Ericksen M, Sharma K, and Ziyadeh FN: Elevated glucose concentration stimulates expression of the type II receptor in glomerular mesangial cells. (abstract). *J. AM. Soc. Nephrol.* 7:1875, 1996.
42. Guh JY, Yang ML, Yanf YY, Chang CC, and Chuang LY: Captopril reverses high-glucose induced growth effects on LLC-PK1 cells partly by decreasing transforming growth factor-b receptor protein expression. *J. AM. Soc. Nephrol.* 7:1207-1215, 1996.
43. Song RH, Singh AK, Alavi N, and Leehey DJ: Decreased collagenase activity of mesangial cells incubated in high glucose media is reversed by neutralizing antibody to transforming growth factor beta. *J Am Soc Neph* 5:972 (abstract), 1994.
44. Sharma K, and Ziyadeh FN: Hyperglycemia and diabetic kidney disease: the case for transforming growth factor-b as a key mediator. *Diabetes* 44:1139-1146, 1995.
45. Park I-S, Kiyomoto H, Abboud S, and Abboud H: Expression of transforming growth factor-b and type IV collagen in early streptozotocin-induced diabetes. *Diabetes* 46:473-480, 1997.
46. Sharma K, and Ziyadeh FN: Renal hypertrophy is associated with upregulation of TGF-b1 gene expression in diabetic BB rat and NOD mouse. *Am J Physiol* 267:F1094-F1101, 1994.
47. Sharma K, Guo J, Jin Y, and Ziyadeh FN: Neutralization of TGF-b by anti-TGF-b antibody attenuates kidney hypertrophy and the enhanced extracellular matrix gene expression in STZ-induced diabetic mice. *Diabetes* 45:522-530, 1996.
48. Pankewycz OG, Guan JX, Bolton WK, Gomez A, and Benedict JF: Renal TGF-beta regulation in spontaneously diabetic NOD mice with correlations in mesangial cells. *Kidney Int* 46:748-58, 1994.
49. Shankland SJ, and Scholey JW: Expression of transforming growth factor-b1 during diabetic renal hypertrophy. *Kidney Int* 46:430-442, 1994.
50. Yang S, Fletcher WH, and Johnson DA: Regulation of cAMP-dependent protein kinase: enzyme activation without dissociation. *Biochem* 34:6267-6271, 1995.
51. Koya D, M.R. J, Lin Y-W, Ishii H, Kuboki K, and King GL: Characterization of protein kinase beta isoform activation on the gene expression of transforming growth factor-b, extracelluar matrix components, and prostanoids in the glomeruli of diabetic rats. *J Clin Med* 100:115-126, 1997.
52. Reckelhoff JF, tygart VL, Mitias MM, and Walcott JL: STZ-inducted diabetes results in decreased activity of glomerular cathepsin and metalloprotease in rats. *Diabetes* 42:1425-1432, 1993.

53. Yamamoto T, Nakamura T, Noble NA, Ruoslahti E, and Border WA: Expression of transforming growth factor beta is elevated in human and experimental diabetic nephropathy. *Proc Natl Acad Sci USA* 90:1814-1818, 1993.
54. Nakamura T, Fukui M, Ebihara I, Osada S, Nagaoka I, Tomino Y, and Koide H: mRNA expression of growth factors in glomeruli from diabetic rats. *Diabetes* 42:450-456, 1993.
55. Bertoluci MC, Schmid H, Lachat J-J, and Coimbra TM: Transforming growth factor-beta in the development of rat diabetic nephropathy- a 10 month study with insulin-treated rats. *Nephron* 74:189-196, 1996.
56. Han DC, Kim YJ, Cha MK, Song KI, Kim JH, Lee EY, Ha H, and Lee HB: Glucose control suppressed the glomerular expression of TGF-b1 and the progression of experimental diabetic nephropathy. *J Am Soc Nephrol* 7:1870 (abstract), 1996.
57. Yamamoto T, Noble NA, Cohen AH, Nast CC, Hishida A, Gold LI, and Border WA: Expression of transforming growth factor-b isoforms in human glomerular diseases. *Kidney Int* 49:461-469, 1996.
58. Yoshioka K, Takemura T, Murakami K, Okada M, Hino S, Miyamoto H, and Maki S: Transforming growth factor-b protein and mRNA in glomeruli in normal and diseased human kidneys. *Lab Invest* 68:154-163, 1993.
59. Iwano M, Atsushi K, Nishino T, Sato H, Nishioka H, Akai Y, Kurioka H, Fuji Y, Kanauchi M, Shiiki H, and Dohi K: Quantification of glomerular TGF-b1 mRNA in patients with diabetes mellitus. *Kidney Int* 49:1120-1126, 1996.
60. Sharma K, Ziyadeh FN, Alzahabi B, McGowan TA, Kapoor S, Kurnik BRC, Kurnik PB, and Weisberg LS: Increased renal production of transforming growth factor-b 1 in patients with type II diabetes. *Diabetes* 46:854-859, 1997.
61. Fukui M, Nakamura T, Ebihara I, Makita Y, Osada S, Tomino Y, and Koide H: Effects of enalapril on endothelin-1 and growth factor expression in diabetic rat glomeruli. *J Lab Clin Med* 123:763-768, 1994.
62. Inaba T, Ishibashi S, Gotoda T, Kawamura M, Morino N, Nojima Y, Kawakami M, Yazaki Y, and Yamada N: Enhanced expression of platelet derived growth factor- beta receptor by high glucose: involvement of platelet derived growth factor in diabetic angiopathy. *Diabetes* 45:507-512, 1996.
63. Throckmorton DC, Brogden AP, Min B, Rasmussen H, and Kashgarian M: PDGF and TGF-b mediate collagen production by mesangial cells exposed to advanced glycation end products. *Kidney Int* 48:111-117, 1995.
64. Doi TT, Vlassara H, Kirstein M, Yamada Y, Striker GE, and Striker L: Receptor-specific increase in extracellular matrix production in mouse mesangial cells by advanced glycosylation end products is mediated via platelet-derived growth factor. *Pro Natl Acad Sci USA* 89:2873-2877, 199
65. Morabito E, Corsico N, and Arrigoni Martelli E: Endothelins urinary excretion in spontaneously diabetic rats: BB/BB. *Life Sciences* 56:13-18, 1995.
66. Nakamura T, Ebihara I, Fukui M, Tomino Y, and Koide H: Effect of a specific endothelin receptor A antagonist on mRNA levels for extracellular matrix components and growth factors in diabetic glomeruli. *Diabetes* 44:895-899, 1995.
67. Takahashi K, Ghatei MA, Lam H-C, O'halloran DJ, and Bloom SR: Elevated plasma endothelin in patients with diabetes mellitus. *Diabetologia* 33:306-310, 1990.
68. Ferri C, Laurenti O, Bellini C, Faldetta MRC, Properzi G, Santucci A, and De Mattia G: Circulating endothelin-1 levels in lean non-insulin-dependent diabetic patients. *Am J Hypertens* 8:40-47, 1995.
69. Wolf G, Mueller E, Stahl RAK, and Ziyadeh FN: Angiotensin II-induced hypertrophy of cultured murine proximal tubular cells by endogenous TGF-b. *J Clin Invest* 92:1366-1373, 1993.
70. Kagami S, Border WA, Miller DE, and Noble NA: Angiotensin II stimulates extracellular matrix protein synthesis through induction of transforming growth factor-b expression in rat glomerular mesangial cells. *J Clin Invest* 93:2431-2437, 1994.
71. Lewis EJ, Hunsicker LG, Bain RP, and Rohde RD: The effect of angiotensin-converting-enzyme inhibition on diabetic nephropathy. *N Engl J Med* 329:1456-1462, 1993.
72. Mogensen CE: Renoprotective role of ACE inhibitors in diabetic nephropathy. *Br Heart J* 72:S38-45, 1994.
73. Ledbetter S, Copeland EJ, Noonan D, Vogeli G, and Hassell JR: Altered steady-state mRNA levels of basement membrane proteins in diabetic mouse kidneys and thromboxane synthase inhibition. *Diabetes* 39:196-203, 1990.

74. Craven PA, Caines MA, and DeRubertis FR: Sequential alterations in glomerular prostaglandin and thromboxane synthesis in diabetic rats: Relationship to the hyperfiltration of early diabetes. *Metabolism* 36:95-103, 1987.
75. Craven PA, and DeRubertis FR: Protein kinase C is activated in glomeruli from streptozotocin diabetic rats. *J Clin Invest* 83:1667-1675, 1989.
76. Gambardella S, Andreani D, Cancelli A, DiMario U, Cardamone I, Stirats G, Cinotti GA, and Pugliese F: Renal hemodynamics and urinary excretion of 6-keto prostaglandin F 1a, and thromboxane B2 in newly diagnosed type I diabetic patients. *Diabetes* 37:1044-1048, 1988.
77. Craven PA, Melhem MF, and DeRubertis FR: Thromboxane in the pathogenesis of glomerular injury in diabetes. *Kidney Int* 42:937-946, 1992.
78. DeRubertis FR, and Craven PA: Contribution of platelet thromboxane production to enhanced urinary excretion and glomerular production of thromboxane and to the pathogenesis of albuminurira in the streptozotocin-diabetic rat. *Metabolism* 41:90-96, 1992.
79. Bruggeman LA, Horigan EA, Horikoshi S, Ray PE, and Klotman PE: Thromboxane stimulates synthesis of extracellular matrix proteins in vitro. *Am J Physiol* 261:F488-F494, 1991.
80. Studer RK, Negrete H, Craven PA, and DeRubertis FR: Protein kinase C signals thromboxane induced increases in fibronectin synthesis and TGF-beta bioactivity in mesangial cells. *Kidney Int* 48:422-430, 1995.
81. Matsuo Y, Takagawa I, Koshida H, Kawabata T, Nakamura M, Ida T, Zhou L, and Marumo F: Antiproteinuric effect of a thromboxane receptor antagonist, S-1452, on rat diabetic nephropathy and murine lupus nephritis. *Pharmacology* 50:1-8, 1995.
82. Hora K, Oguchi H, Furakawa T, Hora K, and Tokunaga S: Effects of a selective thromboxane synthetase inhibitor OKY-046 on experimental diabetic nephropathy. *Nephron* 56:297-305, 1990.
83. Pricci E, Pugliese G, Mene P, Romeo G, Galli G, Casini A, Rotella CM, Di Mario U, and Pugliese F: Regulatory role of eicosanoids in extracellular matrix overproduction induced by long-term exposure to high glucose in cultured rat mesangial cells. *Diabetologia* 39:1055-1062, 1996.
84. Flyvbjerg A, Bornfeldt KE, Marshall SM, Arnqvist HJ, and Orskov H: Kidney IGF-I mRNA in initial renal hypertrophy in experimental diabetes in rats. *Diabetologia* 33:334-338, 1990.
85. Flyvbjerg A, Marshall SM, Frystyk J, Hansen KW, Harris AG, and Orskov H: Octreotide administration in diabetic rats: Effect on renal hypertrophy and urinary albumin excretion. *Kidney Int.* 41:805-812, 1992.
86. Serri O, Beauregard H, Brazeau P, Abribat T, Lambert J, Harris A, and Vachon L: Somatostatin analogue, octreotide, reduces increased glomerular filtration rate and kidney size in insulin-dependent diabetes. *JAMA* 265:888-892, 1991.
87. Quaife C, Mathews L, Pinkert C, Hammer R, Brinster R, and Palmiter R: Histopathology associated with elevated levels of growth hormone and insulin-like growth factor I in transgenic mice. *Endocrinology* 124:40-48, 1989.
88. Goldfarb S, Ziyadeh FN, Kern EFO, and Simmons DA: Effects of polyol-pathway inhibition and dietary *myo*-inositol on glomerular hemodynamic function in experimental diabetes mellitus in rats. *Diabetes* 40:465-471, 1991.
89. DeRubertis FR, and Craven P: Activation of protein kinase C in glomerular cells in diabetes: mechanisms and potential links to the pathogenesis of diabetic glomerulopathy. *Diabetes* 43:1-8, 1994.
90. Fumo P, Kuncio GS, and Ziyadeh FN: PKC and high glucose stimulate collagen a1(IV) transcriptional activity in a reporter mesangial cell line. *Am J Physiol* In Press, 1994.
91. Brownlee M, Vassara H, and Cerami A: Nonenzymatic glycosylation and the pathogensis of diabetes complications. *Ann Int Med* 101:527-537, 1984.
92. Cohen MP, and Ziyadeh FN: Amadori glucose adducts modulate mesangial cell growth and collagen gene expression. *Kidney Int* 45:475-484, 1994.
93. Hoffman B, Sharma K, Ericksen M, and Ziyadeh F: Transcriptional activation of TGF-b1 by high glucose. *J. Am. Soc. Nephrol* 6:1041 (abstract), 1995.
94. Kim S-J, Glick A, Sporn MB, and Roberts AB: Characterization of the promoter region of the human transforming growth factor-b1 gene. *J Biol Chem* 264:402-408, 1989.
95. Negrete H, Studer RK, Craven PA, and DeRubertis FR: Role for transforming growth factor beta in thromboxane-induced increases in mesangial cell fibronectin synthesis. *Diabetes* 44:335-339, 1995.
96. Zhang G, Kazanietz MG, Blumberg PM, and Hurley JH: Crystal structure of the Cys2 activator-binding domain of protein kinase δ in complex with phorbol ester. *Cell* 81:917-924, 1995.

97. Haneda M, Araki S, Togawa M, Sugimoto T, Isono M, and Kikkawa R: Mitogen-activated protein kinase cascade is activated in glomeruli of diabetic rats and glomerular mesangial cells under high glucose conditions. *Diabetes* 46:847-853, 1997.
98. de Groot RP, Auwerx J, Karperien M, Staels B, and Kruijer W: Activation of JunB by PKC and PKA signal transduction through a novel cis-acting element. *Nucleic Acids Res* 19:775-781, 1991.
99. Chung KY, Agarwal A, Uitto J, and Mauviel A: An AP-1 binding sequence is essential for regulation of the human a2(I) collagen promoter activity by transforming growth factor-b. *J Biol Chem* 271:3272-3278, 1996.
100. Shankland SJ, and Scholey JW: Expression of growth-related protooncogenes during diabetic renal hypertrophy. *Kidney Int* 47:782-788, 1995.
101. Kim S-J, Angel P, Lafyatis R, Hattori K, Kim KY, Sporn MB, Karin M, and Roberts AB: Autoinduction of Transforming Growth facor b1 is mediated by the AP-1 complex. *Mol Cell Biol* 10:1492-1497, 1990.
102. Ziyadeh FN, Mogyorosi A, and Kalluri R: Early and Advanced Nonenzymatic glycation products in the pathogenesis of diabetic kidney disease. *Exp Nephrol* 5:2-9, 1997.
103. Yang C-W, Vlassara H, Peten EP, He C-J, Striker GE, and Striker LJ: Advanced glycation end products up-regulate gene expression found in diabetic glomerular disease. *Proc Natl Acad of Sci, USA* 91:9436-9440, 1994.
104. Ha H, Kamanna VS, Kirschenbaum MA, and Kim KH: Role of glycated low density lipoprotein in mesangial extracellular matrix synthesis. *Kidney Int* 52 (suppl 60):s54- s59, 1997.
105. Skolnik EY, Yang Z, Makita Z, Radoff S, Kirstein M, and Vlassara H: Human and rat mesangial cell receptors for glucose-modified proteins: potential role in kidney tissue remodelling and diabetic nephropathy. *J Exp Med* 174:931-939, 1991.
106. Riser BL, Cortes P, Zhao X, Bernstein J, Dumier F, and Narins RG: Intraglomerular pressure and mesangial stretching stimulate extracellular matrix formation in the rat. *J Clin Invest* 90:1932-1943, 1992.
107. Yasuda T, Satoshi K, Homma T, and Harris RC: Regulation of extracellular matrix by mechanical stress in rat glomerular mesangial cells. *J Clin Invest* 98:1991-2000, 1996.
108. Riser BL, Cortes P, Heilig C, Grondin J, Ladsonwofford S, Patterson D, and Narins RG: Cyclic stretching force selectively up-regulates transforming growth factor-beta isoforms in cultured rat mesangial cells. *Am J Pathol* 148:1915-1923, 1996.
109. Ohno M, Cooke JP, Dzau V, J., and Gibbons GH: Fluid shear stress induces endothelial transforming growth factor b-1 transcription and production. Modulation by potassium channel blckade. *J Clin Invest* 95:1363-1369, 1995.
110. Mogensen CE, and Christensen CK: Predicting diabetic nephropathy in insulin-dependent patients. *N Engl J Med* 311:89-93, 1984.

35. BLOOD PRESSURE ELEVATION IN DIABETES: THE RESULTS FROM 24-h AMBULATORY BLOOD PRESSURE RECORDINGS.

Klavs Würgler Hansen, Per Løgstrup Poulsen and Eva Ebbehøj
Medical Department M, Aarhus Kommunehospital, Aarhus, Denmark

Ambulatory blood pressure (BP) measurement permits assessment of BP in the patients own surroundings, during normal daily activities on the job and in the night. Previously semiautomatic monitors were used, which required manually inflation of the cuff [1], or direct (intraarterial) BP measurement [2]. The first true ambulatory 24-h report of indirectly measured BP obtained with a portable and fully automatic monitor was published in 1975 [3].

The application of the technique to diabetic patients was first reported by Rubler in 1982 using an equipment weighing 3.07 kg [4]. The number of studies using ambulatory BP monitoring in diabetic patient in the eighties were moderate and with a few exceptions [4-7] focusing on autonomic neuropathy [8-13].

The knowledge from ambulatory BP measurement in general has recently been reviewed [14-18] and practical guidelines published [18-20]. Including the present one four reviews of ambulatory BP measurement in diabetes have appeared [21-23].

1. METHODOLOGICAL ASPECTS: A GUIDE TO THE CRITICAL READER.

The two most popular ways of obtaining automatic indirect BP records are either by use of an microphone in the cuff or by oscillometric technique [19,24]. Some monitors offers both options. While the manufacturer of the monitor is always stated in papers dealing with ambulatory BP monitoring, the technique is not necessarily described.

No monitor is perfect and even in monitors which have fulfilled national standards, major discrepancies between the monitors and values obtained by sphygmomanometry are observed in some of the patients. Some papers state that individually "calibration" of the monitor to each of the studied patients has been performed (by 3 to 5 simultaneous or sequential measurements). However, it is not possibly to calibrate a fully automatic monitor in strict terms (without returning to the manufacturer) and the word calibration is a misnomer in this context. The difference between auscultatory BP and the monitor can be evaluated in each patient (rather unprecisely) and this difference can either be accepted or not.

If the result of clinic BP measurement is provided it should be observed whether this is obtained by sphygmomanometry or by use of the same monitor as used for ambulatory measurements [25]. Only in the latter case are clinic and ambulatory values directly comparable.

Although more sophisticated methods exist [26,27], the diurnal variation of BP is usually reported as the night/day ratio. Obviously this must be based on individual information of the night period, otherwise the ratio is overestimated [28].

The term "non-dipper" has become a popular short term for a person who do not describe a normal reduction of BP at night. A commonly used definition of a "non-dipper" requires a relative reduction of night blood pressure less than 10 % of the day value for both systolic and diastolic BP [29]. Unfortunately no consensus exist. In addition the proportion of non-dippers also depends on the definition of night and day time which should be based on individiual information of time for going to bed and rising rather than fixed periods.

Patients who are hypertensive by clinic measurements but shows a normal day time BP are designated "white coat hypertensive" [30]. This term is well understood in literature although "isolated clinic hypertension" may be more precise [31]. The effect of the "white coat" was originally described as a transient (5 min) elevation of BP [31]. At present the "white coat effect" is usually calculated as the difference (clinic BP - day time BP) [32]. The proportion of white coat hypertensive subjects in a hypertensive population depends on:

i: The definition of hypertension (usually clinic BP > 140/90 mmHg)

ii: How carefully the hypertensive subjects are identified (if patients are labelled as hypertensive based on only one clinic BP the frequency of white coat hypertension is high, if a several clinic BP measurements -as recommended- are obtained at different occasions before diagnosis, the frequency is lower).

iii: The definition of a normal ambulatory BP (if the cut off limit for a normal ambulatory BP is defined as a day time BP < 131/86 mmHg the frequency of white coat hypertension is lower than for a cut off limit of BP < 140/90 mmHg).

iii: The presence of other selection criteria related to clinic BP level or possible end organ signs. (The frequency of white coat hypertension is higher in a population with mild hypertension than in a population with moderate or severe hypertension even if the white coat effect is higher in the latter group [32]. If a hypertensive population are selected on the basis of criteria which may be related to elevated BP (i.e. albuminuria or retinopathy in diabetes) the proportion of patients who fulfil the criteria for white coat hypertension is assumed to be low).

2. NIDDM AND AMBULATORY BP

2.1 The influence of changes in metabolic control

Shift from sulfonulurea to insulin in poorly controlled elderly NIDDM patient improved glycemic control but ambulatory BP after one year was unaffected perhaps due to weight gain [33].

2.2 Comparison with healthy individuals.

Some discrepancies exist. One study has reported an increase in 24-h systolic (but not diastolic) BP in normoalbuminuric diabetic patients [34]. Two recent studies did not found any difference in 24-h average BP, however the nocturnal reduction of systolic BP was impaired in normoalbuminuric patients [35,36].

If patients (UAE not specified) and healthy subjects were divided into groups with and without hypertension no statistical difference of 24-h BP have been reported [7,37].

2.3 The relation to abnormal albuminuria.

No difference in day time or 24-h BP were noticed between normo- and microalbuminuric patients [34,36,38-41]. In contrast ambulatory BP was reported significantly higher in microalbuminuric patients (90 % males, 50 % non-caucasians) than in normoalbuminuric patients (71 % males, 28 % non-Caucasians) [42]. In NIDDM both ambulatory and clinic BP correlates with UAE roughly to a similar extent [34,42] although one study using albumin/creatinine ratio reported no correlation [43]. Ambulatory BP is higher in patients with diabetic nephropathy than in normoalbuminuric patients [35,44].

Abnormal diurnal BP pattern (high night BP) are seen in patients with microalbuminuria [36,40,41,44-46] and overt diabetic nephropathy [35,44,46]. As in IDDM this abnormality seems closely linked to the presence of autonomic neuropathy [35,36,47].

2.4 The time course of ambulatory BP

In patients receiving standard clinical care including antihypertensive medication, 24-h BP was remarkable stable in both normo- and microalbuminuric patients during an observation period of 4.6 years. Individual changes in both systolic and diastolic 24-h BP were related to changes in UAE [48]. The evolution of UAE did not differ between patients with and without abnormal diurnal BP profile at baseline [48].

2.5 Non-dipper: Autonomic neuropathy, diabetic nephropathy and extracellular volume.

Numerous studies in mixed IDDM and NIDDM populations or unclassified diabetic patients have demonstrated a reduction or (in few patients) even a reversal of the normal nocturnal decline of BP [11-13,49-53] in patients with autonomic neuropathy. Also in homogenous NIDDM diabetic patients several studies demonstrates [35,39,47,54] the association between diabetic nephropathy, signs of autonomic neuropathy or both and a blunted diurnal variation of blood pressure. According to one study expansion of extracellular volume seems not to be involved in reduced nocturnal BP in NIDDM patients with nephropathy [35]. However, a physiological defence against nocturnal volume expansion may explain why a lower night level of aldosteron and a higher level of plasma atrial natriuretic peptide have been reported in "non-dippers", who also had more pronounced signs of autonomic neuropathy than "dippers" [54].

Postprandial hypotension is also a phenomenon observed in patients with autonomic neuropathy [55,56].

2.6 The relation to insulin resistance and sodium-lithium countertransport

Ambulatory systolic BP (and clinic systolic BP) correlated in one study with glucose disposal rate, but not with fasting insulin level [57]. However, this relation was not confirmed in another study (S Nielsen personal communication) [38]. No relation has been found between ambulatory BP and sodium-lithium countertransport [42].

2.7 The relation to diabetic retinopathy

No studies designed for this purpose exist, one study suggest a relation between "non-dipping" status and retinopathy [48].

3. IDDM AND AMBULATORY BP

3.1 The influence of diabetes duration

Two cross sectional study reports a reduction of the nocturnal BP fall in long term normoalbuminuric diabetic patients [58,59].

3.2 The influence of sex

The well known BP difference between healthy males and females seems attenuated in IDDM [59,60].

3.3 The influence of short term changes in metabolic control

This question has so far never been addressed by intervention studies employing ambulatory BP. Clinic BP has been reported lower after short term improvement of diabetic control by insulin pumps (24-h insulin dose unchanged) [61]. Intraarterial BP (10-h day time average) was also reduced after improved glycemic control achieved by increasing insulin dose in most patients [62]. No significant change in clinic BP was observed in a study where poor metabolic control was obtained by reducing insulin dose [63].

3.4 The influence of smoking and type of day (work day/ day-off)

We have compared ambulatory BP in 16 normoalbuminuric smokers and non-smokers without hypertension. Systolic BP was slightly higher (3mmHg day time, 5 mmHg night time) in smokers, but this failed to reach statistical significance [64]. In a larger study encompassing 24 normoalbuminuric smokers and non-smokers diastolic day and night BP was significantly higher (3.9 and 3.5 mmHg respectively) in smokers. In addition a dose response relationship was demonstrated [65]. Notably, this effect of smoking in diabetic individuals contrast the well known finding of a lower night BP in non-diabetic smokers [64,66]. Smoking do not affect the night/day ratio of BP in diabetes [64,65,67].

Day time BP is significantly lower (5 mmHg) on a day off than on a work day [64].

3.5 Comparison with healthy individuals

Most studies [68-73], but not all [74,75] agree that day time BP is indistinguishable between normoalbuminuric diabetic patients and healthy subjects. Also the majority of investigators found no difference in the diurnal BP profile [68,69,72-75]. In contrast one study has reported a slightly reduced nocturnal BP fall [70] and one study has surprisingly described a much higher night/day ratio of BP in normoalbuminuric patients [71]. With this exceptions, the diversities are minor and may be explained by varying diabetes duration or proportion of males/females. Thus, as a rule normoalbuminuric patients have a 24-h BP profile very similar to healthy control subjects (Fig 35-1).

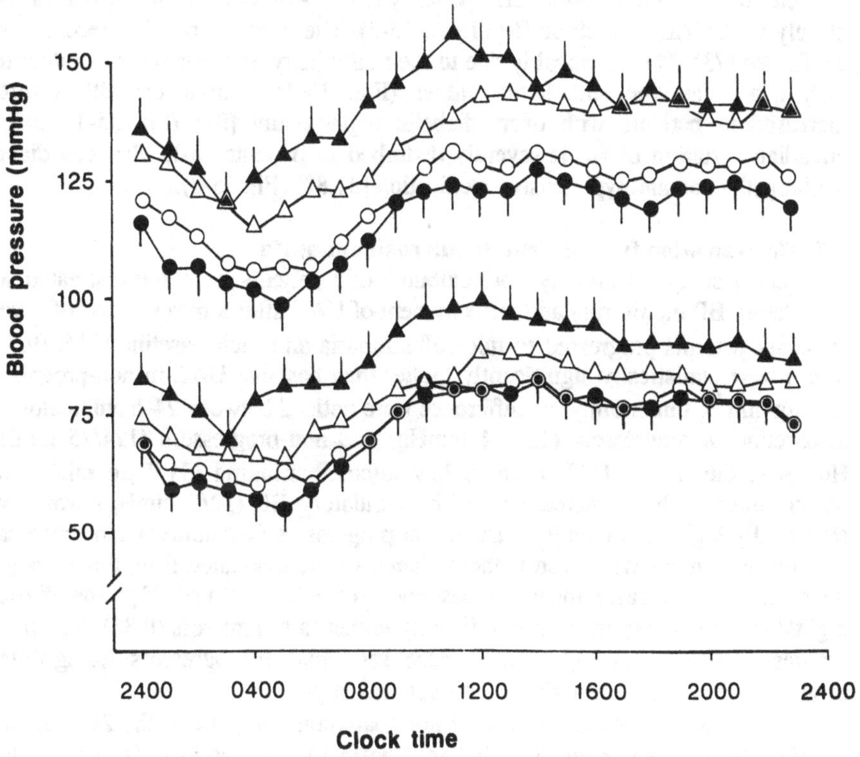

Figure 35-1 Twenty-four hour profile of mean systolic and diastolic BP for type 1 diabetic patients and healthy controls. Diabetic patients with nephropathy and without antihypertensive treatment (n=13, filled triangles), microalbuminuric patients (n=26, open triangles), normoalbuminuric patients (n=26, open circles) and healthy individuals (n=26, filled circles). From [81] with permission.

3.6 The relation to abnormal albuminuria

This subject has recently been reviewed [76]. Ambulatory BP is significantly higher and the diurnal BP pattern is abnormal in consecutively studied patients compared with healthy controls [77]. This largely depends on abnormal albuminuria present in some of the patients [77].

Four studies comparing normo- and microalbuminuric patients as well as healthy controls are summarised in Table 35-1. Ambulatory BP are significantly increased in microalbuminuric as compared with normoalbuminuric patients despite comparable auscultatory clinic BP [68,78]. In some studies day time BP were only numerically but not statistically significantly higher in microalbuminuric patients [74,79,80]. This is probably due to lower number of microalbuminuric patients in these studies. The night/day ratio of diastolic BP is significantly higher in microalbuminuric patients than in healthy individuals [81] and night/day ratio for normoalbuminuric patients is in between (Table 35-1). If the comparison between microalbuminuric and normoalbuminuric patients is restricted to patients in good metabolic control and without any signs of autonomic neuropathy day time BP is still elevated in microalbuminuric patients [73]. Ambulatory BP correlates more closely with UAE than clinic BP (Table 35-2). The phenomenon has recently been confirmed [73]. This is probably due to the multiplicity of measurements rather than their quality as true ambulatory values (Fig. 35-3). Ambulatory BP is further increased in patients with overt diabetic nephropathy [81] (Fig 35-1) and the circadian variation of BP is severely disturbed in patients with advanced diabetic nephropathy and antihypertensive medication [81,82] (Fig 35-2).

3.7 The transition from normo- to microalbuminuria

In a recent study 40 initially normoalbuminuric patients were reinvestigated with ambulatory BP monitoring and measurement of UAE after a mean period of 3 years [83]. Six patients progressed to microalbuminuria and their baseline UAE (9.7 $\mu g\ min^{-1}$) were statistically significantly higher than baseline UAE in non-progressors (5.5 $\mu g\ min^{-1}$). Importantly, no difference were noticed between 24-h ambulatory BP at baseline in progressors (124/74 mmHg) and non-progressors (124/75 mmHg). However, the rise in UAE even to low microalbuminuria (31.7 $\mu g\ min^{-1}$) were accompanied with an increase in 24-h ambulatory BP (12/5 mmHg) which was statistically higher than the increase in non-progressors (4/2 mmHg). No statistically significant changes were seen if these changes were evaluated from the average of three clinic BP measurements at baseline and at follow up [83]. The diastolic night/day ratio at baseline was significantly higher in progressors (0.88) than in non-progressors (0.81), but no further increase was found in progressors during follow-up and the overlap between the two groups was large.

In a cross sectional study of normoalbuminuric patients the 24-h BP were significantly higher in patients with "high" normal UAE than in patients with "low" normal UAE [84,85]. Similar results have been reported in a study comparing "high" normoalbuminuric patients with healthy individuals [86].

These results support the idea that rise in UAE and ambulatory BP can not be separated even in the very early phase of incipient diabetic nephropathy.

3.8 Non-dipper: Autonomic neuropathy, nephropathy and expansion of extracellular volume (EVC)

In IDDM the presence of autonomic neuropathy is clearly associated with impaired reduction of night BP [10,87,88]. Autonomic neuropathy and diabetic nephropathy are closely associated [89-92]. Their relative role for the abnormal diurnal variation in blood pressure is therefore difficult to ascertain. However, the literature gives no examples of a group of IDDM patients with blunted diurnal variation of BP without concomitant signs of autonomic neuropathy either by formal test [87,88] or by increased heart rate [68]. Indeed autonomic dysfunction can be documented even in "high" normoalbuminuric patients if refined test (spectral analysis of heart rate variability) is employed [85]. In contrast an impaired reduction of night BP and increased heart rate is seen in long term diabetic patients who are strictly normoalbuminuric [58,59].

Naturally the question of a possible causative role of autonomic neuropathy for the development of diabetic nephropathy has arisen [93]. The link could be a higher night BP which is more readily transmitted to the glomeruli because of renal vasodilation. Alternatively early autonomic dysfunction may just be part of a syndrome indicative of later diabetic complications in patients with suboptimal glycemic control [85]. A retrospective study in patients with diabetic nephropathy has described a faster decline of renal function in patients with a "non-dipping" BP profile compared with "dippers" [94]. However there was no baseline or follow-up measurement of ambulatory BP, which was measured at one time point only during a 6 year observation period. Since renal function was already reduced in "non- dippers" at the time when the ambulatory BP measurement was performed it is not possible to postulate a cause/effect relationship.

A recent study described expanded ECV even in normoalbuminuric "non-dippers"[95]. Two lines of evidence suggest that homeostasis of ECV is associated with elevated night BP in particular in patients abnormal albuminuria. First plasma aldosteron is reported significantly lower in "non-dipping" patients with incipient diabetic nephropathy, which could be interpreted as a defence again fluid retention [96]. Second, in patients with overt diabetic nephropathy, elevated nocturnal BP is associated with expansion of ECV. This may reflect the result of a nocturnal shift of fluid from the interstitial to the intravascular space [97]. This view has recently been challenged by a study which did not find any association between elevated night BP and ECV in IDDM patients with nephropathy [98].

3.9 The relation to glomerular filtration rate (GFR)

A negative correlation between ambulatory BP and GFR has been described in microalbuminuric patients [74,99].Non dippers with microalbuminuria or overt nephropathy seems not to have a reduced GFR [96-98]. One study in normoalbuminuric patients reported a higher night BP and expanded ECV (23 litre) in patients with glomerular hyperfiltration compared with the group with normofiltration (19 litre) [95]. Despite similar methods (Cr EDTA single shot) ECV is found unexplaningly high in this latter study [95] compared with the two previously mentioned studies dealing with nephropathy (14 litre) [97,98].

3.10 The relation to diabetic retinopathy

Elevated night BP is reported in patients with more advanced signs of diabetic retinopathy. Importantly this association was described in strictly normoalbuminuric patients excluding the confounding effect of diabetic kidney disease [100].

Table 35-1 Four studies comparing ambulatory blood pressure in micro- and normoalbuminuric type 1 diabetic patients and healthy control subjects.

	A Hansen et al. [68]			B Moore et al. [74]			C Benhamou et al. [69]			D Lurbe et al. [79]		
	Controls	Normo	Micro	Controls	Normo	Micro	Controls	Normo	Micro	Controls	Normo	Micro
N (male/female)	34	34	34	36	27	11	12	12	12	45	34	11
Sex (male/female)	24/10	24/10	24/10	19/17	14/13	5/6	7/5	7/5	7/5	20/25	-	-
Age (years)	31	31	30	17	18	19	≈31	≈31	31	23	18	24
Diabetes duration (years)	-	18	18	-	9	14*	-	7	15*	-	5	13*
HbA_{1c} (%)	5.1	8.3	9.1*	-	12.5	12.7	-	7.3	8.8*	-	-	-
Body Mass Index ($kg \cdot m^{-2}$)	23.1	23.7	23.9	-	-	-	≈21.5	≈21.5	21.5	22.2	20.1	24.8
UAE ($\mu g \cdot min^{-1}$)	Three overnight collections			One 24h collection			Three overnight collections			Three 24h collections		
	5.2	5.1	51.7	-	5.3	45.2	-	<15	56	-	4.5	111
Monitor and frequency of measurements	Spacelabs 90202 06.00h-24.00h every 20 min 24.00h-06.00h every 60 min			Spacelabs 90202 06.00h-22.00h every 20 min 22.00h-06.00h every 60 min			Spacelabs 90207 07.00h-17.00h every 15 min 17.00h-07.00h every 30 min			Spacelabs 90207 06.00h-24.00h every 20 min 24.00h-06.00h every 30 min		
Definition of day and night periods	Individually recorded periods			Day (06.00h-22.00h) Night (22.00h-06.00h)			Day (09.00h-19.00h) Night (23.00h-07.00h)			Day (08.00h-22.00h) Night (24.00h-06.00h)		
BP criteria for inclusion of patients	All patients included (no antihypertensive treatment)			<130/85			<140/90			<140/90 or <95 percentile level		
Clinic BP (auscultatory)	119/75	121/77	124/81	-	-	-	118/79	119/78	116/73	121/70	120/69	125/74
Clinic BP (monitor)	125/74	128/74	132/79*	102/54	106/64*	118*/70*	-	-	-	-	-	-
Day time BP	125/77	127/77	136*/82*	117/67	123*/71*	130/76	116/76	118/78	124/81	117/71	117/71	122/72
Night time BP	109/61	112/63	122*/69*	110/59	116*/63*	126*/71*	100/61	103/65	113*/68	113/60	114/60	121*/69*
Night/day ratio (systolic/diastolic)	0.87/0.80	0.88/0.82	0.90/0.85	0.94/0.88[a]	0.94/0.89[a]	0.97/0.93[a]	0.86/0.80[a]	0.88/0.83[a]	0.91/0.84[a]	0.94/0.83	0.93/0.84	0.97/0.94*
day-night BP difference	16/16	15/14	14/13	7/8[a]	7/8[a]	4/5[a]	16/15	15/13	11/13	4/11[a]	3/11[a]	1/3[a]
24h BP	119/71	122/73	131*/78*	116/66	122*/70*	129/75	110/71	112/71	119*/75	114/67	116/66	121/71
Comments	Normoalbuminuric patients individually matched to microalbuminuric patiens for sex, age and diabetes duration			Glycosulated hemoglobin HbA is presented. Clinic BP is not measured with the same monitor as ambulatory blood pressure			Patients were admitted to hospital during the night			No statistical analysis between controls and normoalbuminuric patients have been performed		

Values are numbers or mean except for UAE in study A (geometric mean) and in study C (median). For clarity the level of statistical significance is not indicated more specific and the results of comparison between microalbuminuric patients and healthy controls is not given. *; $p < 0.05$ versus controls (for normoalbuminuric patients) or versus normoalbuminuric patients (for microalbuminuric patients). [a]; the values are derived from original data without access to statistical analysis.

Table 35-2 Correlations between blood pressure and urinary albumin excretion in combined normo- and microalbuminuria type 1 diabetic patients.

	A Hansen et al. [68]	B Moore et al. [74]	C Benhamou et al. [69]	D Lurbe et al. [79]
UAE	Three overnight collections	One 24h collection	Three overnight collections	Three 24h collections
Correlations:	Normo (n=34) and Micro (n=34)	Normo (n=27) and Micro (n=11)	Normo (n=23) and Micro (n=12)	Normo (n=34) and Micro (n=11)
UAE vs. clinic BP (auscultatory)	r=0.21, NS (systolic)	-	r=-0.01, NS (systolic)	r=0.19, NS (MAP)
UAE vs. day time BP	r=0.45, p<0.05 (systolic)	-	r=0.17, NS (systolic)	r=0.35, p<0.05 (MAP)
UAE vs. night time BP	r=0.53, p<0.00001 (systolic)	-	r=0.38, p<0.05 (systolic)	r=0.60, p<0.01 (MAP)
UAE vs. 24h BP	r=0.49, p<0.0001 (systolic)	r=0.40, p<0.01 (systolic) r=0.60, p<0.01 (diastolic)	r=0.29, NS (systolic)	-

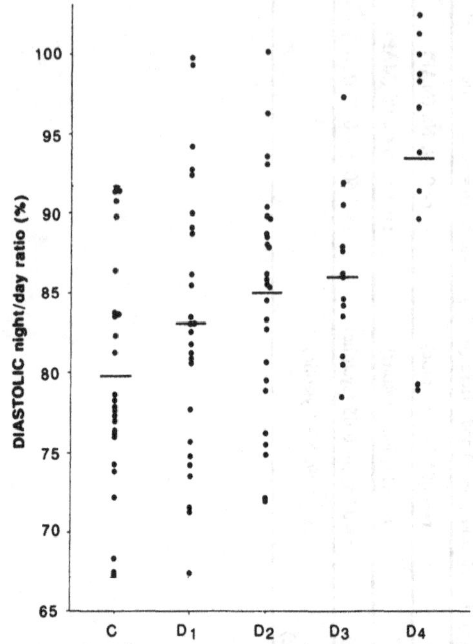

Figure 35-2 Individual night/day ratio for diastolic BP in healthy individuals and type 1 diabetic patients. C= control subjects (n=26), D_1= normoalbuminuric patients (n=26), D_2= microalbuminuric patients (n=26), D_3= patients with diabetic nephropathy without antihypertensive treatment (n=13), D_4= patients with diabetic nephropathy with antihypertensive treatment. From [81] with permission.

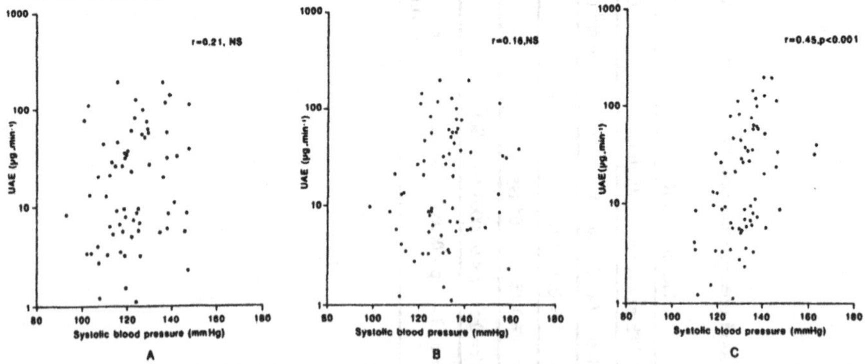

Figure 35-3 The correlation between overnight urinary albumin excretion (UAE, three collections) and BP in normo- and microalbuminuric type 1 diabetic patients. A) systolic clinic BP measured by sphygmomanometry (average of three values) B) systolic ambulatory BP (average of three values) about 11.00 h) C) day time average of systolic ambulatory BP (average of approximately 48 values).The correlation coefficient (Pearson) and significance level are indicated.Partly from [68] with permission.

4. AMBULATORY BLOOD PRESSURE AND INTERVENTION STUDIES

Due to the high reproducibility of ambulatory BP compared with clinic measurements it is an ideal tool for intervention studies [25,101]. The 24-h effectiveness of the intervention can be evaluated, the number of patients needed can be reduced without loosing power and small changes in BP, which would be overlooked by traditional measurements, can be recognised. Ambulatory BP has now been used in several intervention studies in diabetes [43,102-112].

So far there have been no reports of an altered circadian BP profile after antihypertensive treatment in diabetic patients. A shift from morning to evening dose of quinapril [113], perindopril [114] or isradipine [115] has reduced night BP in essential hypertension [113,114] and in renal failure [115]. Evening dose might however result in higher day time BP and adjustment of the dose may be necessary to achieve a well controlled BP in the day time [114].

5. AMBULATORY BLOOD PRESSURE AND CARDIAC MASS

An early study did not find any significant differences in either 24-h BP or cardiac mass NIDDM patients and healthy subjects [6]. Later, increased cardiac mass has been reported in diabetic patients (mixed IDDM and NIDDM) with autonomic neuropathy and associated reduced nocturnal decline of BP as compared with patients without autonomic neuropathy [116]. This may be an effect of autonomic dysfunction per se or the higher nocturnal BP. Similar results has been found in NIDDM patients with nephropathy, who have elevated 24h BP and higher night BP than patients with normoalbuminuria [117].

Left ventricular mass (LVM) and day time diastolic BP were found higher in microalbuminuric than in normoalbuminuric IDDM patients [73]. We have found no significant differences in cardiac mass between microalbuminuric IDDM patients with and without a normal reduction of night BP [96]. In an other study LVM did not differ between white coat hypertensive and normotensive NIDDM patients and LVM was lower in dippers compared to non-dippers (no information about UAE) [118].

6. THE RELATION TO CLINIC BP

When studying young professionally active normotensive subjects the clinic BP is in mean 3- 4 mmHg higher than day time averages [68]. This is the opposite of what is normally seen in about 20-25 % of mildly hypertensive non-diabetic subjects (white-coat hypertension) [30,31]. The clinical implication is that BP is underestimated in some microalbuminuric patients with normal clinic BP.

We have found a markedly lower day time (systolic/diastolic) BP (147.0/ 85.3 mmHg) than clinic BP (162.6 /95.4 mmHg) in 102 consecutive NIDDM and IDDM patients referred to ambulatory BP measurement because of repeated clinic BP > 140/90 mmHg [119]. The frequency of white coat hypertension in normoalbuminuric diabetic patients is about 25 % [119,120]. If patients are selected for the presence of organ lesions related to hypertension (diabetic nephropathy) the proportion of white coat hypertension may be reduced [120]. One study reported a much higher frequency of white coat hypertension (41 %) probably due to a shorter observation period before labelling patients as hypertensive and because patients was designated as "true" normotensive on the basis of 24h BP (containing the lower night BP) rather than day time values [121]. Obviously the reported frequency of white coat hypertension also varies with the definition of a normal ambulatory BP

[30,31] . A widely used definition requires repeated clinic BP > 140/90 and a day time value <135/85 mmHg. An extremely high frequency of white coat hypertension (62 %) was reported in a study measuring clinic BP at one occasion only and using the same cut-off level for establishing the diagnosis of hypertension (clinic mean Due to the high reproducibility of ambulatory BP compared with clinic measurements it is an ideal tool for intervention studies [25,101]. The 24-h effectiveness of the intervention can be evaluated, the number of patients needed can be reduced without loosing power and small changes in BP, which would be overlooked by traditional measurements, can be recognised. Ambulatory BP has now been used in several intervention studies in diabetes [43,102-112].

Due to the high reproducibility of ambulatory BP compared with clinic measurements it is an ideal tool for intervention studies [25,101]. The 24-h effectiveness of the intervention can be evaluated, the number of patients needed can be reduced without loosing power and small changes in BP, which would be overlooked by traditional measurements, can be recognised. Ambulatory BP has now been used in several intervention studies in diabetes [43,102-112].

arterial BP > 100 mmHg) as for identifying those with apparent normal ambulatory BP (day time mean arterial BP < 100 mmHg) [122]. A low frequency (11 %) was reported in NIDDM patients who was categorised as normotensive if day time BP was < 131/86 (women) and < 136/87 (men) [118].

7. AMBULATORY BP AND THE DIABETES CLINIC

In the sixth recommendation of the National Committee for detection and treatment of Hypertension, ambulatory monitoring is approved in certain clinical circumstances [123]. The important problems about establishing a normal reference for ambulatory BP have recently been reviewed thoroughly [124]. Although large individual differences do exist, a clinic BP of 140/90 roughly corresponds to a day time average of 135/85 mmHg [124]. For patients older than 60 years with isolated systolic hypertension the average systolic day time BP is reported much lower (about 20 mmHg) than clinic BP during the placebo run-in phase of the Syst-Eur trial [125]. Since treatment of isolated systolic hypertension significantly reduced the incidence of stroke and cardiovascular events in the SHEP study (Systolic Hypertension in the Elderly Programme) [126] also containing diabetic patients, it is very difficult to suggest a cut off limit for day time BP in this category of patients. In contrast no difference was noted between clinic and day time systolic BP in a small subset of the SHEP population which underwent ambulatory BP monitoring [127]. This discrepancy between the Syst-Eur trial and SHEP trial may relate to the fact that the comparison between clinic and day time BP in the SHEP study was performed after 2 to 3 years enrolment in the study, which may have attenuated the "white coat effect".

Only one study in diabetic patients can give some informations about the level of ambulatory BP, "dipper" or "non-dipper" status and future cardiovascular events [118]. During a follow-up of 3.2 years the rate of cardiovascular events per 100 patient years was 2.0 in clinic and ambulatory normotensive NIDDM patients (n=29), 2.06 in white coat hypertensive patients (n=12), and 7.06 in ambulatory hypertensive patients (n=94) (p<0.001 versus two other groups). Although the absolute number of events in the three groups were low (two,one and 24 events respectively) the data suggest a benign clinical course of white coat hypertensive patients at least in the short term. Furthermore the study showed a higher event rate in female "non-dippers" versus "dippers" [118].

Table 35-3 Suggestions for the clinical use of ambulatory BP in IDDM and NIDDM patients.

	Repeated clinic BP (mmHg)	Value of ambulatory BP monitoring	No indication for initiation or intensification of antihypertensive treatment if day time ambulatory BP (mmHg) is:	Comments
Normo-albuminuria	<140/90 age < 60 years	-	Not relevant	A few patients have a normal clinic BP but an elevated day time BP. The clinical significance is unsettled.
	<160/90 age >60 years	-	Not relevant	
	>140/90 age <60 years	+++	<135/85	The age criteria refers to the St Vincent Declaration [128] and a recent consensus [124]. Other recommendations consider repeated clinic BP>140/90 as hypertensive values irrespective of age [123,130-132].For isolated systolic hypertension, see text.
	>160/90 age >60 years	+++	<140(?)/85	
Micro-albuminuria and diabetic nephropathy without antihypertensive treatment	Not relevant with respect to the indication for ambulatory BP	+	Not relevant	According to recent recommendations, ACE-inhibition should be started irrespective of BP (at least in IDDM) [129]. Ambulatory BP can be performed for comparison after antihypertensive treatment. This is not mandatory.
Micro-albuminuria and diabetic nephropathy with antihypertensive treatment	<130/85	+	<130/85	Some patients who have a normal clinic BP but elevated day time BP (especially on a work day) needs intensified treatment. Treatment may be tailored for patients with nocturnal hypertension.
	>130/85	+++	<130/85	Important to achieve well controlled BP day and night. The goal for clinic and ambulatory BP is even lower for young patients (120/80). Limits for clinic BP refers to[129].
Symptoms of hypotension or autonomic neuropathy	Not relevant with respect to the indication for ambulatory BP	+	Not relevant	Ambulatory BP seldom gives very important additional information not obtained by clinic BP (lying and standing). Since BP measurements are discontinous, it is difficult to draw conclusions from negative findings. A single low BP may be an artifact.

The clinical value of large scale implementation of ambulatory BP monitoring has never been investigated. The value of targeting antihypertensive drug regimen towards high night BP is unexplored. Recommendations for routine clinical work should therefore be rather conservative. The suggested limits for ambulatory BP (Table 35-3) is tentative and should not be over-interpreted. The guidelines will doubtless need corrections based on future studies, which ideally should relate ambulatory BP to end organ damage and to clinical events in antihypertensive drug trials.

8. CONCLUSION

Ambulatory BP is increased in NIDDM and IDDM patients with abnormal albuminuria even in the absence of a detectable difference in clinic BP. An association exist in both NIDDM and IDDM patients between impaired reduction of night BP and the two complications, autonomic neuropathy and diabetic nephropathy. This also counts for the very early phases of diabetic nephropathy in IDDM patients including adolescents [133]. It remains to be elucidated if the abnormal BP variation independently contributes to development of microalbuminuria or to the progression of diabetic nephropathy, or whether this abnormality is merely a cophenomenon found in patients with poor glycemic control and diabetic complications including autonomic neuropathy [93] .

The high reproducibility of ambulatory BP permits registration of small changes in BP which are overlooked by conventional measurement. Large scale longitudinal studies of ambulatory BP and UAE are necessary to characterise the important transition phase from normo- to microalbuminuria. Simultaneous continuous indirect registration of both the sympathovagal balance [134] and BP [135] are perspectives for the future, which probably will add to the understanding of BP variation in diabetes.

The clinical role of ambulatory BP has not been settled. It is seems wise to hesitate with respect to antihypertensive drug treatment of normoalbuminuric diabetic patients with white coat hypertension. The number of these patients who ultimately will become hypertensive by ambulatory BP is unknown and careful observation of BP is essential. Their is an urgent need for more secure guidelines for the use of ambulatory BP including the consequences of specifically addressing antihypertensive treatment towards nocturnal hypertension.

ADDENDUM

Very recently ambulatory BP was compared in normoalbuminuric IDDM patients and healthy controls (n = 55 in each group) [136]. In contrast to a previous comparison [68] (n = 34 in each group) a slightly but significantly higher ambulatory BP was observed in diabetic patients. This could be explained partly by a higher proportion of women (42% versus 29% in the previous study) and partly by increased statistical power due to the larger number of patients. Ambulatory BP (24h and day) was higher in diabetic women than in the control women but no difference (for 24h and day time BP) was observed between diabetic men and control men. The night dip in BP was similar in diabetic and control women but a reduced night dip was reported for diabetic men compared with control men. Diastolic night dip in BP correlated in the total diabetic population with indices of autonomic neuropathy.

The controversy of predisposition to hypertension and development of diabetic nephropathy has recently been addressed by performing ambulatory BP in parents of IDDM patients with and without diabetic nephropathy [137]. The 24h BP was almost identical among the two groups but the frequency of hypertension defined as use of antihypertensive medication or a 24h BP > 135/85 mmHg was significantly higher in parents of patients with nephropathy (57%) than in parents of patients without nephropathy (41%).

REFERENCES

1 Sokolow M, Werdegar D, Kain HK, Hinman AT. Relationship between level of blood pressure measured casually and by portable recorders and severity of complications in essential hypertension. Circulation 1966; 34: 279-298

2 Bevan AT, Honour AJ, Stott FH. Direct arterial pressure recording in unrestricted man. Clin Sci 1969; 36: 329-344

3 Schneider RA, Costiloe JP. Twenty-four hour automatic monitoring of blood pressure and heart rate at work and at home. Am Heart J 1975; 90: 695-702

4 Rubler S, Abenavoli T, Greenblatt HA, Dixon JF, Cieslik CJ. Ambulatory blood pressure monitoring in diabetic males: A method for detecting blood pressure elevations undisclosed by conventional methods. Clin Cardiol 1982; 5: 447-454

5 Osei K. Ambulatory and exercise-induced blood pressure responses in type I diabetic patients and normal subjects. Diabetes Research and Clinical Practice 1987; 3: 125-134

6 Porcellati C, Gatteschi C, Benemio G, Guerrieri M, Boldrini F, Verdecchia P. Analisi ecocardiografica del ventriculo sinistro in pazienti con diabete mellito di tipo II. G Ital Cardiol 1989; 19: 128-135

7 Verdecchia P, Gatteschi C, Benemio G, Porcellati C. Ambulatory blood pressure monitoring in normotensive and hypertensive patients with diabetes (abstract). J Hypertension 1988; 6 (suppl 4): S692-S693

8 Rubler S, Chu DA, Bruzzone CL. Blood pressure and heart rate responses during 24-h ambulatory monitoring and exercise in men with diabetes mellitus. Am J Cardiol 1985; 55: 801-806

9 Guilleminault C, Mondini S, Hayes B. Diabetic autonomic dysfunction, blood pressure and sleep. Ann Neurol 1985; 18: 670-675

10 Reeves RA, Shapiro AP, Thompson ME, Johnsen A-M. Loss of nocturnal decline in blood pressure after cardiac transplantation. Circulation 1986; 73: 401-408

11 Liniger C, Favre L, Adamec R, Pernet A, Assal J-Ph. Profil nyctéméral de la pression artérielle et de la fréquence cardiaque dans la neuropathie diabétique autonome. Schweiz Med Wschr 1987; 117: 1949-1953

12 Hornung RS, Mahler RF, Raftery EB. Ambulatory blood pressure and heart rate in diabetic patients: an assessment of autonomic function. Diabetic Med 1989; 6: 579-585

13 Chanudet X, Bauduceau B, Ritz P, Jolibois P, Garcin JM, Larroque P, Gautier D. Neuropathie végétative et régulation tensionelle chez le diabétique. Arch Mal Coer 1989; 82: 1147-1151

14 The National High Blood Pressure Education Program Coordinating Commitee. National High Blood Pressure Education Program Working Group Report on ambulatory blood pressure monitoring. Arch Intern Med 1990; 150: 2270-2280

15 Stewart MJ, Padfield PL. Blood Pressure measurement: an epitaph for the mercury manometer ? Clin Sci 1992; 83: 1-12

16 Purcell HJ, Gibbs SR, Coats AJS, Fox KM. Ambulatory blood pressure monitoring and circadian variation of cardiovascular disease; clinical and research applications. Int J Cardiol 1992; 36: 135-149

17 Stewart MJ, Padfield PL. Measurement of blood pressure in the technological age. Brit Med Bull 1994; 50: 420-442

18 Pickering TG. Blood pressure measurement and detection of hypertension. Lancet 1994; 344: 31-35

19 Staessen JA, Fagard R, Thijs L, Amery A. A consensus view of the technique of ambulatory blood pressure monitoring. Hypertens 1995; [part 1]: 912-918

20 Pickering TG. Recommendations for the use of home (self) and ambulatory blood pressure monitoring. Am J Hypertens 1995; 9: 11

21 Halimi S, Benhamou PY, Mallion JM, Gaudemaris R, Bachelot I. Intérêt de l'enregistrement de la pression artérielle ambulatoire chez les patients diabétiques. Diabete Metab (Paris) 1991; 17: 538-544
22 White WB. Diurnal blood pressure and blood pressure variability in diabetic normotensive and hypertensive subjects. J Hypertension 1992; 10 (suppl 1): S35-S41
23 Hansen KW. How to monitor blood pressure changes in the diabetes clinic: office, home or 24 h-ambulatory blood pressure recordings. In: Mogensen CE, Standl E (eds). Diabetes Forum Series volume IV. Concepts for the ideal diabetes clinic. Berlin, New York: Walter de Gruyter; 1993; pp. 235-248
24 Hansen KW, Christiansen JS. Research methodologies for recording blood pressure in diabetic patients. In: Mogensen CE, Standl E (eds). Diabetes Forum Series volume V (part 2). Research methodologies in human diabetes. Berlin, New York: Walter de Gruyter; 1994; pp. 113-124
25 Coats AJS, Radaelli A, Clark SJ, Conway J, Sleight P. The influence of ambulatory blood pressure monitoring on the design and interpretation of trials in hypertension. J Hypertens 1992; 10: 385-391
26 Coats AJS, Clark SJ, Conway J. Analysis of ambulatory blood pressure data. J Hypertens 1991; 9 (suppl 8): S19-S21
27 Germano G, Damiani S, Caparra A, Cassone-Faldetta M, Germano U, Coia F, De Mattia G, Santucci A, Balsano F. Ambulatory blood pressure recording in diabetic patients with abnormal responses to cardiovascular autonomic tests. Acta Diabetol 1992; 28: 221-228
28 Hansen KW, Poulsen PL, Mogensen CE. Ambulatory blood pressure and abnormal albuminuria in type 1 diabetic patients. Kidney Int 1994; 45 (suppl.45): S134-S140 (Correction. Kidney Int 45: 1799-1800, 1994)
29 Verdecchia P, Schillaci G, Guerrieri M, Gatteschi C, Benemio G, Boldrini F, Porcellati C. Circadian blood pressure changes and left ventricular hypertrophy in essential hypertension. Circulation 1990; 81: 528-536
30 Pickering TG. White coat hypertension. Curr Opin Nephrol Hypertens 1996; 5: 192-198
31 Mancia G, Zanchetti A. White-coat hypertension: misnomers, misconceptions and misunderstandings. What should we do next ?. J Hypertens 1996; 14: 1049-1052
32 Verdecchia P, Schillaci G, Borgioni C, Ciucci A, Zampi I, Gattobigio R, Sacchi N, Porcellati C. White coat hypertension and white coat effect. Similarities and differences. Am J Hypertens 1995; 8: 790-798
33 Tovi J, Theobald H, Engfeldt P. Effect of metabolic control on 24-h ambulatory blood pressure in elderly non-insulin-dependent diabetic patients. J Hum Hypertens 1996; 10: 589-594
34 Schmitz A, Mau Pedersen M, Hansen KW. Blood pressure by 24 h ambulatory recordings in type 2 (non-insulin-dependent) diabetics. Relationship to urinary albumin excretion. Diabete Metab (Paris) 1991; 17: 301-307
35 Nielsen FS, Rossing P, Bang Lia E, Svendsen TL, Gall M-A, Smidt UM, Parving H-H. On the mechanism of blunted nocturnal decline in arterial blood pressure in NIDDM patients with diabetic nephropathy. Diabetes 1995; 44: 783-789
36 Mitchell TH, Nolan B, Henry M, Cronin C, Baker H, Greely G. Microalbuminuria in patients with non-insulin-dependent diabetes mellitus relates to nocturnal systolic blood pressure. Am J Med 1997; 102: 531-535.
37 Fogari R, Zoppi A, Malamani GD, Lazzari P, Destro M, Corradi L. Ambulatory blood pressure monitoring in normotensive and hypertensive type 2 diabetics. Prevalence of impaired diurnal blood pressure patterns. Am J Hypertens 1993; 6: 1-7
38 Nielsen S, Schmitz O, Ørskov H, Mogensen CE. Similar insulin sensivity in NIDDM patients with normo- and microalbuminuria. Diabetes Care 1995; 18: 834-842
39 Jermendy G, Ferenzi J, Hernandez E, Farkas K, Nadas J. Day -night blood pressure variations in normotensive and hypertensive NIDDM patients with asymptomatic autonomic neuropathy. Diabetes Res Clin Pract 1996; 34: 107-114
40 Berrut G, Fabbri P, Bouhanick B, Lalanne P, Guilloteau G, Marre M, Fressinaud P. Loss of nocturnal blood pressure decrease in non-insulin dependent diabetis subjects with microalbuminuria. Arch Mal Coeur 1996; 89: 1041-1044
41 Lindsay RS, Stewart MJ, Nairn IM, Baird JD, Padfield PL. Reduced diurnal variation of blood pressure in non-insulin-dependent diabetic patients with microalbumnuria. J Hum Hypertens 1995; 9: 223-227

42 Pinkney JH, Foyle W-J, Denver AE, Mohamed-Ali V, McKinlay S, Yudkin JS. The relationship of urinary albumin excretion rate to ambulatory blood pressure and erythrocyte sodium-lithium countertransport in NIDDM. Diabetologia 1995; 38: 356-362

43 Waeber B, Weidmann P, Wohler D, Le Bloch Y. Albuminuria in diabetes mellitus. Relation to ambulatory versus office blood pressure and effects of cilazapril. Am J Hypertens; 9: 1220-1227

44 Iwase M, Kaseda S, Iino K, Fukuhura M, Yamamoto M, Fukudome Y, Yoshizumi H, Abe I, Yoshinari M, Fujishima M. Circadian blood pressure variation in non-insulin-dependent diabetes mellitus with diabetic nephropathy. Diabetes Res Clin Pract 1994; 26: 43-50

45 Fogari R, Zoppi A, Malamani GD, Lazzari P, Albonico B, Corradi L. Urinary albumin excretion and nocturnal blood pressure in hypertensive patients with type II diabetes. Am J Hyp 1994; 7: 808-813

46 Equiluz-Bruck S, Schnack C, Schernthaner G. Nondipping of nocturnal blood pressure is related to urinary albumin excretion in patients with type 2 diabetes mellitus. Am J Hypertens 1996; 9: 1139-1143

47 Nakano S, Uchida K, Kigoshi T, Azukizawa S, Iwasaki R, Kaneko M, Morimoto S. Circadian rhytm of blood pressure in normotensive NIDDM subjects. Its relation to microvascular complications. Diabetes Care 1991; 14: 707-711

48 Nielsen S, Schmitz A, Poulsen PL, Hansen KW, Mogensen CE. Albuminuria and 24-h ambulatory blood pressure in normoalbuminuric and microalbuminuric NIDDM patients. Diabetes Care 1995; 18: 1434-1441

49 Chamontin B, Barbe P, Begasse F, Ghisolfi A, Amar J, Louvet JP, Salvador M. Presion artérielle ambulatoire au cours de l'hypertension arterielle avec dysautonomie. Arch Mal Coer 1990; 83: 1103-1106

50 Felici MG, Spallone V, Maillo MR, Gatta R, Civetta E, Frontoni S, Gambardella S, Menzinger G. Twenty-four hours blood pressure and heart rate profiles in diabetics with and without autonomic neuropathy. Funct Neurol 1991; 6: 299-304

51 Liniger C, Favre L, Assal J-Ph. Twenty-four hour blood pressure and heart rate profiles of diabetic patients with abnormal cardiovascular reflexes. Diabetic Med 1991; 8: 420-427

52 Spallone V, Bernardi L, Ricordi L, Soldà P, Maillo MR, Calciati A, Gambardella S, Fratino P, Menzinger G. Relationship between the circadian rhytms of blood pressure and sympathovagal balance in diabetic autonomic neuropathy. Diabetes 1993; 42: 1745-1752

53 Ikeda T, Matsubara T, Sato Y, Sakamoto N. Circadian variation in diabetic patients with autonomic neuropathy. J Hypertens 1993: 11: 581-587

54 Nakano S, Uchida K, Ishii T, Takeuchi M, Azukizawa S, Kigoshi T, Morimoto S. Association of a nocturnal rise in plasma α-atrial natriuretic peptide and reversed diurnal rhytm in hospitalized normotensive subjects with non-insulin dependent diabetes mellitus. Eur J Endocrinol 1994; 131: 184-190

55 Sasaki E, Kitaoka H, Ohsawa N. Postprandial hypotension in patients with non-insulin-dependent diabetes mellitus. Diabetes Res Clin Pract 1992; 18: 113-121

56 Nakajima S, Otsuka K, Yamanaka T, Omori K, Kubo Y, Toyoshima T, Watanabe Y, Watanabe H. Ambulatory blood pressure and postprandial hypotension. Am Heart J 1992; 124: 1669-1671

57 Pinkney JH, Mohamed-Ali V, Denver AE, Foster C, Sampson MJ, Yudkin JS. Insulin resistance, insulin, proinsulin, and ambulatory blood pressure in type II diabetes. Hypertension 1994; 24: 362-367

58 Rynkiewicz A, Furmanski J, Narkiewicz K, Semetkowska E, Bieniaszewski L, Horoszek-Maziarz S, Krupa-Wojciechowska B. Influence of duration of type 1 (insulin-dependent) diabetes mellitus on 24-h ambulatory blood pressure and heart rate profile (letter). Diabetologia 1993; 36: 577

59 Hansen KW, Poulsen PL, Christiansen JS, Mogensen CE. Determinants of 24-h blood pressure in IDDM patients. Diabetes Care 1995; 18: 529-535

60 Donaldson DL, Moore WV, Chonko AM, Shipman JJ, Wiegmann T. Incipient hypertension precedes incipient nephropathy in adolescents and young adults with type I diabetes (abstract). Diabetes 1992; 42 (suppl 1): 97A

61 Mathiesen ER, Hilsted J, Feldt-Rasmussen B, Bonde-Petersen F, Christensen NJ, Parving H-H. The effect of metabolic control on hemodynamics in short-term insulin-dependent diabetic patients. Diabetes 1985; 34: 1301-1305

62 Richards AM, Donelly T, Nicholls MG, Ikram H, Hamilton EJ, Espiner EA. Blood pressure and vasoactive hormones with improved glycemic control in patients with diabetes mellitus. Clin Exp Hypertens [A] 1989; A11:391-406

63 Mathiesen ER, Gall M-A. Hommel E, Skøtt P, Parving H-H. Effects of short term strict metabolic control on kidney function and extracellular volume in incipient diabetic nephropathy. Diabetic Med 1989; 6: 595-600

64 Hansen KW, Pedersen MM, Christiansen JS, Mogensen CE. Night blood pressure and cigarette smoking: disparate associations in healthy subjects and diabetic patients. Blood Pressure 1994; 3: 381-388

65 Poulsen PL, Ebbehøj E, Hansen KW, Mogensen CE. Effects of smoking on 24-h ambulatory blood pressure and autonomic function in normoalbuminuric IDDM patients. Am J Hypertens (in press)

66 Mikkelsen KL, Wiinberg N, Høegholm A, Christensen HR, Bang LE, Nielsen PE, Svendsen TL, Kampmann JP, Madsen NH, Bentzon MW. Smoking related to 24 hrs ambulatory blood pressure and heart rate. A study in 352 normotensive Danish subjects. Am J Hypertens 1997; 10: 483-491.

67 Sinha RN, Patrick AW, Richardson L, MacFarlane IA. Diurnal variation in blood pressure in insulin-dependent diabetic smokers and non-smokers with and without microalbuminuria. Diabetic Med 1997; 14: 291-295.

68 Hansen KW, Christensen CK, Andersen PH, Mau Pedersen M, Christiansen JS, Mogensen CE. Ambulatory blood pressure in microalbuminuric type 1 diabetic patients. Kidney Int 1992; 41: 847-854

69 Benhamou PY, Halimi S, De Gaudemaris R, Boizel R, Pitiot M, Siche JP, Bachelot I, Mallion JM. Early disturbances of ambulatory blood pressure load in normotensive type 1 diabetic patients with microalbuminuria. Diabetes Care 1992; 15: 1614-1619

70 Peters A, Gromeier S, Kohlmann T, Look D, Kerner W. Nocturnal blood pressure elevation is related to adrenomedullary hyperactivity, but not to hyperinsulinemia, in nonobese normoalbuminuric type 1 diabetic patients. J Clin Endocrinol Metab 1996; 81: 507-512

71 Gilbert R, Philips P, Clarke C, Jerums G. Day-night blood pressure variation in normotensive normoalbuminuric type I diabetic subjects. Diabetes Care 1994; 17: 824-827

72 Khan N, Couper J, Dixit M, Couper R. Ambulatory blood pressure and heart rate in adolescents with insulin-dependent diabetes mellitus. Am J Hyp 1994; 7: 937-940

73 Guglielmi MD, Pierdomenico SD, Salvatore L, Romano R, Tascione E, Pupillo M, Porreca E, Imbastaro T, Cuccurullo F, Mezzetti A. Impaired left ventricular diastolic function and vascular postischemic vasodilation associated with microalbuminuria in IDDM patients. Diabetes Care 1995; 18: 353-360

74 Moore WV, Donaldson DL, Chonko AM, Ideus P, Wiegmann TB, Wiegmann. Ambulatory blood pressure in type I diabetes mellitus. Comparison to presence of incipient nephropathy in adolescents and young adults. Diabetes 41; 1992: 1035-1041

75 Sivieri R, Deandrea M, Gai V, Cavallo-Perin P. Circadian blood pressure levels in normotensive normoalbuminuric type 1 diabetic patients. Diabetic Med 1994; 11; 357-361

76 Hansen KW. Ambulatory blood pressure in insulin-dependent diabetes; the relation to stages of diabetic kidney disease. J Diab Comp 1996; 10:331-351

77 Wiegmann TB, Herron KG, Chonko AM, Macdougall ML, Moore WV. Recognition og hypertension and abnormal blood pressure burden with ambulatory blood pressure recordings in type I diabetes mellitus. Diabetes 1990; 39: 1556-1560

78 Yip J, Mattock MB, Morocutti A, Sethi M, Trevisan R, Viberti G. Insulin resistance in insulin-dependent diabetic patients with microalbuminuria. Lancet 1993; 342: 883-887

79 Lurbe A, Redón J, Pascual JM, Tacons J, Alvarez V, Batlle DC. Altered blood pressure during sleep in normotensive subjects with type I diabetes. Hypertension 1993; 21: 227-235

80 Berrut G, Hallab M, Bouhanick B, Chameau A-M, Marre M, Fressinaud Ph. Value of ambulatory blood pressure in type I (insulin-dependent) diabetic patients with incipient diabetic nephropathy. Am J Hyp 1994; 7: 222-227

81 Hansen KW, Mau Pedersen M, Marshall SM, Christiansen JS, Mogensen CE. Circadian variation of blood pressure in patients with diabetic nephropathy. Diabetologia 1992; 35: 1074-1079

82 Torffvit O, Agardh C-D. Day and night variations in ambulatory blood pressure in type 1 diabetes mellitus with nephropathy and autonomic neuropathy. J Intern Med 1993; 233: 131-137

83 Poulsen PL, Hansen KW, Mogensen CE. Ambulatory blood pressure in the transition from normo- to microalbuminuria. A longitudinal study in IDDM patients. Diabetes 1994; 43; 1248-1253

84 Hansen KW, Pedersen MM, Christiansen, Mogensen CE. Diurnal blood pressure variations in normoalbuminuric type 1 diabetic patients. J Int Med 1993; 234: 175-180

85 Poulsen PL, Ebbehøj E, Hansen KW, Mogensen CE. 24-h blood pressure and autonomic function is related to albumin excretion within the normoalbuminuric range in IDDM patients. Diabetologia 1997; 40: 718-725

86 Page SR, Manning G, Ingle AR, Hill P, Millar-Craig MW, Peacock I. Raised ambulatory blood pressure in type 1 diabetes with incipient microalbuminuria. Diabetic Med 1994; 11; 877-882

87 Spallone V, Gambardella S, Maiello MR, Barini A, Frontoni S, Menzinger G. Relationship between autonomic neuropathy, 24-h blood pressure, and nephropathy in normotensive IDDM patients. Diabetes Care 1994; 17: 578-584

88 Monteagudo PT, Nóbrega JC, Cazarini PR, Ferreira SRG, Kohlmann O, Ribeiro AB, Zanella M-T. Altered blood pressure profile, autonomic neuropathy and nephropathy in insulin-dependent diabetic patients. European J of Endocrinology 1996; 135: 683-688.

89 Dyrberg T, Benn J, Sandahl Christiansen J, Hilsted J, Nerup J. Prevalence of diabetic autonomic neuropathy measured by simple bedside test. Diabetologia 1981; 20: 190-194

90 Zander E, Schulz, Heinke P, Grimmberger E, Zander G, Gottschling HD. Importance of cardiovascular autonomic dysfunction in IDDM subjects with diabetic nephropathy. Diabetes Care 1989; 12: 259-264

91 Mølgaard H, Christensen PD, Sørensen KE, Christensen CK, Mogensen CE. Association of 24-h cardiac parasympathetic activity and degree of nephropathy in IDDM patients. Diabetes 1992; 41: 812-817

92 Mølgaard H, Christensen PD, Hermansen K, Sørensen KE, Christensen CK, Mogensen CE. Early recognition of autonomic dysfunction in microalbuminuria: significance for cardiovascular mortality in diabetes mellitus. Diabetologia 1994; 37; 788-796

93 Hansen KW. Diurnal blood pressure profile, autonomic neuropathy and nephropathy in diabetes. European J of Endocrinology 1997; 136: 35-36

94 Farmer CKT, Goldsmith DJA, Quin JD, Dallyn P, Cox J, Kingswood JC, Sharpstone P. Progression of diabetic nephropathy-Is diurnal blood pressure rhytm as important as absolute blood pressure level. Nephrol Dial Transplant (in press)

95 Pecis M, Azevedo MJ, Gross JL. Glomerular hyperfiltration is associated with blood pressure abnormalities in normotensive normoalbuminuric IDDM patients. Diabetes Care 1997; 20: 1329-1333

96 Hansen KW, Sørensen K, Christensen PD, Pedersen EB, Christiansen JS, Mogensen CE. Night blood pressure: relation to organ lesions in microalbuminuric type 1 diabetic patients. Diabetic Med 1995; 12: 42-45

97 Mulec H, Blohmé G, Kullenberg K, Nyberg G, Bjørck S. Latent overhydration and nocturnal hypertension in diabetic nephropathy. Diabetologia 1995; 38; 216-229

98 Hansen HP, Rossing P, Tarnow L, Nielsen FS, Jensen BR, Parving H-H. Circadian rhytm of arterial blood pressure and albuminuria in diabetic nephropathy. Kidney Int 1996; 50; 579-585

99 Poulsen PL, Juhl B, Ebbehøj E, Klein F, Christiansen C, Mogensen CE. Elevated ambulatory blood pressure in microalbuminuric IDDM patients is inversely associated with renal plasma flow. A compensatory mechanism ? Diabetes Care 1997; 20: 429-432

100 Poulsen PL, Bek T, Ebbehøj E, Hansen KW, Mogensen CE. 24-h ambulatory blood pressure and retinopathy in normoalbuminuric IDDM patients. Diabetologia (1998) 41: 105-110.

101 Hansen KW, Schmitz A, Mau Pedersen M. Ambulatory blood pressure measurement in type 2 diabetic patients: Methodological aspects. Diabetic Med 1991; 8: 567-572

102 Mau Pedersen M, Hansen KW, Schmitz A, Sørensen K, Christensen CK, Mogensen CE. Effects of ACE inhibition supplementary to beta blockers and diuretics in early diabetic nephropathy. Kidney Int 1992; 41: 883-890

103 Wiegmann TB, Herron KG, Chonko AM, MacDougall ML, Moore WV. Effect of angiotensin-converting enzyme inhibition on renal function and albuminuria in normotensive type I diabetic patients. Diabetes 1992; 41: 62-67

104 Nielsen FS, Rossing P, Gall M-A, Skøtt P, Smidt UM, Parving H-H. Impact of lisinopril and atenolol on kidney function in hypertensive NIDDM subjects with diabetic nephropathy. Diabetes 1994; 43; 1108-1113

105 Sundaresan P, Lykos D, Daher A, Diamond T, Morris R, Howes LG. Comparative effects of glibenclamide and metformin on ambulatory blood pressure and cardiovascular reactivity in NIDDM. Diabetes Care 1997; 20: 692-697

106 Hansen KW, Klein F, Christensen PD, Sørensen K, Andersen PH, Møller J, Pedersen EB, Christiansen JS, Mogensen CE. Effects of captopril on ambulatory blood pressure, renal and cardiac function in microalbuminuric type 1 diabetic patients. Diabete Metab (Paris) 1994; 20; 485-493

107 Rossing P, Tarnow L, Boelskifte S, Jensen BR, Nielsen FS, Parving H-H. Differences between nisoldipine and lisinopril on glomerular filtration rates and albuminuria in hypertensive IDDM patients with diabetic nephropathy during the first year of treatment. Diabetes 1997; 46: 481-487

108 Rossing P, Hansen BV, Nielsen FS, Myrup B, Holmer G, Parving H-H. Fish oil in diabetic nephropathy. Diabetes Care 1996; 19: 1214-1219

109 Agardh CD, Garcia Puig J, Charbonnel B, Angelkort B, Barnett AH. Greater reduction of urinary albumin excretion in hypertensive type II diabetic patients with incipient nephropathy by lisinopril than by nifedipine. J Hum Hypertens 1996; 10: 185-192

110 Schneider M, Lerch M, Papiri M, Buechel P, Boehlen L, Shaw S, Risen W, Weidmann. Metabolic neutrality of combined varapamil-trandolapril treatment in contrast to beta-blocker-low-dose chlortalidone treatment in hypertensive type 2 diabetes. J Hypertens 1996; 14: 669-677

111 Rasmussen OW, Thomsen C, Hansen KW, Vesterlund M, Winther E, Hermansen K. Effects on blood pressure, glucose and lipid levels of a high-monounsaturated fat diet compared with a high-carbohydrate diet in NIDDM subjects. Diabetes Care 1993; 16: 1565-1571

112 Nielsen S, Hermansen K, Rasmussen OW, Thomsen C, Mogensen CE. Urinary albumin excretion rate and 24-h ambulatory blood pressure in NIDDM with microalbuminuria: effects of a monounsaturated-enriched diet. Diabetologia 1995; 38; 1069-1075

113 Palatini P, Racioppa A, Raule G, Zaninotto M, Penzo M, Pessina AC. Effect of timing of administration on the plasma ACE inhibitory activity and the antihypertensive effect of quinapril. Clin Pharmacol Ther 1992; 52; 378-383

114 Morgan T, Anderson A, Jones E. The effect on 24h blood pressure control of an angiotensin converting enzyme inhibitor (perindopril) administered in the morning or at night. J Hypertens 1997; 15: 205-211

115 Portaluppi F, Vergnani L, Manfredini R, Uberti ECD, Fersini C. Time-dependent effect of isradipine on the nocturnal hypertension in chronic renal failure. Am J Hyp 1995; 8; 719-726

116 Gambardella S, Frontoni S, Spallone V, Maiello MR, Civetta E, Lanza G, Sandric S, Menzinger G. Increased left ventricular mass in normotensive diabetic patients with autonomic neuropathy. Am J Hyp 1993; 6: 97-102

117 Nielsen FS, Ali S, Rossing P, Bang LE, Svendsen TL, Gall M-A, Smidt UM, Kastrup J, Parving H-H. Left ventricular hypertrophy and systolic dysfunction in non-insulin dependent diabetic patients with and without diabetic nephropathy (abstract). Journal of the American Society of Nephrology 1995; 6: 453

118 Verdecchia P, Porcellati C, Schillaci G, Borgioni, Ciucci A, Gatteschi C, Zampi I, Santucci A, Santucci C, Reboldi G. Ambulatory blood pressure and risk of cardiovascular disease in type II diabetes mellitus. Diab Nutr Metab 1994; 7: 223-231

119 Ebbehøj E, Poulsen PL, Hansen KW, Mogensen CE. White coat effect in diabetes: ambulatory blood pressure in relation to clinic based measurement (abstract). Diabetologia 1997; 40 (suppl 1): A12

120 Nielsen FS, Gæde P, Vedel P, Pedersen O, Parving H-H. White coat hypertension in NIDDM patients with and without incipient and over diabetic nephropathy. Diabetes Care 1997; 20: 859-863

121 Puig JG, Ruilope LM, Ortega R. Antihypertensive treatment efficacy in type II diabetes mellitus. Dissociation between casual and 24-hour ambulatory blood pressure. Hypertension 1995; 26 (part 2): 1093-1099

122 Burgess E, Mather K, Ross S, Josefsberg Z. Office hypertension in Type 2 (non-insulin-dependent) diabetic patients (letter). Diabetologia 1991; 34: 684

123 The Joint National Committee on Detection, Evaluation, and Treatment of High Blood Pressure. The sixth report of the joint national committee on detection, evaluation, and treatment of high blood pressure. Arch Intern Med 1997; 157: 2413-2446

124 O'Brien E, Staessen J. Normotension and hypertension as defined by 24-hour ambulatory blood pressure monitoring. Blood Pressure 1995; 4; 266-282

125 Thijs L, Amery A, Clement D, Cox J, de Cort P, Fagard R, Fowler G, Guo C, Mancia G, Marin R, O'Brien E, O'Malley K, Palatini P, Parati G, Petrie J, Ravogli A, Rosenfeld J, Staessen J, Webster J. Ambulatory blood pressure monitoring in elderly patients with isolated systolic hypertension. J Hypertens 1992; 10; 693-699

126 SHEP Cooperative Research Group. Prevention of stroke by antihypertensive drug treatment in older persons with isolated systolic hypertension. JAMA 1991; 265; 3255-3264

127 Rutan GH, McDonald RH, Kuller LH. Comparison of ambulatory and clinic blood pressure and heart rate in older persons with isolated systolic hypertension. Am J Hypertens 1992; 5; 880-886

128 Viberti GC, Mogensen CE, Passa P, Bilous R, Mangili R. St Vincent declaration, 1994: guidelines for the prevention of diabetic renal failure. In: Mogensen CE (ed). The kidney and hypertension in diabetes mellitus, 2nd ed. Boston, Dordrecht/London: Kluwer; 1994; pp.515-527

129 Mogensen CE, Keane WF, Bennet PH, Jerums G, Parving H-H, Passa P, Steffes MW, Striker GE, Viberti GC. Prevention of diabetic renal disease with special reference to microalbuminuria. Lancet 1995; 346; 1080-1084

130 Consensus statement. Treatment of hypertension in diabetes. Diabetes Care 1993; 16: 1394-1401

131 The national high blood pressure education program working group. National high blood pressure education program working group report on hypertension in diabetes. Hypertension 1994; 23: 145-158

132 The guidelines subcommittee of the WHO/ISH mild hypertension liaison committee. 1993 guidelines for the management of mild hypertension. Hypertension 1993; 22: 392-403

133 Sochett BE, Poon I, Balfe W, Daneman D. Ambulatory Blood Pressure Monitoring in Insulin-Dependent Diabetes Mellitus Adolescents With and Without Microalbuminuria. J Diab Comp 12:18-23.

134 Mølgaard H, Hermansen K. Evaluation of cardiac autonomic neuropathy by heart rate variability. In: Mogensen CE, Standl E (eds). Diabetes Forum Series volume V (part 1). Research methodologies in human diabetes. Berlin, New York: Walter de Gruyter; 1994, pp 219-240

135 Imholz BPM, Langewouters GJ, van Montfrans A, Parati G, van Goudoever J, Wesseling KH, Wieling W, Mancia G. Feasibility of ambulatory, continous 24-hour finger arterial pressure recording. Hypertension 1993; 21: 65-73

136. van Ittersum FJ, Spek JJ, Praet IJA, Lambert J, Ijzerman RG, Fischer HRA, Nikkels RE, Van Bortel LMAB, Donker AJM, Stehouwer CDA. Ambulatory blood pressures and autonomic nervous function in normoalbuminuric type I diabetic patients. Nephrol Dial Transplant 1998; 13:326-332.

137. Fagerudd JA, Tarnow L, Jacobsen P, Stenman S, Nielsen FS, Petterson-Fernholm KJ, Grönhagen-Riska C, Parving H-H, Groop P-H. Predisposition to essential hypertension and development of diabetic nephropathy in IDDM patients. Diabetes 1998; 47: 439-444.

36. LIPIDAEMIA AND DIABETIC RENAL DISEASE

Per-Henrik Groop
Department of Medicine, Helsinki University Central Hospital, Helsinki, Finland

Coronary heart disease (CHD) is not only a major cause of death in the general population but also in IDDM and NIDDM [1]. Whereas in IDDM the increased early cardiovascular morbidity and mortality is largely confined to those with persistent proteinuria [2,3], such complications are frequently seen without signs of renal involvement in NIDDM. The prevalence of CHD and risk of premature death though increases with increasing albuminuria also in NIDDM [4-8]. The same major risk factors (lipid abnormalities) seem to be operative in the diabetic population as in the non-diabetic population [9,10]. However, there are differences in the lipid patterns between IDDM and NIDDM patients, and renal disease further modulates the lipid pattern. A thorough characterisation of the lipid metabolism of these high risk patients is necessary to propose treatment strategies to prevent cardiovascular complications. This chapter will briefly review the present knowledge of the lipid and lipoprotein abnormalities observed in IDDM and NIDDM.

1. LIPID PROFILES AND DIABETES

There is general consensus that IDDM patients without renal disease have an antiatherogenic serum lipoprotein profile [11,12]. This profile is characterised by normal or even subnormal concentrations of total and LDL cholesterol, VLDL triglyceride and elevated HDL cholesterol levels [11]. However, several factors like glycaemic control, mode of insulin administration, genetic factors, obesity and renal disease can modulate the lipoprotein pattern. Glycaemic control especially has an effect on the serum triglyceride level [13].

Nikkilä and Hormila [14] were the first to report the elevation of HDL cholesterol in well or moderately controlled IDDM patients, a finding partly explained by an increase of lipoprotein lipase (LPL) activity in conjunction with peripheral insulin administration. The increase of HDL is associated with a rise in HDL_2 cholesterol [15]. The concentration of apoA-I and apoA-I to apoA-II-ratio has also been reported to be elevated [16]. Laakso et al. [9] observed that HDL cholesterol was lower in normoalbuminuric IDDM patients with CHD than in IDDM patients without CHD, but not significantly lower than in non-diabetic patients with CHD. In insulin-deficient states plasma HDL cholesterol concentration is generally low [11], which is probably due to a low LPL activity and can be corrected by proper insulin treatment.

We studied the spectrum of HDL particles in 86 IDDM patients and 74 nondiabetic subjects [17]. HDL and HDL_2 cholesterol as well as the apoA-I to apoA-II ratio were higher in IDDM than in control subjects and was due to an increased concentration of LpA-I particles [17]. This is an important observation since LpA-I particles are suggested to have a key role in reverse cholesterol transport.

If IDDM patients in general have an antiatherogenic lipid profile, this is not the case in NIDDM. NIDDM is frequently associated with dyslipidaemia, which is characterised by elevations of serum total and VLDL-triglyceride and low HDL cholesterol levels [11,18,19]. LDL cholesterol is usually normal in patients with good glycaemic control [20,21]. The hypertriglyceridaemia is mainly due to increased hepatic synthesis of VLDL particles, particularly the larger triglyceride-rich $VLDL_1$ [11,22,23]. These $VLDL_1$ particles are prone to hepatic removal, and thus escape the VLDL-IDL-LDL cascade before conversion to LDL [24-26]. This may explain the lack of elevation of LDL cholesterol in NIDDM.

In NIDDM the HDL cholesterol concentration is usually 10-20 % lower than in the control population [27] due to a decrease in HDL_2 cholesterol [28,29]. Decreased activities of postheparin plasma LPL [30] and adipose tissue LPL [31] have been described but they do not explain the decreased HDL values [32]. In turn postheparin hepatic lipase (HL) activity has been reported to be elevated [30]. As HDL-triglycerides are generally elevated in NIDDM, the combination of triglyceride-rich HDL and increased HL activity may accelerate the removal of HDL by the liver reducing the HDL concentration [33].

2. LIPIDS IN DIABETIC RENAL DISEASE

ApoB containing triglyceride-rich lipoproteins

IDDM patients with renal disease have increased concentrations of serum total and LDL cholesterol, triglyceride and apoB [34-37]. There is also evidence indicating that these unfavourable changes in the serum lipoproteins are present already at the microalbuminuric stage [38-40]. Whether the lipoprotein changes correlate with the degree of albuminuria is, however, uncertain [34-36]. An elevated serum cholesterol concentration has been shown to be an independent risk factor for death in IDDM patients with renal disease [35].

Few studies have in more detail characterized the triglyceride-rich apoB containing lipoproteins in IDDM patients with elevated albumin excretion rate (AER). We studied 64 IDDM patients with normal AER, 52 with microalbuminuria and 37 with proteinuria matched for age, body weight, disease duration and glycaemic control [12].

The major finding was increased mass concentrations of the IDL fraction in those with elevated AER (figure 36-1). Since substantial evidence indicate that IDL is highly atherogenic [41-44], the increase of IDL mass concentrations is noteworthy and may contribute to the excess CHD risk in these patients. So far IDL has been determined only in one previous study in a small cohort (n=23] of IDDM patients with early nephropathy [45], and these authors did, however, not observe any changes in the IDL concentrations.

Another major observation in our study was that triglyceride, free cholesterol, cholesterol ester and phospholipid concentrations in the VLDL, IDL and LDL fractions as well as total cholesterol, total triglyceride and apoB concentrations were higher in the patients with elevated AER, but notably there were no differences between patients with microalbuminuria and proteinuria (figure 36-2) [12]. We also observed that IDDM patients with microalbuminuria and proteinuria had increased apoB concentrations in the $VLDL_2$ and IDL lipoprotein fractions compared to normoalbuminuric patients [12]. As there is one apoB molecule per particle these data suggested the presence of an increased number of $VLDL_2$ and IDL particles. Of note is that the number of IDL particles is about 6 times higher than the $VLDL_1$ particles and almost 3 times higher than the $VLDL_2$ particles, respectively.

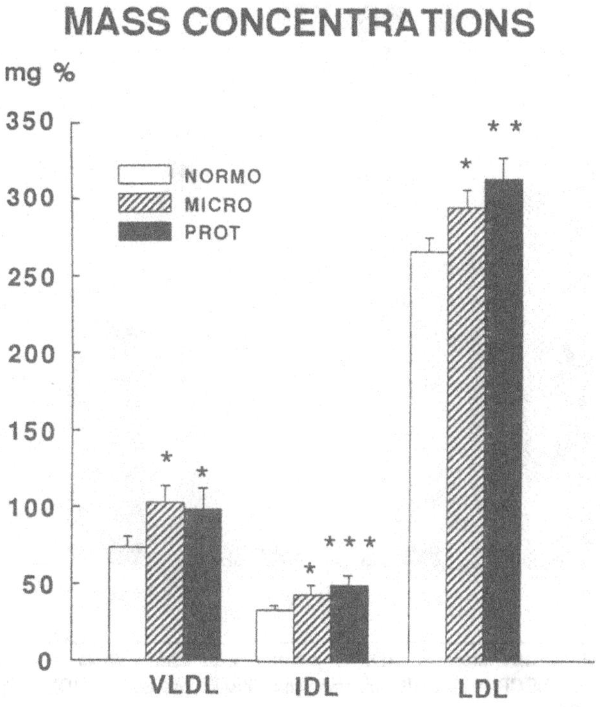

Figure 36-1 Mass concentration of the VLDL-IDL-IDL lipoprotein fractions in IDDM patients with and without renal disease. The sum of all components (cholesterol ester, free cholesterol, triglyceride, phospholipid, protein) in each lipoprotein fraction represents the mass concentration. NORMO=normoalbuminuric, MICRO= microalbuminuric and PROT= proteinuric IDDM patients. *P<0.05, **P<0.01 and ***P<0.001 vs NORMO.

Our data thus confirmed previous studies [34,35,38-40] and also suggested that IDDM patients with renal disease have mild hypertriglyceridaemia in addition to elevation of LDL cholesterol. All these changes are potentially atherogenic and may contribute to the excess of cardiovascular complications seen in such IDDM patients.

In NIDDM patients the impact of renal disease is very similar to that in IDDM in that the lipid profile moves in a more atherogenic direction. Increased levels of total triglyceride and VLDL-triglyceride is a consistent feature in those NIDDM patients with microalbuminuria or proteinuria [46-48]. While most studies have observed an increased total cholesterol concentration [46,47], a recent large study of 1574 Italian NIDDM subjects with various degrees of AER did not detect any differences in total cholesterol levels after adjustment for sex, age and duration of diabetes [48]. The Italian study did unfortunately not include LDL cholesterol measurements, which has been reported normal [46] and elevated [47]. Several studies have shown increased concentrations of apoB in NIDDM patients with renal disease [46,48].

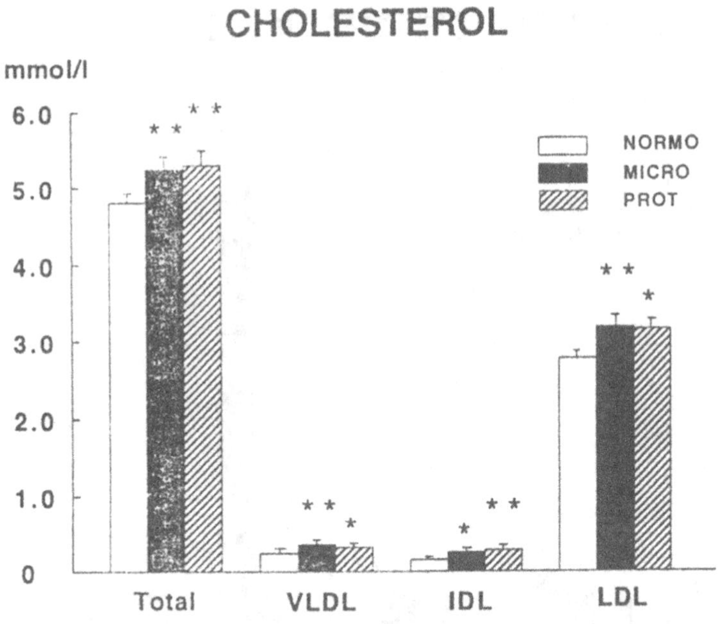

Figure 36-2a Cholesterol concentrations in IDDM patients with and without renal disease. NORMO=normoalbuminuric, MICRO=microalbuminuric and PROT=proteinuric IDDM patients. *P<0.05 and **P<0.01 vs NORMO.

LDL subclasses

Most studies in IDDM patients with renal disease have focused their attention on the lipid and lipoprotein concentrations neglecting the heterogeneity of the lipoprotein particles [34,35,38-40]. LDL consists of a spectrum of particles which vary in size, density, composition and possibly atherogeneity. Two distinct LDL subclass phenotypes can be distinguished according to LDL particle size distribution [49]. Pattern A consists of a major LDL peak with LDL particle diameter larger than 255 Å and of a minor peak with smaller particle size [49], whereas in pattern B the diameter of the major LDL peak is equal to or less than 255 Å [49]. A predominance of the small, dense LDL particles which occur in pattern B is considered to be highly atherogenic [49-51]. Growing evidence indicates that the serum triglyceride concentration is one important determinant of the structural properties of LDL [52].

In order to answer the question, whether elevation of LDL cholesterol in IDDM patients with renal disease is accompanied by changes in LDL size or composition, we studied 57 IDDM patients with normal AER, 46 with microalbuminuria and 33 with proteinuria [53]. The patients were matched for age, BMI, duration of diabetes and glycaemic control. Patients with microalbuminuria or proteinuria had increased LDL mass compared to normoalbuminuric patients [53]. This was mainly due to an increment of small dense LDL. No changes in density distribution or composition of LDL between the three diabetic groups were observed [53]. The increase in LDL mass without major compositional changes therefore suggested that the elevation of LDL in microalbuminuric and proteinuric IDDM patients is primarily due to an increased number of LDL particles. Furthermore, the prevalence of atherogenic small dense LDL particles in the patients with renal disease was closely dependent on plasma triglyceride concentration, although the triglyceride concentrations were within the normal range. It follows that the preponderance of small dense LDL within a range of triglyceride values below the therapeutic target values emphasizes the fact that fasting triglycerides should be maintained as low as possible in IDDM patients with renal disease and at high risk of CHD [53].

Despite of normal LDL concentrations in NIDDM, these patients usually have abnormal composition of the LDL particles. Several studies have indicated an increase in the triglyceride content of LDL particles in NIDDM [54-56], a feature which is independently associated with an increased risk of CHD [56]. Small dense LDL particles were reported to be preponderant in NIDDM [57], but it was not clear whether this was independently related to diabetes or a consequence of hypertriglyceridaemia. A recent study clarified the issue and indicated that the distribution of LDL particles is not regulated by NIDDM per se but its influence on LDL particle size is explained by the ambient concentration of triglyceride as in IDDM patients [53,58]. Although there are no data available concerning LDL particles in NIDDM patients with renal disease, it can be speculated that such patients would have more atherogenic small dense LDL particles due to their increased levels of triglyceride. The clinical implication is that in NIDDM and especially in NIDDM patients with renal disease serum triglyceride should be as low as possible to prevent atherogenic changes in LDL.

HDL metabolism

The data on HDL in IDDM patients with renal disease are inconsistent. In microalbuminuric patients the concentration of total HDL cholesterol has been observed to be lower [35,40], similar [38,39] of even higher [59] than in IDDM patients with normal AER. Consequently, the concentration of HDL_2 cholesterol has been reported to be lower [39] or unchanged [59] in microalbuminuric patients than in normoalbuminuric IDDM patients. Patients with clinical nephropathy have lower plasma HDL

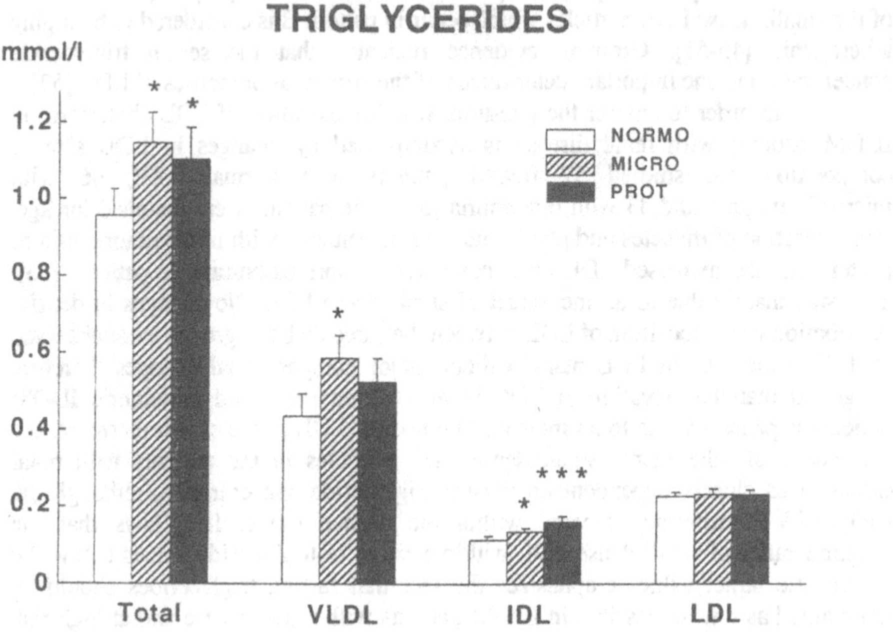

Figure 36-2b Triglyceride concentrations in IDDM patients with and without renal disease. NORMO=normoalbuminuric, MICRO=microalbuminuric and PROT=proteinuric IDDM patients. *P<0.05, **P<0.01 and *** P<0.001 vs NORMO.

cholesterol [35,60] and HDL_2 cholesterol values [60] than normoalbuminuric patients. In our study including 52 microalbuminuric, 37 proteinuric and 64 normoalbuminuric IDDM patients we found no differences in apoA-I, apoA-II or LpA-I or LpA-I:A-II particles, although median HDL and HDL_2 concentration were slightly lower in those with renal disease [61]. Thus, IDDM with renal disease seems to be accompanied by only trivial changes of the HDL metabolism and cannot explain the excess of CHD in these patients [61].

The information about HDL metabolism in NIDDM patients with renal disease is scarce. HDL cholesterol levels have been reported normal [46] or decreased [47] in those with renal disease when compared to those without.

3. LIPOLYTIC ENZYMES IN DIABETIC RENAL DISEASE

Plasma LPL is a key enzyme in the removal of triglyceride-rich apoB containing lipoproteins. Decreased activity of LPL leads to accumulation of triglyceride-rich particles in plasma. Kinetic studies have demonstrated that the enzyme HL participates in the conversion of IDL to LDL [62]. Recent evidence suggest that HL also modulates the properties of circulating LDL particles and thus is an important determinant of the particle distribution within the IDL and LDL densities [63-65].

We studied LPL and HL activities in 64 IDDM patients with normal AER, 52 with microalbuminuria and 37 with proteinuria matched for age, body weight, disease duration and glycaemic control [12]. LPL activity was not different between IDDM patients with or without renal disease. LPL was strongly inversely related to $VLDL_1$-triglyceride as well as to $VLDL_1$ and $VLDL_2$ mass concentration. The data suggested that the removal capacity of triglyceride-rich particles is not impaired in IDDM patients with renal disease and could not explain the elevation of triglyceride in these patients.

HL activity was increased in our IDDM patients with renal disease [12]. Apparently the increase of HL activity should be accompanied by lowering of IDL instead of the elevation of the IDL observed. Since the other removal pathway of IDL is direct uptake into the liver it can be speculated that the direct catabolism of $VLDL_2$ and IDL may be impaired in patients with renal disease. This would also result in increased apoB transport down the delipidation cascade into LDL in the presence of high HL activity. Indeed we have shown that the elevation of LDL in IDDM patients with renal disease is due to increased numbers of LDL particles [53]. However, we cannot exclude the possibility that increases of $VLDL_2$, IDL and LDL are due to enhanced input and consequent flux of apo B down the cascade resulting in increased generation of LDL particles. In fact the observed trends of increases in $VLDL_1$ and $VLDL_2$ despite elevated LPL activity indirectly indicate that the transport of apoB through the whole cascade from $VLDL_1$, through $VLDL_2$ and IDL to LDL is increased. Kinetic studies of apo B using stable isotopes to label endogenously produced $VLDL_1$ and $VLDL_2$ are needed to resolve these tentative options.

In NIDDM the activity of HL is frequently elevated whereas LPL activity is commonly subnormal [11]. This combination favours the formation of small dense atherogenic LDL particles, since high HL facilitates the formation of small dense LDL [58]. There are no data on LPL and HL activities in NIDDM patients with renal disease.

4. LIPOPROTEIN (a)

An increased plasma level of lipoprotein (a) [Lp(a)] has been identified as an independent risk factor for vascular disease in the general population [66-68]. This prompted many investigators to measure Lp(a) in IDDM and NIDDM. Increased Lp(a) levels were reported in IDDM patients with microalbuminuria or macroalbuminuria [69-71], and led to the conclusion that elevation of Lp(a) may contribute to the excess ischaemic heart disease associated with diabetic renal disease. All these studies, however, included rather small and heterogenous groups of patients, and the association was also disputed [72].

We measured Lp(a) in 64 normalbuminuric, 52 microalbuminuric and 37 proteinuric IDDM patients [73]. Microalbuminuric and proteinuric IDDM patients had higher median Lp(a) values (133 and 169 mg/l) than patients with normal AER (73 mg/l). Lp(a) concentrations were not related to AER but independently to diastolic blood pressure, fibrinogen and macroangiopathy. Although Lp(a) tended to be higher in IDDM patients with renal disease, the differences were small and the overlap between groups large. The association between Lp(a), diastolic blood pressure and fibrinogen suggests that Lp(a) could play a role in the pathogenesis of cardiovascular disease. However, Maser et al. [74] failed to observe an association of Lp(a) and CVD in a young cohort of IDDM patients. Therefore, until the role of Lp(a) as a risk factor has been confirmed by prospective studies, available results have to be interpreted with caution.

The available information about Lp(a) levels in NIDDM is also controversial. Ruotolo et al. [75] found no difference in serum apo(a) levels between normoalbuminuric NIDDM patients and control subjects. Also Schernthaner et al. [76] could not detect any difference in mean or median Lp(a) concentrations between patients without nephropathy and non-diabetic subjects. No distinction was, however, made between IDDM and NIDDM in that study. Guillausseau et al. [77] on the other hand found higher levels of Lp(a) in NIDDM compared to healthy subjects, but they did not compare Lp(a) levels in patients with different degrees of AER. Haffner et al. [78] found no difference in Lp(a) levels comparing NIDDM patients with age- and sex-matched non-diabetic control subjects. Patients with Albustix-positive proteinuria had slightly higher Lp(a) levels than those without proteinuria, but the difference was not statistically significant. In contrast, Jenkins et al. [79] found higher apo(a) levels in NIDDM patients with micro- and macroalbuminuria than in control subjects. In a recent case-control study no elevation in apo(a) levels in NIDDM patients with renal disease could be detected [46]. Further studies with larger populations are thus needed to elucidate whether Lp(a) is a risk factor for CHD in NIDDM patients with renal disease.

5. LIPIDS AND PATHOGENESIS OF RENAL DISEASE

There is increasing evidence that changes in lipid profiles could be primary and may even play a pathogenetic role for the initiation and progression of renal disease. Indirect evidence from humans and direct evidence from experimental work in rats support this view. First, it is a well established fact that LCAT deficiency is associated with glomerulosclerosis [80]. Second, lipid deposits and foam cells are frequently found in the glomeruli of humans with renal disease [81]. Third, even at the stage of microalbuminuria without any signs of decline in renal function, multiple lipid abnormalities are observed [12].

Experimental data suggest that lipogenic diets cause glomerular injury and increased urinary protein excretion in rats [82,83]. Interestingly, the glomerular injury caused by such a lipogenic diet was much more extensive, if the rats were made hypertensive by having one kidney clipped [82]. In addition, obese Zucker rats with endogenous hyperlipidaemia present with glomerulosclerosis [84]. Finally, the lipid-lowering agents mevinolin and clofibric acid dramatically reduced both albuminuria and glomerulosclerosis in obese Zucker rats [84]. All these data put together support the view that lipid abnormalities may be primary (possibly genetically determined?) and that they may even play a pathogenetic role in the initiation and progression of diabetic renal disease.

The question arises, can diabetic renal disease be prevented by the use of lipid-lowering agents? A short-term (12 week) study in IDDM patients with overt renal disease, however, did not reveal any beneficial effect on albuminuria despite a striking lipid-lowering effect of simvastatin [86] and similar results were documented by Nielsen et al. in microalbuminuric type 2 diabetes [87]. In contrast, Sasaki et al. [88] observed a reduction (average 60 %) in proteinuria in all 7 hypercholesterolaemic NIDDM patients with micro- and macroalbuminuria treated with pravastatin for 4 weeks. Also Lam et al. found a positive effect in type 2 diabetes [89] which was subsequently disputed [91-93] A new cross-over study also found reduction in microalbuminuria [94]. Thus, the possible importance of hyperlipidaemia in the development and progression of human renal disease still remains to be established. Furthermore, the major end-point for further studies of lipid-lowering treatment should be GFR and evaluation of structural lesions instead of AER.

6. CONCLUSIONS

Diabetic patients with renal disease show a broad spectrum of lipid abnormalities. These changes are characterized by a shift to a more atherogenic lipid profile. Since the patients at the same time carry an increased risk of early cardiovascular morbidity and mortality, it is important and a necessity to pay attention to the lipid and lipoprotein concentrations. Treatment should aim at achieving normal glucose tolerance, which has a favourable effect on the lipid levels, and the use of lipid-lowering agents should be considered.

REFERENCES

1. Pyörälä K, Laakso M, Uusitupa M. Diabetes and atherosclerosis: an epidemiologic view. Diab Metab Rev 1987; 3: 462-524.
2. Borch-Johnsen K, Andersen PK, Deckert T: The effect of proteinuria on relative mortality in type 1 (insulin-dependent) diabetes mellitus. Diabetologia 1985; 28: 590-596
3. Borch-Johnsen K, Kreiner S: Proteinuria: value as predictor of cardiovascular mortality in insulin-dependent diabetes mellitus. BMJ 1987; 294: 1651-1654.
4. Nelson RG, Pettitt DJ, Carraher M-J, Baird HR, Knowler WC. Effect of proteinuria on mortality in NIDDM. Diabetes 1988; 37: 1499-1504.
5. Mogensen CE. Microalbuminuria predicts clinical proteinuria and early mortality in maturity-onset diabetes. N Engl J Med 1984; 310: 356-360.
6. Schmitz A, Vaeth M. Microalbuminuria: A major risk factor in non-insulin dependenrt diabetes. A 10-year follow-up study of 503 diabetic patients. Diabetic Med 5: 126-134, 1988.
7. Mattock MB, Morrish NJ, Viberti GC, Keen H, Fitzgerald A, Jackson G. Prospective study of microalbuminuria as predictor of mortality in NIDDM. Diabetes 1992; 41: 736-741.
8. Nielsen FS, Voldsgaard AI, Gall M-A, Rossing P, Hommel E, Andersen P, Dyerberg J, Parving H-H. Apolipoprotein (a) and cardiovascular disease in Type 2 (non-insulin-dependent) diabetic patiernts with and without diabetic nephropathy. Diabetologia 1993; 36: 438-444.
9. Laakso M, Pyörälä K, Sarlund H, Voutilainen E. Lipid and lipoprotein abnormalities associated with coronary heart disease in patients with insulin-dependent diabetes mellitus. Arteriosclerosis 1986; 6: 679-684.
10. Laakso M, Lehto S, Penttilä I, Pyörälä K. Lipid and lipoproteins predicting coronary heart disease mortality and morbidity in patients with non-insulin-dependent diabetes mellitus. Circulation 1993; 88: 1421-1430.
11. Howard BJ. Lipoprotein metabolism in diabetes mellitus. J Lipid Res 1994; 28: 613-628.
12. Groop PH, Elliott T, Ekstrand A, Franssila-Kallunki A, Friedman R, Viberti GC, Taskinen M-R. Multiple lipoprotein abnormalities in Type-1 diabetic-patients with renal-disease. Diabetes 1996; 45: 974-979.
13. Östlund RE Jr, Semenkovich CF, Schechtman KB. Quantitative relationship between plasma lipids and glycohemoglobin in Type 1 patients. Longitudinal study of 212 patients. Diabetes Care 1989; 12: 332-336.
14. Nikkilä EA, Hormila P. Serum lipids and lipoproteins in insulin-treated diabetes. Diabetes 1978; 27: 1078-1086.

15. Mattock MB, Salter AM, Fuller JH, Omer T, Gohari REI, Redmond SD, Keen H. High density lipoprotein subfractions in insulin-dependent diabetic and normal subjects. Atherosclerosis 1982; 45: 67-79.
16. Eckel RH, Albers JJ, Cheung MC, Wahl PW, Lindgren FT, Bierman EL. High density lipoprotein composition in insulin-dependent diabetes mellitus. Diabetes 1981; 30: 132-138.
17. Kahri J, Groop PH, Viberti GC, Elliott T, Taskinen M-R. Regulation of apolipoprotein A-I-containing lipoproteins in IDDM. Diabetes 1993; 42: 1281-1288.
18. Taskinen M-R. Hyperlipidaemia in diabetes. Clin Endocrinol Metab 1990; 4: 743-775.
19. Taskinen M-R. Quantitative and qualitative lipoprotein abnormalities in diabetes mellitus. Diabetes 1992; 41: Suppl. 2: 12-17.
20. Howard BJ, Abbott WGH, Beltz WF, Harper IT, Fields RM, Grundy SM, Taskinen M-R. Integrated study of low density lipoprotein metabolism and very low density lipoprotein metabolism in non-insulin dependent diabetes. Metabolism 1987; 36: 870-877.
21. Rönnemaa T, Laakso M, Kallio V, Pyörälä K, Marniemi J, Puukka P. Serum lipids, lipoproteins, and apolipoproteins and the excessive occurrence of coronary heart disease in non-insulin-dependent diabetic patients. Am J Epidemiol 1989; 130: 632-645.
22. Taskinen M-R, Packard CJ, Shepherd J: Effect of insulin therapy on metabolic fate of apolipoprotein B-containing lipoproteins in NIDDM. Diabetes 1990; 39:1017-1027.
23. Fisher RM, Coppack SW, Gibbons GF, Frayn KN. Very low density lipoprotein sub-fraction metabolism in normal and obese subjects. Int J Obesity 1993; 17: 263-269.
24. Shepherd J, Packard CJ. Metabolic heterogeneity in very low-density lipoproteins. Am Heart J 1987; 113: 503-508
25. Parhofer KG, Barrett PHR, Bier DM, Schonfield G. Determination of kinetic parameters of apolipoprotein B metabolism using aminoacids labeled with stable isotopes. Clin Chem 1991; 36: 1431-1435.
26. Caslake MJ, Packard CJ, Series JJ, Yip B, Dagen MM, Shepherd J. Plasma triglyceride and low density lipoprotein metabolism. Eur J Clin Invest 1992; 22: 96-104.
27. Taskinen M-R. Hyperlipidaemia in diabetes. In Bailliere's Clinical Endocrinology and Metabolism 1990; 4: 743-775.
28. Taskinen M-R, Välimäki M, Nikkilä EA, Kuusi T, Ehnholm C, Ylikahri R. High density lipoprotein subfractions and postheparin plasma lipases in alcoholic men before and after ethanol withdrawal. Metabolism 1982; 31: 1168-1174.
29. Laakso M, Voutilainen E, Sarlund H, Aro A, Pyörälä K, Penttilä I. Serum lipids and lipoproteins in middle aged non-insulin-dependent diabetics. Atherosclerosis 1985; 56: 271-281.
30. Nikkilä EA, Huttunen JK, Ehnholm C. Postheparin plasma lipoprotein lipase and hepatic lipase in diabetes mellitus. Diabetes 1977; 26: 11-21.
31. Taskinen M-R, Nikkilä EA, Kuusi T, Harno K. Lipoprotein lipase activity and serum lipoproteins in untreated Type 2 (insulin-independent) diabetes associated with obesity. Diabetologia 1982; 22: 46-50.
32. Laakso M, Pyörälä K, Voutilainen E, Marniemi J. Plasma insulin and serum lipids and lipoproteins in middle-aged non-insulin dependent diabetic and non-diabetic subjects. Am J Epidemiol 1987; 125: 611-621.
33. Taskinen M-R, Nestel PJ. »Hypolipidemic agents: their roles in diabetes mellitus.« In *International Textbook of Diabetes Mellitus.* Alberti KGMM, DeFronzo RA, Keen H, Zimmet, eds. John Wiley & Sons, 1992; pp 817-830.
34. Vannini P, Ciavarella A, Flammini M, Bargossi AM, Forlani G, Borgnino LC, Orsoni G: Lipid abnormalities in insulin -dependent diabetic patients with albuminuria. Diabetes Care 1984; 7: 151-154.
35. Jensen T, Stender S, Deckert T. Abnormalities in plasma concentrations of lipoproteins and fibrinogen in Type 1 (insulin-dependent) diabetic patients with increased urinary albumin excretion. Diabetologia 1988; 31: 142-145.
36. Holm J, Hemmingsen L, Nielsen NV. Serum concentrations of lipids and lipoproteins related to degree of albuminuria and low-molecular weight (tubular) proteinuria in insulin-dependent diabetics. Med Sci Res 1989; 17: 945-947.
37. Haaber AB, Kofoed-Enevoldsen A, Jensen T. The prevalence of hypercholesterolaemia and its relationship with albuminuria in insulin-dependent diabetic patients: an epidemiological study. Diabetic Med 1992; 9: 557-561.

38. Dullaart RPF, Groener JEM, Dikkeschei LD, Erkelens DW, Doorenbos H: Increased cholesterylester transfer activity in complicated Type 1 (insulin-dependent) diabetes mellitus - its relationship with serum lipids. Diabetologia 1989; 32: 14-19.
39. Jones SL., Close CF, Mattock MB, Jarret RJ; Keen H, Viberti GC. Plasma lipid and coagulation factor concentrations in insulin-dependent diabetics with microalbuminuria. Br Med J 289: 487-489, 1989.
40. Watts GF, Naumova R, Slavin BM, Morris RW, Houlston R, Kubal C, Shaw KM: Serum lipids and lipoproteins in insulin-dependent diabetic patients with persistent microalbuminuria. Diabetic Med 1989; 6: 25-30.
41. Tatami R, Mabuchi H, Ueda K, Ueda R, Haba T, Kametani T, Ito S, Koizumi J, Ohta M, Miyamoto S, Nakayama A, Kanaya H, Oiwake H, Genda A, Takeda R: Intermediate-density lipoprotein and cholesterol-rich very low density lipoprotein in angiographically determined coronary artery disease. Circulation 1981; 64: 1174-1184.
42. Krauss RM: Relationship of intermediate and low-density lipoprotein subspecies to risk of coronary artery disease. Am Heart J 1987; 113: 578-582.
43. Krauss RM, Lindgren FT, Williams PT, Kelsey SF, Brensike J, Vranizan K, Detre KM, Levy RI: Intermediate-density lipoproteins and progression of coronary artery disease in hypercholesterolaemic men. Lancet 1987; ii: 62-65
44. Steiner G, Schwartz L, Shumak S, Poapst M: The association of increased levels of intermediate-density lipoproteins with smoking and with coronary artery disease. Atherosclerosis 1987; 75: 124-130.
45. Winocour PH, Durrington PN, Bhatnagar D, Ishola M, Mackness M, Arrol S: Influence of early nephropathy on very low density lipoprotein (VLDL), intermediate density lipoprotein (IDL), and low density lipoprotein (LDL) composition. Atherosclerosis 1991; 89: 49-57.
46. Nielsen FS, Voldsgaard AI, Gall M-A, Rossing P, Hommel E, Andersen P, Dyerberg J, Parving H-H. Apolipoprotein (a) and cardiovascular disease in Type 2 (non-insulin-dependent) diabetic patients with and without diabetic nephropathy. Diabetologia 1993; 36: 438-444.
47. Mattock MB, Morrish NJ, Viberti GC, Keen H, Fitzgerald A, Jackson G. Prospective study of microalbuminuria as predictor of mortality in NIDDM. Diabetes 1992; 41: 736-741.
48. Bruno G, Cavallo-Perin P, Bargero G, Borra M, Calvi V, D'Errico N, Deambrogio P, Pagano G. Prevalence and risk factors for micro- and macroalbuminuria in an Italian population-based cohort of NIDDM subjects. Diabetes Care 1996; 19: 43-47.
49. Austin MA, Breslow JL, Hennekens CH, Buring JE, Willet WC, Krauss RM. Low-density lipoprotein subclass patterns and risk of myocardial infarction. JAMA 1988; 260: 1917-1921.
50. Austin MA, Krauss RM. Genetic control of low-density lipoprotein subclasses. Lancet 1986; ii: 592-595.
51. Austin MA, King MC, Vranizan KM, Krauss RM. Atherogenic lipoprotein phenotype. A proposed genetic marker for coronary heart disease. Circulation 1990; 82: 495-506.
52. Deckelbaum RJ, Granot E, Oschry Y, Rose L, Eisenberg S. Plasma triglyceride determines structure-composition in low and high density lipoproteins. Arteriosclerosis 1984; 4: 225-231.
53. Lahdenperä S, Groop PH, Tilly-Kiesi M, Kuusi T, Elliott TG, Viberti GC, Taskinen M-R: LDL subclasses in IDDM patients: relation to diabetic nephropathy. Diabetologia 1994; 37: 681-88.
54. Bagdade JD, Buchanan WE, Kuusi T, Taskinen M-R. Persistent abnormalities in lipoprotein composition in non-insulin-dependent diabetes after intensive insulin therapy. Arteriosclerosis 1990; 10: 232-239.
55. James RW, Pometta D. The distribution profiles of very low density and low density lipoproteins in poorly-controlled male, type 2 (non-insulin-dependent) diabetic patients. Diabetologia 1991; 34: 246-252.
56. Uusitupa MIJ, Niskanen LK, Siitonen O, Voutilainen E, Pyörälä K. Ten-year cardiovascular mortality in relation to risk factors and abnormalities in lipoprotein composition in type 2 (non-insulin-dependent) diabetic and nondiabetic subjects. Diabetologia 1993; 36: 1175-1184.
57. Haffner SM, Mykkänen L, Stern MP, Paidi M, Howard BV. Greater effect of diabetes on LDL size in women than in men. Diabetes Care 1994; 17: 1164-1171.
58. Lahdenperä S, Syvänne M, Kahri J, Taskinen M-R. Regulation of low-density lipoprotein particle size distribution in NIDDM and coronary disease: importance of serum triglycerides. Diabetologia 1996; 39: 453-461.

59. Jay RH, Jones SL, Hill CE, Richmond W, Viberti GC, Rampling MW, Betteridge DJ. Blood rheology and cardiovascular risk factors in type 1 diabetes: relationship with microalbuminuria. Diabetic Med 1991; 8: 662-667.
60. Winocour PH, Durrington PN, Ishola M, Anderson DC, Cohen H: Influence of proteinuria on vascular disease, blood pressure, and lipoproteins in insulin-dependent diabetes mellitus. BMJ 1987; 294: 1648-1651.
61. Kahri J, Groop PH, Elliott T, Viberti GC, Taskinen M-R: Plasma cholesteryl ester transfer protein and its relationship to plasma lipoproteins and apolipoprotein A-I-containing lipoproteins in IDDM patients with microalbuminuria and clinical nephropathy. Diabetes Care 1994; 17: 412-419.
62. Demant T, Carlson LA, Holmquist L, Karpe F, Nilsson-Ehle P, Packard CJ, Shepherd J. Lipoprotein metabolism in hepatic lipase deficiency: studies on the turnover of apolipoprotein B and on the effect of hepatic lipase on high density lipoprotein. J Lipid Res 1988; 29: 1603-1611.
63. Auwerx JH, Marzetta CA, Hokanson JE, Brunzell JD. Large buoyant LDL-like particles in hepatic lipase deficiency. Arteriosclerosis 1989; 9: 319-325.
64. Zambon A., Austin MA, Brown BG, Hokanson JE, Brunzell JD. Effect of hepatic lipase on LDL in normal men and those with coronary artery disease. Arterioscler Thromb 1993; 13: 147-153.
65. Watson TDG, Caslake MJ, Freeman DJ, Griffin BA, Hinnie J, Packard CJ, Shepherd J. Determinants of LDL subfraction distribution and concentrations in young normolipidemic subjects. Arterioscler Thromb 1994; 14: 902-910.
66. Rhoads GG, Dahlén GH, Berg K, Morton NE, Dannenberg AL. Lp(a) lipoprotein as a risk factor for myocardial infarction. JAMA 1986; 256: 2540-2544.
67. Dahlén GH, Guyton JR, Attar M, Farmer JA, Kautz JA, Gotto AM Jr. Association of levels of lipoprotein Lp(a), plasma lipids, and other lipoproteins with coronary artery disease documented by angiography. Circulation 1986; 74: 758-765.
68. Durrington PN, Ishola M, Hunt L, Arrol S, Bhatnagar D. Apolipoproteins (a), A-I and B and parental history in men with early onset ischaemic heart disease. Lancet 1988; i: 1070-1073.
69. Jenkins AJ, Steele JS, Janus ED, Best JD. Increased plasma apolipoprotein (a) levels in IDDM patients with microalbuminuria. Diabetes 1991; 40: 787-790.
70. Kapelrud H, Bangstad H-J, Dahl-Jørgensen K, Berg K, Hanssen KF. Serum Lp(a) lipoprotein concentrations in insulin dependent diabetic patients with microalbuminuria. BMJ 1991; 303: 675-678.
71. Winocour PH, Bhatnagar D, Ishola M, Arrol S, Durrington PN. Lipoprotein (a) and microvascular disease in Type 1 (insulin-dependent) diabetes. Diabetic Med 1991; 8: 922-927.
72. Gall M-A, Rossing P, Hommel E, Voldsgaard AI, Andersen P, Nielsen FS, Dyerberg J, Parving H-H. Apolipoprotein (a) in insulin-dependent diabetic patients with and without diabetic nephropathy. Scand J Clin Lab Invest 1992; 52: 513-521.
73. Groop PH, Viberti GC, Elliott T, Friedman R, Mackie A, Ehnholm C, Jauhiainen M, Taskinen M-R. Lipoprotein (a) in insulin dependent diabetic patients with renal disease. Diabetic Med 1994; 11: 961-967.
74. Maser RE, Drash AL, Usher D, Kuller LH, Becker DJ, Orchard TJ. Lipoprotein (a) concentration shows little relationship to IDDM complications in the Pittsburgh Epidemiology of Diabetes Complications Study Cohort. Diabetes Care 1993; 16: 755-758.
75. Ruotolo G, Zoppo A, Parlavecchia M, Giberti B, Micossi P. Apolipoprotein (a) levels in type 1 and type 2 diabetes mellitus. Acta Diabetol 1991; 28: 158-161.
76. Schernthaner G; Kostner GM, Dieplinger H, Prager R, Mühlhauser I. Apolipoproteins (A-I, A-II, B), Lp(a), lipoprotein and lecithin: cholesterol acetyltransferase activity in diabetes mellitus. Arteriosclerosis 1983; 49: 277-293.
77. Guillausseau P-J, Peynet J, Chanson P, Legrand A, Altman J-J, Poupon J, N'Guyen M, Rousselet F, Lubetski J. Lipoprotein (a) in diabetic patients with and without chronic renal failure. Diabetes Care 1992; 15: 976-979.
78. Haffner SM, Morales PA, Stern MP, Gruber MK. Lp(a) concentrations in NIDDM. Diabetes 1992; 41: 1267-1272.
79. Jenkins AJ, Steele JS, Janus ED, Santamaria JD, Best JD. Plasma apolipoprotein (a) is increased in type 2 (non-insulin-dependent) diabetic patients with microalbuminuria. Diabetologia 1992; 35: 1055-1059.

80. Gjone E. »Familial lecithin: cholesterol acyltransferase deficiency - a new metabolic disease with renal involvement.« In *Advances in Nephrology*, Hamburger, Crosnier, Grunfeld, Maxwell, eds. Chicago: Year Book Medical Publishers, 1981; pp 167-185.
81. Keane WF, Kasiske BL, O'Donnell MP. Lipids and progressive glomerulosclerosis. Am J Nephrol 1988; 8: 261-271.
82. Gröne H-J, Walli A, Gröne E, Niedmann P, Thiery J, Seidel D, Helmchen U. Induction of glomerulosclerosis by dietary lipids. A functional and morphologic study in the rat. Lab Invest 1989; 60: 433-446.
83. Kasiske BL, O'Donnell MP, Lee H, Kim Y, Keane WF. Impact of dietary fatty acid supplementation on renal injury in obese Zucker rats. Kidney Int 1991; 39: 1125-1134.
84. Kasiske BL, Cleary MP, O'Donnell MP, Keane WF. Effects of genetic obesity on renal structure and function in the Zucker rat. J Lab Clin Med 1985; 106: 598-604.
85. Kasiske BL, O'Donnell MP, Cleary MP, Keane WF. Treatment of hyperlipidemia reduces glomerular injury in obese Zucker rats. Kidney Int 1988; 33: 667-672.
86. Hommel E, Andersen P, Gall M-A, Nielsen F, Jensen B, Rossing P, Dyerberg J, Parving H-H. Plasma lipoproteins and renal function during simvastatin treatment in diabetic nephropathy. Diabetologia 1992; 35: 447-451.
87. Nielsen S, Schmitz O, Moller N et al. (1993) Renal function and insulin sensitivity during simvastatin treatment in type 2 (non-insulin-dependent) diabetic patients with microalbuminuria. Diabetologia 36: 1079-1086.
88. Sasaki T, Kuratya H, Nomura K, Utsunomiya K, Ikeda Y. Amelioration of proteinuria with pravastatin in hypercholesterolemic patients with diabetes mellitus. Jpn J Med 1990; 29: 156-163.
89. KSL Lam, Cheng IKP, Janus ED, Pang RWC. Cholesterol-lowering therapy may retard the progression of diabetic nephropahty. Diabetologia (1995) 38: 604-609.
90. Parving H-H. Cholesterol-lowering therapy may retard the progression of diabetic nephropathy. Letter to the editors. Diabetologia 1996; 39: 367-373.
91. Lam KSL. Response from the authors. Diabetologia 1996; 39: 368.
92. Bender R. The effect of cholesterol-lowering therapy on the progression of diabetic nephropathy is unproved. Letter to the editors. Diabetologia 1996; 39: 698-369.
93. Lam KSL, Lauder IJ. Response from the authors. Diabetologia 1996; 39: 369-370.
94. Tonolo G, Ciccarese M, Brizzi P, Puddu L, Secchi G, Calvia P, Atzeni MM, Melis GM, Maioli M. Reduction of albumin excretion rate in normotensive microalbuminuric type 2 diabetic patients during long-term simvastatin treatment. Diabetes Care, Dec. 1997; 20: 1891-1895.

37. MICROALBUMINURIA IN YOUNG PATIENTS WITH TYPE 1 DIABETES.

Henrik Bindesbøl Mortensen
Pediatric Department, Amtssygehuset i Glostrup, Glostrup, Denmark

Diabetic nephropathy is the main cause of the increased morbidity and mortality among patients with Type 1 diabetes[1,2,3] In recent years it has been shown that a slightly elevated urinary albumin excretion rate (microalbuminuria) is an early predictor for later development of manifest diabetic nephropathy [4,5,6,7]. The presence of hypertension in the diabetic individual markedly increases the risk and accelerates the course of the diabetic kidney disease [8,9,10,11] Given the poor prognosis for patients developing manifest diabetic nephropathy emphasize the need for a uniform intervention programme for treatment of microalbuminuria in children and adolescents with Type 1 diabetes.

MEASURE FOR ALBUMIN EXCRETION

In 1989 a nation-wide screening for microalbuminuria in Denmark was performed in 22 paediatric departments treating children with Type 1 diabetes [12]. To assess the prevalence of microalbuminuria in this group of patients, timed overnight urine collection was used. This urine fraction avoids the effect of posture, physical exercise, major blood pressure variations and the acute effect of diet on albuminuria and it is a convenient and practical method for most children. If the urinary albumin excretion rate (AER) was >20 μg min^{-1} in one of the two samples from a diabetic patient, a third sample was taken to determine whether the child had elevated albumin excretion, microalbuminuria. This limit was chosen as the lowest albumin excretion rate predicting diabetic nephropathy on the basis of investigations of the upper 95th percentile for albumin excretion in the control group of 209 healthy children [12]. In the present study the AER was determined by an immunoturbidimetric method which on average gave 13 % higher results than those measured by radioimmunoassay.

Previously Rowe et al [13]. established the upper 95% confidence limit for overnight urine to 12.2 μg min^{-1} in normal children while Davies et al. [14] reported a value related to surface area of 10 μg min^{-1} $1.73m^{-2}$. In another study Gibb et al. [15] estimated the upper 95th centile for overnight albumin excretion rate in

Mogensen, C.E. (ed.), THE KIDNEY AND HYPERTENSION IN DIABETES MELLITUS.

healthy children to 8.2 μg min^{-1} $1.73m^{-2}$.

DEFINITION OF MICROALBUMINURIA AND INCIPIENT NEPHROPATHY

It is now generally accepted that microalbuminuria is present when the AER is in the range of 15 to 150 μg min^{-1} using timed overnight urine collection [16,17]. The corresponding range in 24 hour urine samples is 20 to 200 μg min^{-1} (=30-300 mg $24h^{-1}$) [18] as the AER on average is 25% greater during the day. Incipient diabetic nephropathy is suspected when microalbuminuria is found in at least 2 out of 3 urine samples, preferably within 1 to 6 months period [16]. The within-individual observations of the AER is high [12,19] therefore a minimum of 2 estimations are necessary per individual to determine the true mean value of urine albumin excretion with reasonable confidence.

ALBUMIN EXCRETION RATE AMONG CHILDREN WITH AND WITHOUT DIABETES

The ranges for albumin excretion rate in urine samples collected overnight in both non-diabetic and diabetic children 12 years or less and adolescents from 12 to 19 years are given in Table 37-1. The geometric mean for albumin excretion was significantly elevated ($p<0.001$) in adolescents compared to children for both groups. There were no significant differences ($p>0.05$) in albumin excretion rates between the sexes.

Table 37-1 Timed overnight urinary albumin excretion rates in healthy children and adolescents and in children and adolescents with Type 1 diabetes and AER ≤ 20 μg min^{-1}.

	Children ≤12 years		Adolescents >12-19 years	
	Boys	Girls	Boys	Girls
Normal children				
n	47	30	58	74
AER (μg/l^{-1})	1.28x/÷2.75	1.37x/÷1.97	2.73x/÷2.18[a]	2.23x/÷2.14[a]
Diabetic children				
n	154	124	334	297
AER (μg/min^{-1})	1.70x/÷2.11	1.72x/÷2.07	2.94x/÷2.38[a]	3.16x/÷2.23[a]

Geometric mean x/÷ SD factor.
$p<0.001$ compared with younger age group. Boys vs. girls all NS. [ref. 8, with permission].

These findings are consistent with the recent results reported on night-time collections of urine [13,14]. In non-diabetic adolescents the relationship between AER, body surface area and level of maturity was nearly constant in accordance with the results of Gibb et al [15]. By contrast in diabetic adolescents AER was positively correlated with body surface area and age. This correlation was independent of the current HbA_{1c} level, suggesting that specific metabolic changes other than poor blood glucose control might affect AER, particularly in the diabetic subjects in the pubertal period. Hypersecretion of growth hormone (GH) as a result of altered feedback drive from reduced insulin-like growth factor I (IGF-1) levels and IGF-1 bioactivity have been demonstrated in adolescents with insulin dependent diabetes [20] which may lead to glomerular hyperfiltration [21] and increased risk for development microalbuminuria [22].

TYPE 1 DIABETIC CHILDREN WITH ELEVATED ALBUMIN EXCRETION RATE

A prevalence of 4.3 % for persistent microalbuminuria was revealed in 957 Danish children and adolescents aged from 2 to 19 years with Type 1 diabetes and mean diabetes duration of 6 years [12]. Based on recent literature data the reported prevalence of microalbuminuria in paediatric populations varies from 4.3 to 20% (Table 37-2). The discrepancies in prevalence for persistent microalbuminuria between these studies may partly be explained by differences in age, diabetes duration, blood glucose control, the populations investigated and the screening procedure. However, during the past decade a declining incidence of nephropathy in insulin dependent diabetes mellitus has been observed [27]. In adolescent diabetic patients (above 16 years) the prevalence of microalbuminuria was 13-14 % in accordance with the previous investigations. The prevalence of persistent microalbuminuria in different age groups and in groups with different duration of diabetes are shown in figures 37-1 and 37-2. The occurrence of microalbuminuria is extremely rare before puberty. Two prepubertal children were diagnosed with microalbuminuria in a previous study by Nørgaard et al [24], while Joner et al [26] and Janner et al. [28] reported one case. In our study [12] two other girls were diagnosed, while none were detected in the study of Mathiesen et al [23] or of Dahlquist et al [29]. It still remains controversial whether diabetes duration per se is associated with raised urinary albumin.

Table 37-2 Comparison of prevalence of microalbuminuria in young people with diabetes in different study groups.

Study	**Population (n)**	**Prevalence of microalbuminuria**	**Age group (years)**	**Duration of diabetes (years)**	**Screening procedure**
Mathiesen et al 1986 [23]	clinic (97)	20%	7-18	10	overnight
Nørgaard et al 1989 [24]	clinic (113)	15%	1-18	9	24-h urine
D'Antonio et al 1989 [25]	clinic (62)	21%	5.8-20.9	5	24-h urine
Mortensen et al 1990 [12]	Nation-wide (957)	4.3%	2-19	6	overnight
Joner et al 1992 [26]	Community	12.5%	8-30	10.5	overnight

Some studies have shown a possible association [12,30] while others dispute this [31]. However, this may suggest that young people should be screened for microalbuminuria regardless of diabetes duration, beginning at the very first stage of puberty [12,28].

OVERNIGHT ALBUMIN EXCRETION RATE AND BLOOD GLUCOSE CONTROL

Several previous reports have suggested a relationship between poor blood glucose control and increased urinary albumin excretion [30,32,33,34] We found that only females with microalbuminuria had significantly elevated HbA_{1c} values compared to diabetic patients with normoalbuminuria, in agreement with the results reported by D'Antonio et al [25]. In previous nationwide investigations [35,36] it was shown that blood glucose control is poorer during puberty, particularly in adolescent females compared to males. This observation may be explained by changed hormonal and/or lifestyle factors. An impaired linear growth observed in females with microalbuminuria may also be associated with long-term poor blood glucose in these patients. However, recent studies have suggested [37,38] an association between short stature and diabetic nephropathy particularly in males. Furthermore, from 10 to 25 years duration of the disease males show a threefold increase in prevalence in micro/macroalbuminuria compared to females [39]. The DCCT study [40] demonstrated that improved metabolic control could retard but not prevent the progression of incipient diabetic kidney disease. Recently Krolewski et al [41] reported that the risk of microalbuminuria in patients with Type 1 diabetes increases abruptly above a HbA_{1c} level of 8.1 % suggesting that efforts to reduce the frequency of diabetic nephropathy should be focused on the patients with HbA_{1c} values above this threshold.

OVERNIGHT ALBUMIN EXCRETION RATE AND ARTERIAL BLOOD PRESSURE

The normal range for diastolic blood pressure in diabetic boys and girls aged 8 to 18 years with normoalbuminuria are shown in Figures 37-1,37-2. The Figures also include data from the patients diagnosed with micro- and macroalbuminuria. Ten out of 16 boys had diastolic blood pressure above the upper quartile while eight out of 14 girls with microalbuminuria had diastolic blood pressure above this quartile. Three boys with macroalbuminuria had diastolic blood pressure below the upper quartile while two girls had values above. Consequently 60% of adolescents with microalbuminuria had diastolic blood pressure in the upper quartile for normoalbuminuria [42]. In keeping with this Kordonouri et al [43] reported a relation between diastolic blood pressure and albumin excretion rate in juvenile Type 1 diabetic patients. Thus excess prevalence of raised blood pressure in Type 1 diabetic patients could be explained by the presence of elevated blood pressure in adolescents with micro- and macroalbuminuria as suggested by Nørgaård et al [24].

Re-examination of 15 adolescents with microalbuminuria 2 years after identification revealed that two of these (13%) had developed overt proteinuria during this period. They had initially an overnight albumin excretion rate of 62 and 115.7 μg min^{-1} increasing to 184.4 and 448.3 μg min^{-1}, respectively (unpublished data). Thus without treatment a marked increase in the progression to overt diabetic nephropathy is seen for some individuals. In a study of young diabetic patients all

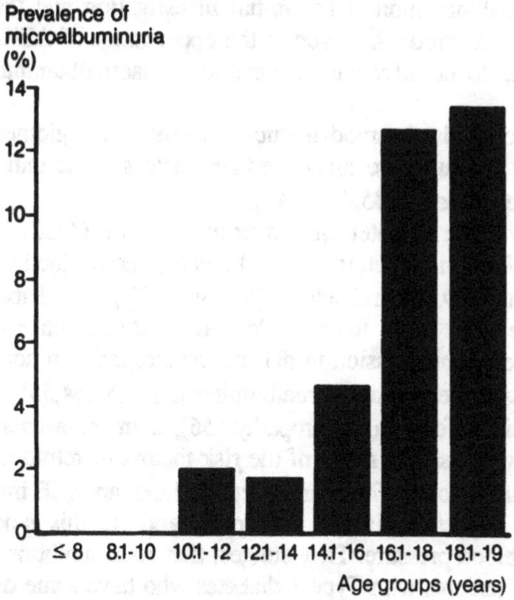

Figure 37-1 The prevalence of microalbuminuria in different age groups in 909 children and adolescents with Type 1 diabetes [8, with permission].

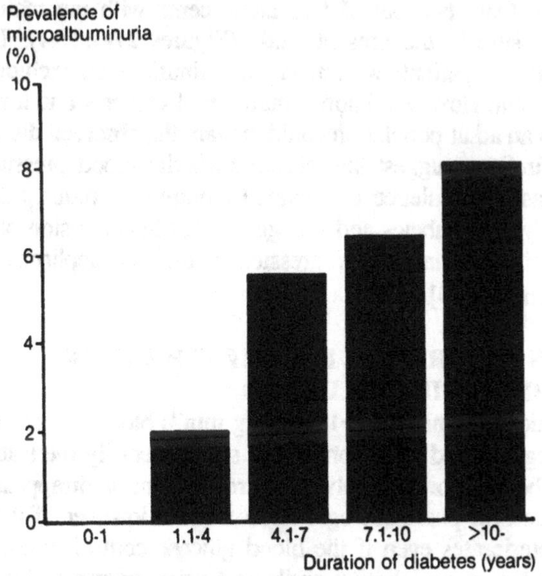

Figure 37-2 The relationship between duration of diabetes and prevalence of microalbuminuria in 909 children and adolescents with Type 1 diabetes [8, with permission].

diagnosed before 15 years of age Bojestig et al. [44] found no relationship between the level of microalbuminuria at the initial investigation and the development of nephropathy. They conclude that even in the upper range of AER excellent glycaemic control seems to be effective in preventing macroalbuminuria and reversing AER to normal.

Altered glomerular haemodynamics with increased glomerular plasma flow and transcapillary pressures are considered key factors in the initiation and progression of diabetic nephropathy [45,46,47,48].

Therapy with an angiotensin converting enzyme (ACE) inhibitor has been shown to lower albumin excretion rate and mean arterial blood pressure in normotensive adolescents [49,50] and adults [51] with Type 1 diabetes and microalbuminuria on the short term. Recently long-term studies have demonstrated that ACE-inhibition delays progression to diabetic nephropathy in normotensive Type 1 diabetic patients with persistent microalbuminuria [52,53,54,55]. Thus ACE inhibitors have beneficial effects in nephropathy [56], a microvascular complication of Type 1 diabetes which shares many of the risk factors of retinopathy. Interestingly, The EUCLID Study Group [57] recently reported that an ACE inhibitor, Lisinopril, has advantageous impact on diabetic retinopathy and that this is not fully accounted for by effects on blood pressure. They suggest that ACE inhibitor therapy should be considered for all patients with Type 1 diabetes who have some degree of retinopathy.

Previous investigations in adults with Type 1 diabetes have shown that at the time of recognition of microalbuminuria the blood pressure is often within the normal range [58], and tends to increase in parallel with the extent of micro-/macroalbuminuria. Only two out of five adolescents with macroalbuminuria had elevated blood pressure in the present study (Figures 27-3,27-4). This may be a selection bias because 2 patients with macroalbuminuria were excluded due to antihypertensive treatment. However, shorter duration of diabetes and lower body mass index compared to an adult population could explain the observed discrepancies.

These findings suggest that elevated arterial blood pressure may be related to the increased prevalence of elevated albumin excretion rate observed in adolescents with Type 1 diabetes and it suggests that hypertension plays an important role for the initiation and the progression of diabetic nephropathy in keeping with previous reports[4,7,10].

INTERVENTION PROGRAMME FOR TREATMENT OF MICROALBUMINURIA IN CHILDHOOD

In children with microalbuminuria (>15-150 μg min^{-1}) blood glucose control should be improved during a period of 6 months and simultaneously the status of microalbuminuria should be monitored closely. If microalbuminuria disappears or improves there is no indication for pharmacologic intervention. However, if the status of microalbuminuria deteriorates even if the blood glucose control improves and blood pressure is within the normal limits, antihypertensive treatment by an ACE-. inhibitor should be instituted. The ACE inhibitors have potential therapeutic advantages over other antihypertensive drugs because they may selectively reduce efferent

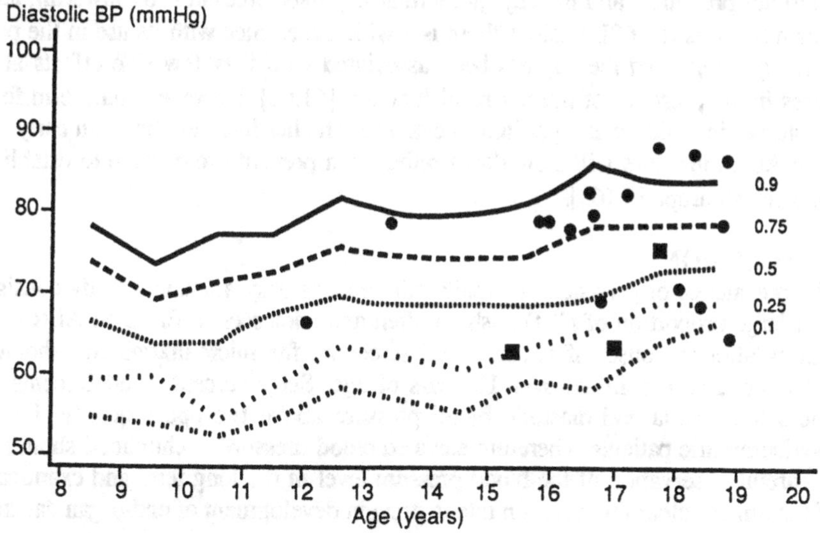

Figure 37-3 Percentile distribution of diastolic blood pressure in 487 boys aged 8 to 18 years with Type 1 diabetes. The dots represent diatolic blood pressure for the 16 boys with microalbuminuria; the squares the three boys with macroalbuminuria [24, with permission].

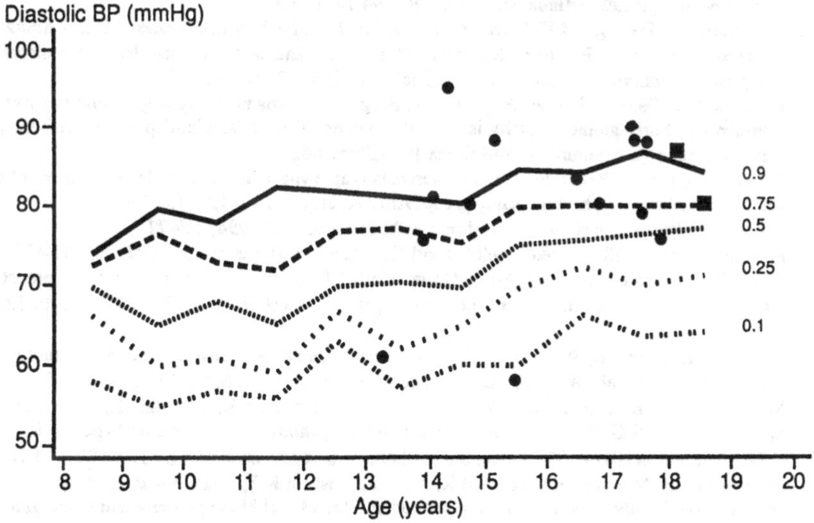

Figure 37-4 Percentile distribution of diastolic blood pressure in 425 girls aged 8 to 18 years with Type 1 diabetes. The dots represent diatolic blood pressure for the 14 girls with microalbuminuria; the squares the two girls with macroalbuminuria [24, with permission].

arteriolar pressures, and thereby glomerular capillary pressures, by lowering angiotensin II levels [59,60]. Besides there is a wide experience with its use in the paediatric age group and therapy has been associated with very few side effects at low doses in the presence of normal renal function [61,62]. However, long-term follow up studies in children are required to evaluate whether intervention at an early stage with ACE-inhibitors will slow down rather than prevent progression to established diabetic nephropathy [63].

CONCLUSION

The prevalence of persistent microalbuminuria was only 4.3% in a study consisting of a large proportion of all Danish children and adolescents. Elevated AER occurs mainly after the onset of puberty, and screening for microalbuminuria should be recommended in children over 12 years of age. Sixty percent of adolescents with microalbuminuria had diastolic blood pressure above the upper quartile for normoalbuminuric patients. Therefore elevated blood pressure in childhood should lead to careful observation of the blood pressure level in the long term and examination of the urinary albumin excretion rate to prevent development of end-organ damage.

REFERENCES

1. Dorman JS, Laporte RE, Kuller LH, Cruickshanks KJ, Orchard TJ,Wagener DK, Becker DJ, Cavender DE, Drash AL. The Pittsburgh insulin-dependent diabetes mellitus (IDDM). Morbidity and mortality study. Mortality results. Diabetes 1984;33:271-276.
2. Borch-Johnsen K, Andersen PK, Deckert T. The effect of proteinuria on relative mortality in Type 1 (insulin dependent) diabetes mellitus. Diabetologia 1985;28:590-596.
3. Borch-Johnsen K, Kreiner S. Proteinuria: value as predictor of cardiovascular mortality in insulin dependent diabetes mellitus Br.Med.J. 1987;294:1651-1654
4. Mogensen CE, Damsgaard EM, Frøland A, Hansen KW, Nielsen S, Pedersen MM, Schmitz A, Thuesen L, Østerby R. Reduced glomerular filtration rate and cardiovascular damage in diabetes: a key role for abnormal albuminuria. Acta Diabetologia 1992; 29: 201-213.
5. Bangstad H-J, Østerby R, Dahl-Jørgensen K, Berg KJ, Hartmann A, Nyberg G, Frahm Bjørn S, Hanssen KF. Early glomerulopathy is present in young, Type 1 (insulin-dependent) diabetic patients with microalbuminuria. Diabetologia 1993;36:523-529
6. Ellis EN, Pysher TJ. Renal disease in adolescents with Type 1 diabetes mellitus: A report of the southwest pediatric nephrology study group. Am J Kidney Dis 1993;22:783-790.
7. Viberti GC. Prognostic significance of microalbuminuria. AJH 1994;7:69-72.
8. Epstein M, Sowers JR. Diabetes mellitus and Hypertension. Hypertension 1992; 19: 403-418.
9. Microalbuminuria Collaborative Study Group, United Kingdom. Risk factors for development of microalbuminuria in insulin-dependent diabetic patients: a cohort study. BMJ 1993; 306: 1235-1239.
10. Mathiesen ER, Rønn B, Storm B, Foght H, Deckert T. The natural course of microalbuminuria in insulin-dependent diabetes: A 10-year prospective study. Diabetic Med 1995;12:482-487.
11. Mangili R, Deferrari G, Di Mario U, Giampietro O, Navalesi R, Nosadini R, Rigamonti G, Spezia R,Crepaldi G, for the Italian Microalbuminuria Study Group. Arterial hypertension and microalbuminuria IDDM: The Italian microalbuminuria study. Diabetologia 1994;37:1015-1024.
12. Mortensen HB, Marinelli K, Nørgaard K, Main K, Kastrup KW, Ibsen KK et al. A nation-wide cross sectional study of urinary albumin excretion rate, arterial blood pressure and blood glucose control in Danish children with Type 1 diabetes. Diabetic Med 1990;7:887-897.
13. Rowe DJF, Hayward M, Bagga H, Betts P. Effect of glycaemic control and duration of disease on overnight albumin excretion in diabetic children. Br Med J 1984;289:957-959.
14. Davies AG, Postlethwaite, Price DA, Burn JL, Houlton CA, Fielding BA. Urinary albumin excretion in school children. Arch Dis Child 1984;59:625-630.

15. Gibb DM, Dunger D, Levin M, Shah V, Smith C, Barratt TM. Early markers of the renal complications of insulin dependent diabetes mellitus. Arch Dis Child 1989;64:984-991.
16. Mogensen CE, Chachati A, Christensen CK, Close CF, Deckert T, Hommel E, Kastrup J, Lefebvre P, Mathiesen ER, Feldt-Rasmussen B, Schmitz A, Viberti GC. Microalbuminuria: An early marker of renal involvement in diabetes. Uremia Invest (1985-86);9:85-95.
17. Feldt-Rasmussen B, Microalbuminuria and clinical nephropathy in Type 1 (insulin-dependent) diabetes mellitus: Pathophysiological mechanisms and intervention studies. Dan Med Bull 1989;36:405-415.
18. Eshøj O, Feldt-Rasmussen B, Larsen ML, Mogensen EF. Comparison of overnight, morning and 24h urine collections in assessment of diabetic microalbuminuria. Diabetic Med 1987;4:531-533.
19. Gibb DM, Shah V, Preece M, Barratt TM. Variability of urine albumin excretion in normal and diabetic children. Pediatr Nephrol 1989; 3:414-419.
20. Taylor AM, Dunger DB, Preece MA, Holly JMP, Smith CP, Wass JAH, Patel S & Tate VE. The growth hormone independent insulin-like growth factor-I binding protein BP-28 is associated with serum insulin-like growth factor-I inhibitory bioactivity in adolescent insulin-dependent diabetics. Clinical Endocrinology 1990; 32: 229-239.
21. Blankestijn PJ, Derkx FHM, Birkenhäger JC, Lamberts SWJ, Mulder P, Verschoor L, Schalekamp MADH, Weber RFA. Glomerular hyperfiltration in insulin-dependent diabetes mellitus is correlated with enhanced growth hormone secretion. J Clin Endocrinol Metab 1993;77:498-502.
22. Chiarelli F, Verrotti A, Morgese G. Glomerular hyperfiltration increases the risk of developing microalbuminuria in diabetic children. Pediatr Nephrol 1995; 9:154-158.
23. Mathiesen ER, Saurbrey N, Hommel E, Parving H.-H. Prevalence of microalbuminuria in children with Type 1 (insulin-dependent) diabetes mellitus. Diabetologia 1986;29:640-643.
24. Nørgaard N, Storm B, Graa M, Feldt-Rasmussen B. Elevated albumin excretion and retinal changes in children with Type 1 diabetes are related to long-term poor blood glucose control. Diabetic Med. 1989;6:325-328.
25. D'Antonio JA, Ellis D, Doft BH, Becker DJ, Drash AL, Kuller LH, Orchard TJ. Diabetic complications and glycemic control. The Pittsburgh prospective insulin-dependent diabetes cohort study status report after 5 yr of IDDM. Diabetes Care 1989;12:694-700.
26. Joner G, Brinchmann-Hansen O, Torres CG, Hanssen KF. A nationwide cross-sectional study of retinopathy and microalbuminuria in young Norwegian Type 1 (insulin-dependent) diabetic patients. Diabetologia 1992;35:1049-1054.
27. Bojestig M, Arnqvist HJ, Hermansson G, Karlberg BE, Ludvigsson J. Declining incidence of nephropathy in insulin-dependent diabetes mellitus. N Engl J Med 1994;330:15-18.
28. Janner M, Eberhard Knill S, Diem P, Zuppinger KA, Mullis PE. Persistent microalbuminuria in adolescents with Type 1 (insulin-dependent) diabetes mellitus is associated to early rather than late puberty. Eur. J Pediatr 1994; 153:403-408.
29. Dahlquist G, Rudberg S. The prevalence of microalbuminuria in diabetic children and adolescents and its relation to puberty. Acta Pædiatr Scand 1987;76:795-800.
30. Rudberg S, Ullman E, Dahlquist G. Relationship between early metabolic control and the development of microalbuminuria - a longitudinal study in children with Type 1 (insulin-dependent) diabetes mellitus. Diabetologia 1993;36:1309-1314.
31. Stephenson MJ, Fuller JH, the EURODIAB IDDM Complications Study Group and, the WHO Multinational Study of Vascular Disease in Diabetes Study Group. Microalbuminuria is not rare before 5 years of IDDM. J Diab Comp 1994; 8:166-173.
32. Bangstad H-J, Østerby R, Dahl-Jørgensen K, Berg KJ, Hartmann A, Hanssen KF. Improvement of blood glucose control in IDDM patients retards the progression of morphological changes in early diabetic nephropathy. Diabetologia 1994;37: 483-490.
33. Powrie JK, Watts GF, Ingham JN, Taub NA, Talmud PJ, Shaw KM. Role of glycaemic control in development of microalbuminuria in patients with insulin dependent diabetes. BMJ 1994;309, 1608-1612.
34. Klein R, Klein BEK, Moss SE, Cruickshanks KJ. Ten-year incidence of gross proteinuria in people with diabetes. Diabetes 1995;44:916-923.
35. Mortensen HB, Hartling SG, Petersen KE, and the Danish study group of diabetes in childhood. A nation-wide cross-sectional study of glycosylated haemoglobin in Danish children with Type 1 diabetes. Diabetic Med 1988;5:871-876.

36. Mortensen HB, Villumsen J, Vølund Aa., Petersen KE, Nerup J and The Danish Study Group of Diabetes in Childhood. Relationship between insulin injection regimen and metabolic control in young Danish Type 1 diabetic patients. Diabetic Med 1992;9: 834-839.
37. Brenner BM, Chertow GM. Congenital oligonephropathy and the etiology of adult hypertension and progressive renal injury. Am J Kidney Dis 1994;23:171-175.
38. Rossing P, Tarnow L, Nielsen FS, Boelskifte S, Brenner BM, Parving H-H. Short stature and diabetic nephropathy. BMJ 1995;310:296-297.
39. Orchard TJ, Dorman JS, Maser RE, Becker DJ, Drash AL, Ellis D, LaPorte RE, Kuller LH. Prevalence of complications in IDDM by sex and duration. Pittsburgh epidemiology of diabetes complications study II. Diabetes 1990; 39: 1116-24.
40. The Diabetes Control and Complications Trial Research Group. The effect of intensive treatment of diabetes on the development and progression of long-term complications in insulin-dependent diabetes mellitus. N Engl J Med 1993;329:977-986.
41. Krolewski AS, Laffel LBM, Krolewski M, Quinn M, Warram JH. Glycosylated hemoglobin and the risk of microalbuminuria in patients with insulin-dependent diabetes mellitus. N Engl J Med 1995; 332: 1251-1255.
42. Mortensen HB, Hougaard P, Ibsen KK, Parving H-H and The Danish Study Group of Diabetes in Childhood. Relationship between blood pressure and urinary albumin excretion rate in young Danish Type 1 diabetic patients: Comparison to Non-diabetic children. Diabetic Med 1994;11:155-161.
43. Kordonouri O, Danne T, Hopfenmüller W, Enders I, Hövener G, Weber B. Lipid profiles and blood pressure: are they risk factors for the development of early background retinopathy and incipient nephropathy in children with insulin-dependent diabetes mellitus? Acta Paediatr;,1996; 85: 43-6.
44. Bojestig M, Arnqvist HJ, Karlberg BE; Ludvigsson. Glycemic control and prognosis in type I diabetic patients with microalbuminuria. Diabetes Care 1996; 19: 313-317.
45. Mogensen CE. Microalbuminuria as a predictor of clinical diabetic nephropathy. Kidney Int 1987; 31: 673-689.
46. Mogensen CE, Christensen CK, Christiansen JS, Boyle N, Pederson MM, Schmitz A. Early hyperfiltration and late renal damage in insulin-dependent diabetes. Pediatr Adolesc Endocrinol 1988; 17: 197-205.
47. Feldt-Rasmussen B, Mathiesen ER, Deckert T, Giese J, Christensen NJ, Bent-Hansen L, Damkjær Nielsen M. Central role for sodium in the pathogenesis of blood pressure changes independent of angiotensin, aldosterone and catecholamines in Type 1 (insulin-dependent) diabetes mellitus. Diabetologia 1987; 30: 610-617.
48. Deckert T, Kofoed-Enevoldsen A, Nørgaard K, Borch-Johnsen K, Feldt-Rasmussen B, Jensen T. Microalbuminuria: implications for micro- and macrovascular disease. Diabetes Care 1992;15:1181-1191.
49. Cook J, Daneman D, Spino M, Sochett E, Perlman K, Balfe JW. Angiotensin converting enzyme inhibitor therapy to decrease microalbuminuria in normotensive children with insulin-dependent diabetes mellitus. J. Pediatr 1990;117:39-45.
50. Rudberg S, Aperia A, Freyschuss U, Persson B. Enalapril reduces microalbuminuria in young normotensive Type 1 (insulin-dependent) diabetic patients irrespective of its hypotensive effect. Diabetologia 1990;33:470-476.
51. Marre M, Chatellier G, Leblanc H, Guyene TT, Menard J, Passa P. Prevention of diabetic nephropathy with enalapril in normotensive diabetics with microalbuminuria. Br Med J 1988; 297: 1092-1095.
52. Mathiesen ER, Hommel E, Giese J, Parving H-H. Efficacy of captopril in postponing nephropathy in normotensive insulin dependent diabetic patients with microalbuminuria. Br Med J 1991; 303: 81-87.
53. Hallab M, Gallois Y, Chatellier G, Rohmer V, Fressinaud P, Marre M. Comparison of reduction in microalbuminuria by enalapril and hydrochlorothiazide in normotensive patients with insulin dependent diabetes. BMJ 1993;306:175-182.
54. Viberti GC, Mogensen CE, Groop LC, Pauls JF, for the European Microalbuminuria Captopril Study Group. Effect of captopril on progression to clinical proteinuria in patients with insulin-dependent diabetes mellitus and microalbuminuria. JAMA 1994;271:275-279.

55. Breyer JA, Hunsicker LG, Bain RP, Lewis EJ, and The Collaborative Study Group. Angiotensin converting enzyme inhibition in diabetic nephropathy. Kidney Int 1994;45:156-160.
56. The Microalbuminuria Captopril Study Group (Barnes DJ, Cooper M, Gans DJ, Laffel L, Mogensen CE, Viberti GC): Captopril reduces the risk of nephropathy in insulin-dependent diabetic patients with microalbuminuria. Diabetologia, 1996; 39: 587-593
57. Charturvedi N, Sjolie A-K, Stephenson JM, Abrahamian H, Keipes M, Castellarin A, Rogulja-Pepeonik Z, Fuller JH, and the EUCLID Study Group. Effect of lisiniopril on progression of retinopathy in normotensive people with Type 1 diabetes. Lancet 1998; 351:28-31.
58. Mathiesen ER, Rønn B, Jensen T, Storm B, Deckert T. Relation between blood pressure and urinary albumin excretion in development of microalbuminuria. Diabetes 1990; 39: 245-249.
59. Zusman RM. Renin- and non-renin-mediated antihypertensive actions of converting enzyme inhibitors. Kidney Int 1984; 25:969-83.
60. Anderson S, Brenner BM. Pathogenesis of diabetic glomerulopathy: Hemodynamic considerations: Diabetes Metab Rev 1988;4:163-177.
61. Frohlich ED, Cooper RA, Lewis EJ. Review of the overall experience of captopril in hypertension. Arch Intern Med 1984;144:1441-44.
62. Mirkin BL, Newman TJ. Efficacy and safety of captopril in the treatment of severe childhood hypertension: report of the International Collaborative Study Group. Pediatrics 1985;75:1091-100.
63. Shield JPH. Microalbuminuria and nephropathy in childhood diabetes. Practical Diabetes 1994;11:146-149.

38. EARLY RENAL HYPERFUNCTION AND HYPERTROPHY IN IDDM PATIENTS INCLUDING COMMENTS ON EARLY INTERVENTION

Margrethe Mau Pedersen
Medical Department M, Aarhus Kommunehospital, Aarhus, Denmark

Diabetic nephropathy is the main cause of reduced survival in insulin-dependent diabetes. Much interest is paid to early alterations in kidney function and structure, since a relationship may exist between such early abnormalities and later development of diabetic nephropathy. A modest increase in urinary albumin excretion, microalbuminuria, has been identified as an early marker of diabetic nephropathy, and therapeutical intervention postponing the onset of overt nephropathy has been introduced. In this chapter the initial renal changes in IDDM, glomerular hyperfunction and renal hypertrophy, will be addressed.

GLOMERULAR HYPERFUNCTION

From the onset of IDDM, kidney function is characterised by elevation of glomerular filtration rate (GFR) and renal plasma flow (RPF) [for recent reviews see 1,2]. Using precise measurements e.g. renal clearance of inulin or iothalamate, it has been found that mean GFR in groups of short-term IDDM patients is increased by 15-25% - to approximately 135-140 ml/min/1.73m^2 during 'usual metabolic control' [3-7]. Before start of insulin treatment, but in the absence of ketoacidosis, glomerular hyperfiltration is even more pronounced, often showing elevations of approximately 40% [8,9]. RPF seems to be elevated synchronously with the increase in GFR, but less pronounced [3,5]. Estimation of RPF from renal clearance of hippuran appears to be a reliable measure also in the diabetic state [10].

During the first one or two decades of diabetes glomerular hyperfunction remains a characteristic feature of kidney function. In cross-sectional studies patients with microalbuminuria - typically developed after 10 to 15 years of diabetes - show more pronounced hyperfiltration than normoalbuminuric patients [7,11]. Until now, however, no prospective studies have described the individual course in GFR during transmission from normo- to microalbuminuria. With further increase in albumin excretion and development of nephropathy, GFR and RPF starts to decline, whereas in patients with persistent normoalbuminuria a moderate degree of glomerular hyperfunction persists [12].

Early renal changes in experimental diabetes in some degree parallel the characteristic glomerular hyperfunction in early stages of human diabetes. As described elsewhere in this book, besides hyperfusion, increased intraglomerular hydraulic pressure is an important factor in hyperfiltration in diabetic animals. In humans the larger increase in GFR than RPF (increased filtration fraction) suggests similar intraglomerular hypertension. However, elevation of the ultrafiltration coefficient due to increased filtration surface, may also offer a mechanism for the increased filtration fraction [13].

RENAL HYPERTROPHY

Kidney volume, estimated from ultrasonic techniques or roentgenographically, like GFR is markedly increased from the debut of diabetes. During initial insulin-treatment, kidney hypertrophy is somewhat reduced. The relative reduction in kidney volume is apparently delayed and smaller than the relative lowering of GFR [14]. The mean size remains elevated by approximately 20-30% during short-term IDDM [5,15-17]. At this stage, kidney volume is strongly correlated to GFR, corresponding to the state in non-diabetic subjects, and in most forms of non-diabetic renal hypertrophy [18]. Later in the course of diabetes this association cannot be found and possibly kidney volume increases further in the microalbuminuric state [19]. Hypertrophy persists also after the onset of overt nephropathy. Morphological studies concerning the initial renal enlargement show glomerular and tubular hypertrophy [20,21]. Subsequent deposition of PAS-positive material in the glomerular tuft and further enlargement of open glomeruli does not play a significant role or the total kidney volume.

DETERMINANTS FOR GLOMERULAR HYPERFUNCTION AND HYPERTROPHY

The pathophysiological mechanisms behind the increased glomerular filtration rate and renal plasma flow are still unclarified. A number of human and animal intervention studies have suggested a specific importance of one particular substance. In table 38-1 such factors with a possible involvement in glomerular hyperfunction are listed. Many factors, however, may represent normal modulators of kidney function influenced by an abnormal metabolic milieu and changes in fluid homeostasis. Furthermore, many of these factors are interrelated and represent different steps in regulatory mechanisms.

The abnormal carbohydrate metabolism no doubt plays a key-role in development of glomerular hyperfunction. An increase in blood glucose concentration apparently is associated with vasodilation in a number of tissues including the glomerular capillaries [22,23]. Suggested mechanisms for this vasodilation include an osmotic effect on cells lining small vessels [24], an increase in production of kallikrein and endothelium-derived-relaxing-factor (EDRF) [25,26], and increased production of vasodilator prostaglandins [27]. Furthermore, the increased amount of filtered and reabsorbed glucose coupled to increased tubular sodium reabsorption may suppress the tubuloglomerular feedback system and thereby contribute to hyperfiltration [25,28]. In human IDDM the influence of elevated blood glucose on GFR and RPF has been elucidated through intervention studies with glucose administration, through studies with intensified insulin treatment, and through cross-sectional studies analysing correlations between metabolic status and kidney function. In IDDM patients a rise in blood glucose by glucose infusion or an oral glucose load increases GFR and RPF in some studies [29-31]. Results, however, have not been completely uniform [32-34], maybe due to different responses in different subgroups of diabetic patients [33,34]. In studies with intensified insulin treatment, a few days of strict metabolic control has not been found to reduce GFR [35], whereas a reduction in GFR was observed during long-term (2 years) insulin pump treatment [36]. In cross sectional studies a correlation between GFR and HbA_{1c} and between intra-individual variation in blood glucose and in RPF has been reported [37,38]. Taken together these studies suggest that the 'acute' glucose level is associated mainly to RPF, whereas long-term metabolic control (e.g. represented by HbA_{1c}) show a closer correlation to GFR. It may be that e.g. biochemical membrane properties are important to the long-term influence of glycemic control of GFR.

Table 38-1. Factors with possible involvement in early diabetic glomerular hyperfunction including suggested intermediary steps.

Metabolic factors:	Blood glucose Long-term glycemic control (HbA_{1c}) Activity of polyol pathway Ketone bodies	[bradykinin, EDRF, prosta-glandins]
Hormonal/peptide substances:	GH, IGF-I Glucagon Insulin (peripheral hyperinsulinemia, hepatic insulinpenia) Atrial natriuretic peptide Kallikrein, bradykinin, kinin Catecholamines (abnormal response) Arginine vasopressin C-peptide	[prostaglandins] [restraining effect from adenosine]
Other vasoactive substances:	Vasodilatory prostaglandins Endothelial derived relaxing factor (EDRF) Nitric oxide	
Dietary factors other than carbohydrates	Protein intake Fat intake	[glucagon, prostaglandins, kallikrein, adenosine, dopamine, nitric oxide]

References : 22-27,29-44,47-54,56-60,64-70.

Another aspect of hyperglycaemia is enhanced glucose metabolism through the polyol pathway in tissues with insulin-independent glucose uptake. High activity of the enzyme aldose reductase leads to sorbitol accumulation and probably to changes in the redox state. These alterations, which appear to be rather closely linked to depletion of myoinositol [39], have been related to development of late diabetic complications in different tissues and recently also to glomerular hyperfiltration [40-42].

An increase in blood concentration of ketone bodies also accompany fairly well-regulated diabetes and intervention studies have suggested this to be of significance for hyperfiltration and hyperfusion [43]. However, no statistical correlation has been demonstrated between the concentration of ketone bodies and GFR or RPF.

Besides the indirect effect of insulin deficiency on renal hemodynamics through the blood glucose level, it has been suggested that inadequate delivery of insulin to the liver is associated with increased production of renal vasoregulatory factors [44]. In diabetic patients conventional insulin treatment with subcutaneous injections give rise to such portal hypoinsulinaemia, while hyperinsulinaemia is found in the systemic circulation [44]. No influence of insulin per se on GFR and RPF has been found [45].

One consequence of hyperglycaemia and peripheral hyperinsulinaemia appears to be an increase in total exchangeable body sodium and extracellular volume expansion [4,46]. Apart from an influence on the tubuloglomerular feedback system, this condition might induce hyperfiltration through a reflectoric increase in atrial natriuretic peptide (ANP).

A significant role for ANP in hyperfiltration is also suggested by experimental studies in animals showing marked reductions in GFR during treatment with anti-ANP serum [27,47] or an ANP-receptor antagonist [48]. In our study on intra-individual variation in kidney function [38] an involvement of ANP in the mechanisms behind human diabetic hyperfiltration was indicated by the finding of a close co-variation between GFR and ANP (figure 38-1).

Growth hormone (GH) and glucagon have long been known to represent possible mediators of diabetic hyperfiltration. Both hormones induce elevation in GFR when injected (through GH not acutely) [49,50]; increased plasma levels of the hormones may be brought about by the diabetic state, and a statistical correlation between plasma levels and GFR has been reported for both hormones [51]. The influence of GH is apparently indirect - acting through insulin-like growth factor I (IGF-I) [52]. Glucagon seems mainly to be of significance for hyperfiltration in poorly regulated diabetic patients [50].

Protein intake plays a special role in diabetic hyperfiltration in the sense that it represents a 'iatrogenic' stimulator of GFR. It is well-know that protein meals and infusion of aminoacids increases GFR [53]. Diabetic diets typically have a protein content of approximately 18-20% of total energy intake compared to a protein intake around 14% in non-diabetic (Danish) subjects [54,55]. By lowering protein intake from 19 to 12% we observed a decrease in mean GFR from 146 to 132 ml/min/-$1.73m^2$ in a group of normoalbuminuric IDDM patients [54]. The type of protein ingested seems to be of importance to the magnitude of influence on GFR [56,57]. Furthermore the content of phosphate may be relevant [58].

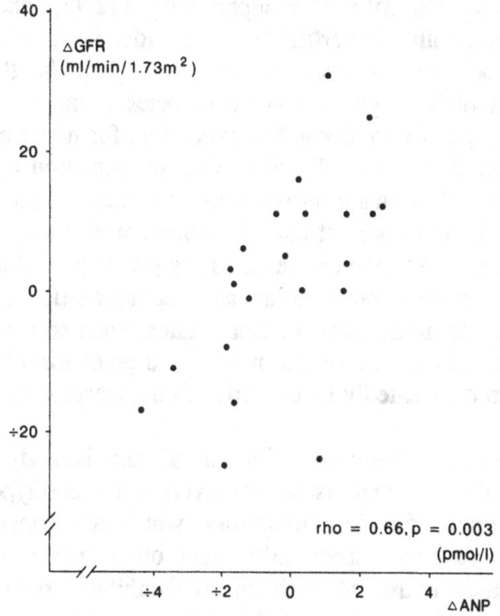

Fig. 38-1 Intra-individual variation in glomerular filtration rate (ΔGFR) in relation to variation in plasma concentration of atrial natriuretic peptide (ΔANP) in 22 patients with IDDM. 0.66 , p=0.003. From Mau Pedersen et al [38, with permission].

With respect to renal hypertrophy glycemic control is a determinant for kidney volume during the early stage of IDDM, as described above. It is unclarified whether kidney volume may still be modulated by alterations in glycemic control after years of diabetes and during the microalbuminuric state [19,59,60]. Knowledge on other pathogenetic factors in renal hypertrophy in human diabetes is limited. Experimental studies points towards GH/IGF-1 as contributors to very early kidney growth [52]. Furthermore, studies in experimental diabetes indicate that renal hypertrophy is closely associated with a depressed protein degradation due to reduced proteinase activity in both glomeruli and tubuli [61,62]. It has been suggested that increased expression of transforming growth factor-ß1 expression [63].

POSSIBLE ROLE OF HYPERFILTRATION AS A RISK MARKER FOR DIABETIC NEPHROPATHY

In certain IDDM patients, glomerular hyperfiltration is especially marked and sustained during many years, and it has been suggested that such hyperfiltration represents a pathogenetic factor for later development of diabetic nephropathy. This suspicion is supported by the apparent analogy between the characteristic early renal hemodynamic changes in human IDDM and in animal models of diabetes. Thus, in experimental diabetes a normalisation of the high GFR or the high intraglomerular hydraulic pressure by pharmacological or dietary means, has attenuated progression of renal disease [71]. In human diabetes retrospective data has suggested that marked hyperfiltration is associated with later nephropathy [12,72], and from a recent prospective study, glomerular hyperfiltration was identified as the only independent predictor for incipient or overt nephropathy [73]. In this study normoalbuminuric adolescent diabetic patients (with diabetes duration >8 years) were followed for 8 years. As possible independent predictors for nephropathy the statistical analysis included the duration of diabetes, albumin excretion rate, blood glucose and HbA_{1c} besides GFR. Also in a group of diabetic children, studied during 10 years, hyperfiltration was found to predict later development of microalbuminuria [74]. However, other studies do not point towards strong predictive value of high GFR [75,76], and a conclusion on hyperfiltration as a pathogenetic factor or a predictor for diabetic nephropathy must await further studies. Such studies need to be designed as long-term prospective and should include a large cohort of patients. GFR should either be measured repeatedly or conditions for measurements should be strictly characterised.

Indirect evidence for a pathogenetic role of abnormal renal hemodynamics is found in the marked slowing of early renal disease observed during antihypertensive treatment. This especially applies for ACE-inhibitors, which are considered to reduce intraglomerular pressure more specifically than other antihypertensives [78,78]. In a recent pilot study treatment with an ACE-inhibitor reduced both albumin excretion and kidney volume in microalbuminuric, normotensive IDDM patients [79].

POSSIBILITIES FOR INTERVENTIONS

An obvious goal for therapeutic intervention is optimizing glycemic control in order to decrease the risk of late complications. Such therapy tend to reduce hyperfiltration. Yet as it appears from above, hyperfiltration *per se* does not constitute an established indication for intervention. It seems rational though, not to prescribe higher protein content in diabetic than in non-diabetic diets to avoid inducing additional hyperfiltration.

Future possibilities for non-glycemic pharmacological intervention include aldose reductase inhibitors, aiming at normalization of the polyol pathway activity [40-42], and treatment with somatostatin analogues [80-82], which may act on GFR through a lowering of GH (or IGF-I) and a suppression of glucagon secretion. Until now these interventions have been tested only in rather short term or small scale studies and the possible long-term benefits awaits further investigations.

Also ACE-inhibitors deserves to be mentioned along with other proposed early interventions. Although these agents have not generally been found to reduce GFR, their ability to reduce the filtration fraction and probably the intraglomerular pressure [83] may prove valuable also before the onset of microalbuminuria [84]. In addition to the hemodynamic effects of ACE-inhibitors, these drugs may also be valuable since they might attenuate growth stimulating effect of ANG II [85].

REFERENCES

1. Mogensen CE. Glomerular hyperfiltration in human diabetes. Diabetes Care 1994; 17: 770-775.
2. Bank N. Mechanisms of diabetic hyperfiltration. Nephrology Forum. Kidney Int 1991; 40: 792-807.
3. Mogensen CE. Glomerular filtration rate and renal plasma flow in short-term and long-term juvenile diabetes mellitus. Scand J Clin Lab Invest 1971; 28: 91-100.
4. Ditzel J, Schwartz M. Abnormally increased glomerular filtration rate in short-term insulin-treated diabetic subjects. Diabetes 1976; 16: 264-267.
5. Christensen JS, Gammelgaard J, Frandsen M, Parving H-H. Increased kidney size, glomerular filtration rate and renal plasma flow in short-term insulin-dependent diabetics. Diabetologia 1981; 20: 451-456.
6. Brøchner-Mortensen J, Ditzel J. Glomerular filtration rate and extracellular fluid volume in insulin-dependent patients with diabetes mellitus. Kidney Int 1982; 21: 696-698.
7. Hansen KW, Mau Pedersen M, Christensen CK, Schmitz A, Christiansen JS, Mogensen CE. Normoalbuminuria ensures no reduction of renal function in type 1 (insulin-dependent) diabetic patients. J Intern Med 1992; 232: 161-167.
8. Mogensen CE. Kidney function and glomerular permeability to macromolecules in juvenile diabetes. Dan Med Bull 1972; 19: 1-36.
9. Christiansen JS, Gammelgaard J, Tronier B, Svendsen PA, Parving H-H. Kidney function and size in diabetics before and during initial insulin treatment. Kidney Int 1982; 21: 683-688.
10. Nyberg G, Granerus G, Aurell M. Renal extraction ratios for ^{51}Cr-EDTA, PAH, and glucose in early insulin-dependent diabetic patients. Kidney Int 1982; 21: 706-708.
11. Christensen CK, Mogensen CE. The course of incipient diabetic nephropathy: studies of albumin excretion and blood pressure. Diabetic Med 1985; 2: 97-102.
12. Mogensen CE, Christensen CK. Predicting diabetic nephropathy in insulin-dependent patients. N Engl J Med 1984; 311: 89-93.
13. Ellis EN, Steffes MW, Coetz FC, Sutherland DER, Mauer SM. Glomerular filtration surface in type 1 diabetes mellitus. Kidney Int 1986; 29: 889-894.
14. Christiansen JS, Frandsen M, Parving H-H. The effect of intravenous insulin infusion on kidney function in insulin-dependent diabetes mellitus. Diabetologia 1981; 20: 199-204.
15. Mogensen CE, Andersen MJF. Increased kidney size and glomerular filtration rate in early juvenile diabetes. Diabetes 1973; 22: 706-713.
16. Mogensen CE, Andersen MJF. Increased kidney size and glomerular filtration rate in untreated juvenile diabetes: Normalization by insulin-treatment. Diabetologia 1975; 11: 221-224.
17. Puig JG, Antón FM, Grande C, Pallardo LF, Arnalich F, Gil A, Vázquez JJ, García AM. Relation on kidney size to kidney function in early insulin-dependent diabetes. Diabetologia 1981; 21: 363-367.
18. Schwieger J, Fine LG. Renal hypertrophy, growth factors, and nephropathy in diabetes mellitus. Semin Nephrol 1990; 10: 242-253.
19. Feldt-Rasmussen B, Hegedüs L, Mathiesen ER, Deckert T. Kidney volume in type 1 (insulin-dependent) diabetic patients with normal or increased urinary albumin excretion: effect of long-term improved metabolic control. Scand J Lab Invest 1991; 51: 31-36.
20. Østerby R, Gundersen HJG. Glomerular size and structure in diabetes mellitus: I. Early abnormalities. Diabetologia 1975; 11: 225-229.
21. Seyer-Hansen K, Hansen J, Gundersen HJG. Renal hypertrophy in experimental diabetes: a morphometric study. Diabetologia 1980; 18: 501-505.
22. Mathiesen ER, Hilsted J, Feldt-Rasmussen B, Bonde-Petersen F, Christensen NJ, Parving H-H. The effect of metabolic control on hemodynamics in short-term insulin-dependent diabetic patients. Diabetes 1985; 34: 1301-1305.
23. Wolpert HA, Kinsley BT, Clermont AC, Wald H, Bursell S-E. Hyperglycaemia modulates retinal hemodynamics in IDDM. Diabetes 1993; 42: A489.
24. Gray SD. Effect of hypertonicity on vascular dimensions in skeletal muscle. Microvasc Res 1971; 3: 117-124.
25. Bank N. Mechanisms of diabetic hyperfiltration. Kidney Int 1991; 40: 792-807.
26. Harvey JN, Edmundson AW, Jaffa AA, Martin LL, Mayfield RK. Renal excretion of kallikrein and eicosanoids in patients with Type 1 (insulin-dependent) diabetes mellitus. Relationship to glomerular and tubular function. Diabetologia 1992; 35: 857-862.

27. Perico N, Benigni A, Gabanelli M, Piccinelli A, Rog M, De-Riva C, Remuzzi G. Atrial natriuretide peptide and prostacyclin synergistically mediate hyperfiltration and hyperperfusion of diabetic rats. Diabetes 1992; 41: 533-538.
28. Blantz RC, Peterson OW, Gushwa L, Tucker BJ. Effect of modest hyperglycaemia on tubuloglomerular feedback activity. Kidney Int 1982; 22: S206-S212.
29. Christiansen JS, Christensen CK, Hermansen K, Pedersen EB, Mogensen CE. Enhancement of glomerular filtration rate and renal plasma flow by oral glucose load in well controlled insulin-dependent diabetics. Scand J Clin Lab Invest 1986; 46: 265-272.
30. Christiansen JS, Frandsen M, Parving H-H. Effect of intravenous glucose infusion on renal function in normal man and in insulin-dependent diabetics. Diabetologia 1981; 21: 368-373.
31. Wiseman MJ, Mangili R, Alberetto M, Keen H, Viberti GC. Glomerular response mechanisms to glycemic changes in insulin-dependent diabetics. Kidney Int 1987; 31: 1012-1018.
32. Mogensen CE. Glomerular filtration rate and renal plasma flow in normal and diabetic man during elevation of blood sugar levels. Scand J Clin Lab Invest 1971; 28: 177-182.
33. Marre M, Dubin T, Hallab M, Berrut G, Bouhanick B, Lejeune J-J, Fressinaud P. Different renal response to hyperglycaemia in insulin-dependent diabetics at risk for, or protected against diabetic nephropathy. Diabetes 1993; 42: A423.
34. Skøtt P, Vaag A, Hother-Nielsen O, Andersen P, Bruun NE, Giese J, Beck-Nielsen H, Parving H-H. Effects of hyperglycaemia on kidney function, atrial natriuretic factor and plasma renin in patients with insulin-dependent diabetes mellitus. Scand J Clin Lab Invest 1991; 51: 715-727.
35. Mathiesen ER, Gall M-A, Hommel E, Skøtt P, Parving H-H. Effects of short-term strict metabolic control on kidney function and extracellular fluid volume in incipient diabetic nephropathy. Diabetic Med 1989; 6: 595-600.
36. Christensen CK, Christiansen JS, Schmitz A, Christensen T, Hermansen K, Mogensen CE. Effect of continuous subcutaneous insulin infusion on kidney function and size in IDDM patients - a two years controlled study. J Diabetes and Its Complications 1987; 1: 91-95.
37. Mogensen CE, Christensen CK, Mau Pedersen M, Alberti KGMM, Boye N, Christensen T, Christiansen JS, Flyvbjerg A, Ingerslev J, Schmitz A, Ørskov H. Renal and glycemic determinants of glomerular hyperfiltration in normoalbuminuric diabetics. J Diabetic Compl 1990; 4: 159-165.
38. Mau Pedersen M, Christiansen JS, Pedersen EB, Mogensen CE. Determinants of intra-individual variation in kidney function in normoalbuminuric insulin-dependent diabetic patients: importance of atrial natriuretic peptide and glycemic control. Clin Sci 1992; 83: 445-451.
39. Greene DA, Lattimer SA, Sima AAF. Sorbitol, phosphoinositides, and sodium-potassium-ATPase in the pathogenesis of diabetic complications. N Engl J Med 1987; 316: 599-606.
40. Mau Pedersen M, Christiansen JS, Mogensen CE. Reduction of glomerular hyperfiltration in normoalbuminuric IDDM patients by 6 mo of aldose reductase inhibition. Diabetes 1991; 40: 527-531.
41. Mau Pedersen M, Mogensen CE, Christiansen JS. Reduction of glomerular hyperfunction during short-term aldose reductase inhibition in normoalbuminuric, insulin-dependent diabetic patients. Endocrinol Metab 1995; 2: 55-62.
42. Passariello N, Sepe J, Marrazzo G, De Cicco A, Peluso A, Pisano MCA, Sgambato S, Tesauro P, D'Onofrio F. Effect of aldose reductase inhibitor (tolrestat) on urinary albumin excretion rate in IDDM subjects with nephropathy. Diabetes Care 1993; 16: 789-795.
43. Trevisan R, Nosadini R, Fioretto P, Avogaro A, Duner E, Iori E, Valerio A, Doria A, Crepaldi G. Ketone bodies increase glomerular filtration rate in normal man and in patients with type 1 (insulin dependent) diabetes. Diabetologia 1987; 30: 214-221.
44. Gwinup G, Elias AN. Hypothesis. Insulin is responsible for the vascular complications of diabetes. Med Hypotheses 1991; 34: 1-6.
45. Christiansen JS, Frandsen M, Parving H-H. The effect of intravenous insulin infusion on kidney function in insulin-dependent diabetes mellitus. Diabetologia 1981; 20: 199-204.
46. Skøtt P, Hother-Nielsen O, Bruun NE, Giese J, Nielsen MD, Beck-Nielsen H, Parving H-H. Effects of insulin on kidney function and sodium excretion in healthy subjects. Diabetologia 1989; 32: 694-699.
47. Ortola FV, Ballermann BJ, Anderson S, Mendez RE, Brenner BM. Elevated plasma atrial natriuretic peptide levels in diabetic rats. Potential mediator of hyperfiltration. J Clin Invest 1987; 80: 670-674.

48. Kikkawa R, Haneda M, Sakamoto K, Koya D, Shikano T, Nakanishi S, Matsuda Y, Shigeta Y. Antagonist for atrial natriuretic peptide receptors ameliorates glomerular hyperfiltration in diabetic rats. Biochem Biophys Res Commun 1993; 193: 700-705.
49. Christiansen JS, Gammelgaard J, Frandsen M, Ørskov H, Parving H-H. Kidney function and size in normal subjects before and during growth hormone administration for one week. Eur J Clin Invest 1981; 11: 487-490.
50. Parving H-H, Christiansen JS, Noer I, Tronier B, Mogensen CE. The effect of glucagon infusion on kidney function in short-term insulin-dependent juvenile diabetics. Diabetologia 1980; 19: 350-354.
51. Hoogenberg K, Dullaart RPF, Freling NJM, Meijer S, Sluiter WJ. Contributory roles of circulatory glucagon and growth hormone to increased renal haemodynamics in type 1 (insulin-dependent) diabetes mellitus. Scand J Clin Lab Invest 1993; 53: 821-828.
52. Flyvbjerg A. »The role of insulin-like growth factor I in initial renal hypertrophy in experimental diabetes.« In *Growth Hormone and Insulin-Like Growth Factor I*. Flyvbjerg A, Ørskov H, Alberti KGMM, eds. John Wiley & Sons Ltd., 1993; pp 271-306.
53. Castellino P, Hunt W, DeFronzo RA. Regulation of renal hemodynamics by plasma amino acid and hormone concentrations. Kidney Int 1987; 32: S-15-S-20.
54. Mau Pedersen M, Mogensen CE, Schönau Jørgensen F, Møller B, Lykke G, Pedersen O. Renal effects from limitation of high dietary protein in normoalbuminuric diabetic patients. Kidney Int 1989; 36: S-115-S-121.
55. Mau Pedersen M, Winther E, Mogensen CE. Reducing protein in the diabetic diet. Diabete Metab (Paris) 1990; 16: 454-459.
56. Jones MG, Lee K, Swaminathan R. The effect of dietary protein on glomerular filtration rate in normal subjects. Clin Nephrol 1987; 27: 71-75.
57. Pecis M, de Azevedo MJ, Gross JL. Chicken and fish diet reduces glomerular hyperfiltration in IDDM patients. Diabetes Care 1994; 17: 665-672.
58. Kraus ES, Cheng L, Sikorski I, Spector DA. Effects of phosphorus restriction on renal response to oral and intravenous protein loads in rats. Am J Physiol 1993; 264: F752-F759.
59. Tuttle KR, Bruto JL, Perusek MC, Lancaster JL, Kopp DT, DeFronzo RA. Effect of strict glycemic control on renal hemodynamic response to amino acids and renal enlargement in insulin-dependent diabetes mellitus. N Engl J Med 1991; 324: 1626-1632.
60. Wisemann MJ, Saunders AJ, Keen H, Viberti GC. Effect of blood glucose control on increased glomerular filtration rate and kidney size in insulin-dependent diabetes. N Engl J Med 1985; 312: 617-621.
61. Shechter P, Boner G, Rabkin R. Tubular cell protein degradation in early diabetic renal hypertrophy. J Am Soc Nephrol 1994; 4: 1582-1587.
62. Schaefer L, Schaefer RM, Ling, Teschner M, Heidland A. Renal proteinases and kidney hypertrophy in experimental diabetes. Diabetologia 1994; 37: 567-571.
63. Shankland SJ, Scholey JW, Ly H, Thai K. Expression of transforming growth factor-ß1 during diabetic renal hypertrophy. Kidney Int 1994; 46: 430-442.
64. Wang YX, Brooks DP. The role of adenosine in glycine-induced glomerular hyperfiltration in rats. J Pharmacol Exp Ther 1992; 263: 1188-1194.
65. Angielski S, Redlak M, Szczepanska KM. Intrarenal adenosine prevents hyperfiltration induced by atrial natriuretic factor. Miner Electrolyte Metab 1990; 16: 57-60.
66. Wang YX, Gellai M, Brooks DP. Dopamine DA1 receptor agonist, fenoldopam, reverses glycine-induced hyperfiltration in rats. Am J Physiol 1992; 262: F1055-F1060.
67. Jaffa AA, Vio CP, Silva RH, Vavrek RJ, Stewart JM, Rust PF, Mayfield RK. Evidence for renal kinins as mediators of amino acid-induced hyperfusion and hyperfiltration in the rat. J Clin Invest 1992; 89: 1460-1468.
68. Friedlander G, Blanchet BF, Nitenberg A, Laborie C, Assan R, Amiel C. Glucagon secretion is essential for aminoacid-induced hyperfiltration in man. Nephrol Dial Transplant 1990; 5: 110-117.
69. Wahren J, Johansson B-L, Wallberg-Henriksson H. Does C-peptide have a physiological role? Diabetologia 1994; 37: Suppl. 2: S99-S107.
70. Bouhanick B, Suraniti S, Berrut G, Bled F, Simard G, Lejeune JJ, Fressinaud P, Marre M. Relationship between fat intake and glomerular filtration rate in normotensive insulin-dependent diabetic patients. Diabete Metab (Paris) 1995; 21: 168-172.

71. Hostetter TH. Diabetic nephropathy. Metabolic versus hemodynamic considerations. Diabetes Care 1992; 15: 1205-1215.
72. Mogensen CE. Early glomerular hyperfiltration in insulin-dependent diabetics and late nephropathy. Scand J Clin Lab Invest 1986; 46: 201-206.
73. Rudberg S, Persson B, Dalqvist G. Increased glomerular filtration rate predicts diabetic nephropathy-results form an 8 year prospective study. Kidney Int 1992; 41: 822-828.
74. Chirelli F, Verrotti A, Morgese G. Glomerular hyperfiltration increases the risk of developing microalbuminuria in diabetic children. Pediatr Nephrol 1995; 9: 154-158.
75. Lervang H-H, Jensen S, Brøchner-Mortensen J, Ditzel J. Does increased glomerular filtration rate or disturbed tubular function early in the course of childhood type 1 diabetes predict the development of nephropathy? Diabetic Med 1992; 9: 635-640.
76. Yip WJ, Jones LS, Wiseman JM, Hill C, Viberti GC. Glomerular hyperfiltration in the prediction of nephropahty in IDDM. Diabetes vol. 45, dec. 1996; 1729-1733.
77. Anderson S. Renal effects of converting enzyme inhibitors in hypertension and diabetes. J Cardiovasc Pharmacol 1990; 15: Suppl. 3: S11-S15.
78. Mau Pedersen M, Christensen CK, Hansen KW, Christiansen JS, Mogensen CE. ACE-inhibition and renoprotection in early diabetic nephropathy. Response to enalapril acutely and in long-term combination with conventional antihypertensive treatment. Clin Invest Med 1991; 14: 642-651.
79. Bakris GL, Slataper R, Vicknair N, Sadler R. ACE inhibitor mediated reductions in renal size and microalbuminuria in normotensive, diabetic subjects. J Diabetic Compl 1994; 8: 2-6.
80. Mau Pedersen M, Christensen SE, Christiansen JS, Pedersen EB, Mogensen CE, Ørskov H. Acute effects of a somatostatin analogue on kidney function in type i diabetic patients. Diabetic Med 1990; 7: 304-309.
81. Serri O, Beauregard H, Brazeau P, Abribat T, Lamber J, Harris A, Vachon L. Somatostatin analogue, octreotide, reduces increased glomerular filtration rate and kidney size in insulin-dependent diabetes. JAMA 1991; 265; 888-892.
82. Jacobs ML, Derkx FH, Stijnen T, Lamberts SW, Weber RF. Effect of long-acting somatostatin analog (Somatolin) on renal hyperfiltration in patients with IDDM. Diabetes Care 1997; 20 (4): 632-636.
83. Mau Pedersen M, Schmitz A, Pedersen EB, Danielsen H, Christiansen JS. Acute and long-term renal effects of angiotensin converting enzyme inhibition in normotensive, normoalbuminuric insulin-dependent diabetic patients. Diabetic Med 1988; 5: 562-569.
84. Pecis M, Azevedo JM, Gross LJ. Glomerular Hyperfiltration is associated with blood pressure abnormalities in normotensive normoalbuminuric IDDM patients. Diabetes Care, vol. 20, no. 8, 1997; 1329-1333.
85. Ichikawa I, Harris RC. Angiotensin actions in the kidney: Renewed insight into the old hormone (Editorial Review). Kidney Int 1991; 40: 583-596.

39. ACE INHIBITION, ANGIOTENSIN II RECEPTOR BLOCKADE, AND DIABETIC NEPHROPATHY

Norman K. Hollenberg, M.D., Ph.D.
Departments of Medicine and Radiology, Brigham and Women's Hospital, Boston, USA

Only a large, rigorous randomized double-blind assessment of a therapeutic candidate compared to the appropriate alternative can prove therapeutic efficacy. One such trial assessed the effect of captopril in patients with insulin-dependent diabetes mellitus (IDDM) who were at risk of nephropathy [1], with results that were sufficiently impressive that the use of captopril quickly became a professional necessity supported by public policy. Moreover, multiple lines of evidence accumulated over a decade suggested that this useful feature of captopril was a class action, extending to all ACE inhibitors. [2,3] In the case of the angiotensin II (Ang II) AT_1 receptor blockers (AT_1 antagonists), we are fortunate in having very early in the development of these agents two ongoing major, high quality trials in patients with NIDDM who are at risk of nephropathy - one involving Irbesartan, the other involving Losartan. Unfortunately, the outcome of these trials is unlikely to be available to us until the coming millennium, and this chapter is due well before!

The issue of the pharmacologic mechanisms by which ACE inhibitors retard the progression of nephropathy lies at the centre of any discussion on whether or not AT_1 antagonists will match their efficacy. Ichikawa, an authority on the renin system and the kidney, marshalled multiple lines of evidence to indicate that much of the salutary actions of ACE inhibitors did not involve Ang II formation, but rather alternative pathways [4]. In a recent editorial, I countered with an alternative view [5] to indicate that the AT_1 receptor blockers held promise beyond what ACE inhibition can offer. What were the arguments?

Ichikawa based his analysis on a range of considerations, the majority of which seem to favour ACE inhibition as these considerations suggest that angiotensin is not important [4] ACE inhibitors can influence alternative pathways that might, in turn, influence extracellular matrix protein degradation and the rate of development of glomerulosclerosis. Macrophage infiltration is also ACE inhibitor responsive. Blocking the AT1 receptor opens the short feedback loop, thereby leading to renin release and increased Ang II formation. With the AT1 receptor blocked, this sequence could lead to unopposed activation of the AT2 receptor -- with unknown but potentially negative consequences. All of these considerations, Ichikawa believed, favour ACE inhibition over Ang II AT1 antagonist action. Perhaps the most important consideration in Ichikawa's analysis involved glomerular hemodynamics, especially glomerular capillary pressure: much of the ACE inhibitor dependent improvement in natural history might reflect the salutary effect of ACE inhibition on glomerular capillary pressure via bradykinin-mediated efferent arteriolar dilatation.

Thus, the kininase action of ACE inhibitors is considered to be crucial, and the reduction in Ang II formation is less important -- or even irrelevant. Conversely, one can make an equally compelling argument for potential efficacy of Ang II antagonists, based on more effective blockade of the renin system [5,6].

Much of the most important data reviewed above were obtained in vitro or in small animal models. If studies in rats never predicted responses in humans, we would probably never do studies in rats -- or at least would not read them. If studies in rats always predicted what would happen in humans, we could not justify studies in humans. Is this an area in which there might be important species differences? I addressed that issue specifically in a recent editorial on ACE inhibition and the kidney [6]. To isolate species differences one has to apply an essentially identical protocol to multiple species. There are species differences. As one example, bradykinin antagonists blunted the renovasodilator response to ACE inhibitors in the dog and in the rat, but not in the rabbit. In accord, an Ang II antagonist blunted ACE inhibitor induced renal vasodilation in the rat and dog very little, but blocked it completely in the rabbit. ACE inhibition increased prostaglandin release in rat and canine kidneys, but not that of the rabbit. In an elegant study Roman, et al [7] showed that in the rat it was medullary perfusion that was especially kinin dependent. Thus, apparent species differences may be primarily anatomical, reflecting the relative contribution of medullary perfusion to total renal blood flow: In this feature humans resemble the rabbit far more than they do the rat or dog [6]. Whatever the explanation one clear message emerges: We cannot extrapolate from studies in a limited range of species, especially the rat, to control mechanisms in humans, even in health and much less so when disease is superimposed.

What of information on the control of the renal circulation in humans, and the mechanisms by which ACE inhibition might influence the renal circulation? Although there are limitations in the approaches that can be employed in humans, several lines of evidence provide an answer. The striking influence of salt intake on the renal vasodilator response to ACE inhibition was recognized early, and supports a dominant role for the Ang II mechanism. This observation is necessary but is not sufficient. More recently, comparative pharmacology has strengthened that conclusion substantially. If the renal vasodilatation induced by ACE inhibitors in humans included a substantial component due to bradykinin, prostaglandins, or nitric oxide, one would anticipate that the renal vasodilator response to renin inhibitors would be substantially less. To our surprise the renal vasodilator response to a renin inhibitor, enalkiren, exceeded expectations from early experience with

ACE inhibitors [6]. To address this issue, we performed a range of follow-up studies. To ascertain whether the observation represented an idiosyncracy associated with one renin inhibitor, we studied a second -- with an identical result. Because of the notorious risk of employing historic controls, we performed a study in which patients received an ACE inhibitor, a renin inhibitor, or vehicle during the same week. This study was coded and double blind. To avoid an idiosyncracy associated with one ACE inhibitor, we employed three, each at the top of the dose response curve. The findings all provided support for a surprising but unambiguous conclusion. Despite the fact that our original premise on the kinin contribution to the renal response to ACE inhibition supported by a wealth of information in animal studies, the renovasodilator response to renin inhibition -- in the neighborhood of 140 ml/min/1.73m^2 -- was substantially larger than the response to ACE inhibition, in the 90-100 ml/min/1.73 m^2 range.

Although the fundamentals of pharmacology would favour as the explanation more effective pharmacological interruption of the renin system at the rate-limiting step, there is an alternative interpretation. As the two renin inhibitors were structurally related, it is possible that they shared a renovasodilator action through a mechanism unrelated to a reduction in Ang II formation. If, indeed, the renin inhibitors operated via the renin cascade, one would anticipate a similar or larger renovasodilator response to Ang II antagonists, in studies performed in the same way. This is precisely what we found. In studies performed with an identical model, protocol and technique, two Ang II antagonists induced a renovasodilator response that matched, or exceeded slightly the response to renin inhibition in healthy humans on a low salt diet [8,9]. From this observation we would draw several conclusions. The renal hemodynamic response to ACE inhibition has underestimated, systematically, the magnitude of the contribution of Ang II to renovascular tone when the renin system is activated. The effectiveness of renin inhibition suggests that this response represents interruption of primarily renin-dependent, additional non-ACE-dependent pathways. In healthy humans, there might be a small contribution from proteolytic pathways that bypass both renin and ACE. In disease, on the other hand, alternative pathways may provide a more substantial contribution [9].

PLASMA-RENIN ACTIVITY, RENAL TISSUE RENIN, AND DIABETES

What evidence is there from studies on the state of the renin system and the contribution of Ang II to renal vascular tone to suggest that angiotensin might be involved in the pathogenesis? When studies on the circulating renin system were first undertaken, the goal was to ascertain whether the hypertension that frequently complicates the course of diabetes could be attributed to the renin system [10]. An unanticipated suppression of the renin system was found in many patients, especially in those with diabetic nephropathy, an observation that has been repeated frequently [11-13]. The low renin state has typically been attributed to organic sclerotic changes in the arteriolar and glomerular region, possibly accentuated by volume expansion and autonomic neuropathy. Several lines of evidence suggest a more interesting, more complex and immediately relevant alteration in the renal tissue renin system in this process. In animal models, multiple studies have shown that renal tissue renin levels, and the message supporting renin production are normal or increased, even in animal models in which PRA is reduced [14-16]. In patients with NIDDM in whom renal function was intact and who were free of evidence of nephropathy, we found an unanticipated abnormality in the control of renin release. In these patients in whom plasma renin activity was normal on challenge with a low salt diet and posture, there was evidence of renin system autonomy [17]. On a low salt diet, renin system activation appeared to be normal and intact as PRA rose normally, and the renal vasodilator response to ACE inhibition with enalapril was identical to normal. Conversely, when the patients received a high salt diet, despite the fact that they showed more positive sodium balance, PRA suppressed less well in patients with NIDDM than in age-matched normal subjects. Moreover, the renal vasodilator response to enalapril on a high salt diet in NIDDM exceeded substantially the response in normal subjects, in whom ACE inhibitor-induced renal vasodilatation is minimal. This vasodilator response in NIDDM was attributable to Ang II based on indirect evidence. At baseline, the renal vascular response to Ang II was already blunted in NIDDM, in keeping with renin system activation. If the renal vasodilator response to enalapril had reflected kinin production, and consequent prostaglandin synthesis or nitric oxide release we would have anticipated further blunting of the response to Ang II. Conversely, if the renal vasodilator response reflected a reduction in Ang II production, we would have anticipated enhancement of the renal vascular response. The dramatic enhancement of responses to Ang II that occurred favored an ACE inhibitor action primarily reflecting reduced Ang II formation.

This indirect evidence is supported further by more recent studies with the Ang II antagonist, Irbesartan [9]. In patients with NIDDM and nephropathy in whom the renin system response to restriction of sodium intake was blunted, the renal vasodilator response to Irbesartan was enhanced, exceeding the response to normal substantially over a range of doses. PRA, suppressed at baseline in the patients with diabetes, responded to the Ang II antagonist with a progressive rise that eventually matched normal. These observations suggest that measures of PRA can be misleading, providing little insight into the state of the intrarenal renin system. Activation of this system in diabetes, perhaps in part due to the effects of hyperglycemia [18] could contribute to pathogenesis.

The final conclusion is that therapeutic trials with Ang II antagonists offer far more promise than did ACE inhibitors, despite the gloomy predictions. They are more effective blockers.

REFERENCES

1. Lewis EJ, Hunsicker LG, Bain RP, and Rohde RD: The effect of angiotensin converting enzyme inhibition on diabetic nephropathy. N Engl J Med 1993;329:1456-1462.
2. Kasiske BL, Kalil RSN, Ma JZ, Liao M, and Keane WF: Effect of therapy on the kidney in patients with diabetes: A meta-regression analysis. Ann Intern Med 1993;118:129-138.
3. Hollenberg NK and Raij L. Angiotensin-converting enzyme inhibition and renal protection. An assessment of implications for therapy. Arch Intern Med 1993;153:2426-2435.
4. Ichikawa I. Will Ang II A1 be renoprotective in humans? Kidney Intern 1996;50:684-692.

5. Hollenberg NK. ACE inhibitors, AT1 receptor blockers, and the kidney. E. Ritz (Ed) Nephrol Dial Transplant 1997;12:381-383.
6. Hollenberg NK and Fisher NK. Renal circulation and blockade of the renin-angiotensin system. Is angiotensin-converting enzyme inhibition the last word? Hypertension 1995; 26:602-609.
7. Roman RJ, Kaldunski ML, Scicli AG, and Carretero OA. Influence of kinins and angiotensin II on the regulation of papillary blood flow. Am J Physiol 1988;255:F690-F698.
8. Price D, DeOliveira J, Fisher N, and Hollenberg N. Contribution of Ang II to renal hemodynamics in healthy men: the renal vascular response to eprosartan, an Ang II antagonist. ASN Program Abstract #A1688 from 29th Annual Meeting in New Orleans, Nov. 3-6. J Am Soc Nephrol 1996;7:1587.
9. Price D, Porter L, DeOliveira J, Fisher N, Gordon M, Laffel L, Williams G, and Hollenberg N. The paradox of the low-renin state: hormonal and renal responses to an Ang II antagonist, Irbesartan, in diabetic nephropathy. ASN Program Abstract #A0591 from 29th Annual Meeting in New Orleans. J Am Soc Nephrology 1996;7:163.
10. Christlieb AR, Kaldany A, and D'Elia JA. Plasma renin activity and hypertension in diabetes mellitus. Diabetes 1976;25:969-974.
11. Bjorck S. The renin-angiotensin system in diabetes mellitus: a physiological and therapeutic study. Scand J Urol Nephrol Suppl 1990;126:1-50.
12. Lush DJ, King JA, and Fray JCS. Pathophysiology of low renin syndromes: sites of renal renin secretory impairment and prorenin overexpression. Kid International 1993;43:983-999.
13. Weidmann P, Ferrari P, and Shaw SG. Renin in Diabetes Mellitus. In: The Renin-Angiotensin System. In: JIS Robertson and MG Nicholls (Ed). Raven Press Ltd., New York, 1991. Chapter 75. pp. 75.1-75.26.
14. Rosenberg ME, Smith LJ, Correa-Rotter R, and Hostetter TH. The paradox of the renin-angiotensin system in chronic renal disease. Kid Internat 1994;45:403-410.
15. Kikkawa R, Kitamura E, Fujiwara Y, Haneda M, and Shigeta Y. Biphasic alteration of renin-angiotensin-aldosterone system in streptozotocin-diabetic rats. Renal Physiol 1986;9:187-192.
16. Anderson S, Jung FF, and Ingelfinger JR. Renal renin-angiotensin system in diabetes: functional immunohistochemical, and molecular biological correlations. Am J Physiol 1993;265:F477-F486.
17. De'Oliveira JM, Price DA, Fisher NDL, Allan DR, McKnight JA, Williams GH, and Hollenberg NK. Autonomy of the renin system in type II diabetes mellitus: Dietary sodium and renal hemodynamic responses to ACE inhibition. Kidney International 1997;52:771-777.
18. Miller JA, Floras JS, Zinman B, Skorecki KL, and Logan AG. Effect of hyperglycemia on arterial pressure, plasma renin activity and renal function in early diabetes. Clin Sci 1996;90:189-195.

40. THE CONCEPT OF INCIPIENT DIABETIC NEPHROPATHY AND EFFECT OF EARLY ANTIHYPERTENSIVE INTERVENTION

Michel Marre, Patrick Fabbri, Gilles Berrut and Béatrice Bouhanick
Unité de Diabétologie, Service de Médecine B, Centre Hospitalier Universitaire, Angers, France

1. INTRODUCTION

Diabetic nephropathy is the main cause for premature death among type 1, insulin-dependent diabetic subjects [1]. To date, aggressive antihypertensive treatment is the main intervention along with better metabolic contact able to improve prognosis of these patients [2]. The term diabetic nephropathy designates glomerular injury attributable to diabetes [3]. As in all glomerular diseases, its diagnosis is based upon three functional abnormalities: proteinuria (mainly albuminuria), elevated blood pressure, and reduced glomerular filtration rate. Technical improvements lead to early detection of glomerular dysfunction in type 1, insulin-dependent diabetic subjects: the first ones were sensitive assays for urinary albumin measurement [4,5]; also sensitive techniques to detect glomerular hyperfiltration early in the course of diabetic renal disease, and only recently automatic blood pressure monitoring to detect minimal blood pressure changes [6,7]. The concept of incipient diabetic nephropathy was validated by 4 follow-up studies of patients whose urinary albumin was measured serially with sensitive techniques [8-11]. These studies indicated that minimal increases in Urinary Albumin Excretion (UAE) (called microalbuminuria) can have a prognostic value. Therefore, the concept of incipient diabetic nephropathy is based upon the premise that persistent microalbuminuria can already indicate initial glomerular injury, and not only glomerular dysfunction as discussed elsewhere.

2. DESCRIPTION AND NATIONAL HISTORY OF INCIPIENT DIABETIC NEPHROPATHY

2.1. Description

2.1.1. UAE

By definition, UAE is elevated in the microalbuminuria range. Although UAE values predictive for diabetic nephropathy varied from 15 to 70 μg/min among the four pilot studies [8-11], a consensus was proposed to define microalbuminuria as UAE ranging 30-300 mg/24h, or 20-200 µg/min, 2 - 3 times over 1 - 6 month period [12]. The Steno group proposed to subdivide into micro- microalbuminuria (30-99 mg/24h) and macro- microalbuminuria (100-300 mg/24h), because the prognosis was poorer for the latter than for the former values [13]. However, these differential prognostic values were not confirmed on an individual basis [14,15].

2.1.2. Blood pressure

The mean blood pressure values of subjects with incipient diabetic nephropathy are higher than those of healthy controls, or of diabetic subjects with normal UAE, but lower than those of subjects with established diabetic nephropathy. There is a good correlation between blood pressure and UAE values. However, diagnosis of incipient diabetic nephropathy cannot be based upon cut-off values for blood pressure, because of large inter-group overlaps. Only the upper limit for blood pressure values can be fixed, namely those defining permanent hypertension: e.g. 140/90 mmHg or more, and/or concurrent hypertensive treatment. This upper limit has practical implications to delineate different causes for microalbuminuria: microalbuminuria with permanent hypertension indicates severe hypertension, but not incipient diabetic nephropathy, and regression lines between blood pressure and UAE are not superimposable for one case and for the other [16].

Automatic devices can improve blood pressure recording precision, but probably not sensitivity to classify subjects with incipient diabetic nephropathy [17]. Nocturnal recordings can ameliorate sensitivity [6,7,17], because a reduction in nocturnal blood pressure decline is characteristic of high blood pressure secondary to glomerular disease [18].

In summary, blood pressure values are not in the permanent hypertension range during incipient diabetic nephropathy; they must be recorded precisely and uniformly for follow-up purposes.

2.1.3. Glomerular filtration rate

In incipient diabetic nephropathy, GFR can be normal, or elevated, but rarely below normal values. The prognostic significance of glomerular hyperfiltration is discussed elsewhere in this book. However, it is not clear by which UAE values within the microalbuminuria range GFR starts declining in normotensive diabetic individuals. Mogensen and Christensen proposed that the initially positive relationship between UAE and GFR values becomes negative for UAE ranges above 30-50 µg/min [11]. In figure 35-1, we traced a parabolic regression line between individual UAE and GFR values obtained in 84 type 1, insulin-dependent diabetic subjects without antihypertensive treatment. The calculated top of the line was found for UAE 34 mg/24h and GFR 130 ml/min/1.73m^2. Hence, it is possible that glomerular filtration surface is reducing from the lowest UAE values within microalbuminuria, even though GFR values are in the normal, or supra-normal ranges. This biphasic relationship between UAE and GFR suggests that the phenomenon observed by Starling [19] on heart muscles is applicable to changes in glomerular function of type 1, insulin-dependent diabetic subjects. This analogy in modelization can have a physical basis, as mesangial cells are of muscular origin.

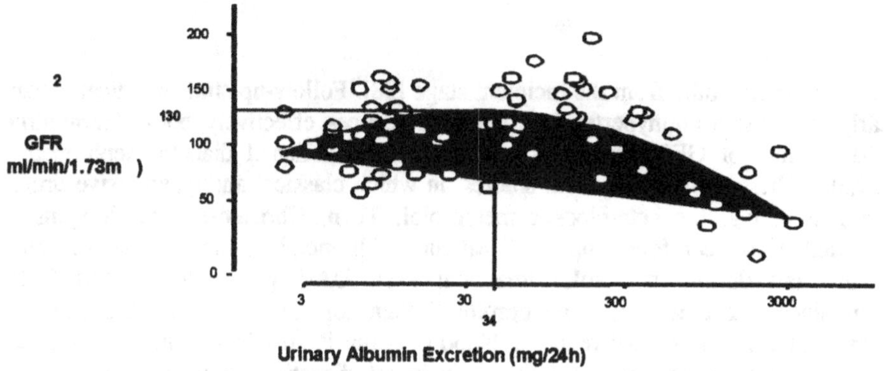

Figure 40-1. Observed relationship between UAE (the mean of 3 consecutive 24-hour urine collections) and GFR (^{51} Cr-EDTA plasma disappearance technique) values measured in 84 consecutive type 1, insulin-dependent diabetic subjects without antihypertensive treatment: $r = 0.576$; $p = 0.0001$; GFR (ml/min/1.73m^2) = 70+78 (SD 16) log UAE (mg/24 h) - 26 (4) [log UAE]^2 - Calculated top of parabolic curve was UAE = 34 mg/24 h and GFR = 130 ml/min/1.73m^2.

2.2. Natural course of incipient diabetic nephropathy

2.2.1. Incidence of diabetic nephropathy

Incidence of persistent microalbuminuria in normotensive type 1, insulin-dependent diabetic subjects was studied by several groups [20,21] over 4 or 5 year-periods. It approximates 1 - 2% cases/year. The main risk factor for microalbuminuria onset is diabetes duration, which is 5 years minimally. It was recently outlined that subjects with microalbuminuria and long diabetes duration may display a better prognosis than those with diabetes duration shorter than 15-17 years [22]. However, this result must be interpreted cautiously, because the slope of UAE progression can vary widely from one individual to another, and because early interventions can alter the course of the disease, especially with ACEIs. Glycaemic control is of paramount importance to prognose microalbuminuria: subjects with HbA1c below 7.5% have a low risk for microalbuminuria [20,21]. Recently, Krolewski et al proposed from follow-up observations that type 1, insulin-dependent diabetic subjects with normoalbuminuria and HbA1c level below 8.1% would have a minimal risk for progression towards microalbuminuria [23]. Accordingly, results from the DCCT indicated that optimized insulin treatment reduced risk for microalbuminuria onset by 21-52% [24].

Genetic factors can affect risk for incipient or established diabetic nephropathy. This is discussed elsewhere in this book .

2.2.2. Duration of incipient diabetic nephropathy

Duration of incipient diabetic nephropathy is not determined precisely from large group follow-up. Some studies indicate a 5-15 year duration [13]. Nonetheless, incidence of established diabetic nephropathy may be high: in control groups of clinical trials performed in normotensive subjects with microalbuminuria, it ranged between 8 and 30% cases/year [14,15,26,27].

3. EFFECT OF EARLY ANTIHYPERTENSIVE INTERVENTION IN INCIPIENT DIABETIC NEPHROPATHY

3.1. Rationale

There is a proportional increase of UAE and of blood pressure during the course of diabetic nephropathy from the incipient stage [28]. Follow-up studies indicated that early, aggressive antihypertensive treatment reduces effectively both albuminuria and the rate of GFR decline in patients with established diabetic nephropathy [29,30]. These were pragmatical studies, in which classical antihypertensive drugs were used, e.g. the beta-blocker metoprolol. Then, Christensen and Mogensen reported a six-year follow-up of 6 patients with incipient diabetic nephropathy before and during metoprolol treatment [31]. UAE was reduced, and GFR maintained unchanged with metoprolol. Taken together, these studies [29-31] supported the concept that reducing blood pressure is an effective mean to reduce microalbuminuria and protect GFR in incipient diabetic nephropathy. However, clinical and experimental data supported that increased UAE results from increased glomerular capillary pressure, which is determined not only by systemic blood pressure, but also by pre./post glomerular vasoconstriction/dilation [32]. This latter determinant is strongly regulated by the activity of the renin-angiotensin-aldosterone system. Beta-blockers can modify glomerular haemodynamics, because they reduce renin secretion, in addition to their actions on cardiac output and blood pressure [33]. In the above mentioned studies [29-31], changes in glomerular haemodynamics were not studied in relation to those of renin secretion.

Conversely, experimental studies to reduce glomerular capillary hypertension of diabetic rats with ACEI lead to prevention of albuminuria and glomerulosclerosis [34], but systolic blood pressure was lower on ACEI than on placebo. Similarly, we set-up a double-blind, placebo-controlled trial demonstrating prevention, or post-pone of diabetic nephropathy with enalapril in normotensive diabetic subjects with microalbuminuria [14]. However, blood pressure was reduced by enalapril compared to placebo, which made interpretation of this trial difficult, since reducing blood pressure reduces UAE in hypertensive subjects [35].

Thus, confusion rose from these two types of observations, because alterations in systemic blood pressure and in glomerular haemodynamics were not controlled simultaneously with changes in activity of the renin angiotensin system. Anderson et al demonstrated later on that ACEI efficacy to prevent albuminuria in diabetic rats was due to both hypotension and reduction of intra-glomerular capillary pressure [36]. In a double-blind, double-dummy, one year parallel trial comparing enalapril to hydrochlorothiazide (two drugs with similar hypotensive effects but symmetrical actions on angiotensin II production) to reduce UAE of normotensive insulin-dependent subjects with microalbuminuria, we demonstrated that reducing systemic blood pressure reduces UAE in the long-term only if the renin-angiotensin system effectiveness is simultaneously blocked [37].

3.2. Eligibility for antihypertensive treatment in incipient diabetic nephropathy

Should subjects with incipient diabetic nephropathy be assigned to antihypertensive treatment on the basis of UAE, or of blood pressure values ? Certainly on the basis of a persistent microalbuminuria, because definition of incipient diabetic nephropathy is based on this biological abnormality. Second, microalbuminuria is probably an early sign of, rather than a factor predictive for diabetic nephropathy [38]. In this connection, UAE >20 µg/min (or 30 mg/24h) is clearly abnormal: more than fifty per cent of healthy subjects excrete less than 5 mg/24h [39]. Also, GFR can start declining from the lowest range of microalbuminuria, as illustrated in figure 40-1. Finally, UAE reduction can be obtained independently of blood pressure reduction, as detailed below.

3.3. Evidence for a superiority of ACEIs over other available hypotensive drugs to reduce UAE in incipient diabetic nephropathy

Several studies indicated that microalbuminuria of normotensive type 1, insulin-dependent diabetic subjects could be reduced by ACEIs, while blood pressure was not modified significantly [15,40]. We reported in a short-term, double-blind study that small doses of ramipril can reduce microalbuminuria as effectively as hypotensive doses. This UAE reduction was obtained independently of blood pressure reduction, but it was related to the degree of ACE inhibition and to changes in filtration fraction [41]. Comparison of enalapril to hydrochlorothiazide to reduce microalbuminuria of normotensive type 1, insulin-dependent diabetic subjects lead to similar conclusions: both drugs were not different for their hypotensive effects, but only enalapril reduced microalbuminuria ; UAE changes were related to those of filtration fraction, not to those of blood pressure [37]. Thus, dose-response curves for the renal and the hypotensive effects of ACEIs may not be superimposable. A meta-regression analysis supports a preferential role for ACEIs to reduce UAE and to protect GFR of diabetic subjects [42]. The Melbourne Diabetic Nephropathy Study Group and a recent Italian study reported no important difference between the ACEI and the calcium-antagonist nifedipine in diabetic subjects with microalbuminuria [43, 44].

3.4. Long-term evolution of GFR in type 1, insulin-dependent diabetic subjects given ACEIs from incipient diabetic nephropathy

Certainly GFR preservation is the only clinically significant outcome for intervention studies in diabetic nephropathy. Microalbuminuria is a surrogate end-point. As outlined above, GFR is normal or still supra-normal during incipient diabetic nephropathy, and GFR reduction is minimal at time of clinical proteinuria onset (See Mogensen, Chapter 3). Also, clinical trials comparing captopril or enalapril to placebo or to metoprolol showed that GFR degradation was reduced by about 50% with ACEIs in type 1, insulin-dependent diabetic subjects with clinical proteinuria [45,46]. The clinical usefulness of ACEIs given from microalbuminuria stage was therefore questionable for type 1, insulin-dependent diabetic subjects with incipient nephropathy. Indeed, GFR evolution was not different between patients on captopril and those on placebo in 2 to 4 year clinical trials [15,26]. Only a marginal difference was found by our group in a one-year trial comparing enalapril to placebo [14]. In a recent two-year trial, Laffel et al reported that creatinine clearance was maintained by captopril compared to placebo in type 1, insulin-dependent diabetic normotensive patients with microalbuminuria [27], and this was confirmed in a recent combined analysis of the two multicenter trials performed with captopril versus placebo for two years [47]. The median GFR slope was -6.4 ml/min/1.73m^2/year in the placebo - treated patients. These data may must be interpreted with caution for methodological reasons, because GFR was estimated from creatinine clearances: in the American trial, baseline GFR values were markedly low (80 ml/min/1.73m^2); second, creatinine clearance can be altered by changes in tubular function provoked by renal vasodilator like ACEIs. However, we found a comparable GFR decline in a recent 4-year follow-up study comparing two treatment strategies with enalapril. Patients' GFR were estimated with the ^{125}I-Iodothalamate constant infusion technique. Those normotensive type 1, insulin-dependent diabetic patients with microalbuminuria given enalapril from microalbuminuria identification kept their GFR unchanged (including those with initial hyperfiltration), while those given enalapril only if they progressed to macroalbuminuria reduced their GFR by 0.62 ml/min/1.73m^2/month. At follow-up, 6 of the 11 patients assigned to late enalapril treatment displayed GFR values <100 ml/min/1.73m^2 (the lower limit of normal values) [48]. Taken together, these recent studies indicate that GFR degradation slope is nearly as high in patients with incipient as in patients with established nephropathy. These longitudinal results fit with the parabolic figure of the relationship between GFR and UAE shown above, and described firstly by Mogensen and Christensen in 1984 [11]. Thus, treatment with ACEIs in proteinuric type 1, insulin-dependent diabetic subjects may be too late to protect their GFR [45]. These results support the current recommendation that ACEIs must be given from microalbuminuria identification in normotensive type 1, insulin-dependent diabetic patients [49]. Recent study by Mathiesen [50] an extention of an earlier study [15] documents preservation of GFR by ACE-I.

3.5. Unanswered questions on the use of ACEIs for diabetic patients with microalbuminuria

First, the above-mentioned data deal with normotensive type 1, insulin-dependent diabetic patients with microalbuminuria. The specific value of ACEIs vs conventional antihypertensive treatment is not demonstrated for kidney function of patients with essential hypertension [51], and this condition can be associated with insulin-dependent diabetes sometimes.

Second, longer-term follow-up studies are required to ascertain if cardiovascular morbidity/mortality is reduced by early ACEIs treatment in these relatively young patients, in addition to the benefit obtained for kidney function.

Third, it not known which are the long-term side-effect attached to the use of ACEIs in young patients [52]. Pharmacovigilant studies are required in this respect.

Fourth, the promising data obtained in type 1, insulin-dependent diabetic patients cannot be applied to type 2, non-insulin-dependent diabetic patients. Only one study reported a benefit for kidney function of normotensive type 2, non-insulin-dependent diabetic patients with microalbuminuria attributable to enalapril compared to placebo [53,54]. However, the type 2, non-insulin-dependent diabetic patients in this study [53,54] were relatively young and thin compared to those commonly encountered in clinical practice. Although such patients are identifiable and may share renal prognosis similar to type 1, insulin-dependent diabetic patients [14], such results cannot be applied to the vast majority of type 2, non-insulin-dependent diabetic patients. Most of them are obese, with hypertension and mixed dyslipidaemia, and the prognostic value of microalbuminuria deals with cardiovascular events [55]. To date, no trial has established a clinical benefit from the preferential use of ACEIs in these patients.

Preventive treatment in normoalbuminuric patient would be interesting but requires long-term intervention [40].

ACKNOWLEDGMENT

We thank Mrs Line GODIVEAU for excellent secretarial assistance.

REFERENCES

1. Andersen AR, Christiansen JS, Andersen JK, Kreiner S, Deckert T. Diabetic nephropathy in type 1 (insulin-dependent) diabetes: an epidemiological study. Diabetologia 1983; 2: 496-501.
2. Mathiesen ER, Borch-Johnsen K, Jensen DV, Deckert T. Improved survival in patients with diabetic nephropathy. Diabetologia 1989; 32: 884-886.
3. Deckert T, Poulsen JE, Larsen M. Prognosis of diabetics with diabetes onset before the age of thirty-one. I- survival, causes of death and complications. Diabetologia 1978; 14: 363-370.
4. Keen H, Chlouverakis C. An immunoassay method for urinary albumin at low concentrations. Lancet 1963; ii: 913.
5. Miles DM, Mogensen CE, Gundersen HJG. Radioimmunoassay for urinary albumin using a single antibody. Scand J Clin Lab Invest 1970; 25: 5-11.
6. Benhamou PY, Halimi S, De Gaudemaris R, Boizel R, Pitiot M, Siche JP, Bachelot I, Mallion JM. Early disturbances of ambulatory blood pressure in normotensive type 1 diabetic patients with microalbuminuria. Diabetes Care 1992; 15: 1614-1619.
7. Hansen KW, Mau Pedersen M, Marshall SM, Christiansen JS, Mogensen CE. Circadian variation of blood pressure in patients with diabetic nephropathy. Diabetologia 1992; 35: 1074-1079.
8. Viberti RC, Hill RD, Jarret RJ, Argyropoulos A, Hahmud U, Keen M. Microalbuminuria as a predictor of clinical nephropathy in insulin dependent diabetes mellitus. Lancet 1982; i: 1430-1432.
9. Parving H-H, Oxenbøll B, Svendsen PAA, Christiansen JS, Andersen AR. Early detection of patients at risk of developing diabetic nephropathy. A longitudinal study of urinary albumin excretion. Acta Endocrinol (Copenh) 1982; 100: 550-555.
10. Mathiesen ER, Oxenbøll B, Johansen K, Svendsen PAA, Deckert T. Incipient nephropathy in type 1 (insulin-dependent) diabetes. Diabetologia 1984; 26: 406-410.
11. Mogensen CE, Christensen CK. Predicting diabetic nephropathy in insulin-dependent patients. N Engl J Med 1984; 311: 89-93.
12. Mogensen CE, Chachati A, Christensen CK, et al. Microalbuminuria: an early marker of renal involvement in diabetes. Uremia Invest 1985-86; 9: 85-95.
13. Feldt-Rasmussen B, Mathiesen ER, Jensen T, Lauritzen T, Deckert T. Effect of improved metabolic control on loss of kidney function in type i (insulin-dependent) diabetic patients: an update of the steno studies. Diabetologia 1991; 34: 164-170.
14. Marre M, Chatellier G, Leblanc H, Guyenne TT, Menard J, Passa P. Prevention of diabetic nephropathy with enalapril in normotensive diabetics with microalbuminuria. BMJ 1988; 297: 1092-1095.
15. Mathiesen ER, Hommel E, Giese J, Parving H-H. Efficacy of captopril in postponing nephropathy in normotensive insulin dependent diabetic patients with microalbuminuria. BMJ 1991; 303: 81-87.
16. Christensen CK, Krusell LR, Mogensen CE. Increased blood pressure in diabetes: essential hypertension or diabetic nephropathy? Scand J Clin Lab Invest 1987; 47: 363-370.
17. Berrut G, Hallab M, Bouhanick B, Chameau AM, Marre M, Fressinaud PH. Value of ambulatory blood pressure monitoring in type 1 (insulin-dependent) diabetic patients with incipient diabetic nephropathy. Am J Hypertens 1994; 7: 222-227.
18. Middeke M, Schrader J. Nocturnal blood pressure in normotensive subjects and those with while coat, primary, and secondary hypertension. BMJ 1994; 308: 630-632.
19. Starling EH. Physiological factors involved in the causation of dropsy. Lancet 1896; i: 1405.

20. Mathiesen ER, Rønn B, Jensen T, Storm B, Deckert T. The relationship between blood pressure and urinary albumin excretion in the development of microalbuminuria. Diabetes 1990; 39: 245-249.
21. Microalbuminuria Collaborative Study Group, United Kingdom. Risk factors for development of microalbuminuria in insulin-dependent diabetic patients: a cohort study. BMJ 1993; 306: 1235-1239.
22. Forsblom CM, Groop PH, Ekstrand A, Groop LC. Predictive value of microalbuminuria in insulin-dependent diabetes of long duration. BMJ 1992; 305: 1051-1053.
23. Krolewski AS, Laffel LM, Krolewski M, Quinn M, Warram JH. Glycosylated hemoglobin and the risk of microalbuminuria in patients with insulin-dependent diabetes mellitus. N Engl J Med 1995; 332: 1251-1255.
24. The Diabetes Control And Complications Trial Research Group. The effect of intensive treatment of diabetes on the development and progression of long-term complications in insulin-dependent diabetes mellitus. N Engl J Med 1993; 329: 977-986.
25. Feldt-Rasmussen B, Mathiesen ER, Deckert T. Effect of two years of strict metabolic control on progression of incipient nephropathy in insulin-dependent diabetes. Lancet 1986; ii: 1300-1304.
26. Viberti GC, Mogensen CE, Groop LC, Pauls JF, for The European Microalbuminuria Study Group. Effect of Captopril on progression to clinical proteinuria in patients with insulin-dependent diabetes mellitus and microalbuminuria. JAMA 1994; 271: 275-279.
27. Laffel LBM, Mc Gill JB, Gans DJ, on behalf of The North American Microalbuminuria Study Group. The beneficial effect of angiotensin converting enzyme inhibition with captopril on diabetic nephropathy in normotensive IDDM patients with microalbuminuria. Am J Med 1995; 99: 497-504.
28. Mogensen CE, Østerby R, Hansen KW, Damsgaard EM. Blood pressure elevation versus abnormal albuminuria in the genesis and prediction of renal disease in diabetes. Diabetes Care 1992; 15: 1192-1204.
29. Mogensen CE. Long-term antihypertensive treatment inhibiting progression of diabetic nephropathy. BMJ 1982; 285: 685-688.
30. Parving H-H, Andersen AR, Smidt UM, Svendsen PAA. Early aggressive antihypertensive treatment reduces the rate of decline in kidney function in diabetic nephropathy. Lancet 1983; i: 1175-1179.
31. Christensen CK, Mogensen CE. Effect of antihypertensive treatment on progression of incipient diabetic nephropathy. Hypertension 1985; 7: Suppl II: 109-113.
32. Brenner BM, Humes HD. Mechanisms of glomerular ultrafiltration. N Engl J Med 1977; 297: 148-154.
33. Keeton T, Campbell WB. The pharmacological alterations of renin release. Pharmacol Rev 1980; 32: 81-227.
34. Zatz R, Meyer TW, Rennke HG, Brenner BM. Predominance of hemodynamic rather than metabolic factors in the pathogenesis of diabetic glomerulopathy. Proc Natl Acad Sci USA 1985; 82: 5963-5967.
35. Parving H-H, Jensen HA, Mogensen CE, Evrin PE. Increased urinary albumin excretion rate in benign essential hypertension. Lancet 1974; i: 1190-1192.
36. Anderson S, Rennke HG, Garcia DL, Brenner BM. Short and long term effects of antihypertensive therapy in the diabetic rat. Kidney Int 1989; 36: 526-536.
37. Hallab M, Gallois Y, Chatellier G, Rohmer V, Fressinaud PH, Marre M. Comparison of reduction in microalbuminuria by enalapril and hydrochlorothiazide in normotensive patients with insulin dependent diabetes. BMJ 1993; 306: 175-182.
38. Mogensen CE. Prediction of clinical diabetic nephropathy in IDDM patients: alternatives to microalbuminuria? Diabetes 1990; 39: 761-767.
39. Marre M, Claudel JP, Ciret P, Luis N, Suarez L, Passa P. Laser immunonephelometry for routine quantification of urinary albumin excretion. Clin Chem 1987; 33: 209-213.
40. The EUCLID Study Group. Randomised placebo-controlled trial of lisinopril in normotensive patients with insulin-dependent diabetes and normoalbuminuria or microalbuminuria. Lancet 1997; 349: 1789-92.
41. Marre M, Hallab M, Billiard A, Le Jeune JJ, Bled F, Girault A, Fressinaud P. Small doses of ramipril to reduce microalbuminuria in diabetic patients with incipient nephropathy independently of blood pressure changes. J Cardiovasc Pharmacol 1991; 18: S165-S168.

42. Kasiske BL, Kalil RS, Ma JZ, Liao M, Keane WF. Effect of antihypertensive therapy on the kidney in patients with diabetes: a meta-regression analysis. Ann Intern Med 1993; 118: 129-138.
43. Melbourne Diabetic Nephropathy Study Group. Comparison between perindopril and nifedipine in hypertensive and normotensive diabetic patients with microalbuminuria. BMJ 1991; 302: 210-216.
44. Crepaldi G, Carta Q, Deferrari G, Mangili R, Navalesi R, Santeusanio F, Spalluto A, Vanasia A, Nosadini R, The Italian Microalbuminuria Study Group in IDDM. Effects of Lisinopril and nifedipine on the progression to overt albuminuria in IDDM patients with incipient nephropathy and normal blood pressure. Diabetes Care, Vol. 21 no. 1, Jan. 1998.
45. Björk S, Mulec H, Johnsen SA, Nyberg G, Aurell M. Renal protective effect of enalapril in diabetic nephropathy. BMJ 1992; 304: 339-343.
46. Lewis EJ, Hunsiker LG, Bain RP, Rohde RD, for The Collaborative Study Group. The effect of angiotensin-converting-enzyme inhibition on diabetic nephropathy. N Engl J Med 1993; 329: 1456-1462.
47. The Microalbuminuria Captopril Study Group. Captopril reduces the risk of nephropathy in IDDM patients with microalbuminuria. Diabetologia 1996; 39: 587-593.
48. Fabbri P, Bouhanick B, Freneau E, Vilayleck B, Berrut G, Fressinaud PH, Marre M. Comparison of two treatment strategies with angiotensin I converting enzyme inhibitors in normotensive IDDM patients with microalbuminuria (Abstract). Diabetes 1995; 44: suppl. 1: 24A.
49. American Diabetes Assocation. Diabetic Nephropathy. Diabetes Care, vol. 21, suppl. 1, jJan. 1998; 50-53.
50. Mathiesen ER, Hommel E, Hansen HP, Parving HH. Preservation of normal GFR with long term captopril treatment in normotensive IDDM patients with microalbuminuria. (Abstract A0546) J Am Soc Nephrol 1997; 8:115A
51. Erley CM, Haefele U, Heyne N, Braun N, Risler T. Microalbuminuria in essential hypertension; reduction by different antihypertensive drugs. Hypertension 1993; 21: 810-815.
52. Azizi M, Rousseau A, Ezan E, Guyene TT, Michelet S, Grognet JM, Lenfant M, Corvol P, Menard J. Acute angiotensin-converting enzyme inhibition increases the plasma level of the natural stem cell regulator N-acetyl-seryl-aspartyl-lysyl-proline. J Clin Invest 1996; 97: 839-844.
53. Ravid M, Savin H, Jutrin I, Bental T, Katz B, Lishner M. Long-term stabilizing effect of angiotensin converting enzyme inhibition on plasma creatinine and proteinuria in normotensive type II diabetic patients. Ann Intern Med 1993; 118: 577-581.
54. Ravid M, Lang R, Rachmani R, Lishner M. Long-term renoprotective effect of angiotensin-converting enzyme inhibition in non-insulin-dependent diabetes mellitus. A 7-year follow-up study. Arch Intern Med 1996; 156: 286-289.
55. Mogensen CE. Microalbuminuria predicts clinical proteinuria and early mortality in maturity-onset diabetes. N Engl J Med 1984; 310: 36-360.

41. CLINICAL TRIALS IN OVERT DIABETIC NEPHROPATHY.

Staffan Björck
Njurmottagningen, Sahlgrenska Sjukhuset, Göteborg, Sweden

There is accumulating data available regarding how overt diabetic nephropathy should be treated to arrest the progressive decline in renalfunction. Some interventions are controversial but improved metabolic control is getting increasing acceptance as a way to improve prognosis also during this stage. There is agreement on that antihypertensive treatment should be aggressive and metaanalyses indicate that ACE-inhibitors offers an advantage. In non-diabetic renal disease intensive antihypertensive treatment adds only little benefit[1]. In contrast to this, several studies have shown that aggressive antihypertensive treatment is probably the most important factor to determine the rate of decline in kidney function in diabetic nephropathy. There are no controlled studies with different target blood pressure in different groups such as in non diabetic renal disease [1]. The evidence that antihypertensive treatment can preserve renal function comes from studies showing a much reduced rate of renal disease progression after effective blood pressure control [2,3]. These studies compare the rate of decline in glomerular filtration rate during intervention with retrospective data which is not ideal since uncontrolled factors might influence the outcome. However, the effect of antihypertensive treatment is so profound that anyone that treats these patients observe that end-stage renal failure is postponed by antihypertensive treatment and that the disease runs an accelerated course during uncontrolled hypertension.

1. DIFFERENCES BETWEEN ANTIHYPERTENSIVE DRUGS.

It has been debated whether all antihypertensive drugs confer the same benefit to the kidneys in diabetic nephropathy. In early uncomplicated type 1 diabetes distinct changes have been found in renal function - see elsewhere in this book. The glomerular filtration rate is increased. The renal blood flow is increased to a smaller extent which result in an increased filtration fraction. These findings might indicate an increase in glomerular filtration pressure. The finding of this early disturbance in renal haemodynamics in a group of patients of which one third develops kidney disease has led to the hypothesis that these haemodynamic alterations are harmful to the kidneys. Since the renin-angiotensin system modulates renal pressures and flows, it has been speculated that angiotensin-converting enzyme inhibition can protect the kidneys by an effect independent of its effect on systemic blood pressure. This class of agents have been shown to increase renal blood flow and decrease filtration fraction while glomerular filtration rate usually remains unchanged which points to a reduction in glomerular pressure [4]. Many studies have tried to determine if there is a specific, blood-pressure independent renal protective effect of angiotensin converting enzyme (ACE)-inhibitors in diabetic nephropathy. The end-points in these studies have been the urinary excretion of proteins and the effect on the natural decrease in renal function. Only a few studies have been large enough or long enough to allow assessment of the effect on development of renal failure.

2. EFFECT ON PROTEINURIA

Reducing blood pressure by any measure leads to a reduction in the urinary excretion of proteins in patients with type 1 diabetes and nephropathy. Therefore, is it difficult to separate an effect of ACE-inhibitors from the non-specific effect of blood pressure reduction. In a short-term study, Taguma et al first showed that captopril treatment induced a reduction in proteinuria even though blood pressure was relatively unchanged [5]. This was an uncontrolled study in patients with concomitant diseases but a dissociation between the hypotensive and the antiproteinuric effect of ACE-inhibitors has also been shown by others [6,7].

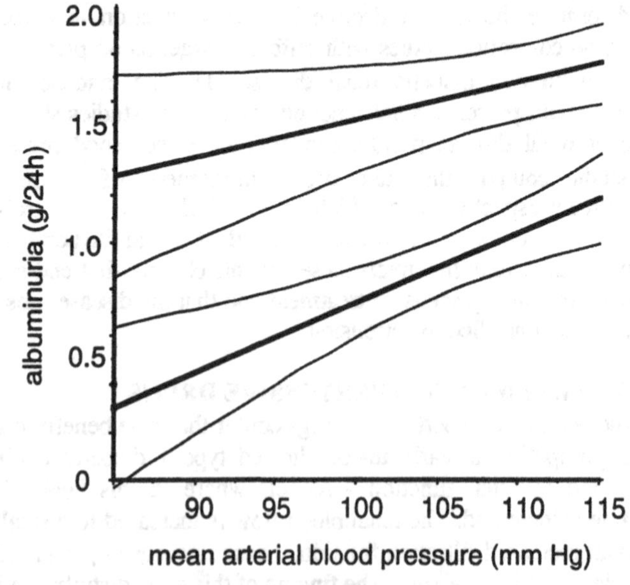

Figure 41-1. Regression lines with 95% confidence intervals for the relationship between supine mean arterial blood pressure and urinary albumin excretion in patients treated with metoprolol (top line) and enalapril (bottom line). Regression lines are based on 417 simultaneous measurements of blood pressure and 24 hour excretions of albumin in 36 patients.

Randomised controlled studies with other classes of antihypertensive drugs serving as controls have been performed with contradictory results. Calcium antagonists for example have been shown to decrease, to have no effect or to increase proteinuria [8-10]. ACE-inhibitors in these studies more consistently reduce proteinuria [10]. In comparisons with betablocking agents, both a superior and an equal antiproteinuric effect has been found [11,12]. Differences between studies regarding experimental design, concomitant treatment, level of blood pressure control and patient selection makes interpretation of results difficult. In two recent meta-regression analyses were concluded that ACE-inhibitors decrease proteinuria independently of changes in blood pressure while reductions in proteinuria with other antihypertensive agents could be explained by changes in blood pressure [13,14]. Non-dihydropyridine calcium antagonists might also confer a special benefit [13]. We have compared the antiproteinuric effect of enalapril and metoprolol on albuminuria in patients with type 1 diabetes and nephropathy [11]. We found that the antiproteinuric effect of enalapril was superior to that of metoprolol. During two years treatment, there was a continuous fall in albuminuria during enalapril treatment but not with metoprolol. The mean reduction in albuminuria was 63% during enalapril treatment while there was no change during metoprolol treatment. In this group of patients, the difference does not seem to be explained by differences in blood pressure.

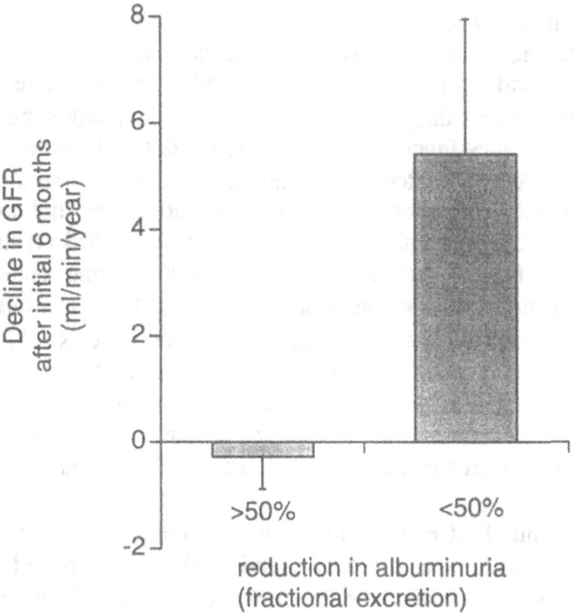

Figure 41-2. Subsequent decline in GFR in 15 patients with diabetic nephropathy observed during mean 4.4 years, divided into two groups depending on initial effect of ACE-inhibition on proteinuria [data from reference 15]

The blood pressure was similar in both groups. The large number of simultaneous determinations of urinary albumin excretion and blood pressure allows a further analysis of the relationship between blood-pressure and albuminuria (figure 41-1). Throughout the range of ordinary blood pressure levels, enalapril-treated patients excrete less albumin than metoprolol-treated patients. In our experience, the initial effect of ACE-inhibitors on proteinuria predicts the renal long-term prognosis [15] (Figure 41-2).

3. LONG-TERM EFFECT ON RENAL FUNCTION.

A few studies have investigated the long-term effect on renal function of ACE-inhibitors. In 1986 we reported on a reduction in the rate of decline in kidney function in captopril-treated patients with diabetic nephropathy despite a rather small effect on treatment resistant hypertension [4]. The study was uncontrolled however, and the study group was small. In our two year study of the effect enalapril or metoprolol we have also investigated the glomerular filtration rate [16]. There was a slower fall rate in glomerular filtration rate in patients treated with enalapril than in those with metoprolol. The study was stopped after two years due to the difference between the groups but the enalapril treated patients have been followed for four years. We have found a stabilisation of renal function during the last years [16]. The main fall in glomerular filtration rate that occurred during the first six months was 7.5±9.8 ml/min/1.73m2. During the following three and a half years the fall was only 0.3±3.9 ml/min/year. The metoprolol treated patients had a decline in renal function of 5.6±5.9 ml/min/year.

Contrary to this Parving et al, in two separate studies on captopril and other antihypertensive agents found that both treatments had a similar effect on proteinuria and rate of decline in kidney function [2,17]. In a carefully controlled study, the rate of decline in kidney function was not different during treatment with a calcium antagonist or an ACE-inhibitor [8]. In this one year study, the authors found a rapid decline in ACE-inhibitor treated patients during the first month followed by a later stabilisation of renal function. Ferder et al, studied creatinine clearance in patients with type 1 diabetes and nephropathy during one year treatment. They found that the renal function remained stable and that albuminuria decreased in the enalapril treated but not in the nifedipine treated patients [18]. The longest reported treatment time is reported by Ravid et al who found that five years treatment of patients with type 2 diabetes and microalbuminuria resulted in unchanged renal function and proteinuria in contrast to the non-ACE-inhibitor treated control group that exhibited a rise in albuminuria and a fall in renal function measured as serum-creatinine 19].

The largest comparison of ACE inhibitors with conventional treatment have been done in 409 patients with type 1 diabetes and nephropathy treated with captopril or placebo [20]. The main outcome measure was doubling of the base-line serum creatinine concentration. It was found that the reduction in the risk of doubling of serum creatinine was 48% in patients treated with a ACE-inhibitor. The groups were slightly different in blood pressure control but when this was statistically corrected for, the risk reduction was still 43%. The large number of patients, enabled assessment of the effect on the end-points death dialysis and transplantation. A 46% risk reduction was found.

In conclusion, ACE inhibitors seem to have an antiproteinuric effect independent of the effect on systemic blood pressure. Clinical studies with the aim to determine if the decline in kidney function can be arrested more effectively with ACE-inhibitors show that so far no class of agents has been shown to be more effective than ACE inhibitors. It has recently been recommended that treatment with these agents should be started even in normotensive patients when microalbuminuria has developed [21].

3.1. Effects of improved blood glucose control.

Intensified treatment with improved blood glucose control has been shown to postpone the onset of microalbuminuria and probably also delay the transition from incipient nephropathy to overt diabetic nephropathy although the latter has been questioned [21,22]. When overt diabetic nephropathy is established, it has been claimed that the progressive course is not influenced by better blood glucose control [23]. From a logical standpoint, this is unlikely. At any stage there should be functioning nephrons and it is difficult to explain why these, at this point should develop resistance to the harmful effects of elevated blood glucose. We have studied a group of patients with overt diabetic nephropathy followed for eight years. In this group of 158 patients, both blood pressure and blood glucose control as determined by mean HbA1c levels turned out to be significantly correlated to decline in renal function ($r=-0.29$ and $r=-0.39$ respectively, $p<0.001$). The same relationship has recently been found in other observational studies during effective blood pressure control [24-26].

3.2 Effect of lipid lowering treatment.

As discussed above there is a rationale for the use of proteinuria as a surrogate end-point for long-term renal effects. In addition, in most nephropathies there is a relationship between proteinuria and renal long-term prognosis irrespective of type of renal disease [27]. Interventions that lower proteinuria universally improve prognosis. From a logical point of view, it does not necessarily have to be that way [28]. If proteinuria merely represents an increased passage of macromolecules over the capillary wall - treatment could be targeted at reduction of this traffic by reduction of proteinuria, for instance by antihypertensive treatment or ACE-inhibition, or at the composition of macromolecules by treatment of lipid abnormalities. Therefore, short-term effects on proteinuria of lipid lowering drugs might be expected not to predict long-term effects on glomerular filtration rate. There are some short-term studies on the effect of statins on renal function in diabetic nephropathy. They usually show no effect on proteinuria or renal function [29,30]. A two years study of lovastatin or placebo showed stable renal function in simvastatin treated patients only but the difference between groups was non-significant [31]. Therefore, we have at present to rely on retrospective data of an association between lipid abnormalities and renal prognosis as indicative of also an intervention effect. In several recent long-term studies, there is a significant correlation between hypercholesterolemia and decline rate in GFR [25,26,28,32]. The demonstration of beneficial vascular effects of increasingly lower cholesterol levels suggest that it will be unethical to have untreated control groups in studies on the renal effects of lipid reduction which will leave us for the future with uncontrolled observational studies only. The much increased cardiovascular risk in these patients however, shows that antihyperlipidemic treatment should be aggressive in these patients, with a beneficial renal effect as a possible additional benefit [33].

4. PROBLEMS RELATED TO STUDIES OF RENAL EFFECTS.

Similar blood pressure levels in study groups are essential for conclusions due to the influence of the blood pressure level both on the proteinuria and on the rate of deterioration in kidney function. Comparisons between different drugs regarding their renal effects are frequently confounded by the difficulty to achieve a similar blood pressure control in the different groups. ACE-inhibitors are often more efficient in reducing blood pressure than other drugs and differences in blood pressure have to be corrected statistically. This makes resultsmore unreliable in small samples. In larger patient samples such calculations become more accurate [20]. In clinical studies, blood pressure determinations are usually done in the supine position in the morning, a few hours after the intake of the medication. The representativity of such isolated measurements may be questioned due to the variability in blood pressure and since differences in duration of action of different drugs may vary. The effects on standing and on supine blood pressure may also differ between drugs. We found that metoprolol was more effective than enalapril in reducing standing blood pressure and we therefore used the mean of supine and standing blood pressure in our evaluation [11]. Twenty-four-hour measurements of blood pressure will probably add to the precision of conclusions. In diabetic nephropathy there is a blunted nocturnal decline in blood pressure. It is largely unknown how different classes of agent affects this blood pressure pattern in overt diabetic nephropathy. We have found a relationship between extracellular volume and lack of decline in nocturnal blood pressure [34].

Proteinuria or albuminuria is frequently used as a measure of the renal effects of antihypertensive drugs. However, changes in proteinuria does not only represent an effect on glomerular function and integrity. It is possible that different antihypertensive agents have different effects on the tubular handling of proteins [9].

Methods to determine renal function differ greatly between studies. Serum creatinine or creatinine clearances are frequently used. Creatinine clearance has reduced accuracy in diabetic nephropathy due to the tubular secretion of creatinine. In a study in patients with overt diabetic nephropathy, creatinine clearance overestimated glomerular filtration rate determined as the clearance of 51CrEDTA with 70% [35]. It is not known whether blood pressure reduction and different drugs can affect this secretion.

In diabetic nephropathy, the effect of interventions may be delayed and the course over many years thus not linear. The use of slopes of change in renal function over time based on linear regression calculations therefore have been questioned. A new technique was recently used by Lewis et al [20]. They used doubling of serum creatinine as endpoint. In their study, there was an approximately 30% cumulative incidence of doubling of baseline serum-creatinine after four years. More recently, in a Danish group of patients recruited more than 16 years ago, the cumulative doubling of baseline serum creatinine was less than 30% after ten years observation. This indicates that doubling of serum creatinine might be a too insensitive method to be used as a marker for renal function deterioration when prognosis is improving unless a selection is done of patients with poorer prognosis. However, the use of doubling of serum creatinine overcomes the problem of linearity in change of renal function over time. This method allows survival statistics to be applied for influence of covariates on the renal outcome. In figure 41-3 is shown an example of a similar method for the analysis of impact of blood pressure on renal prognosis.

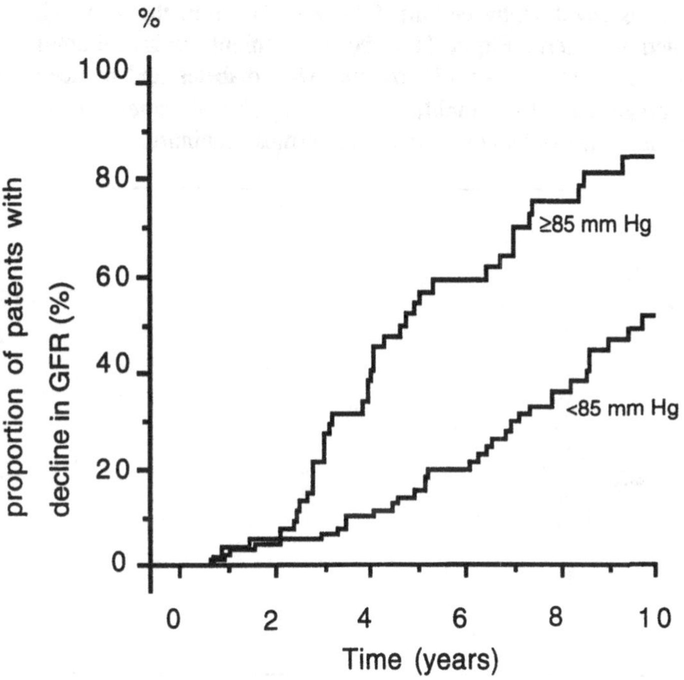

Figure 41-3. 158 patients with type 1 diabetes and nephropathy were observed for mean eight years. The renal end-point was chosen as the loss of 40% from the initial glomerular filtration rate. Patients with diastolic blood pressure <85 mm Hg (upper line) and *85 mm Hg (lower line) were compared. (n=158). Log rank (mantel-Cox) test for difference between groups, chi-square 20.2, $p<0.001$. [data from reference 37].

The use of diuretics has varied markedly between studies. It has been shown that the antiproteinuric effect of ACE-inhibitors is highly dependent on sodium balance and that the activity in the renin-angiotensin system determines the renal haemodynamic response to ACE-inhibitors [36]. The largest reduction in proteinuria was found in a study using high dose diuretic treatment [11].

The follow-up time has to be extensive since the effect of intervention may be delayed [2,11]. Many studies base their conclusions on studies over only weeks or months. In the study by Ravid over 5 years, a distinct separation of the enalapril and the placebo-treated group appeared during the last years [19].

Interest in studies of patients with diabetic nephropathy came into focus when it was demonstrated that blood pressure reduction led to a substantial effect on renal function deterioration and that the poor outlook could be altered [2,3]. At that time the decline rate was 10 to 15 ml/min/year and it was possible to detect effects of intervention in 6 to 14 patients. A problem with future studies is the much improved prognosis necessitating very large studies at great costs. In our experience, many patients also with overt nephropathy and reduced renal function enter a stable phase during intervention making the necessary sample size for randomised comparisons even larger. The majority of our patients, during treatment, get albuminuria below what is traditionally classified as overt nephropathy although they have earlier fulfilled all criteria. Figure 41-4 shows overnight urinary albumin excretion in a cross-sectional analysis of 176 patients with diabetes and reduced renal function (serum-creatinine ≥135 mol/litre). The majority of patients have albuminuria below 200 mol/litre and many patients are normoalbuminuric.

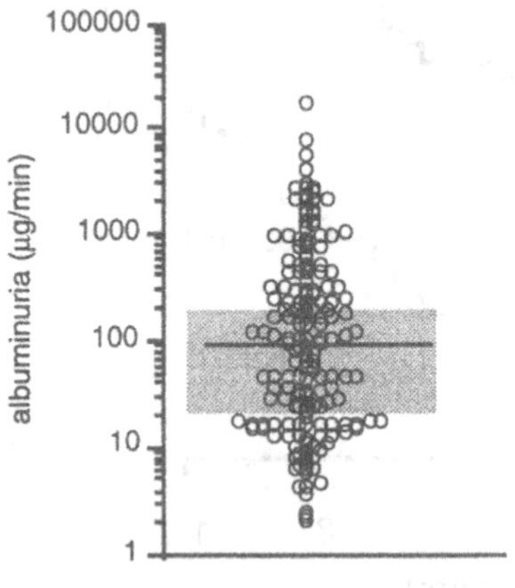

Figure 41-4. Overnight urinary albumin excretion in 176 patients with diabetes and reduced renal function (serum-creatinine ≥135 µmol/litre) Shaded area indicate microalbuminuric range. Geometric mean value is indicated by line. (Björck S et al, unpublished observation.)

In a more carefully controlled population of patients with type 1 diabetes and overt nephropathy observed during eight years, 53% of 158 patients had albuminuria below 200 g/min in overnight urinary samples [37].

Thus, the prognosis have improved very much which will lead to difficulties in getting samples large enough for controlled trials of treatment strategies. Therefore, it is increasingly likely that we have to rely on data generated besides the main outcome measures or on observational data. From several such studies can be concluded that glycemic control, hyperlipidemia and hypertension now must be considered as established progression promoters and that ACE inhibitors are first line agents in diabetich nephropathy provided that diuretic treatment is used according to the clinical situation. Protein intake and smoking might be added to this list of progression promotors.

REFERENCES

1 Klahr S, Levey AS, Beck GJ, Caggiula AW, Hunsicker L, Kusek JW, Striker G. The effect of dietary protein restriction and blood pressure control on the progression of chronic renal disease. N Engl J Med 1993;330: 877-874.

2 Parving H-H, Andersen AR, Smidt UM, Hommel E, Mathiesen ER, Svendsen PA. Effect of antihypertensive treatment on kidney function in diabetic nephropathy. Br Med J 294: 1443-1447, 1987.

3 Mogensen CE. Progression of nephropathy in long-term diabetics with proteinuria and effect of initial anti-hypertensive treatment. Scand J Clin Lab Invest 1976; 36: 383-388.

4 Björck S, Nyberg G, Mulec H, Granerus G, Herlitz H, Aurell M:Beneficial effects of anigiotensin converting enzyme inhibition on renal function in patients with diabetic nephropathy. Br Med J 1986; 293:467-470, .

5 Taguma Y , Kitamoto Y, Futaki G, Ueda H, Monma H, Ishizaki M, Takahashi H, Sekino H, Sasaki Y: Effect of captopril on heavy proteinuria in azotemic diabetics. N Engl J Med 1985, 313: 1617-1620.

6 Rudberg S, Aperia A, Freyschuss U, Persson B. Enalapril reduces microalbuminuria in young normotensive type 1 (insulin-dependent) diabetic patients irrespective of its hypotensive effect. Diabetologia 1990; 33: 470-476.

7 Elving LD, Wetzels JFM, de Nobel E, Hoitsma AJ, Berden JHM. Captopril acutely lowers albuminuria in normotensive patients with diabetic nephropathy. Am J Kidney Dis 1992; 20: 559-563.

8 Bakris GL, Barnhill BW, Sadler R. Treatment of arterial hypertension in diabetic humans: importance of therapeutic selection, Kidney Int 1992; 41: 912-919.

9 Holdaas H, Hartmann A, Lien MG, Nilsen L, Jervell J, Fachald P, Endresen L, Dj seland O, Berg KJ. Contrasting effects of lisinopril and nifedipine on albuminuria and tubular transport functions in insulin dependent diabetics with nephropathy. J Int Med 1991; 229: 163-170.

10 Gansevoort RT, Apperloo AJ, Heeg JE, De Jong PE, De Zeeuw D. The antiproteinuric effect of antihypertensive agents in diabetic nephropathy. Arch Int Med 1992; 152: 2137-2138.

11 Björck S, Mulec H, Johnsen SA, Nordén G, Aurell M. Renal protective effect of enalapril in diabetic nephropathy. BMJ 1992; 304: 339-343.

12 Stornello M, Valvo EV, Scapellato L. Comparative effects of enalapril, atenolol and chlorothalidone on blood pressure and kidney function of diabetic patients affected by arterial hypertension and persistent proteinuria. Nephron 1991; 58: 52-57.

13 Maki DD, Ma JZ, Louis TA, Kasiske BL. Long-term of antihypertensive agents on proteinuria and renal function 1995;155: 1073-1080.

14 Weidmann P, Schneider M, Böhlen L. Therapeutic efficacy of different antihypertensive drugs in human diabetic nephropathy: an updated metaanalysis. Nephrol Dial Transplant 1995;10(suppl 9): 39-45.

15 Mulec H, Johnsén S-A, Carlström J, Björck S. Intial decrease in proteinuria after institution of ACE inhibitor treatment predicts long-term prognosis for kidney function in overt diabet neph. san antonio. J Am Soc Nephrol 1997; 8: 116A.

16 Mulec H, Johnsen S-A, Björck S. Long-term enalapril treatment in diabetic nephropathy. Kidney Int 1994; 45 (suppl 45): S-141-S-144. .

17 Parving H-H, Hommel E, Smidt UM. Protection of kidney function and decrease in albuminuria by captopril in insulin dependent diabetics with nephropathy. Br Med J 1988; 297: 1086-1091.

18 Ferder L Daccordi H, Panzalis M, Inserra F. Angiotensin converting enzyme inhibitors versus calcium antagonists in the treatment of diabetic hypertensive patients. Hypertension 1992; 19 (suppl. 2): II-237-II-242.

19 Ravid M, Savin H, Jutrin I, Bental T, Katz B, Lishner M. Long-term stabilizing effect of angiotensin-converting enzyme inhibition on plasma creatinine and on proteinuria in normotensive type II diabetic patients. Ann Int Med 1993; 118:577-581.

20 Lewis EJ, Hunsicker LG, Bain RP, Rohde RD. The effect of angiotensin converting enzyme inhibition on diabetic nephropathy. N Engl J Med 1993; 329: 1456-1462

21 Mogensen CE, Keane WF, Bennet PH, Jerums G, Parving H-H, Passa P, Steffes MW, Striker GE, Viberti GC. Prevention of diabetic renal disease with special reference to microalbuminuria. Lancet 1995; 346: 1080-4.

22 The Diabetes Control and Complications Trial Research Group: The effect of intensive treatment of diabetes on the development and progression of long-term complications in insulin-dependent diabetes mellitus. N Engl J Med 1993; 329: 977-86.

23 Microalbuminuria collaborative study group: Intensive therapy and progression to clinical albuminuria in patients with insulin dependent diabetes mellitus and microalbuminuria. BMJ 1995; 311: 973-7.

24 Krolewski AS, LMB Lafel, Krolewski M, Quinn M and Warram JH. Glycosylated haemoglobin and the risk of microalbuminuria in patients with insulin-dependent diabetes mellitus. N Engl J Med 1995; 332: 1251-5.

25 H-H, Rossing P, Hommel H, Smidt UM. Angiotensin converting enzyme inhibition in diabetic nephropathy: Ten years experience. Am J Kidney Dis 1995; 26: 99-107.

26 Breyer JA, Bain RP, Evans JK, Nahman NS, Lewis E, Cooper M, McGill J, Berl T, and the collaborative study group: Predictors of renal insufficiency in patients with insulin-dependent diabetes and overt diabetic nephropathy. Kidney Int 1996; 50: 1651-1658.

27 Gerstoft J, Balslov JT, Brahm M, Brun C, J rgensen F, J rgensen HE, Larsen M, Larsen S, Lorenzen I, Lober M, Thomsen AC. Prognosis in glomerulonephritis. II. Regression analysis of prognostic factors affecting the course of renal function and the mortality in 395 patients. Calculation of a prognostic model. Report from a Copenhagen study group of renal diseases. Acta Med Scand 1986; 219: 179-187.

28 Mulec H, Johnsen SA, Björck S. Cholesterol - A renal risk factor in diabetic nephropathy? Am J Kidney Disease 1993; 22: 196-201.

29 Hommel E, Andersen P, Gal M-A, Nielsen F, Jensen B, Rossing P, Dyerberg J, Parving H-H. Plasma lipoproteins and renal function during simvastatin treatment in diabetic nephropathy. Diabetologia 1992; 35: 447-451.

30 Nielsen S, Schmitz O, Moller N, Porksen N, Klausen IC, Alberti KG, 0Mogensen CE. Renal function and insulin sensitivity during simvastatin treatment in type 2 (non-insulin-dependent) diabetic patients with microalbuminuria.Diabetologia 1993; 36(10): 1079-86

31 Lam KSL, Cheng IKP, Janus ED, Pang RWC. Cholesterol-lowering therapy may retard the progression of diabetic nephropathy. Diabetologia 1995; 38: 604-609.

32 Ravid M, Neuman L, Lishner M. Plasma lipids and the progression of nephropathy in diabetes mellitus type II: Effect of ACE inhibitors. Kidney Int 1995; 47: 907-910.

33 Pyorala K, Pedersen TR, Kjekshus J, Faergeman O, Olsson AG, 0Thorgeirsson G. Cholesterol lowering with simvastatin improves prognosis of diabetic patients with coronary heart disease. A subgroup analysis of the Scandinavian Simvastatin Survival Study (4S) :Diabetes Care 1997; 20: 614-20

34 Mulec H, Blohmé G, Kullenberg K, Nyberg G, Björck S. Latent overhydration and nocturnal hypertension in diabetic nephropathy. Diabetologia 1995; 38: 216-220.

35 Nordén G, Björck S, Granérus G, Nyberg G: Renal function estimation in diabetic nephropathy - evaluation of five methods. Transplantation proceedings 1986; 18: 1645-1646.

36 Heeg JE, De Jong PE, van der Hem GK, de Zeeuw D. Efficacy and variability of the antiproteinuric effect of ACE inhibition by lisinopril. Kidney Int 1989; 36: 272-279.

37 Mulec H, Blohmé G, Grände B, Björck S. The Effect of Metabolic Control on Rate of Decline in Renal Function in Insulin Dependent Diabetes Mellitus with Overt Diabetic Nephropathy. Nephrol Dial Transplant in press.

42. ANTIHYPERTENSIVE TREATMENT IN NIDDM, WITH SPECIAL REFERENCE TO ABNORMAL ALBUMINURIA

Mark E Cooper, MB BS PhD FRACP
Paul G McNally, MD MRCP
Department of Medicine, University of Melbourne, Austin & Repatriation Medical Centre (Repatriation Campus), West Heidelberg Australia, and Leicester Royal Infirmary NHS Trust, Leicester, United Kingdom

The deleterious effects of systemic blood pressure on glomerular structure were reported more than twenty years ago in a patient with NIDDM and unilateral renal artery stenosis, in which characteristic nodular diabetic glomerulosclerosis was present in the non-ischaemic kidney only [1]. To date the impact of antihypertensive therapy on renal injury in NIDDM has received less attention than in IDDM. This is despite the cumulative incidence of persistent proteinuria and microalbuminuria in NIDDM subjects being comparable in frequency to IDDM subjects of similar duration [2, 3]. The clinical relevance of these figures is reflected by statistics which now show that over 50% of patients entering renal replacement programs have NIDDM [4-7]. Furthermore, in NIDDM the relationship between nephropathy and hypertension is more complex than in IDDM, since hypertension is not necessarily linked to the presence of renal disease, and often precedes the diagnosis of diabetes.

This review focuses on the role of antihypertensive agents in NIDDM subjects with abnormal albuminuria (microalbuminuria and macroalbuminuria), the significance of albuminuria in NIDDM and the consequences of treatment with these agents.

1. THE USE OF ANTIHYPERTENSIVE AGENTS IN NIDDM SUBJECTS WITH ESTABLISHED DIABETIC NEPHROPATHY (TABLE 42-1)

The impact of angiotensin converting enzyme inhibitors (ACEI), calcium channel blockers (CCB) and conventional antihypertensive agents on renal function has been evaluated in both normotensive and hypertensive NIDDM subjects with persistent proteinuria and variable degrees of renal impairment [8-26]. Administration of low dose enalapril (5 mg/day) for 6-12 months to normotensive subjects with persistent

Table 42-1. The effect of antihypertensive agents on albuminuria, renal function and blood pressure in hypertensive NIDDM subjects with established nephropathy.

Agent	Duration	n	AER (%)*	GFR	BP	Reference
Captopril	6 months	12	→	→	↓	Valvo et al [17]
Captopril (C) Nicardipine (N) C&N	4 weeks	12	↓(-48) ↓(-61) ↓(-75)	→ → →	↓ ↓ ↓	Stornello et al [10]
Enalapril Chlorthalidone Atenolol Placebo	6 weeks	12	↓(-37) → ↓ →	→ → → →	↓ ↓ ↓ →	Stornello et al [12]
Captopril	6 months	9	↓(-62)	→	↓	Stornello et al [9]
Diltiazem Lisinopril	18 weeks	8	↓(-38) ↓(-43)	→ →	↓ ↓	Bakris [15]
Nifedipine Diltiazem	6 weeks	14	↑(+89) ↓(-52)	↓ →	↓ ↓	Demarie and Bakris [16]
Lisinopril Diltiazem Frus & Atenolol	18 months	10 10 10	↓(-42) ↓(-45) ↓	→ → ↓	↓ ↓ ↓	Slataper et al [24]
Lisinopril Atenolol	36 months	17 19	↓(-55) ↓(-15)	↓ ↓	↓ ↓	Nielsen et al [18]
Ramipril Nitrendipine	6 months	19 19	↓(-28) →	→ →	↓ ↓	Fogari et al [20]
Enalapril Nifendipine	12 months	18 12	↓(-87) →	→ →	↓ ↓	Ferder et al [21]
Enalapril Nifedipine	52 weeks	7 10	↓(-71) →	→ →	↓ ↓	Chan et al [19]
Captopril Isaradipine	6 months	15 16	↓(-30) ↑(+50)	→ →	↓ ↓	Guasch et al [26]
Captopril Hydralazine	18 months	24 18	↓(-27) →	→ →	↓ ↓	Liou et al [23]
Lisinopril (L) Verapamil (V) L+V G+H	12 months	8 8 8 6	↓(-59) ↓(-50) ↓(-78) →	↓ ↓ ↓ ↓	↓ ↓ ↓ ↓	Bakris et al [22]
Captopril Nifedipine	6 months	10 10	↓(-50) →(+18)	↓ →	↓ ↓	Romero et al [25]
Verapamil (V) Atenolol	>4 years	18 16	↓(-60) ↓(-20)	↓ ↓↓	↓ ↓	Bakris et al [14]
Lisinopril (L) Atenolol V or Diltiazem	5 years	18 16 16	↓(-25) → ↓(-18)	↓ ↓↓ ↓	↓ ↓ ↓	Bakris et a l [13]

AER, Albumin excretion rate. GFR, glomerular filtration rate. BP, Blood pressure. Frus, Frusemide. G+H, Guanfacine + Hydrochlorothiazide. * In some of these studies proteinuria rather than AER was measured.

proteinuria reduced albuminuria without affecting systemic or renal haemodynamics [8, 11]. Similarly, in hypertensive NIDDM subjects with persistent proteinuria studied for periods of up to 6 months, ACEI [9, 15] and certain CCB [10, 15, 16] reduced albuminuria. Comparable responses were also obtained with the beta-blocker, atenolol, but not with the thiazide diuretic, chlorthalidone, despite similar reduction in blood pressure [12]. However, administration of captopril to NIDDM subjects with moderate renal impairment for up to 6 months failed to alter albuminuria or renal haemodynamics, despite satisfactory blood pressure control [17]. Parving's group has reported a disparity in effects on albuminuria and renal function [18]. Whereas lisinopril was more effective than atenolol in reducing albuminuria, both agents were similar in efficacy in terms of rate of decline in GFR. A number of recent studies have confirmed that ACE inhibitors are superior to other antihypertensive agents including the dihydropyridine CCB including nifedipine [19, 21, 25] and nitrendipine [20] as well as the vasodilator, hydralazine [23], in reducing albuminuria in hypertensive NIDDM subjects with macroproteinuria.

There have been significant differences in the effect on albuminuria obtained with various CCB, which has been attributed by Bakris and coworkers to the particular class of CCB [15, 16, 22, 24]. Bakris [15] initially demonstrated in hypertensive, nephrotic NIDDM subjects that diltiazem, a benzothiazepine CCB, had a comparable response to lisinopril in decreasing albuminuria. This author has also reported an anti-proteinuric effect with the CCB, verapamil [22]. In contrast, nifedipine, a dihydropyridine CCB, given for 6 weeks to 14 hypertensive NIDDM patients with baseline renal impairment, precipitated an increase in albuminuria and a deterioration in renal function, despite equivalent blood pressure reduction to diltiazem [16]. A similar lack of efficacy of the dihydropyridine class of CCB has been reported by other groups [19-21]. In a recent study in African American NIDDM subjects with hypertension and macroproteinuria, isradipine was associated with an increase in proteinuria whereas captopril reduced proteinuria [26].

Slataper et al have reported in a randomized parallel group study comparing diltiazem, lisinopril and conventional therapy (atenolol and frusemide) in hypertensive NIDDM subjects with marked albuminuria (> 2.5 g/24 hours) and renal insufficiency (creatinine clearance < 70 ml/min/1.73 m2) [24] that after 18 months of therapy the rate of decline of glomerular filtration rate was attenuated with either diltiazem or lisinopril when compared to the conventional therapy group despite comparable blood pressure reduction [24]. The beneficial changes on glomerular filtration rate were paralleled by changes in albuminuria with significant reductions in the diltiazem and lisinopril groups, but no change in the conventionally treated group.

More recently, Bakris et al have reported the findings of 2 studies in hypertensive NIDDM subjects with macroproteinuria followed for over 4 years [13, 14]. In both studies, the beta blocker atenolol was associated with a more rapid decline in GFR and less efficacy in terms of reduction in albuminuria than the non-dihydropyridine CCBs, verapamil and diltiazem [13, 14] or the ACE inhibitor, lisinopril [14].

table 42-2. The effect of antihypertensive agents on albuminuria, renal function and blood pressure in NIDDM with normo- and microalbuminuria

Patients	Agent	Duration of study	n	Δ in AER (%)	Δ in GFR	Δ in BP	Reference
Micro HT	Indapamide	36 mths	10	↓(-64)	→	↓	Gamardella et al [30]
Normo HT	Captopril	36 mths	25	→	→	↓	Lacourcière et al [31
	M or HCTZ		28	→	→	↓	
Micro HT	Captopril		9	↓(-65)	→	↓	
	M or HCTZ		12	→	→	↓	
Normo HT	Enalapril (E)	12 mths	18	→	→	↓	Chan et al [19]
	Nifidipine (N)		24	→	→	↓	
Micro HT	Enalapril		16	↓(-70)	→	↓	
	Nifidipine		15	→	→	↓	
Micro HT+NT	Captopril	12 wks	9	↓(-21)	N/D	↓	Flack et al [28]
	Indapamide		9	↓(-27)	N/D	↓	
Micro HT+NT	Ramipril (R)	6 mths	54	↓(-27)	N/D	↓	Trevisan et al [35]
	Placebo		54	↓(+28)	N/D	→	
Micro HT	E+N	48 mths	11	↓(-42)	→	↓	Sano et al [33]
	Nifidipine		13	↑(+29)	→	↓	
Micro NT	Enalapril		12	↓(-47)	→	↓	
	Untreated		12	→	→	→	
Normo HT	Nicardipine	4 wks	6	→	→	↓	Baba et al [38]
Micro HT	Nicardipine	4 wks	6	↓(-29)	→	↓	
Micro NT	Nifedipine	12 mths	13	→	→	→	MDNSG [32]
	Perindopril		11	→	→	→	
Micro HT	Enalapril	12 mths	8	↓(-28)	↑	↓	Ruggenenti et al [34]
	Nitrendipine		8	↓(-17)	↑	↓	
Micro HT	Lisinopril	12 mths	156	↓(-37)	→	↓	Agardh et al [37]
	Nifedipine		158	→	→	↓	
Micro HT	Cilazipril	3 yrs	9	↓(-27)	↓	↓	Velussi et al [36]
	Amlodipine		9	↓(-31)	↓	↓	
Micro HT	Enalapril	12 mths	23	↓(-16)	→	↓	Fogari et al [40]
	Amlodipine		22	↓(-18)	↑	↓	
Micro HT	Nivaldipine	6 mths	8	↓(-40)	N/D	↓	Sumida et al [41]
Micro HT	Quinapril	8 wks	10	↓(-50)	N/D	↓	Dominguez et al [27]
Micro HT	R ± Felodipine	12 mths	46	→	→	↓	Schnack et al [39]
	A ± HCTZ		45	↑	↓	↓	
Micro NT	Captopril	6 mths	13	↓(-36)	→	↓	Romero et al [42]
	Untreated		13	→	→	→	
Micro NT	Enalapril	5 yrs	49	→	→	→	Ravid et al [44]
	Placebo		45	↑(+152)	↓	→	
Micro NT	Enalapril	5 yrs	52	↓(-64)	→	→	Ahmad et al [45]
	Placebo		51	↑(+60)	→	→	

2. THE USE OF ANTIHYPERTENSIVE AGENTS IN HYPERTENSIVE NIDDM WITH NORMOALBUMINURIA AND MICROALBUMINURIA (TABLE 42-2).

The use of antihypertensive therapy in NIDDM subjects with hypertension and microalbuminuria has been evaluated by an increasing number of investigators over the last decade [19, 27-41]. Gambardella and coworkers [30] showed that indapamide 2.5 mg daily did not alter albuminuria or glomerular filtration rate over a 24 month period in hypertensive, normoalbuminuric patients despite a significant reduction in blood pressure. In contrast, in the microalbuminuric patients indapamide reduced albuminuria after 6 months and this effect was sustained at 36 months [29, 30]. A double blind study compared captopril with conventional therapy (metoprolol and hydrochlorothiazide) in normoalbuminuric and microalbuminuric hypertensive NIDDM subjects over a 3 year period [31]. Both regimens reduced blood pressure without altering albuminuria in the normoalbuminuric NIDDM subjects. However, their findings in hypertensive NIDDM patients with microalbuminuria indicated that despite a comparable reduction in blood pressure, only the ACEI induced a persistent decline in albuminuria during the 36 months of therapy. Although these findings suggested that the ACEI conferred a beneficial renoprotective effect long-term, these data are potentially biased by the fact that the conventionally treated group had a lower baseline glomerular filtration rate than the captopril treated group (87 versus 99 ml/min) and hence, possibly a greater potential to progress to macroalbuminuria. Also, the lack of a placebo group makes it difficult to determine if the effects of the conventional treatment could still represent a beneficial effect.

Schnack et al have recently reported that ramipril ± felodipine stabilised albuminuria. By contrast, atenolol ± diuretic treatment was associated with an increase in urinary albumin excretion [39]. Furthermore, the ramipril treated group had stable renal function whereas the group receiving beta blockers had a decline in GFR. A reduction in albuminuria by ACE inhibition has also been observed by a number of other investigators [19, 27, 28, 34-37, 40].

In the Melbourne Diabetic Nephropathy Study, nifedipine was shown to produce a similar response to perindopril in decreasing albuminuria over 12 months in the NIDDM subjects with microalbuminuria [32]. Nicardipine, another dihydropyridine CCB, reduced albuminuria over 4 weeks in microalbuminuric patients but this finding was not observed in patients with macroproteinuria [38]. It has been reported by Chan et al that the ACE inhibitor, enalapril, was more effective than nifedipine in reducing albuminuria in a group of hypertensive microalbuminuric subjects [19]. Recently, several new studies have been reported which have compared calcium channel blockade with ACE inhibition in hypertensive microalbuminuric NIDDM subjects [34, 36, 37]. In a study over 3 years, in a relatively small number of subjects, amlodipine was as effective as the ACE inhibitor, cilazapril in reducing albuminuria with both treatment groups having similar declines in renal function [36]. A similar effect of reducing AER has been recently reported with the CCB, nivaldipine [41]. Similar efficacy between enalapril and amlodipine in 50 hypertensive NIDDM subjects with microalbuminuria has recently been reported by Fogari et al [40]. However, in a much larger multi-centre study of over 300 subjects, the ACE inhibitor, lisinopril, reduced albuminuria over 12 months whereas nifedipine failed to significantly influence urinary albumin excretion [37].

3. THE USE OF ANTIHYPERTENSIVE AGENTS IN NORMOTENSIVE NIDDM WITH MICROALBUMINURIA (TABLE 42-2)

The possibility that early therapy will postpone or retard progression of renal injury in diabetes has led to the use of antihypertensive agents in normotensive subjects. Albuminuria over a 6 month period was reduced in a group of normotensive NIDDM patients with microalbuminuria treated with captopril, whereas the untreated group had no change in albuminuria [42]. In the Melbourne study [32] there was no change in albuminuria after 12 months treatment with either nifedipine or perindopril in normotensive microalbuminuric patients, despite a small but significant reduction in blood pressure (4 mmHg). Nonetheless, on stopping therapy at 12 months a dramatic increase in albuminuria was detected in the NIDDM but not in the IDDM subjects (Figure 42-1), which was independent of mode of treatment [43].

The inability of either agent to reduce albuminuria in the normotensive cohort coupled with the rapid rise after stopping therapy needs to be considered in the setting of the natural history of microalbuminuria. Albuminuria would be anticipated to rise by an average rise of 20 to 50 per cent if left untreated for 12 months in microalbuminuric NIDDM subjects. This phenomenon of a rapid rise in albuminuria was not as clearly apparent in the IDDM patients and may indicate a difference in the underlying etiology and pathogenesis of albuminuria in NIDDM as compared to IDDM.

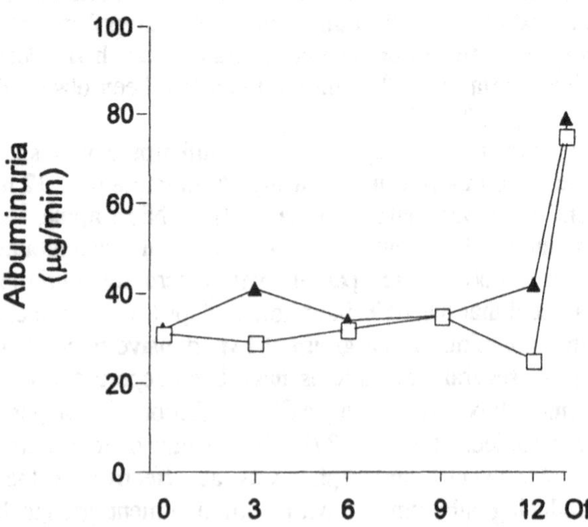

Figure 42-1. Effects of perindopril (□, n=11) or nifedipine (▲, n=13) on albuminuria (geometric means) over 12 months of treatment and after 1 month off treatment (Off) in normotensive microalbuminuric NIDDM patients from the Melbourne Diabetic Nephropathy Study, adapted from [46].

It is possible that there are differences in the sensitivity to structural damage incurred from blood pressure between IDDM and NIDDM.

Flack et al have also reported no difference in the ability to decrease albuminuria between indapamide and captopril [28]. However, in that cross-over study, several of the subjects were borderline hypertensive.

The first long-term (5 years) placebo controlled double blind randomized study to evaluate the effect of an antihypertensive agent in normotensive, microalbuminuric NIDDM subjects with normal renal function (as assessed by a serum creatinine < 123 μmol/l) was reported by Ravid et al [44]. During the first year of treatment albuminuria decreased in the enalapril treated group from an initial mean of 143 mg/24 hours to a mean of 122 mg/24 hours. Thereafter, a small but steady increase in albuminuria occurred in the enalapril treated patients to 140 mg/24 hours after 5 years. Conversely, in the placebo treated patients a gradual increase in albuminuria occurred from a baseline of 123 to 310 mg/24 hours over the 5 years. Albuminuria exceeded 300 mg/24 hours in only 6/49 (12.2%) of the enalapril group compared to 19/45 (42.2%) of the placebo treated group. Renal function remained unchanged in the enalapril group during the first 2 years of follow up, but from the third year a small but non-significant decrease was evident, in the order of 1% after 5 years, in contrast to 13% in the placebo treated group. Although the assessment of renal function (assessed by 100/serum creatinine) was rather crude this is the first long-term study to demonstrate both an antiproteinuric effect of an ACE inhibitor in normotensive NIDDM patients with microalbuminuria and preservation of renal function. A follow up report after 7 years of treatment has confirmed a renoprotective effect of ACE inhibition in this cohort [47]. Sano et al have observed in a 4 year study that enalapril treatment reduced albuminuria whereas placebo treatment was associated with no change in albuminuria in a group of normotensive, microalbuminuric NIDDM patients [33]. Similar effects on albuminuria have been observed in a 6 month study by an Italian multi-centre group using the ACEI, ramipril [35].

Recently, Ahmad et al have reported similar effects on albuminuria after 5 years of ACE inhibitor therapy in a group of Indian normotensive NIDDM subjects with microalbuminuria [45]. Enalapril treatment was associated with a reduction in albuminuria whereas in the placebo group there was a progressive rise in urinary albumin excretion. Of particular interest was the finding that these effects were observed in the absence of a discernible difference in blood pressure between the two groups. Whether these effects of ACE inhibitors in normotensive patients will also be observed with other antihypertensive agents such as CCBs is the subject of a new placebo controlled study by the Melbourne Diabetic Nephropathy Study Group [48].

4. THE ROLE OF ANGIOTENSIN II RECEPTOR ANTAGONISTS

Although most studies involving agents which interrupt the renin-angiotensin system have used ACE inhibitors, the advent of angiotensin II (AII) receptor antagonists such as losartan provides a more specific approach to inhibit the actions of AII without influencing other hormonal systems such as bradykinin [49]. As yet, it is not clear if this new class will confer similar renal protection to ACE inhibitors

[50]. Recently, several small studies have been performed in hypertensive and diabetic patients [51, 52]. In a study of elderly Chinese hypertensive subjects, some of whom had diabetes, losartan reduced albuminuria whereas the calcium channel blocker, felodipine, was ineffective [51]. A similar finding has been suggested from a preliminary analysis of a multi-centre study in European NIDDM subjects comparing amlodipine to losartan [52]. The AII antagonist but not amlodipine reduced albuminuria. The relevance of these findings is now being explored with several large clinical trials in progress to assess the renoprotective effects of AII receptor antagonists in NIDDM patients with macroproteinuria.

5. ROLE OF COMBINATION THERAPY

It has been proposed that the combination of a calcium antagonist with a converting enzyme inhibitor should result in a greater reduction in urinary protein excretion and slowed morphological progression of nephropathy [53]. Bakris et al have compared the renal hemodynamic and antiproteinuric effects of a calcium antagonist, verapamil, and an ACE inhibitor, lisinopril, alone and in combination in three groups of non-insulin dependent diabetic subjects with documented nephrotic range proteinuria, hypertension, and renal insufficiency [22]. Patients treated with the combination of a calcium antagonist and an ACE inhibitor manifested the greatest reduction in albuminuria. In addition, the decline in GFR was the lowest in this group. Similar findings are suggested by another study performed in microalbuminuric subjects using the combination of verapamil and cilazapril [54]. Sano et al have shown that the addition of enalapril to nifedipine conferred an additional effect in decreasing albuminuria in a group of microalbuminuric NIDDM subjects [33]. A recent preliminary report by Bakris et al has suggested that the combination of verapamil and trandolapril, administered in a fixed dose combination, is more effective at reducing proteinuria than either drug alone, despite similar effects on blood pressure [55]. Similar findings have now been reported by Fogari et al who have shown that benazepril plus amlodipine tended to be more effective than benazepril alone in reducing albuminuria in microalbuminuric, hypertensive NIDDM patients [56]. The above findings with combination therapy provide an exciting approach for optimizing antihypertensive therapy in diabetic patients with renal disease.

6. THE USE OF ANTIHYPERTENSIVE AGENTS IN PATIENTS WITH NIDDM.

The choice of an antihypertensive agent in the management of abnormal albuminuria in NIDDM depends not only on its potential renoprotective effect but must take into consideration other factors which could be deleterious to the patient. Microalbuminuria in the NIDDM patient is more closely linked to subsequent death from cardiovascular disease than from nephropathy [57]. Therefore, it is important that any antihypertensive intervention in the NIDDM patient with abnormal albuminuria does not exacerbate existing hypertriglyceridaemia or further reduce HDL-cholesterol, lipid abnormalities associated with NIDDM [58]. Furthermore, reduced sensitivity to insulin after administration of thiazides and various beta-blockers may be detrimental [59]. However, more recent studies suggest that low dose diuretics do not have deleterious effects on plasma glucose or lipid levels [60]. In contrast, improved insulin sensitivity is seen after captopril [59] and doxazocin [61] and minimal or neutral effects are observed with CCB [62]. Also, in contrast to beta-blockers and thiazide diuretics, neither CCB nor ACEI affect glucose tolerance deleteriously [62]. The effects of the AII receptor antagonists such as losartan have not been as extensively studied but they appear to have either no effect [63] or a beneficial effect on insulin sensitivity [64].

7. WHICH AGENT TO USE?

The limited evidence so far published on the effects of antihypertensive agents in NIDDM with abnormal albuminuria concur with findings in IDDM [65]. Both ACEI and CCB may possess beneficial effects over and above simple blood pressure control, although in most studies the small numbers of subjects included may have introduced a Type II statistical error. Several meta-analyses of trials involving patients with either IDDM or NIDDM have demonstrated the salutary effects of ACEI on proteinuria and renal function compared to other classes of antihypertensive agent, whether or not the patients had IDDM or NIDDM, hypertension, normoalbuminuria, microalbuminuria or macroproteinuria [66, 67]. These analyses have suggested that ACE inhibitors have an ability to reduce proteinuria independent of their hypotensive effects. However, a recent update of one of these meta-analyses has suggested that at maximal hypotensive doses no significant difference was observed in the anti-proteinuric effects of ACE inhibitors and other antihypertensive drugs [68].

8. ABNORMAL ALBUMINURIA IN NIDDM: WHAT DOES IT SIGNIFY?

Microalbuminuria predicts not only nephropathy in NIDDM subjects but also is a strong predictor of all-cause mortality, particularly from cardiovascular diseases [57].

Therefore, the effects of these antihypertensive agents must include assessment of cardiovascular endpoints as reported in the ABCD study where there was evidence of a superiority of enalapril over nisoldipine in terms of reduced cardiovascular events [69]. Of particular interest is the recent finding from the FACET study suggesting that fosinopril was associated with less cardiovascular events than amlodipine in a study of 380 hypertensive NIDDM subjects [70]. These studies suggest that ACE inhibitors confer cardioprotective effects which are not as clearly evident with dihydropyridine CCBs. However, this requires further confirmation from additional studies such as the ALLHAT trial now in progress which includes 40,000 subjects, one third with diabetes [71].

Although the principal endpoint in evaluating the influence of an antihypertensive agent on renal function in diabetes is its ability to alter the progression of the disease, it is clear that abnormally elevated albuminuria is also associated with progressive renal injury [72]. Although many of the short-term trials that have been performed in subjects with NIDDM only document a reduction in albuminuria in the absence of a change in glomerular filtration rate, longterm studies in IDDM subjects suggest that the severity of proteinuria also correlates with the rate of progression of renal disease [73]. A similar link between the level of albuminuria and decline in renal function has been reported in a study of hypertensive NIDDM patients [74]. Nonetheless, studies involving renal structural assessment are warranted to more accurately determine the response to antihypertensive agents.

Finally, although the focus of treatment of NIDDM subjects with early and overt renal disease has been on antihypertensive therapy one cannot ignore the role of glycaemic control. In natural history studies, it has been shown that glycaemic control is a major determinant of the rate of progression of albuminuria, not only in IDDM but also in NIDDM subjects [75]. Furthermore, a recent study in Japanese NIDDM subjects has shown that intensified insulin therapy over a 6 year period prevented the progression of diabetic microvascular complications including nephropathy [76]. These findings are similar to those reported from the DCCT study performed in IDDM subjects [77]. It is anticipated that further information on the role of glycaemic control in the development of diabetic complications in NIDDM subjects will become available over the next 12 months from the UK Prospective Diabetes Study [78]. However, strong evidence for the important role of improved glycemic control in preventing microvascular complications already exists [79].

REFERENCES

1. Berkman J, Rifkin H. Unilateral nodular diabetic glomerulosclerosis (Kimmelstiel-Wilson).Report of a case. Metabolism Clin Exp 1973; 22: 715-722.
2. Nelson RG, Knowler WC, McCance DR, Sievers ML, Pettitt DJ, Charles MA, Hanson RL, Liu QZ, Bennett PH. Determinants of end-stage renal disease in Pima Indians with type 2 (non-insulin-dependent) diabetes mellitus and proteinuria. Diabetologia 1993; 36: 1087-93.
3. Ritz E, Stefanski A. Diabetic nephropathy in type II diabetes. Am J Kidney Dis 1996; 27: 167-194.
4. Grenfell A, Bewick M, Snowden S, Watkins PJ, Parsons V. Renal replacement for diabetic patients: experience at King's College Hospital 1980-1989. Q J Med 1992; 85: 861-74.
5. Held PJ, Port FK, Webb RL, Wolfe RA, Garcia JR, Blagg CR, Agodoa LY. The United States Renal Data System's 1991 annual data report: an introduction. Am J Kidney Dis 1991; 18: 1-16.
6. Pugh JA, Medina RA, Cornell JC, Basu S. NIDDM is the major cause of diabetic end-stage renal disease. More evidence from a tri-ethnic community. Diabetes 1995; 44: 1375-80.
7. Cowie CC. Diabetic renal disease: racial and ethnic differences from an epidemiologic perspective. Transplant Proc 1993; 25: 2426-30.
8. Stornello M, Valvo EV, Puglia N, Scapellato L. Angiotensin converting enzyme inhibition with a low dose of enalapril in normotensive diabetics with persistent proteinuria. J Hypertension 1988; 6(suppl 4): S464-S466.
9. Stornello M, Valvo E, Vasques E, Leone S, Scapellato L. Systemic and renal effects of chronic angiotensin converting enzyme inhibition with captopril in hypertensive diabetic patients. J Hypertension 1989; 7 (suppl 7): S65-S67.
10. Stornello M, Valvo EV, Scapellato L. Hemodynamic, renal, and humoral effects of the calcium entry blocker nicardipine and converting enzyme inhibitor captopril in hypetensive Type II diabetic patients with nephropathy. J Cardiovasc Pharmacol 1989; 14: 851-855.
11. Stornello M, Valvo EV, Scapellato L. Angiotensin converting enzyme inhibition in normotensive type II diabetics with persistent mild proteinuria. J Hypertension 1989; 7 (suppl 6): S314-S315.
12. Stornello M, Valvo EV, Scapellato L. Comparative effects of enalapril, atenolol and chlorthalidone on blood pressure and kidney function of diabetic patients affected by arterial hypertension and persistent proteinuria. Nephron 1991; 58: 52-7.

13. Bakris GL, Copley JB, Vicknair N, Sadler R, Leurgans S. Calcium channel blockers versus other antihypertensive therapies on progression of NIDDM associated nephropathy. Kidney International 1996; 50: 1641-1650.
14. Bakris GL, Mangrum A, Copley JB, Vicknair N, Sadler R. Effect of calcium channel or beta-blockade on the progression of diabetic nephropathy in African Americans. Hypertension 1997; 29: 744-750.
15. Bakris GL. Effects of diltiazem or lisinopril on massive proteinuria associated with diabetes mellitus. Ann Intern Med 1990; 112: 701-702.
16. Demarie BK, Bakris GL. Effects of different calcium antagonists on proteinuria assocaited with diabetes mellitus. Ann Intern Med 1990; 113: 987-988.
17. Valvo EV, Bedogna V, Casagrande P, Antiga L, Zamboni M, Bommartini F, Oldrizzi L, Rugiu C, Maschio G. Captopril in patients with type II diabetes and renal insufficiency: systemic and renal hemodynamic alterations. Am J Med 1988; 85: 344-348.
18. Nielsen FS, Rossing P, Gall MA, Skott P, Smidt UM, Parving HH. Long-term effect of lisinopril and atenolol on kidney function in hypertensive NIDDM subjects with diabetic nephropathy. Diabetes 1997; 46:1182-8.
19. Chan JC, Cockram CS, Nicholls MG, Cheung CK, Swaminathan R. Comparison of enalapril and nifedipine in treating non-insulin dependent diabetes associated with hypertension: one year analysis. BMJ 1992; 305: 981-5.
20. Fogari R, Zoppi A, Pasotti C, Mugellini A, Lusardi P, Lazzari P, Corradi L. Comparative effects of ramipril and nitrendipine on albuminuria in hypertensive patients with non insulin dependent diabetes mellitus and impaired renal fundtion. J Hum Hypertens 1995; 9: 13-15.
21. Ferder L, Daccordi H, Martello M, Panzalis M, Inserra F. Angiotensin converting enzyme inhibitors versus calcium antagonists in the treatment of diabetic hypertensive patients. Hypertension 1992; 19: II237-42.
22. Bakris GL, Barnhill BW, Sadler R. Treatment of arterial hypertension in diabetic humans: importance of therapeutic selection. Kidney Int 1992; 41: 912-9.
23. Liou HH, Huang TP, Campese VM. Effect of long-term therapy with captopril on proteinuria and renal function in patients with non-insulin-dependent diabetes and with non-diabetic renal diseases. Nephron 1995; 69: 41-8.
24. Slataper R, Vicknair N, Sadler R, Bakris GL. Comparative effects of different antihypertensive treatments on progression of diabetic renal disease. Arch Intern Med 1993; 153: 973-80.
25. Romero R, Salinas I, Lucas A, Teixido J, Audi L, Sanmarti A. Comparative effects of captopril versus nifedipine on proteinuria and renal function of type 2 diabetic patients. Diabetes Res Clin Pract 1992; 17: 191-8.
26. Guasch A, Parham M, Zayas CF, Campbell O, Nzerue C, Macon E. Contrasting effects of calcium channel blockade versus converting enzyme inhibition on proteinuria in african americans with non-insulin-dependent diabetes mellitus and nephropathy. Journal of the American Society of Nephrology 1997; 8: 793-798.
27. Dominguez LJ, Barbagallo M, Kattah W, Garcia D, Sowers JR. Quinapril reduces microalbuminuria in essential hypertensive and in diabetic hypertensive subjects. Am J Hypertens 1995; 8: 808-14.
28. Flack JR, Molyneaux L, Willey K, Yue DK. Regression of microalbuminuria: results of a controlled study, indapamide versus captopril. J Cardiovasc Pharmacol 1993; 22 Suppl 6: S75-7.
29. Gambardella S, Frontoni S, Felici MG, Spallone V, Gargiulo P, Morano S, G M. Efficacy of antihypertensive treatment with indapamide in patients with non-insulin-dependent diabetes and persistent microalbuminuria. Am J Cardiol 1990; 65: 46H-50H.
30. Gambardella S, Frontoni S, Lala A, Felici MG, Spallone V, Scoppola A, Jacoangeli F, Menzinger G. Regression of microalbuminuria in type II diabetic, hypertensive patients after long-term indapamide treatment. Am Heart J 1991; 122: 1232-8.
31. Lacourciere Y, Nadeau A, Poirier L, Tancrede G. Captopril or conventional therapy in hypertensive type II diabetics. Three-year analysis. Hypertension 1993; 21: 786-94.
32. Melbourne Diabetic Nephropathy Study Group. Comparison between perindopril and nifedipine in hypertensive and normotensive diabetic patients with microalbuminuria. Br Med J 1991; 302: 210-6.

33. Sano T, Kawamura T, Matsumae H, Sasaki H, Nakayama M, Hara T, Matsuo S, Hotta N, Sakamoto N. Effects of long-term enalapril treatment on persistent micro-albuminuria in well-controlled hypertensive and normotensive NIDDM patients. Diabetes Care 1994; 17: 420-4.
34. Ruggenenti P, Mosconi L, Bianchi L, Cortesi L, Campana M, Pagani G, Mecca G, Remuzzi G. Long-term treatment with either enalapril or nitrendipine stabilizes albuminuria and increases glomerular filtration rate in non-insulin-dependent diabetic patients. American Journal of Kidney Diseases 1994; 24: 753-761.
35. Trevisan R, Tiengo A. Effect of low-dose ramipril on microalbuminuria in normotensive or mild hypertensive non-insulin-dependent diabetic patients. North-East Italy Microalbuminuria Study Group. Am J Hypertens 1995; 8: 876-83.
36. Velussi M, Brocco E, Frogato F, Zolli M, Muollo B, Maioli M, Carraro A, Tonolo G, Fresu P, Cernigoi AM, Fioretto P, Nosadini R. Effects of cilazapril and amlodipine on kidney function in hypertensive NIDDM patients. Diabetes 1996; 45: 216-222.
37. Agardh C-D, Carcia-Puig J, Charbonnel B, Angelkort B, Barnett AH. Greater reduction of urinary albumin escretion in hypertensive type II diabetic patients with incipient nephropathy by lisinopril than by nifedipine. J Human Hypertens 1996; 10: 185-192.
38. Baba T, Tomiyama T, Murabayashi S, Takebe K. Renal effects of nicardipine, a calcium antagonist, in hypertensive Type 2 (non-insulin-dependent) diabetic patients with and without nephropathy. Eur J Clin Pharmacol 1990; 38: 425-429.
39. Schnack C, Hoffmann W, Hopmeier P, Schernthaner G. Renal and metabolic effects of 1-year treatment with ramipril or atenolol in niddm patients with microalbuminuria. Diabetologia 1996; 39: 1611-1616.
40. Fogari R, Zoppi A, Malamani GD, Lusardi P, Destro M, Corradi L. Effects of amlodipine vs enalapril on microalbuminuria in hypertensive patients with type II diabetes. Clinical Drug Investigation 1997; 13: 42-49.
41. Sumida Y, Yano Y, Murata K, Goto H, Ura H, Ezaki J, Tsutsumi S, Shirayama K, Misaki M, Shima T. Effect of the calcium channel blocker nivaldipine on urinary albumin excretion in hypertensive microalbuminuric patients with non-insulin-dependent diabetes mellitus. Journal of International Medical Research 1997; 25: 117-126.
42. Romero R, Salinas I, Lucas A, Abad E, Reverter JL, Johnston S, Sanmarti A. Renal function changes in microalbuminuric normotensive type II diabetic patients treated with angiotensin-converting enzyme inhibitors. Diabetes Care 1993; 16: 597-600.
43. Jerums G, Allen TJ, Tsalamandris C, Cooper ME, Melbourne Diabetic Nephropathy Study G. Angiotensin Converting Enzyme inhibition and Calcium Channel Blockade in incipient diabetic nephropathy. Kidney Int 1992; 41: 904-911.
44. Ravid M, Savin H, Jutrin I, Bental T, Katz B, Lishner M. Long-term stabilizing effect of angiotensin-converting enzyme inhibition on plasma creatinine and on proteinuria in normotensive type II diabetic patients. Ann Intern Med 1993; 118: 577-81.
45. Ahmad J, Siddiqui MA, Ahmad H. Effective postponement of diabetic nephropathy with enalapril in normotensive type 2 diabetic patients with microalbuminuria. Diabetes Care 1997; 20: 1576-1581.
46. Cooper ME, Doyle AE. The management of diabetic proteinuria. Which antihypertensive agent? Drugs Aging 1992; 2: 301-9.
47. Ravid M, Lang R, Rachmani R, Lishner M. Long-term renoprotective effect of angiotensin-converting enzyme inhibition in non-insulin-dependent diabetes mellitus. A 7-year follow-up study. Arch Intern Med 1996; 156: 286-9.
48. Melbourne Diabetic Nephropathy Study Group, Cooper ME, Allen T, Jerums G, DeLuise M, Alford F, Doyle AE. Effects of different antihypertensive agents on normotensive microalbuminuric type I and type II diabetic patients. Proc XIIth International Congress of Nephrology 1993; Jerusalem: 424.
49. Johnston CI. Angiotensin receptor antagonists: focus on losartan. Lancet 1995; 346: 1403-7.
50. Ichikawa I, Madias NE, Harrington JT, King AS, Singh A, Levey AS. Will angiotensin II receptor antagonists be renoprotective in humans? Kidney International 1996; 50: 684-692.

51. Chan JCN, Critchley J, Tomlinson B, Chan TYK, Cockram CS. Antihypertensive and anti-albuminuric effects of losartan potassium and felodipine in chinese elderly hypertensive patients with or without non-insulin-dependent diabetes mellitus. American Journal of Nephrology 1997; 17: 72-80.
52. Os I. Losartan vs. amlodipine in hypertensive patients with NIDDM. Proc 15th International Congress of Nephrology Symposium 'Emerging therapeutic intervention with AII antagonism in diabetic nephropathy' 1997.
53. Brown SA, Walton CL, Crawford P, Bakris GL. Long-term effects of antihypertensive regimens on renal hemodynamics and proteinuria. Kidney Int 1993; 43: 1210-8.
54. Fioretto P, Frigato F, Velussi M, Riva F, Muollo B, Carraro A, Brocco E, Cipollina MR, Abaterusso C, Trevisan M, Crepaldi G, Nosadini R. Effects of angiotensin converting enzyme inhibitors and calcium antagonists on atrial natriuretic peptide release and action and on albumin excretion rate in hypertensive insulin-dependent diabetic patients. Am J Hypertens 1992; 5: 837-46.
55. Bakris G, Weir M, De Quattro V, Rosendorff C, McMahon G. Renal effects of a long acting ACE inhibitor, trandolapril (T) or nondihydropyridine calcium blocker, verapamil (V) or in a fixed dose combination in diabetic nephropathy: A randomized double blind placebo controlled multicenter study. Nephrology 1997; 3 (Suppl 1): S271.
56. Fogari R, Zoppi A, Mugellini A, Lusardi P, Destro M, Corradi L. Effect of benazepril plus amlodipine vs benazepril alone on urinary albumin excretion in hypertensive patients with type II diabetes and microalbuminuria. Clinical Drug Investigation 1997; 13: 50-55.
57. Mogensen CE. Microalbuminuria predicts clinical proteinuria and early mortality in maturity-onset diabetes. N Engl J Med 1984; 310: 356-60.
58. Garber AJ, Vinik AI, Crespin SR. Detection and management of lipid disorders in diabetic patients. A commentary for clinicians. Diabetes Care 1992; 15: 1068-74.
59. Lind L, Pollare T, Berne C, Lithell H. Long-term metabolic effects of antihypertensive drugs. Am Heart J 1994; 128: 1177-83.
60. Harper R, Ennis CN, Heaney AP, Sheridan B, Gormley M, Atkinson AB, Johnston GD, Bell PM. A comparison of the effects of low- and conventional-dose thiazide diuretic on insulin action in hypertensive patients with NIDDM. Diabetologia 1995; 38: 853-9.
61. Giordano M, Matsuda M, Sanders L, Canessa ML, DeFronzo RA. Effects of angiotensin-converting enzyme inhibitors, Ca2+ channel antagonists, and alpha-adrenergic blockers on glucose and lipid metabolism in NIDDM patients with hypertension. Diabetes 1995; 44: 665-71.
62. Stein P, Black H. Drug treatment of hypertension in patients with diabetes mellitus. Diabetes Care 1991; 14: 425-448.
63. Laakso M, Karjalainen L, Lempiainenkuosa P. Effects of losartan on insulin sensitivity in hypertensive subjects. Hypertension 1996; 28: 392-396.
64. Moan A, Hoieggen A, Nordby G, Eide IK, Kjeldsen SE. Effects of losartan on insulin sensitivity in severe hypertension - connections through sympathetic nervous system activity. Journal of Human Hypertension 1995; 9: 50.
65. Mathiesen ER, Hommel E, Giese J, Parving H-H. Efficacy of captopril in postponing nephropathy in normotensive insulin dependent diabetic patients with microalbuminuria. Br Med J 1991; 303: 81-7.
66. Kasiske BL, Kalil RS, Ma JZ, Liao M, Keane WF. Effect of antihypertensive therapy on the kidney in patients with diabetes: a meta-regression analysis. Ann Intern Med 1993; 118: 129-38.
67. Bohlen L, de Courten M, Weidmann P. Comparative study of the effect of ACE-inhibitors and other antihypertensive agents on proteinuria in diabetic patients. Am J Hypertens 1994; 7: 84s-92s.
68. Weidmann P, Schneider M, Bohlen L. Therapeutic efficacy of different antihypertensive drugs in human diabetic nephropathy: an updated meta-analysis. Nephrol Dial Transpl 1995; 10(suppl): 39-45.
69. Estacio RO, Jeffers BW, Hiatt WR, Biggerstaff SL, Gifford N, Schrier RW. The effect of nisoldipine as compared with enalapril on cardiovascular outcomes in patients with non-insulin-dependent diabetes and hypertension. N Engl J Med 1998; 338: 645-652.

70. Tatti P, Pahor M, Byington RP, DiMauro P, Guarisco R, Strollo F, for the FACET study group. Results of the Fosinopril AMlodipine Cardiovascular Events Trial (FACET) in hypertensive patients with non-insulin dependent diabetes mellitus (NIDDM). Proc American Heart Association, Orlando 1997.
71. Cutler JA. Calcium channel blockers for hypertension – Uncertainty continues. N Engl J Med 1998; 338:679-681.
72. Remuzzi G, Bertani T. Is glomerulosclerosis a consequence of altered glomerular permeability to macromolecules? Kidney Int 1990; 38: 384-394.
73. Rossing P, Hommel E, Smidt UM, Parving HH. Impact of arterial blood pressure and albuminuria on the progression of diabetic nephropathy in IDDM patients. Diabetes 1993; 42: 715-9.
74. Lebovitz HE, Wiegmann TB, Cnaan A, Shahinfar S, Sica DA, Broadstone V, Schwartz SL, Mengel MC, Segal R, Versaggi JA, et al. Renal protective effects of enalapril in hypertensive NIDDM: role of baseline albuminuria. Kidney Int Suppl 1994; 45: S150-5.
75. Gilbert RE, Tsalamandris C, Bach L, Panagiotopoulos S, O'Brien RC, Allen TJ, Goodall I, Young V, Seeman E, Murray RML, Cooper ME, Jerums G. Glycemic control and the rate of progression of early diabetic kidney disease: a nine year longitudinal study. Kidney Int 1993; 44: 855-859.
76. Ohkubo Y, Kishikawa H, Araki E, Miyata T, Isami S, Motoyoshi S, Kojima Y, Furyoshi N, Shichiri M. Intensive insulin therapy prevents the progression of diabetic microvascualr complications in Japanese patients with non-insulin-dependent diabetes mellitus: a randomized prospective 6-year study. Diabetes Res Clin Pract 1995; 28: 103-117.
77. Diabetes Control and Complications Trial Research Group. The effect of intensive treatment on the development and progression of long-term complications in insulin-dependent diabetes mellitus. New Engl J Med 1993; 329: 977-86.
78. Turner R, Cull C, Holman, United Kingdom Prospective Study 17:A 9-Year Update of a Randomized, Controlled Trial on the Effect of Improved Metabolic Control on Complications in Non-insulin-dependent diabetes Mellitus. Ann Intern Med 1996; 124: 136-145.
79. Gaster B, Hirch IB. The effects of improved Glycemic control on complications in type 2 diabetes. Arch Intern Med, 1998, 158: 134-140.

ADDENDUM REGARDING RENOVASCULAR HYPERTENSION AND RENAL ARTERY STENOSIS (especially NIDDM)

Co-author: Bryan Williams

Since diabetes is associated with accelerated atherosclerosis, it has been presumed that it is a state of increased prevalence of renal artery stenosis (RAS). This is of clinical relevance since ACE inhibitors, which can precipitate renal failure in the setting of bilateral RAS [1], are widely used in diabetic patients for nephropathy, heart failure and hypertension. Autopsy studies have suggested that RAS may be increased in diabetic patients [2] but it is likely that the pathologically detected stenoses are not functionally significant.

Only a few studies have been performed to screen for RAS in hypertensive diabetic patients. Ritchie et al have reported in a cross-sectional study of hypertensive NIDDM subjects that RAS is commonly detected [3]. However, more detailed functional studies performed by this group suggested that the RAS was haemodynamically insignificant and unlikely to be a significant cause of hypertension in the majority of patients. In a recent study by Parving et al [personal communication] in aptients with NIDDM and overt nephropathy who had a mean age of 60 years, no clinical evidence of RAS was noted during treatment with an ACE inhibitor or beta blocker.

At present, there are no specific recommendations from any of the appropriate societies with respect to screening for RAS in diabetic patients. Since there is no convincing evidence to suggest that diabetic patients with hypertension have a much higher prevalence of RAS than non-diabetic, hypertensive patients we recommend that the presence of diabetes *per se* is not a justification for routine screening for RAS. Nevertheless, there are clearly clinical features which are associated with an increased prevalence of RAS. RAS is more common with ageing, male gender, history of smoking, in those subjects with evidence of peripheral and coronary vascular disease and in those subjects with hypertension refractory to treatment [4, 5]. This patient profile should alert the clinician to the possibility of RAS. Where a strong clinical suspicion of RAS exists, it would be prudent to investigate the patient prior to commencing ACE inhibitor therapy [6, 7]. These investigations might include renal ultrasound and renal artery doppler studies or functional studies such as renal isotopic scanning, depending on local expertise. Renal angiography is usually reserved for confirmation of the diagnosis in those in whom intervention is being contemplated. In the vast majority of diabetic patients however, these investigations are not warranted prior to the prescription of ACE inhibitor therapy. Prior to, and within a week of commencing ACE inhibitors, serum creatinine and potassium should be measured to determine whether there has been an acute deterioration in renal function secondary to bilateral RAS [1]. This often occurs rapidly after the introduction of ACE inhibitors and is usually reversible if detected immediately. An acute deterioration in renal function after commencing ACE inhibition does not necessarily imply the presence of RAS as this clinical scenario often occurs in the setting of volume depletion, particularly with concurrent diuretic therapy. It is suggested that at this stage similar caution is exerted with the introduction of angiotensin II receptor antagonists such as losartan to diabetic patients [8].

In conclusion, an appropriate level of clinical vigilance and simple clinical assessment of hypertensive diabetic patients should identify most of those at risk of RAS and allow the safe use of agents which interrupt the renin-angiotensin system such as ACE inhibitors and AII antagonists in diabetic patients.

REFERENCES

1. Hricik DE, Browning PJ, Kopelman R, Goorno WE, Madias NE, Dzau VJ. Captopril induced functional renal insufficiency in patients with bilateral renal-artery stenoses or renal-artery stenosis in a solitary kidney. N Engl J Med 1983; 308: 373-376.
2. Sawicki PT, Kaiser S, Heinemann L, Frenzel H, Berger M. Prevalence of renal artery stenosis in diabetes mellitus--an autopsy study. J Intern Med 1991; 229: 489-92.
3. Ritchie CM, McGrath E, Hadden DR, Weaver JA, Kennedy L. Renal artery stenosis in hypertensive diabetic patients. Diab Med 1988; 5: 265-267.
4. Jean WJ, al Bitar I, Zwicke DL, Port SC, Schmidt DH, Bajwa TK. High incidence of renal artery stenosis in patients with coronary artery disease. Cathet Cardiovasc Diagn 1994; 32: 8-10.
5. Isaksson H, Danielsson M, Rosenhamer G, Konarski Svensson JC, Ostergren J. Characteristics of patients resistant to antihypertensive drug therapy. J Intern Med 1991; 229: 421-6.

6. Robinson ACJ, Kong C, Henzen C, Pacy P, Chong P, Gedroyc W, Elkeles RS, Robison S. Magnetic resonance angiography and renal artery stenosis in hypertensive patients with type 2 diabetes (Abstract). Diabetologia 1996; 39: Suppl 1: A36.
7. Courreges JP, Bacha J, Maraoui M, Taurines H, Paris F, Aboud E. Renal artery stenosis prevalence in non insulin dependant diabetes (NIDDM) and hypertension. (Abstract) Diabetologia 1995; 38, Suppl 1: A269.
8. Johnston CI. Angiotensin receptor antagonists: focus on losartan. Lancet 1995; 346: 1403-7.

43. THE COURSE OF INCIPIENT AND OVERT DIABETIC NEPHROPATHY: THE PERSPECTIVE OF MORE OPTIMAL INSULIN TREATMENT

Bo Feldt-Rasmussen
Medical Department P, Rigshospitalet, Copenhagen, Denmark

The long-term objective of insulin treatment of insulin dependent diabetes mellitus (IDDM) is prevention of late complications. Through the years it has been a widely accepted hypothesis that development of such microvascular complications should be, at least in part, due to the lack of good glycemic control. This hypothesis has been unduely hard to prove but results from a number of small scaled interventionstudies and the result of the larger scaled American Diabetes Control and Complication Trial (DCCT) has now decisively documented, that development and progression of diabetic complications is closely associated with poor glycemic control. The design and outcome of a number of these studies will be presented and discussed in this chapter as will the practical consequences of this newly gained knowledge.

1. THE CONCEPT OF MICROALBUMINURIA

Much of our recent knowledge has been obtained because it is now possible in a very early stage to identify patients at risk of clinical diabetic nephropathy as recently reviewed in a number of dissertations and elsewhere [1-6]. The proteinuria of clinical diabetic nephropathy is classically defined as a total urinary proteinexcretion of 0.5 g per 24 h or more, equivalent to a urinary albumin excretion rate (UAER) of approximately 300 mg/24h or 200 μg/min. It has been documented that a UAER raised above a certain lower level is a good predictor of the development of clinical diabetic nephropathy. Patients at high risk of diabetic nephropathy have a UAER above the normal range but below that of clinical nephropathy. In 1986 a general consensus was made stating that this range of microalbuminuria should be defined as a UAER between 30 to 300 mg/24 h (20 to 200 μg/min) in a 24h or a short term, timed urine collection [7]. At early onset of nephropathy (UAER just above 300 mg/24 h) when the GFR is mainly within the normal range, an annual decline in GFR of approximately 3 to 4 ml/min can be demonstrated. Furthermore patients with microalbuminuria share a number of cardiovascular risk factors with patients with nephropathy [1-7]. Therefore the variations of the UAER have been an important end-point to study in many of the recent studies of effects of glycemic control in diabetes.

2. EFFECT OF IMPROVED GLYCEMIC CONTROL ?

2.1 The Scandinavian Experience

Following the introduction of intensified insulin treatment regimens with multiple injections or continuous subcutaneous infusion of short-acting insulins, it became possible to establish and maintain a long-term improvement of the glycemic control. On this basis a number of prospective randomized studies of the effect of improved glycemic control on development and progression of late diabetic complications were initiated as recently reviewed [8,9]. Among the early but smaller scaled studies including from 36 to 91 patients, three Scandinavian studies will be briefly summarized.

In the Steno studies 1 and 2, a total of 70 patients with IDDM had been included and randomized to either unchanged conventional insulin treatment or to intensified treatment using portable insulin infusion pumps [10-12].

The long-term glycemic control given as the mean of all HbA_{1c} readings during the entire follow up period had been significantly improved in the insulin infusion groups during the 5 to 8 years of follow-up:

HbA_{1c} at entry - HbA_{1c} mean of all; (insulin infusion group vs control group), (%)) Steno I: 2.0±0.6 versus 0.7±1.2; Steno 2: 1.8±1.2 versus 0.4±1.3 ($p<0.01$). In Steno I with the longest follow-up, the decline rate of glomerular filtration rate was reduced from -3.7 (-5.4 to -2.0) (mean, 95% confidence interval) to - 1.0 (-2.1 to -0.1) ml/min/1.73m^2 ($p<0.05$). More patients had progressed to clinical nephropathy during conventiona l insulin treatment than in the insulin infusion groups. Also among the 19 patients with an initial UAER in the high range from 100 to 300 mg/24h, a significant treatment effect was observed. Thus clinical nephropathy (10/10 versus 2/9, $p<0.01$) and arterial hypertension (7/10 vs 1/9, $p<0.01$) were diagnosed more often in the the conventional treatment group.

In the Oslo study [13-15] 45 IDDM patients had been included. In general the patients had less severe microangiopathy than the patients of the Steno Studies. After four years of continuous subcutaneous insulin infusion, UAER was reduced from 26±3 (SEM) to 16±5 mg/24h ($2p<0.01$). No change was observed in the conventional treatment group: 21±4 to 22±6 mg/24h. After 4 years the randomization had been broken. The follow up after 7 years analyzed the patients according to their long-term glycemic level in terms of 7 year mean HbA_1 values [14]. None of the patients received antihypertensive treatment and the protein intake had been unchanged. The patients increasing their UAER by more than 300 mg/24h had significantly higher HbA_1 values during the 7 years of study. The diastolic blood pressure was unchanged in patients with a mean HbA_1<10%, but increased slightly in patients with HbA_1 >10% (NS). The changes in glomerular filtration rates were not associated to the glycemic control, but the changes had only been minor in the study groups with a mean change of -1.1 ml/min/year or less [14].

In the Stockholm Study [16,17,18] all the patients had to have a poor glycaemic control at entry. The control was improved by means of intensified treatment regimens without the use of insulin infusion pumps. Ninetyfive patients had been included and randomized to an unchanged regimen (n=51) or intensified treatment (n=44). They all had non-proliferative retinopathy and a normal s-creatinine and had been followed for 5 years or more. Antihypertensive treatment was added if needed but was not accounted for in the paper [16]. Eight in the control group developed diabetic nephropathy in contrast to none in the intensified treatment group ($p<0.05$). The changes in UAER was related to the mean HbA_{1c} levels in a dose-related manner. Manifest nephropathy after 3 years was seen almost exclusively in patients with HbA_{1c} levels above 9%. The glomerular filtration rate decreased by a mean of 7 ml/min during three years of study with no differences between the groups (intensified treatment group: 122±3 to 115±3 ml/min, $p<0.05$).

In a ten-year follow-up, endothelial function was measured as flow-mediated dilation of the right brachial artery. Also the carotid arteries were scanned for plaques, intima-media thickness was measured and arterial wall stiffness was calculated [18]. Patients with lower HbA_{1C} generally had better endothelial function and less stiff arteries [18].

A meta regression analysis of the results from 16 prospective randomized studies including the Scandinavian studies was performed [8]. In these studies, the mean reduction of HbA_{1c} had been 1.45% (as an example, a reduction of HbA_{1c} from 9.2% to 7.8%). After more than two years of intensified therapy the risk of retinopathy progression was lower (odds ratio 0.49 (95% confidence interval 0.28-0.85, $p=0.011$). The risk of nephropathy progression was also decreased significantly (odds ratio 0.34 (0.20-0.58, $p<0.001$). The incidence of severe hypoglycemia was increased by 9.1 episodes per 100 patient years in the intensively treated patients. The incidence of diabetic ketoacidoses increased by 12.6 episodes per 100 patient years (95 confidence interval 8.7-16.5) in the patients treated with continuous subcutaneous insulin infusion.

2.2 The Diabetes Control and Complication Trial (DCCT). The American Experience

The DCCT study is a multicenter study performed in the period 1983 to 1993. The data were published in New England Journal of Medicine in september 1993 [19]. It comprised 1441 IDDM patients of whom only 19 patients dropped out. They had been randomized to either conventional insulin treatment with 1 to 2 daily insulin injections or to intensified treatment with more than 3 daily injections. This group also had to measure blood-glucose 4 times a day (and the adherence to this regimen had been documented). If so wished they could choose to be treated with portable insulin infusionpumps. The aims were:

1. To study if intensified treatment can prevent development of retinopathy (primary intervention of complications, 726 patients).
2. To study if intensified treatment can delay or stop the progression of retinopathy (secundary prevention of complications, 715 patients).

Other indicators of diabetic complications as for instance the UAER and blood pressure were carefully monitored as well.

The main results were:

The mean HbA_{1c} at baseline had been 8.8 and 9.0% in the study groups. In the intensified treatment group the mean HbA_{1c} was maintained at about 7.0% throughout the study i.e. for a mean of 6.5 years. The upper reference level of HbA_{1c} was 6.05%. Only 5% of the patients on intensified treatment were consistently treated to a level below or equal to that level.

Intensified treatment had reduced the risk of developing the first microaneurism by 27% (95% confidence interval; 11-40) (primary intervention) and of developing moderate retinopathy by 76% (62-85) (secondary intervention). In the secondary intervention study, the risk of progression to severe non-proliferative - or proliferative retinopathy had been reduced by 47% (14-67). A positive correlation between HbA_{1c} and development of retinopathy was observed (Figure 43-1). This was taken by the authors to indicate that any reduction of HbA_{1c} should reduce the risk of retinopathy. The figure may to my mind however also be taken as an indication of the existence of a cut off point of HbA_{1c} of about 7.5% below which very little extra protection against complications can be obtained.

In the intensified treatment groups, the risk of *developing* microalbuminuria (UAER >40 mg/24h) were reduced by 39% (21-52) and for *developing* clinical nephropathy (UAER >300 mg/24h), by 54% (19-74). A recent subanalysis of 73 patients with microalbuminuria at entry showed no difference in the rate of *progression* to clinical albuminuria which occurred in eight patients in each group [20].

The risk reductions of development and progression of neuropathy was 60 % (38-74).

The most serious side-effects of intensified treatment had been the risk of severe hypoglycaemia which had been increased by a factor 3.5. An inverse correlation between HbA_{1c} and severe hypoglycaemia was observed (figure 43-2). The risk of ketoacidoses were similar in the groups, 1.8 versus 2.0 cases per 100 patient year respectively.

In a more recent publication it was shown that also in the DCCT study, intensive glycemic control had extended the time of demonstrable islet function [21].

2.3 Microalbuminuria collaborative study group. The UK Experience

From 1984 to 1993 in the UK a randomized controlled multicentre study of intensive versus conventional therapy was performed [22]. Seventy patients with IDDM and microalbuminuria in the range of 30 μg/min-200 μg/min (overnight urine) were included and followed for a medium of 5 years (2-8 years). Mean HbA_1 which initially was similar (10.3% vs, 9.8%) fell significantly in the intensive therapy group only. The difference was maintained for three years with an absolute difference of about 1% between the groups. It could be questioned whether this small improvement of the glycaemic control is sufficient to rule out effects of improved control. Progression to clinical proteinuria occurred in six patients in each group. The Study Group concluded: Arterial blood pressure rather than glycated haemoglobin concentration seems to be the main predictor of progression of microalbuminuria.

3. INTENSIFIED INSULIN TREATMENT. PRACTICAL GUIDELINES

The intensified treatment regimens operates with at least three important principles

First, frequent or continuous administration of fast-acting insulins and little or no (infusionpumps) use of intermediate or long-acting insulins. The advantages of this is (a) small differences between the administered and absorbed amounts of insulin over 24 h, (b) postprandial insulin peaks and (c) a stable overnight insulin level (at least when administered by insulin infusionpumps).

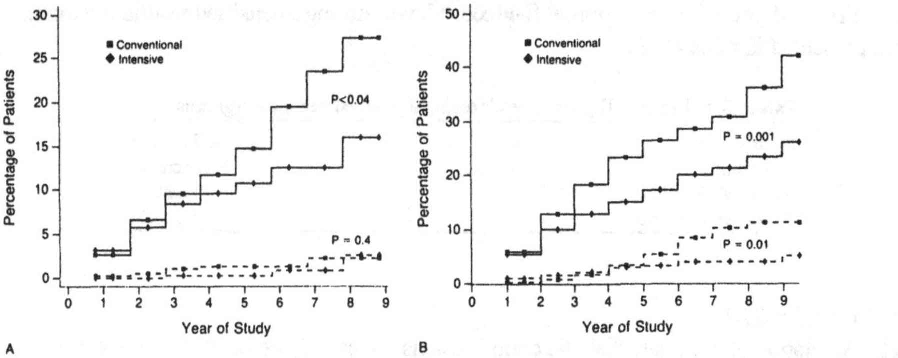

Figure 43-1 Cumulative incidence of urinary albumin excretion ≥ 300 mg per 24 hours (dashed line) and ≥40 mg per 24 hours (solid line) in patients with IDDM receiving intensive or conventional therapy. In the primary-prevention cohort (Panel A), intensive therapy reduced the adjusted mean risk of microalbuminuria by 34% (P<0.04). In the secondary-intervention cohort (Panel B), patients with urinary albumin excretion of ≥ 40 mg per 24 hours at baseline were excluded from the analysis of the development of microalbuminuria. Intensive therapy reduced the adjusted mean risk of albuminuria by 56% (P=0.01) and the risk of microalbuminuria by 43% (P=0.001), as compared with conventional therapy.

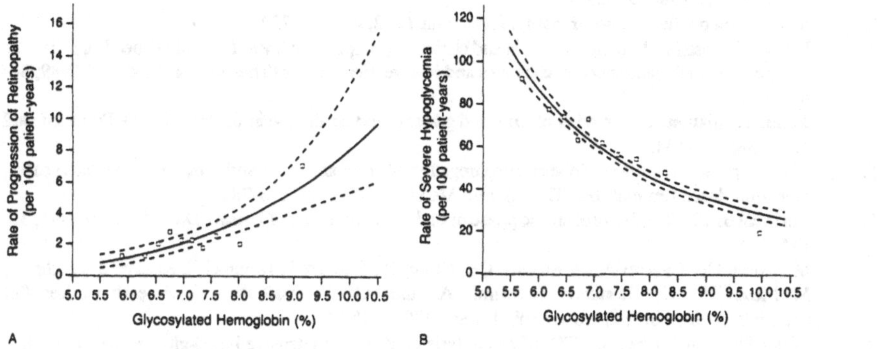

Figure 43-2 Risk of sustained progression of retinopathy (panel A) and rate of severe hypoglycaemia (panel B) in the patients receiving intensive therapy, according to their mean glycosylated haemoglobin values during the trial. In panel A, the glycosylated haemoglobin values used were the mean of the values obtained every six months. In panel B, the mean of the monthly values was used. Squares indicate the crude rates within deciles of the mean glycosylated haemoglobin values during the trial; each square corresponds to more than 400 patient-years. The solid lines are regression lines estimated as a function of the log of the mean glycosylated haemoglobin value in panel A and the log of the lines are regression lines estimated as a function of the log of the mean glycosylated haemoglobin value in panel A, and the log of the glycosylated haemoglobin value in panel B; the dashed lines are 95 per cent confidence intervals.

<u>Second</u>, frequent blood glucose readings before meals and bedtime, making it possible to adjust the injected amount of insulin, not only according to experience (size and character of meal, physical exercise etc.) but also according to actual glycemic level, and,

Third, educational programmes making possible all the above.

Practical guidelines for optimal B-glucose levels during intensified insulin treatment are presented in table 43-1.

Table 43-1. Target of B-glucose levels during intensified treatment regimens.

Fasting	4-7 mmol/l
Postprandial	5-10 mmol/l
Avoid values below	3 mmol/l
Avoid values above	10 mmol/l

4. CONCLUSION

The development of all late diabetic complications are closely associated with the quality of long-term glycemic control, and improving the control significantly reduces the risk of complications. There are indications that also progression of established lesions may benefit from improved glycemic control although this is still debated [18,20]. Optimizing glycaemic control and other treatment modalities after myocardial infarction is an important new area for improving the prognosis of patients with diabetes mellitus [23].

REFERENCES

1. Rosenstock J, Raskin P. Early diabetic nephropathy: Assesment and potential therapeutic interventions. Diabetes Care 1986; 9: 529-545.
2. Symposium on diabetic nephropathy. Kidney Int 1992; 41: 717-729.
3. Feldt-Rasmussen B. Microalbuminuria and clinical nephropathy in Type 1 (insulin-dependent). diabetes mellitus: Pathophysiological mechanisms and intervention studies (Thesis). Dan Med Bull 1989; 36: 405-415.
4. Jensen T. Albuminuria-a marker of renal and general vascular disease in IDDM (Thesis). Dan Med Bull 1991; 38: 134-144.
5. Mathiesen ER. Prevention of diabetic nephropathy: Microalbuminuria and perspectives for intervention in insulin-dependent diabetes (Thesis). Dan Med Bull 1993; 40: 273-285.
6. Christensen CK. The pre-proteinuric phase of diabetic nephropathy (Thesis). Dan Med Bull 1991; 38: 145-159.
7. Mogensen CE, Chacati A, Christensen CK, Close CF, Deckert T, Hommel E, Kastrup J, Lefebre P, Mathiesen ER, Feldt-Rasmussen B, Schmitz A, Viberti GC. Microalbuminuria: An early marker of of renal involvement in diabetes. Uremia Invest 1986; 9: 85-95.
8. Wang PH, Lau J, Chalmers TC. Meta-analysis of effects of intensive blood-glucose control on late complications of Type 1 diabetes. Lancet 1993; 341: 1306-1309.
9. Hanssen KF, Dahl-Jørgensen K, Lauritzen T, Feldt-Rasmussen B, Brinchmann-Hansen O, Deckert T. Diabetic control and microvascular complications: The near-normoglycaemic experience. Diabetologia 1986; 29: 677-684.
10. Lauritzen T, Frost-Larsen K, Larsen HW, Deckert T, Steno Study Group. Two years experience with continuous subcutaneous insulin infusion in relation to retinopathy and neuropathy. Diabetes 1985; 34 suppl 3: 74-79.
11. Feldt-Rasmussen B, Mathiesen ER, Deckert T. Effect of 2 years of of strict metabolic control on progression of incipient nephropathy in insulin-dependent diabetes. Lancet 1986; i: 1300-1304.
12. Feldt-Rasmussen B, Mathiesen ER, Jensen T, Lauritzen T, Deckert T. Effect of improved metabolic control on loss of kidney function in insulin-dependent diabetic patients. Diabetologia 1991; 34: 164-170.
13. Dahl-Jørgensen K, Hanssen KF, Kierulf P, Bjøro T, Sandvik L, Aagenaess Ø. Reduction of urinary albumin excretion after 4 years of continuous subcutaneous insulin infusion in insulin-dependent diabetes mellitus. Acta Endocrinol 1988; 117: 19-25.

14. Dahl-Jørgensen K, Bjøro T, Kierulf P, Sandvik L, Bangstad HJ, Hanssen KF. The effect of long-term stict glycemic control on kidney function in insulin-dependent diabetes mellitus: seven years result from the Oslo Study. Kidney Int 1992; 41; 920-923.
15. Bangstad H-J, Østerby R, Dahl-Jørgensen K, et al. Early glomerulopathy is present in young Type 1 (insulin-dependent) diabetic patients with microalbuminuria. Diabetologia 1993; 36: 523-529.
16. Reichard P, Berglund B, Britz A, Cars I, Nilsson BY, Rosenqvist U. Intensified conventional insulin treatment retards the microvascular complications of insulin-dependent diabetes mellitus (IDDM). The Stockholm Diabetes Intervention Study after five years. J Int Med 1991; 230: 101-108.
17. Reichard P, Nilsson BY, Rosenqvist U. The effect of long-term intensified insulin treatment on the development of microvascular complications of diabetes mellitus. N Engl J Med 1993; 329: 304-309.
18. Jensen-Urstadt KJ, Reichard PG, Rosfors JS, Lindblad JS, Lindblad LEL, Jensen-Urstadt MT. Early atherosclerosis is retarded by improved long-term blood glucose control in patients with IDDM. Diabetes 1996; 45: 1253-1258.
19. The Diabetes Control an Complication Trial Research Group. The effect of intensive treatment of diabetes on the development and progression of long-term complications in insulin-dependent diabetes mellitus. N Engl J Med 1993; 329: 977-986.
20. Diabetes Control and Complications (DCCT) Research Group. Effect of intensive therapy on the development and progression of diabetic nephropathy in the diabetes control and complications trial. Kidney Int 1995; 42: 1703-1720.
21. Steffes M, Tamburlane W, Becker D, Palmer J, Cleary P for the DCCT research group. The effect of intensive diabetes treatment on residual beta cell function in the Diabetes Control and Complications Trial (DCCT) Abstract. Diabetes 1996; 46 suppl. 2: 18A.
22. Microalbuminuria Collaborative Study Group, United Kingdom. Intensive therapy and progression to clinical albuminuria in patients with insulin dependent diabetes mellitus and microalbuminuria. BMJ 1995; 311: 973-977.
23. Malmberg K, Rydén L, Efendic S, Herlitz J, Nicol P, Waldenström A, Wedel H, Welin L on behalf of the Digami Study Group. Randomized trial of insulin-glucose infusion followed by subcutaneous insulin treatment in diabetic patients with acute myocardial infarction (DIGAMI study): Effects on mortality at 1 year. JACC 1995; 26: 57-65.

44. NON-GLYCAEMIC INTERVENTION IN DIABETIC NEPHROPATHY: THE ROLE OF DIETARY PROTEIN INTAKE

James D. Walker
Department of Diabetes, Royal Infirmary of Edinburgh, Edinburgh, Scotland

By the time clinical diabetic nephropathy is diagnosed by persistent proteinuria and a declining glomerular filtration rate (GFR), treatment options to preserve renal function are limited. Improving glycaemic control at this stage of the disease process is difficult and has little influence on the rate of decline of the GFR [1-3] whereas treatment of a raised blood pressure (BP) is more efficacious [4-8]. Dietary protein restriction has long been known to influence renal function [9] and numerous studies have tested the effect of dietary protein restriction in various renal diseases [10]. Additionally in animal models of chronic renal failure dietary protein restriction lessens proteinuria, mesangial expansion and glomerulosclerosis and preserves GFR [11-14]. This chapter discusses the influence of dietary protein on renal function and examines the effects of the therapeutic manoeuvre of restricting dietary protein in diabetic nephropathy.

DIETARY PROTEIN AND RENAL FUNCTION

Normal humans

Vegans who eat less total protein than omnivores (0.95 vs. 1.29 g/kg/day) and 100% of their protein intake is the form of vegetable protein, have glomerular filtration rates that are 11% lower than matched omnivores [15]. In addition, urinary albumin excretion and blood pressure levels are lower [15]. A similar effect of diet on blood pressure is seen after a 6 week period of a lacto-ovo-vegetarian diet in healthy habitually omnivorous subjects independent of changes in weight and sodium or potassium intake [16]. In normal humans consuming a usual diet GFR increases by 7-18% and urinary albumin excretion by 100-300% in response to a meat meal of 80 g of protein as lean cooked beef [17,18]. In contrast a 3 week period of low-protein diet (LPD) (43 g/day) causes a 14% reduction in baseline GFR, a 9% reduction in renal plasma flow (RPF) and a 50% reduction in the urinary albumin excretion rate [17].

In diabetic patients

Normoalbuminuric insulin-dependent patients completing 3 weeks of LPD (45

Mogensen, C.E. (ed.), THE KIDNEY AND HYPERTENSION IN DIABETES MELLITUS.

g/day) had a reduction in GFR with no difference in RPF and thus a reduction in filtration fraction (FF) (FF=GFR/RPF) [19]. This contrasts to the effect of LPD on FF in non-diabetics [17]. Glycaemic control and blood pressure levels were unchanged while the fractional clearance of albumin was lower on LPD. A larger study involving 35 normoalbuminuric insulin-dependent diabetic patients investigated the response to a 100 g/1.73 m^2 protein load in the form of a meat meal [18]. The area under the glomerular filtration rate curve rose more in normals than in the diabetic patients by a factor of 3.8. The impaired response of glomerular filtration rate to the meat meal in the diabetic patients was not due to differences in absorption of the meal since plasma levels of branched-chain amino acids were not different between normals and diabetics. Possible mechanisms of the differing responses included glucagon-mediated increases in the vasodilatory prostaglandins, prostaglandin E_2
and 6-keto prostaglandin $F_{1\alpha}$, which were impaired in diabetics.

A similar study employing a cross-over design tested the renal effects of 10 days of a diet of 0.9 g/kg/day or 1.9 g/kg/day of dietary protein. GFR and FF were lower on the diet containing the lesser amount of protein with a more marked fall in GFR in those patients with glomerular hyperfiltration (GFR >127 ml/min) [20].

At the stage of microalbuminuria a reduction in GFR, urinary albumin excretion rate and fractional clearance of albumin was seen after 3 weeks of a low-protein diet (47 g/day) [21]. These changes were independent of changes in glycaemia or blood pressure. In insulin-dependent diabetic patients with diabetic nephropathy 3 weeks of LPD was associated with an improvement in glomerular permselectivity while no differences were seen in renal haemodynamics (GFR, RPF, and FF) between the two diet periods [22,23]. The reabsorption rate of B_2 microglobulin was similar in both diet periods, suggesting that tubular function was not influenced by the different diets.

Thus in both normals and diabetic subjects with microalbuminuria and glomerular hyperfiltration, short-term dietary protein restriction leads to a reduction in albuminuria and GFR whereas in diabetic patients with proteinuria although urinary protein loss is diminished in the short-term, this intervention has no effects on renal haemodynamics.

MEDIATORS OF RENAL EFFECTS OF DIETARY PROTEIN

In order to define some of the determinants of the change in glomerular filtration rate in response to different dietary protein intakes, Krishna and colleagues administered a 1 g of protein/kg body weight as beef steak, to 9 healthy males [24]. The renal haemodynamic studies were repeated on three separate occasions after pretreatment with either placebo, indomethacin (to inhibit renal prostaglandin synthesis) or enalapril (to inhibit angiotensin II synthesis). Following placebo GFR increased by 29% with an accompanying increase in RPF and a fall in renal vascular resistance (RVR). Pretreatment with indomethacin attenuated the rise in the GFR (12% rise) whereas treatment with enalapril was not different to placebo. Urinary excretion rates of prostaglandin E_2 fell significantly in the indomethacin group, levels of plasma renin activity were increased in the enalapril group while plasma noradrenaline and adrenaline were unchanged in all groups. From these data it appears that the protein-mediated elevation in glomerular filtration is in part associated with prostaglandin levels. In diabetic patients the attenuated glucagon response to a protein challenge may mediate the reduced prostaglandin effect [18].

The effects of similar amounts of animal and vegetable protein ingestion on renal haemodynamics were investigated in a short-term study of 10 normal males [25]. GFR, RPF and the fractional clearance of albumin were all lower on the vegetable protein diet while renal vascular resistance (RVR) was higher compared to the animals protein diet. In a separate experiment, seven normal subjects were given an 80 g protein load of animal protein (lean cooked beef) and subsequently 80 g of diluted soya powder (vegetable protein). While an elevation in GFR and RPF and a reduction in RVR was seen after animal protein no changes occurred after soya. The incremental glucagon area was greater for meat than soya and whereas the vasodilatory prostaglandin 6-keto $PGF_{1\alpha}$ rose significantly after the animal protein, it did not change after soya challenge. From these data, it appears that the same quantity of vegetable protein causes different renal effects compared to animal protein, and that this difference is associated with a smaller glucagon and vasodilatory prostaglandin response. These hormonal mediators have been also implicated from a study in which infusion of somatostatin diminished the renal response to amino-acid infusion [26].

Elevated levels of plasma renin activity on high protein diets have been observed in man and experimental animals [22,27]. This difference could not be explained in terms of differences in sodium or potassium intakes, which were identical between the two diets. As prostaglandins are known to mediate renin release [27,28] the elevated levels of prostaglandins may have caused the elevated renin levels. Although there were no changes in mean arterial pressure between the two diet periods the elevated renin levels may have resulted in increased levels of angiotensin II to cause constriction of both the afferent and efferent glomerular arterioles. The role of angiotensin II in the physiological and pathophysiological response to low-protein feeding may be important since in the rat captopril reverses the reduced GFR and RPF and increased renal vascular resistance seen with LPD [29].

Other mediators in addition to glucagon, prostaglandin and the renin/angiotensin/ aldosterone system may be involved in the renal response to dietary protein. Recently increased levels of mRNA for PDGF-A and -B chains and TGF-ß genes have been shown to correlate with glomerulosclerosis in a rat model [30]. Low-protein feeding reduced the prevalence of glomerulosclerosis and attenuated the abnormally high expression of the PDGF-A and -B and TGF-ß genes. These data suggest that growth factors may play a role in the development of glomerulosclerosis and can be modulated by LPD.

LONG-TERM CLINICAL STUDIES OF LOW-PROTEIN DIETS IN PATIENTS WITH DIABETIC NEPHROPATHY

Some studies designed to test the effects of a diet restricted in protein in insulin dependent patients with diabetic nephropathy have used creatinine clearance or the reciprocal of the serum creatinine to assess renal function (table 44-1). This is not an accurate or precise measure of GFR compared to isotopic clearance methods, such as the plasma clearance of ^{51}Cr EDTA, which give nearly identical values to inulin clearances. In addition changes in the creatine pool and creatinine intake seen in low-protein diet studies further render such measurements unreliable for the assessment of GFR [31-35].

Study designs have varied. Evanoff used patients as their own control [36]. After a 12 month observation period a LPD of 0.6 g/kg/day was instituted and, using creatinine clearance and the reciprocal of the serum creatinine to assess renal functional response, 11 patients were studied for 2 years [35]. The period of LPD was associated with a slowing in the rate of decline of the reciprocal of the serum creatinine and no change in the creatinine clearance levels during the 2 years of study. However, 9 of the 11 patients had antihypertensive agents initiated during the study and systolic blood pressure levels fell significantly. No attempts were made to correct for the substantial fall in systolic blood pressure (about 20 mmHg) and it is therefore difficult to separate the effects of the blood pressure reduction from those of LPD making interpretation of the effects of LPD in this study difficult. Using the same study design Barsotti followed 8 patients with more severe renal impairment for 16 months on a normal protein diet (NPD) (1.2 to 1.4 g/kg/day) and then instituted a more restrictive protein prescription of 0.25 to 0.35 g/kg/day with essential amino acid supplementation for a mean duration of 17 months [37]. Urinary urea and urinary protein levels fell during the diet, body weight, triceps skin thickness, mid-arm muscle circumference and plasma albumin levels were unchanged and insulin requirements fell despite an increase in the carbohydrate intake. The rate of decline of creatinine clearance was slowed on LPD in a heterogeneous manner.

A 6 month controlled study involving 7 patients in a LPD and 9 in a control group revealed no changes in creatinine clearance but a reduction in urinary albumin excretion on LPD [38]. The majority of patients in both groups had serum creatinine levels that were within the normal range indicating well preserved renal function and thus it was not surprising that no change in creatinine clearances were observed in this short-term study. A more recent study employing the same study design with 11 patients in each group, with more impairment of GFR, demonstrated that during a six month follow-up LPD stabilised the decline in GFR and reduced the degree of proteinuria from 2.15 to 1.13 g/day [39]. Importantly, GFR was measured isotopically and blood pressure was similar in both the NPD and LPD patients.

A larger controlled trial that employed an isotopic clearance method for measurement of GFR demonstrated a significant reduction in the rate of decline of GFR after 37 months on a low-protein diet (0.72 g/kg/day) compared to a control group on a normal protein diet (1.08 g/kg/day) for this period [40]. Blood pressure was lower in the group on the low-protein diet but when included as an independent variable in a stepwise regression analysis with change in glomerular filtration rate as the dependent variable, it was found to exert no significant effect. Interestingly, the rate of decline of GFR was only significantly different between the patients on the two diets when those with initial glomerular filtration rates above 45 ml/min were considered. This may be taken to suggest that dietary intervention should be introduced early in the course of diabetic nephropathy before significant reductions in glomerular filtration rate occur. There was no indication that the LPD had any nutritional adverse effect. Serum cholesterol and triglyceride levels were increased during the LPD period but the changes failed to reach statistical significance.

The only other prospective study employing an isotopic clearance method to assess GFR investigated the effect of LPD in 19 insulin-dependent diabetic patients with nephropathy. Patients were followed for 29 months on NPD (1.11 g/kg/day) and subsequently for 33 months on LPD (0.66 g/kg/day). GFR decline was slowed by an average of 0.47 ml/min/month (figure 44-1) and the rise in albuminuria halted independent of changes in glycaemia or blood pressure [41]. The effect of LPD on the decline in GFR was heterogeneous with 10 of the 19 patients exhibiting a significant slowing yet in the remaining 9 the rate was either non-significantly slower or in some cases faster. No identified factors separated the responders from the non-responders. This study quantitated and emphasised the heterogeneity of the GFR response with has also been observed in a trial of antihypertensive therapy in patients with diabetic nephropathy [5].

A recently published meta-analysis of the effect of dietary protein restriction on the progression of renal disease has included patients with diabetic nephropathy [42]. The studies identified for the meta-analysis included 4 presently summarised in table 40-1 [38-41] and a study involving microalbuminuric patients [43]. The relative risk for progression of renal disease in insulin-dependent diabetic patients on a low-protein diet was 0.56 (95% confidence intervals 0.40 to 0.77). A reduced relative risk was also seen in cases of non-diabetic renal disease treated with a low-protein diet [42]. The validity of this metanalysis has recently been questioned by Parving [43].

PROBLEMS WITH LOW-PROTEIN DIETS

Two main problems are associated with the prescription of a LPD namely protein/calorie malnutrition and compliance [44,47]. Protein intakes below 0.6 g/kg/day have been associated with protein malnutrition [45,46] and the aim of a LPD should be reduce protein intake to a non-harmful yet achievable level by the majority of patients. Despite increased carbohydrate intake, necessary to compensate for the calorie reduction caused by a reduction in dietary protein, energy intake has been reported to fall and a small degree of weight loss occur on LPD in some studies [37,41]. However, stable or increased serum albumin levels and no change in mid-arm muscle circumference are reassuring parameters and suggest that the levels of protein reduction in reported studies are not associated with muscle loss and protein malnutrition [40,41].

Compliance is a prerequisite for this form of treatment and 2 recent studies, one involving patients with diabetes and microalbuminuria, have demonstrated how difficult this can be to achieve. Locatelli, in a large study, prescribed a LPD of 0.6 g/kg/day yet the achieved level of protein intake was 0.83 g/kg/day [47] - not a low-protein diet. In patients with diabetes and microalbuminuria only 7 of 14 patients achieved the prescribed protein reduction of <0.8 g/kg/day during a 2 year study [44]. The reasons for the poor level of compliance in this study may include the lack of concern of the patients about their renal condition at this early stage of renal disease.

Table 44-1. Clinical studies of low protein diet in insulin-dependent patients with diabetic nephropathy

AUTHOR / YEAR	STUDY DESIGN	DIETARY PRESCRIPTION	DIETARY ASSESSMENT	GFR ASSESSMENT	DURATION OF LPD	OUTCOME
Raal, 1994	Randomised controlled, 22 pts.	0.8 g/kg/day in pts. 1.6 g/kg/day in controls		Plasma clearance of ^{51}Cr EDTA	6 months	Decrease in TUP in LPD group GFR fell at 1.3 ml/min/mo in NPD group. No change in LPD group.
Zeller, 1991	Randomised controlled, 68 pts.	0.72 g/kg/day in pts. 1.08 g/kg/day in controls	Weighed food records Urinary urea nitrogen	Iothalamate clearances	37 months	Iothalamate clearances 0.26 ml/min/mo in pts. 1.01 ml/min/mo in controls MBP 102 in pts., 105 in controls
Walker, 1989	Self controls 19 tps.	1.1 g/kg/day on NPD→0.66 g/kg/day on LPD	Weighed food records Urinary urea nitrogen	Plasma clearance of ^{51}Cr EDTA	29 months on NPD 33 months on LPD	GFR 0.61 ml/min/mo on NPD, 0.14 ml/min/ mo on LPD MBP 106 on NPD, 102 on LPD
Evanoff, 1989	Self controls 11 pts.	1.2 g/kg/day on NPD→0.95 g/kg/ day on LPD	Dietary recall urinary urea nitrogen	Creatinine clearance l/serum creatinine	24 months	Δ l/serum creatinine -0.18/yr on NPD -0.03/yr on LPD Systolic BP 147 LPD□126 NPD
Barsotti, 1988	Self controls 8 pts.	1.3 g/kg/day on NPD 0.3 g/kg/day on LPD (supplemented with essential amino- and ketoacids)	Urinary urea nitrogen	Creatinine clearance	17 months	Decrease in TUP Increase in TPP Rate of decline in CrCl on NPD 1.38 ml/min/ mo on LPD 0.03 ml/ min/mo
Ciavarella , 1987	Randomised controlled 16 pts.	0.71 g/kg/day in pts. 1.44 g/kg/day in controls	Dietary interview Blood urea nitrogen Urinary urea nitrogen	Creatinine clearance	4.5 months	Decrease in AER in LPD group

AER = Urinary albumin excretion rate; TUP = Urinary total protein excretion rate; LPD = Low protein diet; CrCl = Creatinine clearance; NPD = Normal protein diet; TPP = Total plasma protein level; Δ = Delta (change in); All blood pressure values are in mmHg; MBP = Mean blood pressure

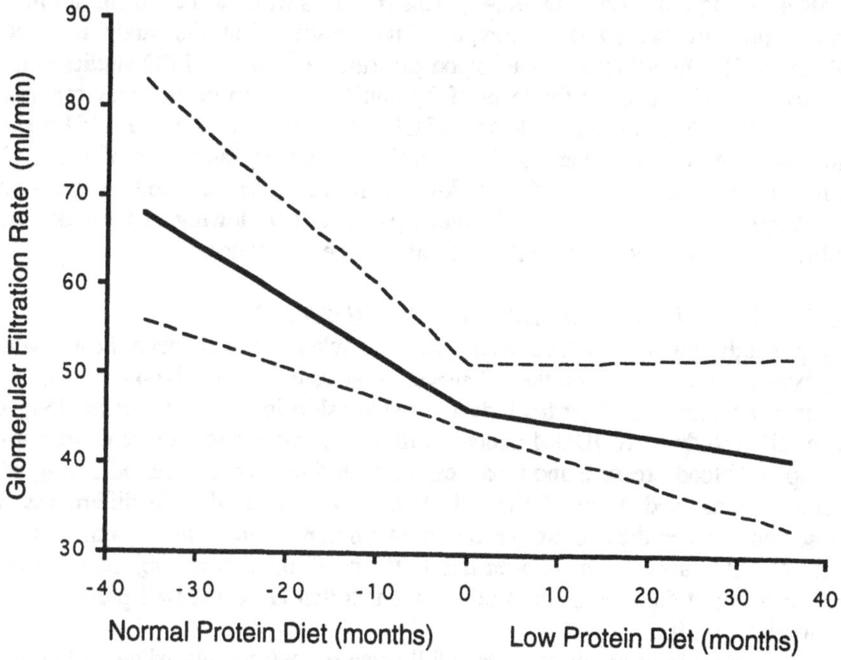

Figure 44-1. GFR decline (mean - solid line and 95% confidence intervals - dashed lines) in 19 insulin-dependent diabetic patients with nephropathy on a normal and subsequently a low protein diet. [Data taken from reference 41].

Compliance with, or more correctly adherence to, a low protein diet has recently been debated following the publication of a study investigating the effect of a LPD on the progression of chronic renal failure in children [48] in which the protein content of LPD was greater than 25% of the WHO recommended amount [49]. Thus whether such a trial can analyse the effect of a LPD on the progression of chronic renal failure is open to question [50]. Secondary analysis [51] of the Modification of Diet in Renal Disease study [52] demonstrates a close correlation between achieved protein intake and the rate of decline of the GFR suggesting that if the intervention is correctly adhered to the achieved results are more promising.

BLOOD PRESSURE TREATMENT AND DIETARY PROTEIN RESTRICTION IN DIABETIC NEPHROPATHY

No study has tested the effects of blood pressure reduction and dietary protein restriction in diabetic nephropathy. In non-diabetic renal disease evidence for an additive effect is provided by a short-term study of 17 patients in whom addition of enalapril to a LPD resulted in a further decrease in proteinuria and a reversal of some acute renal haemodynamic changes associated with LPD [53]. In diabetic patients with nephropathy, the 2 clinical trials that used isotopic clearances to assess GFR found that the small reduction in mean blood pressure on LPD exerted a very small effect on the change in GFR [40,41]. In these studies mean blood pressure was only 4 mmHg lower on LPD [40,41]. This contrasts with the 12 mmHg fall in mean blood pressure caused by antihypertensive treatment in the study reported by Parving [5]. The achieved mean blood pressure level in the LPD studies was 102 mmHg a level similar to the level of 99 mmHg achieved in the study reported by Parving [5]. The reduction in the rate of GFR decline associated with LPD is similar to that seen with treatment of hypertension. However, as levels of mean blood pressure on NPD were considerably lower than the untreated blood pressures levels of Parving's patients (106 vs. 112 mmHg) the further slowing of GFR decline on LPD argues for an additional effect of this therapeutic manoeuvre.

DIETARY SALT AND DIABETIC NEPHROPATHY

Surprisingly few studies have investigated the relationship between dietary salt and diabetic nephropathy given the extensive literature on salt and blood pressure in the general population and particularly the relationship in the renal patient [54]. One controlled study of 16 IDDM patients with nephropathy and mild renal impairment compared blood pressure and renal responses during a 4 week period during which subjects consumed 92 or 199 mmol of sodium a day [55]. No differences were observed between the two groups in term of blood pressure or renal parameters. This lack of difference may have been due to the small number of subjects studied, the relatively short duration of the study or the fact that GFR was well preserved in the individuals studied.

Dietary sodium intake tends to fall when patients are placed on a LPD. In one study with IDDM mean urinary sodium excretion fell significantly from 178 on a usual protein diet to 143 mmol/day on a LPD [41]. Thus the prescription of a LPD will in itself cause a reduction in salt intake.

In clinical practice all patients with diabetes are assessed by dietician and a part of this assessment details the dietary salt intake and advice is given when indicated. In those with significant renal functional impairment the advice on dietary sodium restriction will be more specific.

CONCLUSIONS AND IMPLICATIONS

There is now enough evidence to strongly support the hypothesis that a reduction in the dietary intake of protein retards the rate of decline of renal functional loss in cases of established diabetic nephropathy in patients with insulin-dependent diabetes mellitus, but generally more work needs to be done [56]. Subjecting a patient to this dietary regime should not be undertaken lightly and needs full co-operation of the patient and full involvement of a nutritionist experienced in this field. GFR response to LPD appears to be heterogeneous thus making it is vital to assess whether an individual is benefiting from the intervention. Patients who remain heavily proteinuric (>6 g/day) despite adequate blood pressure control and treatment with an angiotensin-converting enzyme inhibitor should be strongly considered for LPD therapy. It would thus be prudent for such patients to have a run-in period on their usual diet and therapy with 3 isotopic measurement of GFR to establish a baseline rate of decline against which the response to LPD can be compared. Protein restriction of 0.6 g/kg/day appears to have no untoward nutritional effect.

Interestingly nutritional intake of protein continue to be generally high among diabetic patients [57].

REFERENCES

1. Bending JJ, Pickup JC, Viberti GC, Keen H. Glycaemic control in diabetic nephropathy. BMJ 1984; 288: 1187-1191.
2. Bending JJ, Viberti GC, Watkins PJ, Keen H. Intermittent clinical proteinuria and renal function in diabetes: evolution and the effect of glycaemic control. BMJ 1986; 292: 83-86.
3. Viberti GC, Bilous RW, Mackintosh D, Bending JJ, Keen H. Long term correction of hyperglycaemia and progression of renal failure in insulin-dependent diabetes. BMJ 1983; 286: 598-602.
4. Mogensen CE. Long-term antihypertensive treatment inhibiting progression of diabetic nephropathy. BMJ 1982; 285: 685-688.
5. Parving H-H, Andersen AR, Smidt UM, Hommel E, Mathiesen ER, Svendsen PA. Effect of antihypertensive treatment on kidney function in diabetic nephropathy. BMJ 1987; 294: 1443-1447.
6. Björck S, Mulec H, Johnsen SA, Nyberg G, Aurell M. Contrasting effects of enalapril and metoprolol on proteinuria in diabetic nephropathy. BMJ 1990; 300: 904-907.
7. Björck S, Mulec H, Johnsen SA, Nordén G, Aurell M. Renal protective effect of enalapril in diabetic nephropathy. BMJ 1992; 304: 339-343.
8. Mogensen CE. Angiotensin converting enzyme inhibitors and diabetic nephropathy. Their effects on proteinuria may be independent of their effects on blood pressure. BMJ 1992; 304: 327-328.
9. Folin P. Laws governing the chemical composition of urine. Am J Physiol 1905; 13: 66.
10. Fouque D, Laville M, Boisell JP, Chifflet R, Labeeuw M, Zech PY. Controlled low protein diets in chronic renal insufficiency: meta-analysis. BMJ 1992; 304: 216-220.
11. Nath KA, Kren SA, Hostetter TH. Dietary protein restriction in established renal injury in the rat. J Clin Invest 1986; 78: 1199-1205.
12. Hostetter TH, Meyer TW, Rennke HG, Brenner BM. Chronic effects of dietary protein in the rat with intact and reduced renal mass. Kidney Int 1986; 30: 509-517.
13. El Nahas AM, Paraskevakou H, Zoob S, Rees AJ, Evans DJ. Effect of dietary protein restriction on the development of renal failure after subtotal nephrectomy in rats. Clin Sci 1983; 65: 399-406.
14. Mauer SM, Steffes MW, Azar S, Brown DM. Effect of dietary protein content in streptozotocin-diabetic rats. Kidney Int 1989; 35: 48-59.
15. Wiseman MJ, Hunt R, Goodwin A, Gross JL, Keen H, Viberti GC. Dietary composition and renal function in healthy subjects. Nephron 1987; 46: 37-42.
16. Rouse IL, Armstrong BK, Beilin LJ, Vandongen R. Blood pressure-lowering effect of a vegetarian diet: controlled trial in normotensive subjects. Lancet 1983; i: 5-10.
17. Viberti GC, Bognetti E, Wiseman MJ, Dodds R, Gross JL, Keen H. Effect of protein-restricted diet on renal response to a meat meal in humans. Am J Physiol 1987; 253: F388-F393.
18. Fioretto P, Trevisan R, Valerio A, et al. Imparied renal response to a meat meal in insulin-dependent diabetes: role of glucagon and prostaglandins. Am J Physiol 1990; 258: F675-F683.
19. Wiseman MJ, Bognetti E, Dodds R, Keen H, Viberti GC. Changes in renal function in response to protein restricted diet in type I (insulin-dependent) diabetic patients. Diabetologia 1987; 30: 154-159.
20. Rudberg S, Dahlquist G, Aperia A, Persson B. Reduction of protein intake decreases glomerular filtration rate in young Type 1 (insulin-dependent) diabetic patients mainly in hyperfiltering patients. Diabetologia 1988; 31: 878-883.
21. Cohen D, Dodds R, Viberti GC. Effect of protein restriction in insulin dependent diabetics at risk of nephropathy. BMJ 1987; 294: 795-798.
22. Rosenberg ME, Swanson JE, Thomas BL, Hostetter TH. Glomerular and hormonal responses to dietary protein intake in human renal disease. Am J Physiol 1987; 253: F1083-F1090.
23. Bending JJ, Dodds RA, Keen H, Viberti GC. Renal response to restricted protein intake in diabetic nephropathy. Diabetes 1988; 37: 1641-1646.

24. Krishna GP, Newell G, Miller E, Heeger P, Smith R, Polansky M, Kapoor S, Hoeldtke R. Protein-induced glomerular hyperfiltration: role of hormonal factors. Kidney Int 1988; 33: 578-583.
25. Kontessis P, Jones SL, Dodds RA, et al. Renal, metabolic and hormonal responses to ingestion of animal and vegetable proteins. Kidney Int 1990; 38: 136-144.
26. Castellino P, Giordano C, Perna A, DeFronzo RA. Effects of plasma amino acid and hormonal levels on renal hemodynamics in humans. Am J Physiol 1988; 247: F444-F449.
27. Paller MS, Hostetter TH. Dietary protein increases plasma renin and reduces pressor reactivity to angiotensin II. Am J Physiol 1986; 251: F34-F39.
28. Oates JA, Whorton AR, Gerkens JF, Branch RA, Hollifield JW, Frolich JC. The participation of prostaglandins in the control of renin release. Fed Proc 1979; 38: 72-74.
29. Fernandez-Repollet E, Tapia E, Martinez-Maldonado M. Effects of angiotensin-converting enzyme inhibition on altered renal hemodynamics induced by low protein diet in the rat. J Clin Invest 1987; 80: 1045-1049.
30. Fukui M, Nakamura T, Ebihara I, Nagaoka I, Tomino Y, Koide H. Low-protein diet attenuates increased gene expression of platelet-derived growth factor and transforming growth factor-ß in experimental glomerulosclerosis. J Lab Clin Med 1993; 121: 224-234.
31. Perrone RD, Madias NE, Levey AS. Serum creatinine as an index of renal function: new insights into old concepts. Clin Chem 1992; 38: 1933-1953.
32. Crim MC, Calloway DH, Margen S. Creatinine metabolism in man: creatine and creatinine excretions with creatine feeding. J Nutr 1975; 105: 428-438.
33. Crim MC, Calloway DH, Margen S. Creatinine metabolism in men: creatine pool size and turnover in relation to creatine intake. J Nutr 1976; 106: 371-381.
34. Shemesh O, Globetz M, Kriss JP, Meyers BD. Limitations of creatinine as a filtration marker in glomerulopathic patients. Kidney Int 1985; 28: 30-38.
35. Walker JD, Dodds RA, Bending JJ, Viberti GC. Monitoring kidney function in diabetic nephropathy. Diabetologia 1995; 38: 252.
36. Evanoff G, Thompson C, Brown J, Weinman E. Prolonged dietary protein restriction in diabetic nephropathy. Arch Intern Med 1989; 149: 1129-1133.
37. Barsotti G, Ciardella F, Morelli E, Cupitsti A, Mantovanelli A, Giovenetti S. Nutritional treatment of renal failure in Type 1 diabetic nephropathy. Clin Nephrol 1988; 29: 280-287.
38. Ciavarella A, Di Mizio GF, Stefoni S, Borgniino L, Vannini P. Reduced albuminuria after dietary protein restriction in insulin-dependent diabetic patients with clinical nephropathy. Diabetes Care 1987; 10: 407-413.
39. Raal FJ, Kalk WJ, Lawson M, Esser JD, Buys R, Fourie L, Panz VR. Effect of moderate dietary protein restriction on the progression of overt diabetic nephropathy: a 6-mo prospective study. Am J Clin Nutr 1994; 60: 579-585.
40. Zeller K, Whittaker E, Sullivan L, Raskin P, Jacobson HR. Effect of restricting dietary protein on renal failure in patients with insulin-dependent diabetes mellitus. N Engl J Med 1991; 324: 78-84.
41. Walker JD, Bending JJ, Dodds RA, Mattock MB, Murrells TJ, Keen H, Viberti GC. Restriction of dietary protein and progression of renal failure in diabetic nephropathy. Lancet 1989; ii: 1411-1414.
42. Pedrini MT, Levey AS, Lau J, Chalmers TC, Wang PH. The effect of dietary protein restriction on the progression of diabetic and non-diabetic renal disease: a meta-analysis. Ann Intern Med 1996; 124: 627-632.
43. Parving H-H. Effects of dietary protein in renal disease (letter). Ann Intern Med 1997; 126: 330-331.
44. Dullaart RPF, Van Doormaal JJ, Beusekamp BJ, Sluitter WJ, Meijer S. Long-term effects of protein-restricted diet on albuminuria and renal function in IDDM patients without clinical nephropathy and hypertension. Diabetes Care 1993; 16: 483-492.
45. Lucas PA, Meadows JH, Roberts DE, Coles GA. The risks and benefits of a low protein-essential amino acid-keto acid diet. Kidney Int 1986; 29: 995-1003.
46. Goodship THJ, Mitch WE. Nutritional approaches to preserving renal function. Adv Intern Med 1988; 33: 37-56.

47. Locatelli F, Alberti D, Graziani G, Buccianti G, Redaelli B, Giangrande A. Prospective, randomized, multicentre trial of effect of protein restriction on progression of chronic renal insufficiency. Lancet 1991; 337: 1299-1304.
48. Wingen AM, Fabian-Bach C, Schaefer F, Mehls O. Randomised multicentre study of a low-protein diet on the progression of chronic renal failure in children. Lancet 1997; 349: 1117-1123.
49. Ledermann S, Shaw V, Trompeter R. Low-protein diet on the progression of chronic renal failure (letter) Lancet 1997; 350:146.
50. Locatelli F. Low-protein diet on the progression of chronic renal failure (letter). Lancet 1997; 350:145.
51. Levey AS, Adler S, Caggiula AW et al. Effects of dietary protein restriction on the progression of advanced renal disease in the modification of diet in renal disease study. Am J Kidney Dis. 1996; 27: 652-663.
52. Klahr S, Levey AS, Beck GJ et al. The effects of dietary protein restriction and blood pressure control on the progression of chronic renal disease. N Engl. J Med 1994; 330: 877-884.
53. Ruilope LM, Casal MC, Praga M, et al. Additive antiproteinuric effect of converting enzyme inhibition and a low protein intake. J Am Soc Nephrol 1992; 3: 1307-1311.
54. Ritz E, Matthias S. What you should know about blood pressure in renal disease. Proc. R Coll Physicians Edinb. 1997; 27: 449-462.
55. Mulhauser I, Prange K, Sawicki PT, Bender R, Dworschak A, Berger M. Effects of dietary sodium on blood pressure in IDDM patients with nephropathy. Diabetologia 1996; 39: 212-219.
56. Maschio G. Low-protein diet and progression of renal disease: an endless story. Nephrol Dial Transplant 1995; 10: 1797-1800.
57. Toeller M, Klischan A, Heitkamp G, Schumacher W, Milne R, Buyken A, Karamanos B, Gries FA and the EURODIAB IDDM Complications Study Group. Nutritional intake of 2868 IDDM patients from 30 centres in Europe. Diabetologia 1996; 39: 929-939.

45. MICROALBUMINURIA AND DIABETIC PREGNANCY

Carl Erik Mogensen and Joachim G. Klebe
Medical Department M and Department of Gynecology/Obstetric, Aarhus Kommunehospital, Aarhus, Denmark

Renal and vascular damage, including blood pressure elevation, is often involved in complications of diabetic pregnancy. Therefore, sensitive methods for measuring elevated urinary protein excretion, especially of albumin (so-called microalbuminuria) [1-3], might be useful in early prediction of complications in diabetic as well as nondiabetic pregnancy. This is the case in nonpregnant diabetics [3-9], in whom microalbuminuria is a sensitive marker of generalized subclinical vascular disturbance and damage [6] and in whom it predicts overt nephropathy [3-6] as well as proliferative retinopathy [7]. In a normal pregnancy, increases in UAER are either absent or very limited [10-12]. However, certain low-molecular weight plasma protiens may increase in excretion rate [13]. There are certainly increases in albumin uria when preeclampsia is present [14,23]. This chapter deals with the pattern of urinary albumin excretion rate in diabetic pregnancy as studied with a sensitive radioimmunoassay for albumin using 24-h urine samples. Patients with overt nephropathy are discussed in Chapter 42

1. PATIENTS, METHODS, AND CLASSIFICATIONS

We studied 52 insulin-dependent diabetic patients consecutively. One patient was pregnant twice. Patients were studied every second week when attending the clinic for general obstetric control. About 10% of the diabetics were seen at prepregnancy consultations. In all pregnant diabetics, values were available from week 16. Blood glucose, HbA_{1c}, blood pressure, and urinary albumin excretion (UAE) (on 24-h urine samples collected at home) were determined [15].

No increase in UAE is seen either early or late in the course of normal pregnancy. In our laboratory, 330 normal pregnant women showed values of 3.0 μg/min ×/÷ 1.8 week 20 (geometric mean ×/÷ tolerance factor) (figure 45-1), corresponding to or lower than those in nonpregnant normals [15,16], and also no increase was seen late in pregnancy (weeks 38-41) in normal women (5.5 μg/ml ×/÷ 1.6 in morning urine samples, $n = 35$).

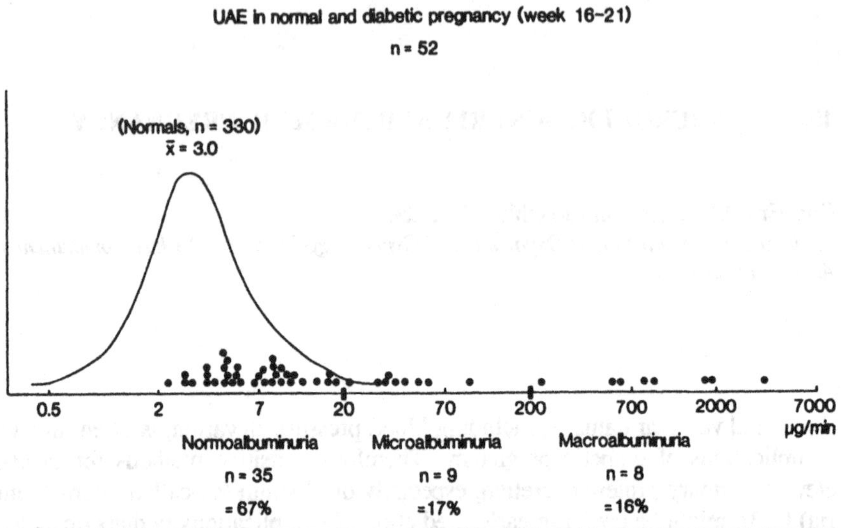

Figure 45-1. Urinary albumin excretion rate in normal and diabetic pregnancy (weeks 16-21). The *solid line* show the distribution curve for normal pregnancies ($n = 330$), and the *dots* indicate diabetics ($n = 52$).

1.1. Classification of patients

Patients were classified according to a newly proposed classification system for renal involvement in insulin-dependent diabetics [17], as outlined elsewhere in this book.

Group I included patients with diabetes diagnosed during pregnancy. Group II comprised patients with normal UAE around week 16 (≤20 µg/min). This group had to be subdivided into groups IIa and IIb since a number of patients later in pregnancy showed values higher than 20 µg/min (IIb). Group III included patients with microalbuminuria early in pregnancy (UAE 20.1-200 µg/min), and group IV included patients with clinical proteinuria, which corresponds to approximately >200 µg/min in UAE. According to this system, the 52 patients were classified as follows: I, 4; IIa, 17; IIb, 14; III, 9; and IV, 8 patients. Pertinent clinical data are presented in table 45-1, including age, duration of diabetes, initial blood pressure, and mean HbA_{1c} values, as well as information on retinal lesions and complications in general.

2. URINARY ALBUMIN EXCRETION DURING PREGNANCY

Figure 45-2 shows the longitudinal course of UAE in the group IIb, as just described. Mean values are shown, with the exception of data from three pregnancies in two patients with a complicated course. In four pregnancies (one in group IIa, two in group IIb, and one in group III), early or late intrauterine death was of recorded. One patient in group IIb developed preeclampsia. In one patient in group IIa with foetus mortus no change in UAE was seen. As table 45-1 14 shows, (45%) 31 patients changed from normoalbuminuria to microalbuminuria during

Table 45-1 Patient data including number of patients, mean age, duration of diabetes, blood pressure, HBA_{1c} values and retinopathy data creatinine clearance, number of total death, %caesarean section, and mean birth weight

Patient data	*n*	Mean age (years)	Mean known duration of diabetes	Initial MAP (mmHg)	Mean HbA_{1c} values	Retinopathy (NIL/S/P)[a]	Creatinine clearance[b] ml/min	Fetal death (*n*)	% Caesarean section	Mean birth weight (g)
I Diabetes diagnosed during pregnancy	4	26±2	-	77±8	6.0±1.4	4/0/0	111	0	0	3867
IIa Normoalbuminuria	17	27±4	13±7	81±9	6.8±1.0	8/8/1	122	1	30	3570
IIb Normo→Micro-alb.	14	25±4	11±6	85±10	6.2±0.7	7/6/1	130	2	69	3425
III Microalbuminuria	9	27±7	14±6	91±6	7.1±1.1	0/8/1	98	1	37	3505
IV Macroalbumin initially	8	26±3	16±7	100±10	6.9±1.0	1/1/6	82	0	87	2633

[a]S, simplex retinopathy; and P, proliferative retinopathy.
[b]Late in pregnancy.

pregnancy, a phenomenon generally not seen in normal pregnancy. Patients with microalbuminuria remained stable unless intrauterine death occurred. Urinary track infection unrelated to change in UAE occurred in two patients. In other studies the prevalence of microalbuminuria appears. Early in diabetic pregnancy, the prevalence of microalbuminuria appears to be the same as in non-pregnant diabetic women; however, increases in albuminuria are often seen as the pregnancy continues [18-20]. In diabetic individuals, further increases in albuminuria during a pregnancy appear to signal a more complicated course of pregnancy [10,11], but further studies are need in this area.

2.1. Blood pressure and creatinine clearance in the course of pregnancy

Figure 45-3 shows values of mean arterial pressure (MAP), defined as diastolic pressure plus one-third of pulse pressure, early (week 16) and late in pregnancy (the week before delivery). A tendency toward MAP increase in the last trimester is seen in all groups, but this increase becomes significant in only group IIb, which was characterized by an increase in UAE during pregnancy. Initial MAP increased throughout all of the groups. Creatinine clearance remained stable in all patients, except in one patient in group IV whose clearance decreased dramatically (95→31 ml/min).

2.2. Urinary albumin excretion groups and White classification

Data are presented in table 45-2. No difference in the White classification is seen between groups IIa and IIb.

3. URINARY ALBUMIN EXCRETION IN THE MANAGEMENT OF DIABETIC PREGNANCY

This consecutive study shows that marked abnormalities in UAE are seen both early and late in the course of diabetic pregnancy. In many patients, an abnormal increase in UAE was seen during pregnancy (i.e., in 45% of patients with normal values around week 20). Such increases were generally not seen in normal pregnancy [21-23], also in accordance with our normal material. In several cases, UAE changes in the subclinical range were associated with a complicated course of pregnancy. We observed four pregnancies with late intrauterine death, and one with late abortion, a rather high percentage in 53 consecutive diabetic pregnancies. In normal pregnancies, the number is very small, around 0.5%, but it remains one of the significant problems in the management of diabetic pregnancy [24,25], where the figure now is generally around 1%-2%. The three pregnancies in two patients with early or late intrauterine death showed a gradual and marked increase in UAE in the preceding weeks, as seen from figure 45-2.

The increase in UAE may represent a form of subclinical preeclampsia with development of microalbuminuria and, alter, macroalbuminuria in some cases (i.e., more than 200 μg/min). Decreased placental blood flow is seen in diabetic pregnancy and in preeclampsia, which is also associated with increased frequency of late intrauterine death [26,27]. Preeclampsia is seen more often in diabetic pregnancy than in nondiabetic pregnancy [25]. In fact, one patient in group IIb did develop the clinical picture of preeclampsia. New prognostic markers, with possible therapeutic implications, are clearly needed so that the frequency of deleterious

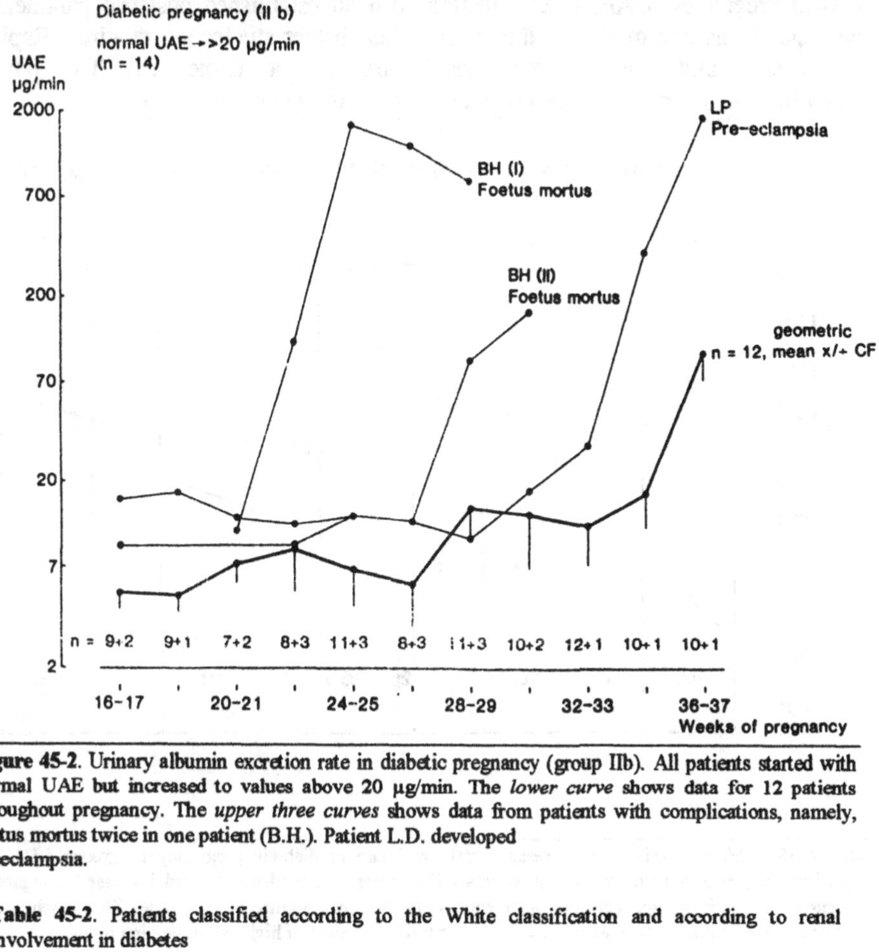

Figure 45-2. Urinary albumin excretion rate in diabetic pregnancy (group IIb). All patients started with normal UAE but increased to values above 20 µg/min. The *lower curve* shows data for 12 patients throughout pregnancy. The *upper three curves* shows data from patients with complications, namely, foetus mortus twice in one patient (B.H.). Patient L.D. developed preeclampsia.

Table 45-2. Patients classified according to the White classification and according to renal involvement in diabetes

		White classes				
	Total	A	B	C	D	F/R
I	4		4			
IIa	17		3	3	10	1
IIb	14		3	2	8	1
III	9				8	1
IV	8		1(?)			7

(?) Nondiabetic renal disease

complications in diabetic pregnancy can be reduced to a level not higher than that in normal pregnancy. UAE, in conjunction with an established obstetric parameter, may qualify as one marker in this respect, but further studies are required. Rapid, inexpensive, and sensitive immunoassay are now available [28]. The White classification, subgrouping diabetic patients according to complication

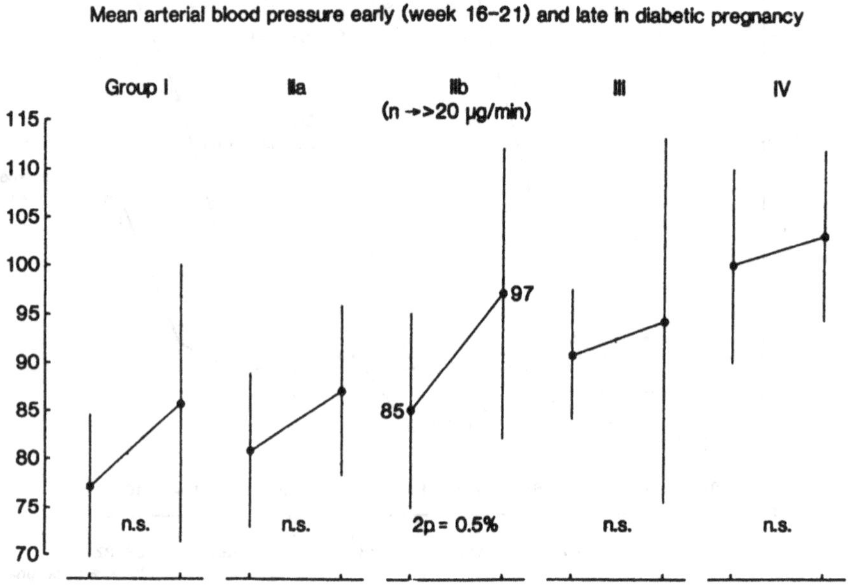

Figure 45-3. Mean arterial blood pressure early and late in diabetic pregnancy in groups I-IV. A significant increase is seen throughout groups I-IV. There is a tendency toward increase throughout pregnancy in each group, but this difference only became significant in group IIb, which was characterized by initial normal albumin excretion, but development of high values late in pregnancy (>20 μg/min).

and duration of disease, is widely used in most centers. This classification is very useful, but additional information may be obtained by classifying patients accordingto UAE. Thus, patients starting with normal excretion rates who later develop increased UAE may be more prone to complications. This will not be detected by using the White classification criteria. It should also be borne in mind that many patients, e.g., in White classification D, show a normal albumin excretion rate throughout pregnancy and thus will not be prone to develop complications (group D is defined as insulin-dependent diabetes diagnosed between the age of 0-10 years, diabetes duration of more than 20 years, or background retinopathy). The present classification of diabetic patients in pregnancy is in accordance with a new classification system regarding renal changes in nonpregnant patients [17], and this system may also be useful in pregnant diabetics [29]. Large-scale studies on abnormal albuminuria in diabetic pregnancy are now being undertaken. The significance of renal growth during diabetic pregnancy needs to be further evaluated [30].

REFERENCES

1. Mogensen CE. Microalbuminuria as a predictor of clinical diabetic nephropathy. Kidney Int 1987; 31: 673-689.
2. Viberti GC, Mackintosh D, Bilous RW, Pickup JC, Keen H. Proteinuria in diabetes mellitus: role of spontaneous and experimental variation of glycaemia. Kidney Int 1982; 21: 714-720.
3. Mogensen CE, Christensen CK. Predicting diabetic nephropathy in insulin-dependent patients. N Engl J Med 1984; 311: 89-93.
4. Viberti GC, Hill RD, Jarrett RJ, Argyropoulos A, Mahmud U, Keen H. Microalbuminuria as a predictor of clinical nephropathy in insulin-dependent diabetes mellitus. Lancet 1982; i: 1430-1432.
5. Parving H-H, Oxenbøll B, Svendsen PAa, Christiansen JS, Andersen AR. Early detection of patients at risk of developing diabetic nephropathy: a longitudinal study of urinary albumin excretion. Acta Endocrinol (Copenh) 1982; 100: 550-555.
6. Mathiesen ER, Oxenbøll B, Johansen K, Svendsen PAa, Deckert T. Incipient nephropathy in type 1 (insulin-dependent) diabetes. Diabetologia 1984; 26: 406-410.
7. Vigstrup J, Mogensen CE. Proliferative diabetic retinopathy: at risk patients identified by early detection of microalbuminuria. Acta Ophthalmol 1985; 63: 530-534.
8. Feldt-Rasmussen B. Increased transcapillary escape rate of albumin in type 1 (insulin-dependent) diabetic patients with microalbuminuria. Diabetologia 1986; 29: 282-286.
9. Feldt-Rasmussen B, Mathiesen E, Deckert T. Effect of two years of strict metabolic control on the progression of incipient nephropathy in insulin-dependent diabetes. Lancet 1986; ii: 1300-1304.
10. Mogensen CE, Klebe JG. »Microalbuminuria and diabetic pregnancy.« In *The Kidney and Hypertension in Diabetes Mellitus*. Mogensen CE, ed. Boston, Dordrecht, London: Kluwer Academic Publishers, 1994; pp 381-388.
11. Mogensen CE, Hansen KW, Klebe J, Christensen CK, Schmitz A, Mau Pedersen M, Pedersen EB, Jespersen B, Petersen RS, Christiansen JS, Schmitz O, Damgaard EM, Frøland A. »Microalbuminuria: Studies in diabetes, essential hypertension, and renal diseases as compared with the background population.« In *Advances in Nephrology*. Grünfeld JP, ed. Chicago: Mosby Year Book, 1991; 20: 191-228.
12. Misiani R, Marchesi D, Tiraboschi G, Gualandris L, Pagni R, Goglio A, Amuso G, Muratore D, bertuletti P, Massazza M. Urinary albumin excretion in normal pregnancy and pregnancy-induced bypertension. Nephron 1991; 59: 416-422.
13. Bernard A, Thielemans N, Lauwerys R, van Lierde M. Selective increase in the urinary excretion of protein 1 (Clara cell protein) and other low molecular weight proteins during normal pregnancy. Scand J Clin Lab Invest 1992; 52: 871-878.
14. Brown MA, Wang M-X, Buddle ML, Carlton MA, Cario GM, Zammit VC, Whitworth JA. Albumin excretory rate in normal and hypertensive pregnancy. Clin Sci 1994; 86: 251-255.
15. Miles DW, Mogensen CE, Gundersen HJG. Radioimmunoassay for urinary albumin using a single antibody. Scand J Clin Lab Invest 1970; 26: 5-11.
16. Mogensen CE. »Microalbuminuria and kidney function in diabetes: Notes on methods, interpretation and classification.« In *Methods in Diabetes Research, volume II: Clinical Methods*. Clarke WL, Larner J, Pohl SL, eds. New York, Chichester, Brisbane, Toronto, Singapore: John Wiley & Sons, 1986; pp 611-631.
17. Mogensen CE, Chachati A, Christensen CK, Close CF, Deckert T, Hommel E, Kastrup J, Lefebvre P, Mathiesen ER, Feldt-Rasmussen B, Schmitz A, Viberti GC. Microalbuminuria: an early marker of renal involvement in diabetes. Uremia Invest 1985-86; 9: 85-95.
18. Biesenbach G, Zazgornik J, Stöger H, Grafinger P, Hubmann R, Kaiser W, Janko O, Study U. Abnormal increases in urinary albumin excretion during pregnancy in IDDM women with pre-existing microalbuminuria. Diabetologia 1994; 37: 905-910.

19. Biesenbach G, Zazgornik J. Incidence of transient nephrotic syndrome during pregnancy in diabetic women with and without pre-existing microalbuminuria. BMJ 1989; 299: 366-367.
20. McCance DR, Traub AI, Harley JMG, Hadden DR, Kennedy L. Urinary albumin excretion in diabetic pregnancy. Diabetologia 1989; 32: 236-239.
21. Pedersen EB, Rasmussen AB, Johannesen P, Lauritsen JG, Kristensen S, Mogensen CE, Sølling K, Wohlert M. Urinary excretion of albumin, beta-2-microglobulin and light chains in preeclampsia, essential hypertension in pregnancy and normotensive pregnant and non-pregnant control subjects. Scand J Clin Lab Invest 1982; 41: 777-784.
22. Lopez-Espinoza I, Dhar H, Humphreys S, Redman CWG. Urinary albumin excretion in pregnancy. Br J Obstet Gynaecol 1986; 93: 176-181.
23. Irgens-Møller L, Hemmingsen L, Holm J. Diagnostic value of microalbuminuria in preeclampsia. Clin Chim Acta 1986; 157: 295-298.
24. Freinkel N, Dooley SL, Metzger BE. Care of the pregnant woman with insulin-dependent diabetes mellitus. N Engl J Med 1985; 131: 96-101.
25. Pedersen J. *The Pregnant Diabetic and Her Newborn*, 2nd ed. Copenhagen: Munksgaard, 1977.
26. Redman DWG. The definition of pre-eclampsia. Scand J Clin Lab Invest 1984; 44: Suppl. 169: 7-14.
27. Gregorini G, Perico N, Remuzzi G. »2. Pathogenesis of preeclampsia«. In *The Kidney in Pregnancy*. Andreucci VE, ed. Boston: Martinus Nijhoff, 1986; pp 13-33.
28. Mogensen CE, Poulsen PL, Heinsvig EM. »Abnormal albuminuria in the monitoring of early renal changes in diabetes.« In *Concepts for the Ideal Diabetes Clinic. Diabetes Forum Series, Volume 4*. Mogensen CE, Standl E, eds. Berlin, New York: Walter de Gruyter, 1993; pp 289-313.
29. Klebe JG, Mogensen CE, Christensen T. »Nephropathy in Pregnancy.« In *Carbohydrate Metabolism in Pregnancy and the Newborn IV*. Sutherland HW, Stowers JM, Pearson DWM, eds. London, Berlin, Heidelberg, New York, Paris, Tokyo: Springer Verlag, 1989; pp 173-187.
30. Lauszus FF, Klebe JG, Rasmussen OW, Klebe TM, Dørup J, Christensen T. Renal growth during pregnancy in insulin-dependent diabetic women. Acta Diabetol 1995; 32: 225-229.

46. DIABETIC NEPHROPATHY AND PREGNANCY

John L. Kitzmiller, MD, C. Andrew Combs, MD, Ph.D
Division of Maternal-Fetal Medicine, Good Samaritan Hospital, San José, California, USA

The potential problems of diabetic nephropathy and pregnancy require the anticipation of preconception care. Every practitioner who cares for adolescent and adult diabetic women has an obligation to recognize that these women may become pregnant, that most of the risks to mother and offspring are related to poor glycemic control, and that the risks may be reduced through special programs that achieve meticulous metabolic balance before conception and thoughout pregnancy.

With diabetic nephropathy (DN) as with diabetes in general, in recent years the most common cause of perinatal morbidity and mortality is major congenital malformations [1]. A major advance is the demonstration that most malformations can be prevented by institution of strict metabolic control before conception in women with DN [2-4]. Every diabetic woman should have instruction in contraception [5,6], and should be intensively treated or referred to a specialized center when pregnancy is considered. The encouragement by diabetes care practitioners is a major factor in preventing unplanned pregnancies [7,8].

Until recently, women with DN were generally advised to avoid pregnancy because there was a low probability of a healthy infant and a chance that nephropathy would worsen. Although advances in obstetrical and neonatal care have improved the outlook, nephropathy in pregnancy still presents a challenging situation requiring coordination between the patient, obstetrician, perinatologist, diabetologist, nephrologist, ophthalmologist, neonatologist, nurse-educator, dietician, social worker, and other personnel. As reviewed in this chapter, women with nephropathy remain at high risk for many pregnancy complications in addition to congenital malformations, including superimposed preeclampsia or accelerated hypertension, preterm delivery, fetal growth restriction, and cesarean delivery. Good glycemic balance and control of hypertension are necessary to reduce these complications and to slow the expected decline in renal function during and after pregnancy.

EVALUATION BEFORE CONCEPTION

An outline of preconception management of women with established diabetes is included in table 46-1. Evaluation for diabetic microvascular disease and hypertension are critical. Creatinine clearance (CrC1) as an estimate of GFR, and the degree of microalbuminuria (**incipient DN**, 30-299 mg/24 hrs) [9] or clinical total proteinuria (**overt DN**, > 300 mg/24 hrs albumin, <500 mg/24 hrs total protein) [9] should be quantified, preferably with a 24-hour specimen [10,11,12]. If nephropathy is diagnosed, the patient should be thoroughly

Table 46-1 Management of diabetic nephropathy before and during pregnancy

At all times
Prevent hyperglycaemia
Control hypertension
Low protein diet
Restrict exercise

Prior to pregnancy
Measure renal function
Ophthalmologic exam
Cardiovascular evaluation
(history, exam, EKG)
Thyroid evaluation
Hepatitis B surface antigen
Serologic testing for syphilis
Counselling and education

First prenatal visit
Measure renal function
Ophthalmologic exam
sonogram for dating

Second trimester
Measure renal function (12, 24 weeks)
Maternal serum alphafetoprotein (15-18 weeks)
Detailed sonogram with fetal echocardiogram (18-20 weeks)

Third trimester
Monthly sonogram
Weekly nonstress test (26 weeks)
Ophthalmologic exam
Measure renal function (36 weeks)
Delivery planning

counselled regarding possible complications of pregnancy and her own probability of reduced life expectancy. She must then decide whether to attempt pregnancy.

Antihypertensive therapy is indicated for most patients with microalbuminuria or overt nephropathy. Agents should be used which are safe in early pregnancy. *Angiotensin converting-enzyme (ACE) inhibitors are contraindicated during pregnancy* because they may be teratogenic [13] and are associated with neontal renal failure [14,15]. This is unfortunate because there are extensive data, reviewed elsewhere in this volume, indicating that ACE-inhibitors retard the development and progression of nephropathy. The hypothesis that use of ACE-inhibitors in the preconception period will also decrease complications in the subsequent pregnancy [16] should be tested in controlled trials in women with excellent glycemic control. In a study of 8 women with presumed DN, Jovanovic found that normoglycemia achieved by early pregnancy also resulted in stable renal function and low complication rates [17]. Diltiazem and other calcium-entry blockers are probably best avoided during the first trimester since some indicate an association with fetal limb defects [18]. Agents believed to be relatively safe for pregnancy include alpha-methyldopa, prazocin, clonidine, and beta-adrenergic antagonists.

Ophthalmologic examination is especially important for women with nephropathy because most also have diabetic retinopathy. Rapid normalization of blood glucose may cause worsening of retinopathy [19]. With background or proliferative retinopathy, allow a few months to normalize blood glucose before pregnancy. Proliferative retinopathy, should be in remission or laser-treated before pregnancy. In women with background retinopathy at the beginning of pregnancy, there is a 6-10% risk of development of neovascularization during gestation [20,21].

The association of DN with cardiovascular disease [22] gives concern in evaluating patients for pregnancy, since there has been a high mortality in diabetic women with coronary artery disease [23]. There are no studies of the coronary vessels in diabetic women preparing for pregnancy. However, Manske et al found little coronary disease among diabetic patients >45 years old with end-stage renal disease if diabetes duration was less than 25 years, and there were no ST-T wave changes on ECG [24]. Therefore, pregnancy should be safe if these conditions are met. Otherwise, coronary angiography should be considered, since maternal-fetal outcome after coronary artery bypass grafts has been good [25].

Glycaemic control is achieved with a monitored meal plan and intensive insulin therapy. The diet prescription for pregnancy is 25-35 kcal/kg ideal body weight. With nephropathy, protein intake should be restricted, but 60 g/day is probably required for fetal development. The preferred insulin regimen includes a mix of short and intermediate-acting human insulins or continuous subcutaneous insulin infusion therapy. The optimal doses and timing are determined by self-monitored capillary blood glucose determinations before and after each meal. The targets for capillary blood glucose control before and during pregnancy are premeal values of 3.9-5.6 mM (70-100 mg/dL) and peak postprandial values of 5.6-7.2 mM (100-129 mg/dL) [1].

COURSE OF NEPHROPATHY DURING PREGNANCY

GFR rises by 40-80% in normal pregnancy, as reflected by increasing creatinine clearance and decreasing serum creatinine [24]. With diabetic nephropathy, however, the normal rise in CrCl is seen in only about one-third of patients, as summarized in table 46-2 [17,27,28]. In another third, CrCl actually decreases, probably reflecting the underlying natural progression of nephropathy or accelerating hypertension. Jovanovic found that prevention of hyperglycaemia and hypertension allowed a normal rise in CrC1 during pregnancy in 8 diabetic women with sub-par values prior to conception [17].

Table 46-2 Changes in creatinine clearance in 44 women with diabetic nephopathy with measurements in both first and third trimester of pregnancy[a]

	First trimester	Third trimester		
CrC1	n(%)	Increased >25%	Stable	Decreased>15%
>90 ml/min	14 (32%)	3 (21%)	5 (36%)	6 (43%)
60-89 ml/min	20 (45.5%)	9 (45%)	6 (30%)	5 (25%)
<60 ml/min	10 (22.5%)	2 (20%)	6 (60%)	2 (20%)
Total	44 (100%)	14 (32%)	17 (39%)	13 (29%)

Data stratified by CrC1 in first trimester: normal, moderate reduction, and severe reduction. Data pooled from Kitzmiller et al [27], Jovanovic and Jovanovic [17], and Reece et al [28].

An increase in kidney volume can be measured by ultrasound in pregnancies in normal controls [29] and in insulin-dependent diabetic women [30]. In the latter group the expansion occurs in spite of strict glycaemic control, and the increase correlates with CrC1 but not with albuminuria, BP levels, or with the placental hormone hPL. Renal expansion is less in pregnant women with diabetic nephropathy, but renal volume did not decline as expected 4 months postpartum in this group in one study [30]. Interestingly, development of persistent microalbuminuria was most likely in the group with normoalbuminuria and relatively small renal volumes in early pregnancy.

The excretion of albumin increases slightly in *normal pregnancy* [31-33], while total urinary protein excretion increases by 40-200% albeit to <300 mg/24hrs [34,35], presumably due to increased GFR and decreased tubular reabsorption (table 46-3) [12,35,36]. Therefore the charge- and pore size-specific glomerular barrier to filtration of albumin seems to remain intact. In *diabetic women without microalbuminuria* in early pregnancy, urinary albumin excretion increases slightly in the second trimester and sometimes greatly in the third trimester, while urinary total protein excretion can rise to >300 mg/24hrs [37-39]. Of course, some cases of this proteinuria may be explained by mild preeclampsia, which always muddles the view of changes in renal function in pregnant diabetic women. With *microalbuminuria before pregnancy in diabetic women*, the increase in albumin and total protein excretion during gestation is even greater (table 46-3) [40-42]. (Many [40,42-44] but not all investigators [45] have proposed that microalbuminuria in early pregnancy predicts preeclampsia.) These gestational changes in total proteinuria mean that most clinical studies of DN in pregnancy have probably included women with undetected microalbuminuria prior to conception who happened to progress to mild macroproteinuria (400-600 mg total protein/24 hrs) in early pregnancy, and thus were inappropriately counted as patients with mild DN. With definite *clinical diabetic nephropathy*, albuminuria and total proteinuria often increases dramatically, even without associated hypertension, frequently exceeding 10 g/day in the third trimester. Though some of this increase may reflect the underlying progression of nephropathy, protein excretion usually subsides after delivery [25,26].

Table 46-3 Proteinuria before, during and after normal and type 1 diabetic pregnancies without clinical nephropathy.

	Before	3rd trimester	4*-6**mo PP
11 nl controls *			
ur alb (mg/d)	9	12	13
ur total prot (mg/d)	117*	262	174
7 normoalb type 1**			
ur alb	12	71	13
ur total prot	73	417	96
7 microalb type 1**			
ur alb	80	478	114
ur total prot	233	2350	239

* Roberts et al: Am J Physiol 270:F338, 1996; UAE 9 mg/d 12 mo PP
TPE 177 "" "" ""
** Biesenbach, Zasgornik: Br Med J 299:366, 1989

Maternal characteristics identified in early pregnancy in 225 cases of DN reported in 1981-1996 include ~ 50% frequencies of proliferative retinopathy, anemia, and hypertension. There were 45% of cases with reduced CrC1 (<80 ml/min), and 15% with serum creatinine (Cr) > 134 uM (table 46-6) [17,27,28,46-53]. Minimal proteinuria (<1 gm total protein/24 hrs before 20 weeks gestation) was detected in many of the women, so these cases are suspected not to be "true" DN, therefore the above frequencies probably should be higher. Of 146 diabetic women with >1 gm total protein/24 hrs in early pregnancy, 57 had impaired renal function at that stage of gestation (Cr>134 uM or CrC1 <80 ml/min), and 37% showed a further decline of >15% during later pregnancy.

Diabetic nephropathy can progress to end-stage renal disease during pregnancy, although this is unusual. Of 195 women followed after pregnancy and summarized in table 46-4, none progressed to end-stage disease during pregnancy. There is some experience with both haemodialysis and peritoneal dialysis in pregnancy [54,55]. Complications of dialysis include preeclampsia, placental abruption and stillbirth. The latter two are related to large shifts in extravascular volume and may be less common with peritoneal dialysis [54]. Because of the high complication rate, pregnancy is probably contraindicated if the serum creatinine is above 177 uM or creatinine clearance is below 50 ml/min, at least until renal transplantation can be performed.

EFFECTS OF PREGNANCY ON THE NATURAL HISTORY OF DN

For years, there has been a hypothetical concern that the physiologic hyperfiltration of pregnancy might damage the glomeruli and accelerate the postpartum progression of diabetic nephropathy to end-stage renal disease. However, the few data available that directly address this hypothesis do not support it. Three studies assessed renal function after pregnancy in women with nephropathy [27,51,56]. All three found that creatinine clearance declined an average of about 10 ml/min per year , no different than the average rate in men and women with diabetic nephropathy without pregnancy [57].

In the pooled series of 195 women experiencing pregnancies with DN and having renal function assessed 1-10 years afterwards, 23% were in renal failure and 5.6% had died (table 46-4). Not surprisingly, the frequency of progression to renal failure after pregnancy was 49% in the group of women with impaired renal function in early pregnancy, compared to 7% if Cr was <134 μM or CrCl was >80 ml/min early gestation (table 46-5) [17,27,28,46-53]. Other authors have questioned whether experiencing pregnancy hastens the progression of diabetic nephropathy. The speed of progression to end-stage disease is little or not different whether a pregnancy is terminated in the first trimester or carried into the third trimester [27]. Miodovnik observed that increased parity did not increase the risk of renal failure after pregnancy [51], and the EURODIAB type 1 complications survey found that parity did not increase the incidence of micro- or macroalbuminuria [57].

Table 46-4 Course of renal parameters during and after pregnancy in women with diabetic nephropathy. Data pooled from references 27,28, 48-53.

	Hypertension	Ur Prot > 5 gm/d	Decr CrCl Incr Cr	Renal Failure	Death
Early preg	42%	9%	34%	0	0
Late preg	71%	26%	26%	0	0
Follow-up	60%	17%	43%	23%**	5.6%

* 195 women x 1-10 yrs, median 2.6 yrs

Table 46-5 Course of diabetic nephropathy during and after pregnancy comparing patients with preserved vs impaired renal function in early pregnancy. Data pooled from references 27,28,48,49,50. Note the limited number of cases with severe azotemia in early pregnancy.

	Initial renal function		Cr
	Preserved	Impaired*	>177
Number	70	57	(6)
Decline during pregnancy	12 (17%)	21 (37%)	(1)
Renal failure after preg**	4 of 57 (7%)	37 of 55 (49%)	(3)
Died	2 (3.5%)	5 (9.1%)	(0)

* Cr >100 uM, CrCl >80 ml/min
** 1-10 yrs.

Purdy et al thought that 5 of 11 women with DN and moderate renal insufficiency had an accelerated rate of decline in renal function during pregnancy, but in the follow-up for a mean of 2 years postpartum the group of 11 had slightly less decline in inverse Cr than 11 similar patients without pregnancy [52]. Mackie and colleagues [53] and Kaaja et al 59] also found no evidence for accelerated decline of renal function after pregnancy compared to non-pregnant patients. Therefore the medical practice of discouraging pregnancy in women with DN based on presumed increased threats to renal function has no basis on published experience.

DIABETIC NEPHROPATHY AND PERINATAL OUTCOME

In spite of the dramatic improvements in perinatal outcome over the last 25 years in pregnancies of diabetic women [60], complications remain more frequent when DN is present. Examining the pooled results of the 13 clinical series published in 1981-96 (table 46-6) [16,17,27,28,46-53,61], of 265 infants born to women with DN, nearly 2/3 were preterm deliveries prior to 37 weeks gestation, 72.5% were delivered by caesarean section, and respiratory distress syndrome was diagnosed in 24.5% of liveborn infants. Fetal growth restriction was noted in 14.3%, and the major correlates of small size for dates were the degree of maternal hypertension and impaired renal function [27,28,49]. Major congenital malformations were diagnosed in 7.55% of the 265 infants. The frequencies of these perinatal complication were similar in 90 pregnancies reported in 1981-88 compared to 175 reported in 1992-96 (table 46-6). Perinatal mortality rates were 5.55/1000 and 34.3/1000 in the earlier and later group, respectively. Overall, 95.8% of infants survived to leave the neonatal intensive care unit.

It must be noted that these clinical results may be somewhat worse in women with "true" clinical DN, since at least 16% of the pooled cases probably had only microalbuminuria prior to pregnancy, because they were included in the DN series based on <1 gm/day total protein excretion in the first trimester. Limiting the analysis of perinatal mortality to 223 cases with >1gm/day total urinary protein excretion in the first trimester, perinatal mortality rates were 54.8/1000 in 1982-88 compared to 71.4/1000 in 1992-96. Major congenital malformations and severe fetal growth restriction were responsible for most of the perinatal deaths.

Table 46-6 Diabetic nephropathy and perinatal outcome in two eras in which perinatal technology was utilized. Data pooled from references 17,27,28,46-53.

Year of report	1981-88	1992-96
Infants	90	275
Perinatal survival	94.4%	96.6%
Fetal growth restriction	13.3%	14.9%
Preterm delivery	57.8%	64.6%
Caesarean delivery	68.9%	74.3%
Respiratory distress syndrome	25.6%	24.2%
Major congenital malformations	7.8%	7.7%

The relationship of perinatal morbidity to the severity of diabetic nephropathy is illustrated in table 46-7. Selecting out cases from the pooled series with sufficient detail for analysis [27,28,48,49], 19 women had >1 gm/day total urinary protein with preserved renal function in early pregnancy, compared to 41 proteinuric diabetic women with CrCl<80 ml/min. or serum Cr>134uM. Not surprisingly, the latter group had much higher rates of fetal growth restriction, preeclampsia, fetal distress causing delivery, and serious prematurity (table 46-7). These data can be used for counseling women with DN prior to pregnancy.

Table 46-7 Perinatal outcome related to renal status in early pregnancy in women with diabetic nephropathy. Data combined from cases reported in references 27,28,48,49.

		Initial Renal Function	
	Prot 0.3-0.9gm/d	Preserved	Impaired*
Number	18	19	41
Fetal growth restriction	1 (6%)	1 (5%)	11 (27%)
Preeclampsia	2 (11%)	4 (21%)	15 (37%)
Fetal distress	1 (6%)	4 (21%)	12 (29%)
Fetal death	1	1	1
Deliv 24-33 w	4 (22%)	5 (26%)	18 (38%)
Uncomplicated	10 (56%)	6 (32%)	9 (24%)

*Cr >1.2 or CrCl <80 ml/min

Superimposed preeclampsia is a leading cause of prematurity in women with diabetes [62,63] and DN. The condition is suspected when there is an increase in blood pressure and proteinuria in the third trimester. With pre-existing nephropathy, it may not be possible to clinically distinguish "true" preeclampsia from a "simple" worsening of hypertension and proteinuria. The distinction is important because the former is best treated by delivery whereas the latter is treated with bed rest and hypertensive agents. Edema and hyperuricemia are common in patients with renal disease and therefore are not useful in the differential diagnosis. Occasionally, thrombocytopenia or elevated transaminases are found and these support a diagnosis of superimposed preeclampsia. As a practical matter, it is generally necessary to observe the patient at hospital bed rest, with or without antihypertensive therapy. Hypoalbuminemia commonly results from excessive proteinuria and leads to generalized edema. The edema can be treated with diurecties. It is controversial whether albumin infusions are beneficial or useless. The decision to deliver the infant must balance the gestational age, the severity of the maternal condition, and indicators of fetal well-being.

Maternal anemia results from both decreased erythropoietin production by damaged glomeruli and the physiologic hemodilution of pregnancy. The degree of anemia is related to the severity of nephropathy as reflected in lower creatinine clearance and is not usually associated with abnormal iron studies [27]. Exogenous erythropoietin can be considered to treat anemia unresponsive to iron and folate replacement [64,65].

As noted, fetal growth delay is related to maternal hypertension. Serial sonography is indicated to evaluate fetal growth. In addition, fetal heart rate monitoring or biophysical assessment should be employed because growth restriction or fetal hyperglycemia-hypoxia-acidosis [66] is frequently associated with evidence of fetal distress. For women with clinical DN, begin weekly nonstress testing at 26 weeks' gestation and twice-weekly testing at 34 weeks, earlier if there is growth delay. Vaginal delivery is preferred if there is no evidence of fetal distress and no obstetric contraindication. However, as noted in table 46-6, there was a remarkably high caesarean rate with DN, the reasons for which are not entirely elucidated.

PREGNANCY AFTER RENAL TRANSPLANTATION

Ogburn et al compiled the experience of nine diabetic women from several centres who had pregnancy after renal transplantation for DN [67]. All were managed with prednisone and azathioprine. No transplant rejections occurred during pregnancy. Complications were frequent, including preeclampsia in six, fetal distress in six, and preterm delivery in all. Armenti and the US Transplant Pregnancy Registry reported 28 pregnancies in diabetic renal transplant recipients [68]. Rejection was observed in 4% and graft dysfunction in 11%. Preeclampsia was diagnosed in 17% although 59% had hypertension – 47% of the infants had neonatal complications. Combined kidney-pancreas transplants prior to pregnancy have been reported several times [69], and Armenti and colleagues also reported 12 pregnancies after combined transplants [68]. In this group 25% had preeclampsia while 83% were hypertensive. Two-thirds of these gravidas were treated for some type of infections.

There has been hypothetical concern that pregnancy may adversely affect renal graft survival. However, two recent studies with long-term follow-up found no difference in graft survival or function between women who became pregnant and matched controls who did not [70,71].

REFERENCES

1. Kitzmiller JL, Buchanan TA, Kjos S et al. Preconception care of diabetes, congenital malformations, and spontaneous abortions. Technincal review. Diab Care 1996; 19: 514-541.
2. Fuhrmann K, Reiher H, Semmler K, Glockner E. The effect of intensified conventional insulin therapy before and during pregnancy on the malformation rate in offspring of diabetic mothers. Exp Clin Endocrinol 1984; 83:173-177.
3. Damm P, Molsted-Pedersen L. Significant decrease in congenital malformations in newborn infants of an unselected population of diabetic women. Am J Obst Gynec 1989; 161:1163-7
4. Kitsmiller JL, Gavin LA, Gin GD, et al. Preconception care of diabetes. Glycemic control prevents congenital anomalies. JAMA 1991; 265:731-736.
5. StJames PJ, Younger MD, Hamilton BD, Waisbren SE. Unplanned pregnancies in diabetic women. Diab Care 1993; 16:1572-8.
6. Kjos SL. Contraception in diabetic women. Obst Gynecol Clinics North Amer 1996; 23:243-57.
7. Janz NK, Herman WH, Becker MP, et al. Diabetes and pregnancy: factors associated with seeking pre-conception care. Diab Care 1995; 18:157-65.
8. Holing E, Beyer CS. Why don't women with diabetes plan their pregnancies? Diab 1997; 46, suppl. 1:15A.
9. Mogensen CE, Chachati A, Christensen CK et al. Microalbuminuria: an early marker for renal involvement in diabetes. Uremia Invest 1985-86; 9:85-95.
10. Combs CA, Wheeler BC, Kitzmiller JL. Urinary protein/crearinine ratio before and during pregnancy in women with diabetes mellitus. Am J Obstet Gynecol 1991; 165:920-923.
11. Stehouwer CDA, Fischer HRA, Hackeng WHL, et al. Diurnal variation in urinary protein excretion in diabetic nephropathy. Nephrol Dial Transplant 1991; 6:238-243.
12. Quadri KHM, Bernardini J, Greenberg MD, et al. Assessment of renal function during pregnancy using a random urine protein to creatinine ratio and Cockcroft-Gault ratio.Amer J Kid Dis. 1994; 24:416-420.
13. Piper JM, Ray WA, Rosa FW. Pregnancy outcome following exposure to angiotensinconverting enzyme inhibitors. Obst Gynec 1992; 80:429-32.
14. Rosa FW, Bosco LA, Graham CF et al. Neonatal anuria with maternal angiotensinconverting enzyme inhibition. Obst Gynec 1989; 74:371.
15. Hanssens M, Keirse MJNC, Vankelecom F, Van Assche FA. Fetal and neonatal effects of treatment with angiotensin-converting enzyme inhibitors in pregnancy. Obstet Gynecol 1991;78: 128-135.

16. Hod M, van Dijk DJ, Karp M, et al. Diabetic nephropathy and pregnancy: the effect of ACE inhibitors prior to pregnancy on maternal outcome. Neph Dial Transpl 1995; 10: 2328-33.
17. Jovanovic R, Jovanich L. Obstetric management when normoglycemia is maintained in diabetic pregnant women with vascular compromise. Am J Obstet Gynecol 1984; 149: 617-623.
18. Magee LA, Conover B, Schick B, et al. Exposure to calcium channel blockers in human pregnancy: a prospective, controlled, multicentre cohort study. Teratol 1994; 49:372-6.
19. Brinchmann-Hansen O, Dahl-Jørgensen K, Hanssen KF, et al. Effects of intensified insulin treatment on various lesions of diabetic retinopathy. Am J Ophthalmol 1985; 100:644-9.
20. Klein BEK, Moss SE, Klein R. Effect of pregnancy on progression of diabetic retinopathy. Diab Care 1990; 13:34-40.
21. Chew EY, Mills JL, Metzger BE et al. The diabetes and early pregnancy study. Metabolic control and progression of retinopathy. Diab Care 1995; 18:631-7.
22. Jensen T, Borch-Johnson K, Kofoed-Enevoldsen A, Deckert T. Coronary heart disease in young type 1 (insulin-dependent) diabetic patients with and without diabetic nephropathy: incidence and risk factors. Diabetologia 1987; 30:144-8.
23. Reece EA, Egan JFX, Coustan DR, et al. Coronary artery disease in diabetic pregnancies. Amer J Obst Gynec 1986; 154:150-1.
24. Manske CL, Thomas W, Wang Y, Wilson RF. Screening diabetic transplant candidates for coronary artery disease: identification of a low risk subgroup. Kidney Intl. 1993; 44:617-21.
25. Salomon NW, Page US, Oskies JE et al. Diabetes mellitus and coronary artery bypass: short term risk and long term prognosis. J Thorac Cardiovasc Surg 1983; 85:264-8.
26. Krutzen E, Olufsson P, Back SE, Nilsson-Ehle P. Glomerular filtration rate in pregnancy: a study in normal subjects and in patients with hypertension, preeclampsia and diabetes. Scand J Clin Lab Invest 1992; 52: 387-392..
27. Kitzmiller JL, Brown ER, Phillipe M, et al. Diabetic nephropathy and perinatal outcome. Am J Obstet Gynecol 1981; 141: 741-751.
28. Reece EA, Coustan DR, Hayslett JP, et al. Diabetic nephropathy: pregnancy performance and fetomaternal outcome. Am J Obstet Gynecol 1988; 159:56-66.
29. Christensen T, Klebe JG, Berthelsen V, Hansen HE. Changes in renal volume during normal pregnancy. Acta Obst Gynec Scand 1989; 68:541-3.
30. Lauszas FF, Klebe JG, Rasmussen OW, et al. Renal growth during pregnancy in insulin-dependent diabetic women. A prospective study of renal volume and clinical variables. Acta Diabetol 1995; 32:225-9.
31. Pedersen EB, Rasmussen AB, Johannsen P, et al. Urinary excretion of albumin, beta-2-microglubulin and light chains in preeclampsia, essential hypertension in pregnancy, and normotensive pregnant and non-pregnant control subjects. Scand J Clin Lab Investig 1981; 41:777-84.
32. Lopez-Espinoza I, Humphreys S, Redman CWG. Urinary albumin excretion in pregnancy. Br J Obst Gynec 1986; 93:176-81.
33. Wright A, Steele P, Bennett JR et al. The urinary excretion of albumin in normal pregnancy. Br J Obstet Gynaecol 1987; 94:408-412.
34. Cheung CK, Lao T, Swaminathan R. Urinary excretion of some proteins and enzymes during normal pregnancy. Clin Chem 1989; 35: 1978-1980.
35. Higby K, Suiter CR, Phelps JY, et al. Normal values of urinary albumin and total protein excretion during pregnancy. Am J Obst Gynec 1994; 171: 984-9.
36. Roberts M, Lindheimer MD, Davison JM. Altered glomerular permselectivity to neutral dextrans and heteroporous membrane modeling in human pregnancy. Am J Physiol 1996; 270:F338-43.
37. McCance DR, Traub AI, Harley JMG, et al. Urinary albumin excretion in diabetic pregnancy. Diabetologia 1989; 32:236-9.
38. Biesenbach G, Zasgornik J. Incidence of transient nephrotic syndrome during pregnancy in diabetic women with and without pre-existing microalbuminuria. Br Med J 1989; 299: 366-7.
39. MacRury SM, Pinion S, Quin JD, et al. Blood rheology and albumin excretion in diabetic pregnancy. Diabetic Med 1995; 12:51-5.
40. Winocour PH, Taylor RJ. Early alterations of renal function in insulin-dependent diabetic pregnancies and their importance in predicting preeclamptic toxaemia. Diabetes Res 1989; 10:159-164.

41. Biesenbach G, Zasgornik J, Stoger H et al. Abnormal increases in urinary albumin excretion during pregnancy in IDDM women with preexisting albuminuria. Diabetologia 1994; 37: 905-10.
42. Combs CA, Rosenn B, Kitzmiller JL, et al. Early-pregnancy proteinuria in diabetes related to preeclampsia. Obstet Gynecol 1993; 82: 802-807.
43. Bar J, Hod M, Erman A, et al. Microalbuminuria as an early predictor of hypertensive complications in pregnant women at high risk. Am J Kidney Dis 1996; 28: 220-5.
44. Das V, Bhargava T, Das SK, Pandey S. Microalbuminuria: a predictor of pregnancy-induced hypertension. Br J Obst Gynec 1996; 103-928-30.
45. Konstantin-Hansen KF, Hesseldahl H, Moller Pedersen S. Microalbuminuria as a predictor of preeclampsia Acta Obst Gynec Scand 1992; 71: 341-6.
46. Dicker B, Feldberg, Peleg, et al. Pregnancy complicated by diabetic nephropathy. J Perin Med 1986; 14:299-306.
47. Grenfell A, Brudenell JM, Doddridge MC, Watkins PJ. Pregnancy in diabetic women who have proteinuria. Quart J Med 1986; 59: 379-386.
48. Biesenback G, Stoger H, Zazgornik J. Influence of pregnancy on progression of diabetic nephropathy and subsequent requirement of renal replacment therapy in female type 1 diabetic patients with impaired renal function. Nephrol Dial Transplant 1992; 7: 105-109.
49. Kimmerle R, Zass R-P, Cupisti S, et al. Pregnancies in women with diabetic nephropathy: long-term outcome for mother and child. Diabetologia 1995; 38: 227-235.
50. Gordon M, Landon MB, Samuels P, et al. Perinatal outcome and long-term follow-up associated with modern management of diabetic nephropathy? Am J Obstet Gynecol 1996; 174:1180-91.
51. Miodovnik M, Rosenn BM, Khoury JC, et al. Does pregnancy increase the risk for development and progression of diabetic nephropathy? Am J Obstet Gynecol 1996; 174:1180-91.
52. Purdy LP, Hantsch CE, Molitsch ME, et al. Effect of pregnancy on renal function in patients with moderate-to-severe diabetic renal insufficiency. Diab Care 1996; 19: 1067-74.
53. Mackie ADR, Doddridge MC, Gamsu HR et al. Outcome of pregnancy in patients with insulin-dependent diabetes mellitus and nephropathy with moderate renal impairment. Diabetic Med 1996; 13: 90-96.
54. Yasin SY, Bey Doun SN. Hemodialysis in pregnancy. Obst Gynec Surv 1988; 43: 655-68.
55. Hou S. Pregnancy in women requiring dialysis for renal failure. Am J Kidney Dis 1987; 9:368-375.
56. Reece EA, Winn HN, Hayslett JP, et al. Does pregnancy alter the rate of progression of diabetic nephropathy? Am J Perinat 1990; 7: 193-7.
57. Mogensen CE. Progression of nephropthy in long-term diabetics with proteinuria and effect of initial antihypertensive treatment. Scand J Clin Lab Invest 1976; 36: 383-7.
58. Chartuvedi N, Stephenson JM, Fuller JH, et al. The relationship between pregnancy and long-term maternal complications in the EURODIAB IDDM complications study. Diabetic Med 1995; 12:494-9.
59. Kaaja R, Sjoberg L, Hellstedt T et al. Long-term effects of pregnancy on diabetic complications. Diabetic Med 1996; 13: 165-9.
60. Kitzmiller JL. Sweet success with diabetes. The development of insulin therapy and glycemic control for pregnancy. Diab Care 1993; 16 (suppl 3): 107-21.
61. Holley JL, Bernadini J, Quadri KHM, et al. Pregnancy outcomes in a prospective matched control study of pregnancy and renal disease. Clinical Nephrol 1996; 45: 77-82.
62. Greene MF, Hare JW, Krache M, et al. Prematurity among insulin-requiring diabetic gravid women. Am J Obst Gynec 1989; 161: 106-11.
63. Garner PR, D'Alton ME, Dudley DK, et al. Preeclampsia in diabetic pregnancies. Am J Obst Gynec 1990; 163: 505-8.
64. Yankowitz J, Piraino B, Laifer A, et al. Use of erythropoietin in pregnancies complicated by severe anemia of renal failure. Obst Gynec 1992; 80: 485-8.
65. Hou S, Orlowski J, Pahl M, et al. Pregnancy in women with end-stage renal disease: treatment of anemia and premature labor. Am J Kidney Dis 1993; 21: 16-22.
66. Salvesen DR, Higueras MT, Brudenell M, et al. Doppler velocimetry and fetal heart studies in nephropathic diabethic. Am J Obst Gynec 1992; 167: 1297-1303.
67. Ogburn PL, Jr, Kitzmiller JL, Hare JW, et al. Pregnancy following renal transplantation in class T diabetes mellitus. JAMA 1986; 225:911-5.

68. Armenti VT, McGrory CH, Cater J, et al. The national transplantation registry: comparison between pregnancy outcomes in diabetic cyclosporine-treated female kidney recipients and CyA-treated female pancreas-kidney recipients. Transpl Proc 1997; 29: 669-70.
69. Skannal DG, Miodovnik M, Dungy-Poythress LJ, First MR. Successful pregnancy after combined renal-pancreas transplantion: a case report and literature review. Am j Perinatol 1996; 13: 383-7.
70. Davison JM. The effect of pregnancy on kidney function in renal allograft recipients. Kidney Int. 1985; 27:74-9.
71. First MR, Combs CA, Weiskittel P, Miodovnik M. Lack of effect of pregnancy on renal allograft survival or function. Transplantion 1995; 59:472-6.

47. EVOLUTION WORLDWIDE OF RENAL REPLACEMENT THERAPY IN DIABETES

Rudy W. Bilous, MD FRCP
Middlesbrough General Hospital, Middlesbrough, Cleveland, UK

INTRODUCTION

The numbers of patients entering renal replacement therapy (RRT) with diabetic nephropathy as their primary disease continues to rise worldwide, although there is some suggestion that the rate of increase may be declining in the USA[1]. However, long term survival of patients on RRT remains much less good for diabetic compared to non-diabetic recipients [2], although short term (one year) mortality adjusted for age has declined by 39% in the decade 1984-94 in the USA [3].

It must be remembered that much of these data are extracted from registers of patients who have been accepted onto RRT programmes, they are therefore an underestimate of the true prevalence of renal failure in diabetes as many patients will not survive until end stage renal disease (ESRD). Secondly, some registers are much less comprehensive, with ascertainment rates as low as 55% of patient questionnaires in Europe [2]. Finally, methods of reporting differ between registers. The USRDS data retrieval only begins after patients have survived 90 days of RRT [4] whereas data from Europe and Japan relate to entry onto RRT [2,5].

Nonetheless reported differences and contrasts in the incidence and outcome between countries raise intriguing questions about both the pathophysiology of diabetic nephropathy and optimum management of ESRD in diabetes [6,7]. The following areas will be covered in turn:

1. Evolution of acceptance of diabetic patients on RRT.
2. Impact of age, type of diabetes and ethnicity of subject population.
3. Mode and outcome of RRT used to treat diabetic patients.
4. Suggested management strategies.

Mogensen, C.E. (ed.), THE KIDNEY AND HYPERTENSION IN DIABETES MELLITUS.

EVOLUTION OF ACCEPTANCE OF DIABETIC PATIENTS ON RRT

The USRDS has shown a year on year increase in the incidence of new diabetic patients entering RRT to 40.4% of the total enrolled in 1995 (27,851 of 68,870 patients) [1]. This represents a rate of 103 per million population (pmp). Overall prevalence seems to be showing a decline in the rate of increase; however, in 1982, diabetic patients would comprise only 3% (21pmp) patients on RRT in an average dialysis centre, whereas nationally the figures were 26.1% (188pmp) in 1991 and 31.4% (303pmp) in 1995 [1].

In Japan in 1994, the incidence of diabetes as a cause of RRT requiring haemodialysis (HD), (which represents 92.7% of all RRT), was 31.2% (60pmp) and the prevalence was 18.2% (209pmp) total population, which is more than double the figure for 1984 (8.2%) [5].

In Europe, recent data collection is much less complete than previously [2] and it is hard to draw firm conclusions across frontiers since 1992. However, where the data are confirmed by national registers, it is still possible to detect more recent trends. In 1978 overall prevalence of diabetes as the primary renal disease was 3.8%, compared to 13% in 1989 and 17% (50pmp) in 1992 [8]. These prevalence figures hide a wide range in international and within country incidence rates, however; Austria recording 21pmp, Denmark 14pmp, and the Netherlands 8.5pmp; whereas in the UK the national figure was 6pmp, with one inner-city unit in London recording 34pmp in 1993. Thus although overall prevalence of diabetes in RRT patients is similar in Europe and Japan, the absolute numbers in terms of pmp are far less and local variations suggest that future large increases are likely.

IMPACT OF AGE, TYPE OF DIABETES AND ETHNICITY OF POPULATION

Part of the explanation for the increasing numbers of diabetic patients on RRT has been a relaxation of age limits for entry [2]. Diabetes prevalence increases dramatically with age and one of the major risk factors for the development of nephropathy is duration of disease. Thus it is no surprise that as the average age of acceptance onto RRT has increased from 45.8 years in 1977 to 57.4 years in 1992 in Europe, and the number of new patients commencing RRT over 65 years at acceptance increased from 9 to 37% of the total over the same period of time [2], that the proportion with diabetes has jumped dramatically. In Japan the mean age rose from 49.2 to 57.3 years over the period 1984-94 [5], and in the USA the increase was slightly less dramatic from approximately 56 years in 1986 to 60 years in 1995 [1].

Although the cumulative incidence and rates of development of nephropathy are similar for both types of diabetes [9], a smaller proportion of patients with type 2 enter RRT, probably because of excess cardiovascular mortality prior to developing ESRD [10]. However, as there are numerically many more patients with type 2 diabetes, they represent a greater and growing proportion of the diabetic patients on RRT. The precise figures are not certain however, as the USRDS does not code for type of diabetes and those registers that do, such as the

EDTA Registry, have been shown to be very imprecise in the assignation of patients [11,12]. Using a carefully designed algorithm for the diagnosis of diabetes type, Cowie et al [13] found an increased probability of developing ESRD over a 10 year period of 5.82% in type 1 but only 0.5% in type 2 African-American and Europid patients. However, there was a suggestion of an increasing incidence in type 2 patients over the decade 1974-83. The proportion of patients with carefully defined type 2 diabetes on RRT varies from 50-90% in Europid populations worldwide [14].

It is difficult to separate the impact of type of diabetes from ethnic factors. In Japan for example, >90% of patients on RRT have type 2 diabetes [5] but this is a reflection of the remarkably low incidence of type 1 nationally. Many ethnic groups have high prevalences of both type 2 diabetes and nephropathy [5], and countries with minorities with these characteristics will reflect an over preponderance in their RRT population. For example, in 1993 diabetic Aboriginal patients in Australia and Maori/Pacific Islanders in New Zealand receiving RRT were 85% and 83% type 2 respectively, compared to Europid proportions of 48 and 55% in the same countries [14]. The USRDS reports that incidence of ESRD for all causes in 1993-5 for African Americans was 758, for Native Americans 640, and for Asian/Pacific Islanders 327pmp per year, compared to 180pmp per year for Europids [1]. Furthermore, although the incidence in 1995 of Native Americans with diabetic ESRD was just 2.4% of the total diabetic patient population, this accounted for 63% of all Native Americans receiving RRT. The figures for Asians/Pacific Islanders were similarly discrepant at 3% and 39.9%; whereas those for African Americans were 28.3 and 36.4%; and for Europids 65.4 and 38% respectively. The incidence rates of treated ESRD for diabetes for the period 1991-3 in pmp per year were 322, 89, 224, and 57 for Native Americans, Asian/Pacific Islanders, African Americans and Europid patients respectively [1]. Cowie et al [13] found an increased ratio of probability of developing ESRD in African Americans of 1.62 and 3.93 for type 1 and type 2 diabetes respectively when compared to Europids.

In the UK there has been a dramatic increase in ESRF in patients from Southern Asia (India, Pakistan, Bangladesh, Sri Lanka) and the West Indies, such that in 1991-2 these patients were accepted onto RRT at a rate of 239 and 220 pmp respectively [16], with diabetes as a major cause in both groups. The reported risk for developing diabetic ESRD is up to fourteen-fold in South Asians compared to Europid patients in Leicester [15]. Interestingly South Asian patients also have an increased risk of approximately five-fold for non-diabetic ESRD [15]. Recently it has been estimated that the proportion of patients from Southern Asia and the Caribbean requiring RRT in the UK will rise from 39 to >50% by the year 2001 [16].

The reasons for the increased incidence of diabetes and its complications in ethnic minorities are not understood and are currently the source of intense controversy, particularly the low birth weight - thrifty phenotype hypothesis [17].

Whatever the cause, the consequence will be rapidly increasing numbers of patients with diabetic ERSD worldwide for the foreseeable future.

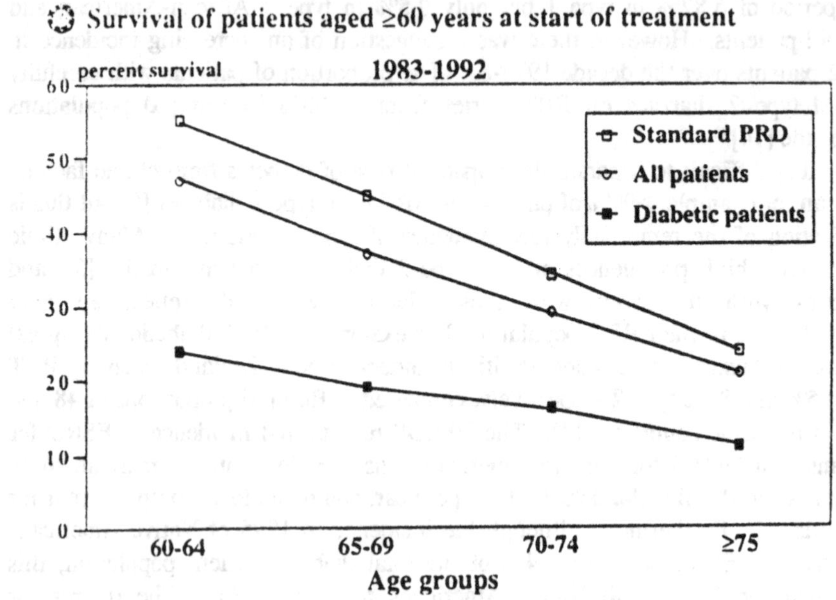

Figure 47-1 Comparison of percent 5 year survival in patients with standard (non-diabetic) primary renal disease (PRD) with diabetic patients broken down by age at commencement of RRT for the decade 1983-92. [Reproduced from ref. 2 with permission of the EDTA Registry and the publishers.]

MODE OF TREATMENT AND OUTCOME

There is a wide range of preferred RRT options for diabetic ESRD worldwide for reasons that are cultural/religious (e.g. low transplantation rates in Japan) [6], financial (e.g. higher rates of haemodialysis (HD) in some European countries because of its link to government remuneration), and medical (e.g. theoretical advantages of CAPD v. HD) [18]. No randomised control trials have ever been performed, perhaps for obvious reasons, thus it is hard to draw firm conclusions about preferred treatment.

In the USA in 1995, 18% of diabetic patients with ESRD had a functioning transplant (Tx). 69% were on HD and 12% were on a form of peritoneal dialysis (PD) [19]. For Europe in 1992 the figures were 15%, 68% and 32% respectively, with considerable variation between countries [8]. For example, in the UK in 1991, 50% were on PD, 35% on HD and 15% had a functioning graft. For France and Scandinavia the proportions were <10% and 33%, 65% and 37%, and 25% and 30% for PD, HD and Tx respectively. In Japan in 1994, 96% of diabetic patients were on HD and 4% on PD [5].

Table 47-1 Worldwide incidence and prevalence of ESRD in patients with diabetes mellitus.

COUNTRY	POPULATION STUDIED	YEAR OF OBSERVATION	PREVALENCE PER MILLION POP.		INCIDENCE PER MILLION POP.		% TYPE 2 DIABETES	REF.
			ALL CAUSES	DIABETES	ALL CAUSES	DIABETES		
USA	NATIONAL	1995	967	303	253	104	59	1
	EUROPID	1993-5 ALL CAUSES 1991-3 DIABETES			180	57		1
	NATIVE AMERICAN				640	322		1
	AFRICAN-AMERICAN				758	224		1
	ASIANS/PACIFIC ISLANDERS				327	89		1
JAPAN	NATIONAL	1994	1149	209	194	60	>90	5
EUROPE (EDTA)		1994	312	61	59	10		6
AUSTRALA	NATIONAL	1993	427	33	65	10	61	14
	EUROPID		374	23	54	7	48	
	ABORIGINAL		1129	335	338	125	85	
NEW ZEALAND	NATIONAL	1993	406	58	65	20	79	14
	EUROPID		311	16	37	4	55	
	MAORI/PACIFIC ISLANDERS		648	273	166	91	83	

In most reported series, survival is best in those diabetic patients receiving a kidney transplant [3,8], but this almost certainly reflects a degree of patient selection. Short term survival for diabetic patients has gradually increased in the USA over the decade until 1994 [3]. For the first time, the incident death rate in 1994 declined below that recorded for causes of ESRD other than hypertension and glomerulonephritis to 27 per hundred patient years [3]. This represents a reduction of 39% from the death rate of 44 per hundred patient years recorded in 1984. Prevalent death rates in 1995 range from approximately 75 per thousand patient years for 15-19 year olds, to >300 per thousand patient years for 60-64 year olds, and >400 per thousand patient years for >70 year olds. These rates were highest for Europid patients [3]. For non-diabetic patients, the rates were approximately 40, 200, and >300 per thousand patient years for 15-19, 60-64, and >70 year olds respectively.

From 1993-5 for never transplanted patients aged 20-44 years, the death rate was approximately twice as high in diabetic compared to non-diabetic patients (160.7 v. 83.3 per thousand patient years), but this was five times the rate seen in diabetic subjects with a functioning transplant (31.4 per thousand patient years); and this in turn was almost three times the rate in non-diabetic transplant recipients over the same period (11.9 per thousand patient years). The major cause of death in these diabetic patients was cardiovascular disease (49% for never transplanted, 30% for functioning transplant v. 29% and 22% for non-diabetic patients respectively) [20]. Five year survival rates for diabetic patients are not given separately in this report.

In Japan 5 and 10 year survival for diabetic patients on HD from 1983 onwards was 47% and 21% respectively, compared to 71% and 53% for patients with chronic glomerulonephritis [5]. Detailed causes of death are not provided, and the data are not broken down by age.

In Europe the latest information on survival relates to >60 year olds on treatment from 1983-92 [2]. For diabetic patients, five year survival rates were 23% for 60-64 year olds and 18% for 70-74 year olds compared to 56% and 36% for non-diabetic ESRD respectively. Cardiovascular causes of death again predominated but there was not a great difference between diabetic and non-diabetic >60 year olds (59 v. 55%) [2]. Five year survival rates in patients on dialysis in Northern European countries are broadly similar despite different proportions of modality of treatment of RRT, but diabetic patients in Southern Europe (Italy, Spain and Portugal) do significantly better than those in the North, whatever the treatment [2]. A similar phenomenon has been reported for Hispanic compared to Europid diabetic patients in Texas [21]. The reasons are not entirely clear but may be a reflection of the lower incidence of cardiovascular disease, perhaps secondary to dietary factors, seen in these groups.

The survival rates for Japanese patients on HD [22] are better than for Europe [2] and the USA [3] and this may be a reflection of the longer time and consequently more effective dialysis in the Japanese patients [6]. Currently, studies are ongoing to explore this proposition. Longer survival in Japanese patients may also be explained by their lower risk of cardiovascular disease.

Because of the increased rate of cardiovascular death in diabetic patients on all modalities of RRT, some centres are advocating full vascular investigation prior to ESRD with coronary angiography in high risk subjects [23]. These workers have reported improved survival in patients who undergo coronary artery bypass grafting prior to renal transplantation [24].

SUGGESTED MANAGEMENT STRATEGIES

One of the key factors determining outcome of RRT for all patients is clinical status at entry. This is particularly true for diabetic patients in whom there is often considerable co-morbidity. The guidelines for referral suggested by the kidney working group of the St Vincent Declaration include joint assessment by nephrologist and diabetologist once serum creatinine exceeds 200μmol/l [25]. A recent report from a German centre suggests that in practice many patients are presenting in established renal failure [26]. In addition, specific treatments of proven worth such as angiotensin converting enzyme inhibitors drugs, and good blood pressure control were either absent or inadequate. No mention in this report was made of cholesterol lowering therapy or aspirin use. A major priority for all of us looking after diabetic patients with renal complications is to improve on these figures. Only then are we likely to see further significant improvements in survival.

CONCLUSIONS

Incidence of diabetic ESRD is increasing world-wide, particularly in Southern Asian, Afro-Caribbean, Native American, Hispanic, and Pacific Islander populations. Rates in North American Europid subjects may be slowing down.

Acceptance of diabetic patients onto RRT is consequently increasing with a prevalence of around 300 pmp in the USA. European rates are much less than this but growing.

Survival on RRT is less good for diabetic patients who tend to have much higher death rates from cardiovascular disease.

Early referral and aggressive management of vascular risk factors and established arterial disease is recommended.

REFERENCES

1. United States Renal Data System 1997 - Annual Data Report. II Incidence and prevalence of ESRD. Am. J. Kid. Dis. 1997; 30: suppl 1: S40-53.
2. Valderrabano F, Berthoux F C, Jones E H P, Mehls O. Report on management of renal failure in Europe XXV, 1994. Endstage renal disease and dialysis report. Nephrol. Dial. Transplant 1996; 11: suppl 1: 2-21.
3. United States Renal Data System 1997 - Annual Data Report. V Patient mortality and survival. Am. J. Kid. Dis. 1997; 30: suppl 1: S86-106.
4. United States Renal Data System 1997 - Annual Data Report. XIII Analytical methods. Am. J. Kid. Dis. 1997; 30: suppl 1: S195-213.

5. Shinzato T, Nakai S, Akiba T et al. Current status of renal replacement therapy in Japan: results of the annual survey of the Japanese society for dialysis therapy. Nephrol. Dial. Transplant 1997; 12: 889-898.
6. Valderrabano F. Renal replacement therapy. What are the differences between Japan and Europe? Nephrol. Dial. Transplant 1996; 11: 2151-2153.
7. United States Renal Data System 1997 - Annual Data Report. XII International comparisons of ESRD therapy. Am. J. Kid. Dis. 1997; 30: suppl 1: S187-94.
8. Valderrabano F, Jones E H P, Mallick N P. Report on management of renal failure in Europe XXIV, 1993. Nephrol. Dial. Transplant 1995; 10: suppl 5. 1-25.
9. Hasslacher C, Ritz E, Wahl P, Michael C. Similar risks of nephropathy in patients with type I and type II diabetes mellitus. Nephrol. Dial. Transplant 1989; 4: 859-863.
10. Lippert J, Ritz E, Schwarzbeck A, Schneider P. The rising tide of endstage renal failure from diabetic nephropathy type II - an epidemiological analysis. Nephrol. Dial. Transplant 1995; 10: 462-467.
11. Catalano C, Postorino M, Kelly P J et al. Diabetes mellitus and renal replacement therapy in Italy: prevalence, main characteristics and complications. Nephrol. Dial. Transplant 1995; 788-96.
12. Zmirou D, Benhamou P-Y, Cordonnier D, Borgel F, Balducci F, Papoz L, Halimi S. Diabetes mellitus prevalence among dialysed patients in France (UREMIDIAB Study). Nephrol. Dial. Transplant 1992; 7: 1092-1097.
13. Cowie C C, Port F K, Wolfe R A, Savage P J, Moll P P, Hawthorne V M. Disparities and incidence of diabetic endstage renal disease according to race and type of diabetes. N. Engl. J. Med. 1989; 321: 1074-1079.
14. Ritz E, Stefanski A. Diabetic nephropathy in type II diabetes. Am. J. Kid. Dis. 1996; 27: 167-194.
15. Buck K, Feehally J. Diabetes and renal failure in Indo-Asians in the UK - A paradigm for the study of disease susceptibility. Nephrol. Dial. Transplant 1997; 12: 1555-1557.
16. Raleigh V S. Diabetes and hypertension in Britain's ethnic minorities: implications for the future of renal services. BMJ 1997; 314: 209-213.
17. Barker D J P, Hales C N, Fall C H D, Osmond C, Phipps K, Clark P M S. Type II (non-insulin dependent) diabetes mellitus, hypertension and hyperlipidaemia (syndrome X); relation to reduced foetal growth. Diabetologia 1993; 36: 62-67.
18. Khanna R. Dialysis considerations for diabetic patients. Kidney Int. 1993; 43: suppl 40: S 58-S64.
19. United States Renal Data System 1997 - Annual Data Report. III Treatment modalities for ESRD patients. Am. J. Kid. Dis. 1997; 30: suppl 1: S54-66.
20. United States Renal Data System 1997 - Annual Data Report. VI Causes of death. Am. J. Kid. Dis. 1997; 30: suppl 1: S107-S117.
21. Medina R A, Pugh J A, Monterrosa A, Cornell J. Minority advantage in diabetic endstage renal disease survival on haemodialysis: due to different proportions of diabetic type? Am. J. Kid. Dis. 1996; 28: 226-234.
22. Shinzato T, Nakai S, Akiba T et al. Survival in long term haemodialysis patients: results from the annual survey of the Japanese society for dialysis therapy. Nephrol. Dial. Transplant 1997; 12: 884-888.
23. Manske C L, Thomas W, Wang Y, Wilson R F. Screening diabetic transplant candidates for coronary artery disease: identification of a low risk sub-group. Kidney Int. 1993; 44: 617-621.
24. Manske C L, Wang Y, Rector T, Wilson R F, White C W. Coronary revascularisation in insulin dependent diabetic patients with chronic renal failure. Lancet 1992; 340: 998-1002.
25. Viberti G C, Mogensen C E, Passa P, Bilous R, Mangili R. St Vincent Declaration, 1994: Guidelines for the prevention of diabetic renal failure. In, The kidney and hypertension in diabetes mellitus, second ed, Mogensen C E ed. Boston, Dordrecht, London: Kluwer Academic Publishers, 1994; pp 515-527.
26. Pommer W, Bressel F, Chen F, Molzahn M. There is room for improvement of pre-terminal care in diabetic patients with endstage renal failure - the epidemiological evidence in Germany. Nephrol. Dial Transplant. 1997; 12: 1318-20

48. HEMODIALYSIS IN TYPE I AND TYPE II DIABETIC PATIENTS WITH ENDSTAGE RENAL FAILURE

Eberhard Ritz, Antony Raine†, Daniel Cordonnier
Klinikum der Universität Heidelberg, Medizinische Klinik Heidelberg, Germany, Centre Hospitalier Régional, et Universitaire de Grenoble, Grenoble, France

INTRODUCTION

In the early days of hemodialysis efforts to treat and rehabilitate uremic diabetics were largely unsuccessful [1] until dialysis procedures and volume control had become more effective. Although diabetics have a poorer outcome than non-diabetics, survival has improved progressively, e.g. in the US adjusted first year mortality decreasing from 46% in 1982 to 30% in 1992 [2], although long-term survival is still very unsatisfactory, e.g. at 5 years 45% in type I and 10% in type II diabetics according to a recent German multicenter study [3]. Nevertheless it is no longer justified to deny admission to renal replacement therapy to the diabetic patient [4].

1. EPIDEMIOLOGY

In many countries, endstage renal failure (ESRF) in diabetic patients (in most patients presumably from diabetic glomerulosclerosis) has meanwhile become the single most important cause of ESRF in many countries [5, 6]. In Europe, there has been a constant increase in the absolute number and proportion of diabetics entering renal replacement programs [7]. It has meanwhile become the single most important cause of ESRF in Germany. In 1996, diabetics accounted for 58% admissions for renal replacement therapy in Heidelberg. This compares with 38% in US whites [5]. In Heidelberg, 90% of admissions for renal replacement therapy were for type II diabetes. Although wide differences exist between countries in Northern and Southern Europe, possibly related to differences in life style and in genetic predisposition, admission rates for diabetic ESRF are on the rise in

† Deceased October 14th, 1995

Southern Europe as well. For instance, a 10-fold increase during the last decade has recently been reported from Spain [8]. Remarkably low incidence rates, i.e. 20%, are still reported from Australia [9]. A striking difference between metropolitan France (6.9%) and overseas territories (Guadeloupe 15%, Tahiti 34%) may reflect racial differences in the propensity to develop diabetes and diabetic nephropathy [10], as has been described for the black population in the USA [11]. In the past, the renal risk in type II diabetes has clearly been underappreciated [12]. Misclassification has also occurred in many studies, since the use of insulin was equated with type I diabetes [7,10,12]. Cordonnier et al. [10] noted that the relative proportion of type I diabetics decreased by 50% when patients were re-examined by diabetologists and when C-peptide measurements were performed. Similar misclassification has also been recognised in Italy: 35% were classified as type II by the registry, but 57% by a specific questionnaire [13]. While virtually all patients with type I diabetes entering renal replacement programs suffer from diabetic nephropathy, a certain proportion of type II diabetics, ranging from 20% [12] to 50% [10], was reported to suffer from standard primary renal diseases. Several studies showed pronounced ischemic lesions of the kidney of patients with type II diabetes in contrast to those with type I. Isolated ischemic nephropathy, or ischemic nephropathy, superimposed upon Kimmelstiel Wilson lesions, may differ with respect to evolution of renal failure and may also differ with respect to the response to antihypertensive medication. It is also important that a substantial proportion of patients with type II diabetes enter terminal renal failure subsequent to an episode of acute renal failure from administration of contrast media, cardiac events or septicemic episodes [6].

2. SURVIVAL AND CAUSES OF DEATH

The recent US data report [5] gives death rates in diabetic dialysis patients of 100-300 deaths/1000 patient years for the ages 20-70 years compared to 30-200 in non-diabetic patients. In a matched case control study we found that actuarial 5 year survival in diabetics was worse than in matched non-diabetic patients [14] and this difference has not diminished in recent years [3]. The causes of death are mostly cardiovascular [15] as shown in table 48-1, which is very often completely asymptomatic. Survival is roughly similar on hemodialysis and CAPD. While in the European series, a slightly better survival on CAPD was found for elderly patients in general and for elderly diabetics specifically [16], the US Renal Data System shows generally better survival on CAPD for the younger patients and slightly worse survival for elderly diabetic patients [17]. If one wishes to improve survival in diabetic patients on renal replacement therapy, it is imperative to reduce the cardiovascular death and death from infection. Septicemia is not negligable as a cause. Today, septicemia originates from foot gangrene and rarely from infected vascular access [15].

3. PREDICTORS OF SURVIVAL

It is clearly important to identify the high risk patient in order to target appropriate preventive measures. Cardiac death is strongly predicted by a history of vascular disease, specifically myocardial infarction or angina pectoris [3,15,18]. Proliferative retinopathy and polyneuropathy are also predictive, possibly through causing imbalance of autonomic cardiac innervation [15,19]. Biochemical predictors are lipoprotein concentrations [20], particularly low apolipoprotein A [3] and low molecular weight isoforms of LP(a) [21], smoking [18,22] and, interestingly, poor glycemic control, both on CAPD [23] and hemodialysis [24]. Cardiac death rate is higher in patients with left ventricular concentric hypertrophy or ischemic heart disease [18,25], the presence of which is significantly higher than in non-diabetic patients. The recent molecular studies showed that the risk of cardiac events is particularly higher in individuals with the D/D (deletion) genotype of the ACE gene [26].

4. METABOLIC CONTROL ON RENAL REPLACEMENT THERAPY

Using the euglycemic clamp technique, DeFronzo documented impaired efficacy of insulin in uremic subjects [27] and this was partially improved with institution of maintenance hemodialysis. This observation suggests that putative dialyzable inhibitors of insulin action are removed by dialysis. Peptidic inhibitors of non-insulin-mediated glucose uptake have also been identified in the ultrafiltrate of dialysis patients [28]. In clinical practice, the need for insulin decreases upon institution of maintenance hemodialysis, although complexities arise because of the prolongation of insulin half life in anephric patients and the confounding effects of reduced food intake (anorexia of renal failure) and of refeeding (after commencement of hemodialysis).

Table 48.1 Causes of death (57 months after start of dialysis). [15].

Type I	Type II (n=67)		(n=129)	
Dead	29	(=40%)	80	(=43%)
Myoc.infarction	8/29		12/80	
Sudden death	7/29		13/80	
		62% CV		(60% CV)
Cardiac other	3/29		17/80	
Stroke	0/29		6/80	
Septicemia	7/29		11/80	
Interruption of treatment	2/29		8/80	
Other	2/29		13/80	

Most nephrologists prefer to dialyse against glucose (200 mg/dl) to achieve better stabilisation of plasma glucose concentrations. This strategy allows patients to stay on their regular insulin schedules and take their regular meals irrespective of dialysis sessions. Diabetic control is occasionally rendered difficult by diabetic gastroparesis and the tendency of gastric motility to deteriorate acutely during dialysis sessions. Despite all these complexities, efforts to aim at good glycemic control received a strong rationale by the recent observation that glycemia predicts survival of diabetic patients on CAPD [23] and on hemodialysis [24].

5. DIABETIC COMPLICATIONS ON RENAL REPLACEMENT THERAPY

In contrast to previous experience [1] de novo amaurosis has become rare in the diabetic on dialysis. In a series of 200 diabetics entering hemodialysis from 1987-1989, no single case experienced loss of vision in an eye whose vision had been normal when entering hemodialysis [15]. With appropriate laser treatment and control of blood pressure, previous concerns about hemorrhagic retinal complications as a result of dialysis-related anticoagulation are no longer justified. Diabetic polyneuropathy, specifically autonomic polyneuropathy with cystopathy, gastroparesis and intestinal dysmotility have emerged as major problems on dialysis. The observation that polyneuropathy is preditive of cardiac death suggests that imbalanced autonomic innervation of the heart also contributes to arrhythmia and sudden death. This suspicion gains further credence from the observation that 3% of patients dying from myocardial infarction vs. 18% of survivors had been on betablockers, the agents of choice for treating imbalanced autonomic innervation and this has recently led to the postulate to administer betablockers more liberally [29]. Detection of cystopathy and latent urinary tract infection is important when patients are prepared for renal transplantation. Ischemic heart disease has emerged as a major threat to the dialysed diabetic. The issue is further compounded by the fact that this complication is often clinically silent. Studies of Weinrauch [30] and subsequently others [3,18,21] identified hemodynamically significant coronary stenosis in approximately 30% of prospective diabetic recipients of renal allografts. There is discussion whether routine coronary angiography should routinely be performed even in asymptomatic diabetics prior to renal transplantation. High risk patients can be recognized by relatively simple algorithms [31]. In a small number of patients, Manske et al. [32] documented that survival was superior in diabetic patients with CHD who had surgical intervention than in those who remained on medical therapy. The conclusions are obvious and call for aggressive diagnosis and management. In the future the main problem will be to interfere with the development of coronary heart disease in the predialytic phase, since ischemic heart disease is already prevalent when patients enter renal replacement therapy.

The reocclusion rate after PTCA is disappointing; i.e. 70% after one year [33], but long-term prognosis with bypass surgery appears to be more encouraging. No controlled information is available on the use of stents. Uncontrolled observations suggest that symptomatic ischemic heart disease is strikingly ameliorated when hemoglobin levels are raised by treatment with recombinant human erythropoietin [34]. Left ventricular hypertrophy and diastolic left ventricular malfunction are early and very common complications [35] and may contribute to arrhythmia and circulatory instability during dialysis sessions [36]. Amputation because of neuropathic or ischemic foot lesions is required in approximately 8% of dialysed diabetic patients over three years. Pre-existing arterial occlusive disease and a history of smoking are potent predictors. Ischemic foot lesions benefit strikingly from treatment with rhEPO. Interestingly, in transplanted diabetics the rate of amputation tends to be higher, possibly because of the use of steroids and/or cyclosporin. A controlled study on the potential effect of lipid lowering has not been performed, but this issue is currently under investigation in a large prospective trial using Atorvastatin.

It is commonly stated, that vascular access is more difficult in diabetics. Venous hypoplasia is very common in elderly female diabetics and in polymorbid patients veins are often thrombosed from preceding i.v. therapy. Otherwise, however, we have not found that fistula problems are more frequent in diabetics than in non-diabetic patients. It is useful to monitor arterial blood flow by Duplex sonography. In case of low arterial flow, a high anastomosis in the elbow region is recommended. It is advisable to create the fistula prophylactically once the creatinine clearance is approximately 20 ml/min, since "maturation" of the fistula takes decidedly longer in the diabetic patient.

6. TRANSPLANTATION IN THE DIABETIC PATIENT

There is agreement that medical rehabilitation for the diabetic uremic patient is best after transplantation [37,38]. Recent US data [39] show that while the relative survival benefit from transplantation over hemodialysis is marginal for patients with glomerulonephritis, it becomes dramatic for the diabetic. This applies not only to the younger type I, but increasingly also to the elderly type II diabetic, if patients with severe vascular disease are excluded [40]. Outcome from transplantation in diabetics is poorer (fig. 48-1), but results are continuously improving and an increasing number of patients is asking for transplantation. This is true both for type I (simultaneous pancreas and kidney graft) and for type II (kidney alone). The latter are not necessarily very old and very handicapped. In the French Uremidiab Study [41,42], 40 of the French type II diabetics on dialysis were less than 50 year of age and their own perception of the handicap was not different from that of diabetic patients without nephropathy or non-diabetic dialysed patients. So far cases of preemptive transplantation i.e. prior to the stage of dialysis dependency have remained anecdotal. Successful pancreas transplants undoubtedly improve the quality of life. Whether they have a positive influence on delayed diabetic complications is currently uncertain, although duration of follow-up may not have been sufficient to proof the point. There is very suggestive evidence for amelioration of autonomic polyneuropathy. Combined kidney/pancreas transplantation has become a relatively safe procedure and as a consequence, the numbers have recently increased substantially [37].

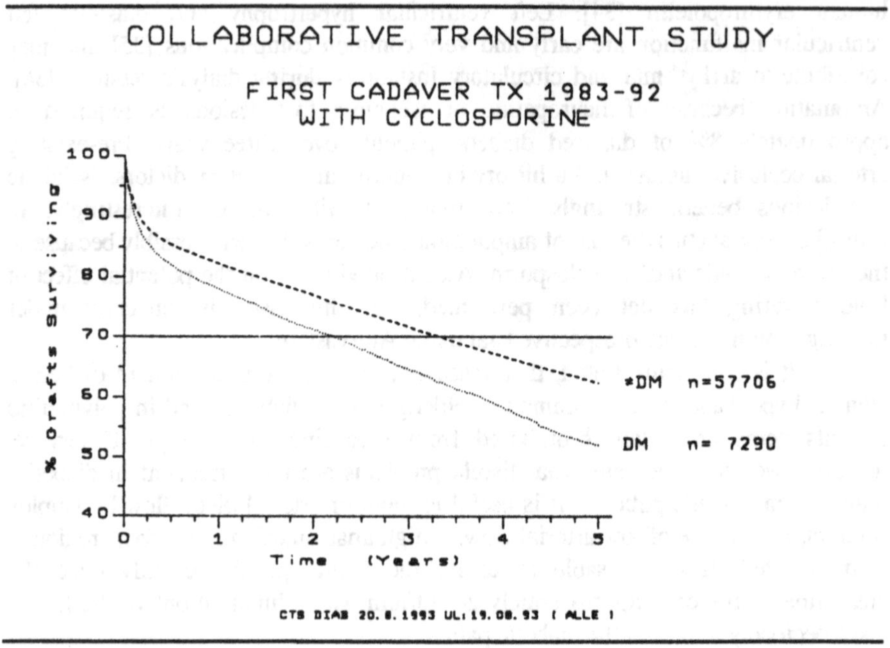

Fig. 48-1 Renal graft survival in patients with type 1 diabetes. (First graft). According to the CTS study (combined transplantation study, courtesy Professor Opelz, Heidelberg.)

SUMMARY

The number of diabetic patients entering renal replacement programs is increasing in all Western countries. Hemodialysis is the preferred modality of treatment, hemofiltration and CAPD being used only in a minority. The proportion of patients undergoing renal or combined renal and pancreatic transplantation is rising encouragingly. Survival in diabetic compared to non-diabetic patients is worse for all renal replacement modalities. This is mainly due to cardiovascular death. Cardiac death is predicted by a history of vascular disease, echocardiographic abnormalities, smoking and lipid abnormalities. Common clinical problems in the dialysed diabetic include difficulties in metabolic control, visual disturbance, sequelae of autonomic polyneuropathy, amputation and vascular access.

REFERENCES

1. Ghavamian M, Gutch CG, Kopp KF, Kolff WJ. The sad truth about hemodialysis in diabetic nephropathy. JAMA 1972; 222: 1386-1389
2. Brunner FP et al. Survival on renal replacement therapy: data from the EDTA registry. Nephrol Dial Transplant 1988; 1: 109-122
3. Koch M, Kutkuhn B, Grabensee B, Ritz E. Apolipoprotein A, fibrinogen, age, and history of stroke are predictors of death in dialysed diabetic patients: a prospective study in 412 subjects. Nephrol Dial Transplant 1997; 12: 2603-2611
4. Pirson Y. The diabetic patient with ESRD: how to select the modality of renal replacement. Nephrol Dial Transplant 1996; 11: 1511-1514
5. Annual Data Report. United States Renal Data System, April 1997

6. Lippert J, Ritz E, Schwarzbeck A, Schneider P. The rising tide of endstage renal faiulre from diabetic nephropathy type II - an epidemiological analysis. Nephrol Dial Transplant 1995; 10: 462-467
7. Raine AEG. Epidemiology, development and treatment of endstage renal failure in non-insulin dependent diabetics in Europe. Diabetologia 1993; 36: 1099-1104
8. Rodriguez JA, Clèries M, Vela E and Renal Registry Committee. Diabetic patients on renal replacement therapy: anqalysis of Catalan Registry Data. Nephrol Dial Transplant 1997; 12: 2501-2509
9. Nineteenth Report of the Australia and New Zealand Dialysis and Transplant Registry (ANZDATA) 1996 (Disney APS, ed.)
10. Cordonnier DJ, Zmirou D, Benhamou PY, Halimi S, Ledoux F, Guiserix J. Epidemiology, development and treatment of endstage renal failure in Type 2 (non-insulin-dependent) diabetes. The case of mainland France and of overseas French territories. Diabetolgia 1993; 36: 1109-1112
11. Cowie CC, Port FK, Wolfe RA, Savage PJ, Moll PP, Hawtorne VM. Disparities in incidence of diabetic end-stage renal disease according mto ravce and type of diabetes. N Engl J Med 1989; 321: 1074-1079
12. Ritz E, Nowack R, Fliser D, Koch M, Tschöpe W. Type II diabetes: Is the renal risk adequately appreciated? Nephrol Dial Transplant 1991; 6: 679-682
13. Catalano C, Postorino M, Kelly PJ, Fabrizi F, Emnia G, Goodship TH. Diabetes melliltus and renal replacement therapy in Italy: prevalence, main charcteristics and complications. Nephrol Dial Transplant 1990; 5: 788-796
14. Ritz E, Strumpf C, Katz F, Wing AJ, Quellhorst E. Hypertension and cardiovascular risk factors in hemodialysed diabetic patients. Hypertension 1985; 7: 118-125
15. Koch M, Thomas B, Tschöpe W. Survival and predictors of death in dialysed diabetics. Diabetologia 1993; 36: 1113-1117
16. Majorca R, et al. A six year comparison of patient and technique survivals in CAPD and HD. Kidney Int 1988; 34: 518-524
17. United States Renal Data System. Annual Data Report. Am J Kidn Dis 1991; 18: Suppl 2
18. Foley RN, Culleton BF, Parfrey PS, Harnett JD, Kent GM, Murray DC, Bare PE. Cardiac disease in diabetic endstage renal disease. Diabetologia 1997; 40: 1307-1312
19. Kikkawa A, Arimura T, Haneda M, Nkshio T, Katsunori S, Yagisawa M, Shigeta Y. Current status of type II (non-insulin-dependent) diabetic subjects on dialysis therapy in Japan. Diabetologia 1993; 36: 1105-1108
20. Tschöpe W, Koch M, Thomas B, Ritz E. Serum lipids predict cardiac death in diabetic patients on maintenance hemodialysis. Nephrol 1992; 64: 354-358
21. Koch M, Kutkuhn B, Trenkwalder E, Bach D, Grabensee B, Dieplinger H, Kronenberg F. Apolipoprotein B, fibrinogen, HDL cholesterol, and apolipoprotein(a) phenotypes predict coronary artery disease in hemodialysis patients. J Am Soc Nephrol 1997; 8: 1889-1898
22. McMillan MA, Briggs JD, Junor BS. Outcome of renal replacement therapy in patients with diabetes mellitus. Bit Med J 1990; 301: 540-544
23. Yu CC, W MS, W CH, Yang CW, Huang JY, Hong JJ, Chian CYF, Leu ML, Huang CC. Predialysis glycemic control is an independent predictor of clinical outcome in typoe II diabetics on continuous ambulatory peritoneal dialysis. Periton Dial Internat 1997; 17: 262-268
24. Wu MS, Yu CC, Wang CW, Wu CH, Haung JY, Hong JJ, Fan Chiang CY, Huang CC, Leu ML. Poor predialysis glycemic control is a predictor of mortality in type II diabetic patients on maintenance hemodialysis. Nephrol Dial Transplant 1997; 12: 2105-
25. Foley RN, Parfrey PS. Cardiac disease in the diabetic dialysis patient. Nephrol Dial Transplant (in press)
26. Fujisawa T, Ikegami H, Shen GG. Angiotensin I converting enzyme polymorphism is associated with myocardial infarction, but not with retinopathy or nephropathy, in NIDDM. Diabetes Care 1995; 18: 983-985
27. DeFronzo Ra, Alvestrand A, Smith D, Hendler E, Waren J. Insulin resistance in uremia. J Clin Invest 1981; 67: 563-568
28. Hörl WH, Haag-Weber M, Georgopoulos A, Block LH. The physicochemical characterization of a novel polypeptide present in uremic serum that inhibits the biological activity of polymorphonuclear cells. Proc Natl Acad Sci 1990; 87: 6353-6357
29. Zuanetti G, Maggioni AP, Keane W, Ritz E. Nephrologists neglect administration of betablockers to dialysed diabetic patients. Nephrol Dial Transplant 1997; 12: 2497-2501

30. Weinrauch LA, D'Elia JA, Healy RW. Asymptomatic coronary artery disease angiography in diabetic patients before renal transplantation. Ann Intern Med 1978; 88: 346-348
31. Manske CL, Thomas W, Wang Y, Wilson RF. Screeding diabetic transplant candidates for coronary artery disease: Identification of a low risk subgroup. Kidney Int 1993; 44: 617-621
32. Manske CL, Wang Y, Rector T, Wilson RF, White CW. Coronary revascularisation in insulin-dependent diabetic patients with chronic renal failure. Lancet 1992; 340: 998-1002
33. Rinehart AL, Herzog CA, Collins AJ, Flack JM, Ma JZ, Opsahl JA. Greater risk of cardiac events after coronary angioplasty (PTCA) than bypass grafting (CABG) in chronic dialysis patients. J Am Soc Nephrol 1992; 3: 389(a)
34. Wizemann V, Kaufmann J, Kramer W. Effect of erythropoietin on ischemia tolerance in anemic hemodialysis patients with confirmed coronary artery disease. Nephron 1992; 62: 161-165
35. Uusitupa M et al. Relationship of blood pressure and left ventricular mass to serum insulin levels in newly diagnosed NIDDM (type II) and in non-diabetic subjects. Diabetes Res 1987; 4: 19-25
36. Ritz E, Ruffmann K, Rambausek M, Mall G, Schmidly M. Dialysis hypotension - is it related to diastolic left ventricular malfunction? Nephrol Dial Transplant 1987; 2: 193-197
37. Ringe B, Braun F. Pancreas transplantation: where do we stand in Europe in 1997? Nephrol Dial Transplant 1997; 12: 1100-1104
38. Rischen-Vos J, van der Woude FJ, Tegzess AM,. Zwinderman AH, Gosszen HC, van den Akker PJ, van Es LA. Increased morbidity and mortality in patients with diabetes mellitus after kidney transplantation as compared with non-diabetic patients. Nephrol Dial Transplant 1992; 7: 433-437
39. Port FK, Wolfe RA, Mauger EA, Berlin DP, Jian K. Comparison of survival probabilities for dialysis patients vs cadaveric renal transplant recipients. JAMA 1993; 270: 1339-1343
40. Hirschl MM, Derfler K, Heinz G, Sunder-Plassmann G, Waldhäusl W. Longterm follow-up of renal transplantation in type I and type II diabetic patients. Clin Invest 1992; 70: 917-921
41. Borgel F, Benhamou PY, Zmirou D, Balducci F, Halimi S, Cordonnier A. Assessment of handicap in chronic dialysis diabetic patients (Uremidiab Study). Scand J Rehab Med 1992; 24: 203-208
42. Zmirou D, Benhamou PY, Cordonnier D, Borgel F, Balducci F, Papoz L, Halmi S. Diabetes mellitus prevalence among dialysis patients in France (Uremidiab Study). Nephrol Dial Transplant 1992; 7: 1092-1097

49. CONTINUOUS AMBULATORY PERITONEAL DIALYSIS IN UREMIC DIABETICS

Elias V. Balaskas and Dimitrios G. Oreopoulos
Peritoneal Dialysis Unit, University of Toronto, The Toronto Hospital, Toronto, Ontario, Canada

During the last 15 years, there has been an impressive increase in the number of patients with end-stage renal disease (ESRD) due to diabetic nephropathy[1]. Diabetic nephropathy has become the leading cause of ESRD in such countries as United States, Canada, Japan, Scandinavia and much of Western Europe, accounting for 30% of new patients and 26% of U.S. dialysis and transplant patients[2,3]. In the recent USRDS 1997–Annual Data Report, 37.4% of total treated ESRD patients for 1991 to 1995 years are diabetics with an incidence of 94 patients/million pop./ year and a prevalence of 274 patients /million pop/year, for 1993 to 1995 years[4]. Hemodialysis (HD), continuous ambulatory peritoneal dialysis (CAPD) and renal transplantation are standard therapies for these patients. Despite encouraging results with renal transplantation which offers a better quality of life and perhaps longer survival than dialysis[5,6] the majority are treated with dialysis, mainly because of the advanced age of most diabetics and the lack of kidney donors. When transplantation is not available or is not medically feasible, dialysis therapy becomes inevitable for many of these patients while waiting for renal transplant. The choice of dialysis therapy depends on such factors as nephrologist's bias, existence of comorbid disease treatment availability and other medical and social factors[2]. CAPD, which offers some advantages in the diabetic, was proposed, from early on, as the preferred dialytic treatment[7]. Now, CAPD is the first choice in dialytic treatment for ESRD in diabetes in Australia, New Zealand, England, Canada and some regions of the United States[2].

1. INDICATIONS AND CONTRAINDICATIONS

CAPD has both medical and social benefits and most patients with diabetes are eligible for it. This technique enables patients to stay at home, can be rapidly taught as home dialysis regimen and allows flexibility in treatment and increased ability to enjoy normal activities, giving such social benefits as care at home, long distance travel and uninterrupted employment[8,9]. The medical benefits of CAPD include [8]: (1) slow and sustained ultrafiltration and a relative absence of rapid fluid and electrolyte changes, (2) ease of blood pressure control, (3) preservation of residual renal function for long periods, (4) easy peritoneal access, (5) good glycaemic control with intraperitoneal (IP) insulin administration, and (6) steady–state biochemical parameters. Moreover, CAPD is ideal for those awaiting transplantation because it requires only a short training period and provides satisfactory support in the immediate post-transplant period[10]. Since this method provides more stable biochemical parameters and avoids the rapid fluctuations in extracellular fluid volume and blood pressure, minimising cardiovascular stress, it may be better for patients with significant cardiovascular disease[11]. CAPD becomes imperative for those patients who live a long distance from the dialysis center; among the latter, even if they are not ideal candidates for CAPD, it should be given a trial before recommending change of domicile.

However, patients with previous recurrent peritonitis, severe visual impairment, or any physical disability that limits dexterity (if they do not have a helper at home) are not appropriate candidates. Even in those patients with a helper, the daily "grind" of exchanges extracts a cost as well, leading to patient and caregiver burnout[11,12]. Elderly patients may have a learning disability and need a helper who is willing to take the responsibility. Unfortunately, long–term studies of CAPD in patients with diabetic nephropathy have demonstrated that the micro- and macrovascular disease of diabetes mellitus continues after initiation of CAPD, leading to ongoing problems with cardiovascular disease, malnutrition, autonomic neuropathy, retinopathy and peripheral vascular disease[13-22]. CAPD, especially if it is accompanied by hypotension may aggravate the symptoms of patients with generalised vascular disease, particularly with involvement of the iliac and femoral vessels. Previous extensive abdominal surgery, low-back pain, history of diverticulitis, polycystic kidney disease, chronic recurrent pancreatitis and chronic obstructive pulmonary disease (COPD) are not necessarily contraindications to CAPD, especially if there are no other contraindications. Finally, severe inflammatory bowel disease, low peritoneal membrave transport, severe active psychotic or depressive disorder and those with intellectual impairment with no helper are contraindications and patients with these disorders should not be assigned to CAPD[2].

2. MODALITY OF TREATMENT

CAPD is a continuous process in which 2 to 3 litres of a commercial dialysate is exchanged 3 to 5 times per day through a subcutaneously tunnelled intraperitoneal catheter. The most widely used of these catheters is the Tenckhoff of which there are many modifications, but the most commonly used of them are Swan Neck Missouri (SNM) and the Oreopoulos–Zellermann or Toronto Western Hospital (TWH) catheters. Modifications of the Tenckhoff catheter have reduced considerably the incidence of pericatheter leak, one–way obstruction, and catheter–tip displacement from pelvic cavity [23]; however, exit–site infection remains the main problem.

The choice of peritoneal catheter implantation technique (bedside or insertion by peritoneoscopic or surgical technique), which varies from center to center depends on local surgical practice. Preinsertion patient preparation, insertion technique, subcutaneous tunnel creation, post–operative care, catheter break–in procedure and subsequent catheter and exit–site care in diabetics are similar to those in non–diabetic patients[24]. However, usually CAPD technique is modified to accommodate individual patient handicaps such as visual impairment and extremity amputation. Devices such as Ultraviolet Box, Splicer, Oreopoulos–Zellermann connector, Y–transfer set with a UV system, and Injecta–Aid have helped visually or otherwise handicapped diabetics to continue independent lives [24,25].

Glucose is an effective osmotic agent in dialysate for generating ultrafiltration during CAPD and an average of 100–150grams of glucose are absorbed per day. However, glucose and its degradation products (some forms of aldehyde) may be associated with toxic effects on peritoneum and undesirable metabolic complications, including obesity, hyperinsulinaemia, hypertriglyceridaemia and premature atherosclerosis.

Because of these problems many have attempted to substitute glucose as another alternate, low or high molecular weight, osmotic agents, such as amino acids, xylitol, glycerol, sorbitol, dextrans, gelatin, poyanions, peptides and polyglucose, but have been foiled by adverse effects, cumulative systemic effects or prohibitive cost [26,27], except for amino acid solutions, which are used in some malnourished CAPD patients and one glucose polymer (icodextrin–20.000 daltons molecular weight) with some degree of clinical use[27]. Thus, glucose remains the preferred osmotic agent.

Frequently, diabetic patients with ESRD have many comorbid conditions such as severe cardiovascular disease and eye complications and may be better off if they start dialysis early, at a creatinine clearance of about 10ml/min, in the hope of preventing or slowing the progression of diabetic complications [15,28,29]. Furthermore, an increased tubular secretion of creatinine in these patients may make creatinine clearance an unreliable index of glomerular filtration rate (GFR)[30]

3. BLOOD SUGAR CONTROL AND INSULIN ADMINISTRATION DURING CAPD

Strict glucose control during CAPD minimises gastroparesis and may slow progression of other diabetic complications such as retinopathy and neuropathy[11]. The aim of the treatment is to achieve at most times a fasting blood sugar below 140mg/dl, and postmeal levels below 200mg/dl and a glycosylated haemoglobin(HbA_{1c}) of 9% or below. Haemoglobin A1c levels in these patients must be interpreted with caution since carbamylated haemoglobin formation increases in uremia and both substances have a similar chromatographic motility. Thus, haemoglobin A 1c levels will falsely elevate when chromatographic methods of measurement are used[31]. In CAPD patients, blood sugar can be controlled by diet, oral hypoglycaemic agents, IP or subcutaneous (SC) insulin administration or combination of these. The choice of the route of insulin administration depends on such factors as individual patient variations, preferences, and responsiveness[32].

For diabetics on CAPD, insullin can be administered via the IP or SC route and both methods have their own advantages and disadvantages[33]. It seems that the IP route gives better blood glucose control as assessed by mean blood glucose, mean amplitude of glycaemic excursions and glycosylated haemoglobin[7,8,28,29,33–36]. Several insulin dosage schedules have been described[29,32,33,35–37].

The absorption kinetics of intraperitoneally administrered isnulin and that secreted physiologically by the islet cells share several physiological similarities. Insulin secreted by the pancreas is transported to the liver via the portal vein and thereafter, 50% of the portal venous insulin is extracted by the liver before reaching the systemic circulation[38]. In the basal state, the ratio of insulin in the portal/peripheral blood is 3:1 and, in response to administered glucose or amino acids, may reach to 9:1. This high concentration of insulin in the liver, which promotes metabolic modulation of absorbed nutrients, may be important in the normal glucose homeostasis[32]. IP insulin administration allows for continuous delivery of the hormone at a basal rate. Absorption of IP insulin occurs preferentially by diffusion across the visceral peritoneum into the portal circulation and directly across the capsule of the liver[37,39] simulating physiological insulin secretion; this suggests that the metabolism of insulin may be more physiological when the hormone is delivered into the peritoneal space than by systemic injection.

IP insulin absorption continues until the end of the dwell and promotes the control of glycaemia throughout the entire period. Insulin levels in the serum peak 15 to 45 minutes after administration into an empty peritoneal cavity, 90 to 120 minutes when isnulin is added to the dialysis solution, but only approximately 50% of the insulin instilled into the peritoneal cavity is absorbed after an 8 hours dwell time[38–41]. The addition of IP insulin has no effect on solute clearances, ultrafiltration volume, or glucose absorption from the dialysate[40,42] and no one has reported a connection between the IP insulin administration and development of sclerosing peritonitis.

The glucose absorbed from dialysate (80–250g/day) and the incomplete absorption (<50%) of the insulin delivered intraperitoneally increase the insulin requirements of diabetic patients on CAPD. There are great interindividual variations (18–283units/day) in IP insulin requirements but usually, the daily IP dose is more than twice the pre–CAPD SC dose[36,41,42]. The total daily dose of insulin is divided among all four exchanges but to avoid nocturnal hypoglycaemia, the dose added to the overnight dwell is reduced. Each exchange with IP insulin should be carried out before meals to achieve peak insulin absorption at the time of food intake and thus minimise prostprandial hyperglycaemia. More insulin is added to each additional hypertonic dialysis incorporated into the daily program. In the case of the blind patient who cannot add isnulin to the dialysate bags, insulin can be mixed with the dialysis solution up to 24 hours before use without significant isnulin absorption onto the plastic bags[43].

One can achieve adequate control of blood glucose with both (IP and SC) methods of insulin administration. SC route may be preferred in patients with frequent episodes of hyper–or hypoglycaemia, excessive IP requirements and inability to add insulin to the dialysate bags and in patients on automated peritoneal dialysis (APD) [33,34]. However, IP insulin delivery is associated with fewer glycaemic excursions, so that during the day, the differences between low and high glucose values are lower than that seen with SC insulin[44]. Insulin – mediated glucose uptake is closer to normal in CAPD patients treated with IP insulin than in HD patients treated with SC insulin[45]. In a retrospective study, at every time interval for as long as 15 months, blood glucose levels were significantly lower in CAPD patients taking IP insulin compared to both CAPD and HD patients taking SC insulin[46].

It has been reported that IP insulin administration is associated with lipoprotein profiles of lower atherogenic potential, correcting a key step in reverse cholesterol transport in diabetics[47,48]. Intraperitoneal insulin can suppress hepatic glucose production with a relative lower degree of hyperinsulinaemia compared to that given by the SC route[49,50]; this is important because increased peripheral insulin levels may be directly related to an increased risk of atherosclerosis[51]. It has been reported, in non–uremic type I diabetics, lipoprotein composition becomes more atherogenic, and these abnormalities could be reversed by IP insulin administration[47,48]. However, a recent study in 8 type I diabetic patients on CAPD treated with both SC and IP insulin for at least three months, showed better glycaemic control and insulin sensitivity during IP insulin period, but unfavorable changes of serum lipids (decreased HDL–cholesterol, increased LDL–cholesterol and LDL/HDL ratio)[36].

IP insulin delivery avoids SC injections, and some of the causes of glycaemic lability such as degradation in the subcutaneous tissues and variations in absorption; this assures good patient compliance[38,52]. During episodes of peritonitis, IP insulin requirements are increased or decreased, depending upon the relative importance of increased insulin absorption and reduced carbohydrate intake due to anorexia versus increased glucose absorption and the infection–related hypercatabolism state[32.53].

In CAPD patients, the influence of IP insulin in the progression of target–organ disease is difficult to determine because of the advanced stage of diabetic complications when dialysis is started; however it seems clear that short–term metabolic control with IP insulin is better than that with SC insulin[8]. Subcapsular liver steatonecrosis[54,55] and malignant omentum syndrome[56] have been reported with IP insulin but more studies are needed to assess these complications.

Despite the reported increased incidence of peritonitis with IP insulin administration in diabetics on CAPD [57], a survery by the National CAPD Registry showed similar peritonitis rate for patients using SC and IP insulin[58]. Also, a recent study from the Italian Co–operative Peritoneal Dialysis Study Group showed no difference in peritonitis rate between diabetics on CAPD treated with IP and SC insulin administration and IP insulin administration was not associated with an increased probabiltiy of first peritonitis episode[16], as it was confirmed by others[36]. The benefits of IP insulin warrant its use in diabetic patients in order to further minimise long–term complications in this population[35].

From these data, it seems that IP insulin administration offers some metabolic and long–term benefits for diabetic patients compared to SC insulin delivery and may be one reason to choose CAPD over HD.

4. CARDIOVASCULAR DISEASE

The most common causes of death in ESRD patients are cardiac arrest, acute myocardial infarction and other cardiac problems, accounting for 50% of mortality in patients aged 45–64 years[18] and, as recent data (USRDS 1997 Annual Data Report) showed, 43.6% of mortality for all dialysis patients[59]. Regardless of the type of dialysis (HD or CAPD/CCPD) diabetics had two to threefold higher death rates than non– diabetics for myocardial infarction and other cardiac causes of death[18,59]. In recent studies reported that the high mortality due to cardiovascular disease in CAPD patients can be explained by a high prevalence of risk factors for cardiac disease or pre–existing heart desease at the starting of dialysis[21,60]. Also, diabetics had a significantly higher frequency of hypertension, cardiac disease, and peripheral vascular disease than non–diabetics[21]. Risk factors for cardiovascular disease in diabetic patients do not differ from those that increase the risks for non–diabetic patients and include a positive family history for heart disease, hyperlipidaemia, hypertension, lack of exercise, cigarette smoking, low HDL–cholesterol, increased platelet adhesiveness, elevated fibrinogen, and probably the level of glucose control[61].

The role of glucose control in the increased cardiovascular risk in the diabetics CAPD patients deserves further study, but a recent study reported that glycaemic control before starting dialysis is a predictor of survival for type II diabetics on CAPD in whom action with poor glycaemic control predialysis is associated with increased morbidity and shortened survival[62]. Also, it has been reported in a recent study that serum arachidonic acid (AA) levels were significantly higher in all CAPD patients (diabetics and nondiabetics) in comparison to healthy controls and diabetic patients without late complications[63]. In contrast, the serum eicosapentaenoic acid (EPA) concentrations were significantly lower in the CAPD groups, mainly in type I diabetic CAPD patients, leading to a higher AA/ EPA factor, resulting in the presence of a reduced prostaglandin I_2 biosynthesis and a higher formation rate of potentially proatherogenic metabolites such as thromboxane A_2, a vasoconstricting and platelet aggregating agent. Thus, the lack of EPA may be one reason for the lipid abnormalities, being indirectly responsible for the higher risk for atherosclerosis and the quotient AA/EPA could possibly be used as a marker of atherogenicity in the future[63].

Because of the high incidence of cardiovascular disease and the increased chance of silent myocardial infarction in diabetic patients on dialysis, investigation for cardiac disease is warranted even though the patient may be asymptomatic[11]. Non–invasive screening tests, as echocardiography to evaluate left ventricular function and to detect left ventricular hypertrophy, and cardiac radionuclide imaging (thallium 201) to detect perfusion defects, are effective[11]. Coronary arteriography should be used in symptomatic patients or those in whom perfusion defects have been detected[31].

Some authors have reported benefits using beta–adrenergic blockade and aspirin in diabetic CAPD patients with established coronary artery disease to prevent reinfarction. The use of beta–adrenergic blockers reduced significantly cardiac related death and nonfatal reinfarction both in diabetic and non–diabetic population[64,65]. There were no complications such as hypoglycaemic unawareness, diminished reflex tachycardia, and potentiation of hypoglycaemia, which are generally seen with doses higher than those that provide protection against cardiac death[66]. Aspirin has also been shown to significantly reduce cardiovascular mortality[67] and it was used safely even in patients with early retinopathy[68].

5. BLOOD PRESSURE CONTROL

Although no comparative studies have been done between CAPD and HD diabetic patients regarding blood pressure control, it is generally accepted that this control is better on CAPD; the continuous ultrafiltration and sodium removal without wide and rapid fluctuations (in fluid removal) produces a stable dry body weight, maintaining a relatively constant euvolemic state[69,70]. Thus, the reduction in blood pressure starts with the initiation of CAPD, continues to decrease over the next few months and correlates well with the reduction in body weight, emphasising the importance of fluid volume in the pathogenesis of hypertension in ESRD[8,69,70]. Blood pressure control is satisfactory in at least three quarters of all CAPD patients [71], and often can be achieved without drugs[8,34].

During the course of CAPD, some patients may become sodium depleted due to a combination of dialysate sodium loss and restricted sodium consumption[8]. Total body sodium depletion can lead to hypotension, especially in patients with diabetic autonomic neuropathy and/or with cardiac dysfunction[8]. Blood pressure control is generally an advantage of CAPD versus HD, but in the individual diabetic it may be a disadvantage, since improved blood pressure control can cause symptomatic orthostatic hypotension[72]. In this case, the physician may discontinue use of antianginals or afterload–reducing agents, but these drugs are useful in the routine treatment of coronary artery disese and cardiomyopathy. These medication changes are potentially responsible for some of the increased myocardial infarction and death rates seen in CAPD patients reported previously[59,73].

In diabetic patients, particularly those with significant cardiovasular disease, rapid fluid removal during a HD session can lead to hypotension resulting in ischemic symptoms and complications; rapid infusion of saline or colloid solution is needed to correct this transient hypotension and maintain blood pressure. On the other hand, the continuous nature of CAPD produces a slow rate of ultrafiltration; one to two litres are removed over a 24–hour period without large and rapid fluctuations of intravascular volume. However, CAPD patients can develop gangrene if hypotension persists. It has been reported that control of blood pressure in this population (CAPD and HD) may well depend on patient compliance and physician interest, rather than modality alone[61]. Also, there are some unanswered questions about blood pressure control and treatment: Are there potential differences in outcome of patients based on the specific antihypertensive agents chosen to treat the hypertension? Do agents that are either renoprotective or cardioprotective influence outcomes in these patients? Only future studies of risk factors including blood pressure and blood pressure treatment as potential variables may will clearly demonstrate their role in determing outcomes[61].

The above factors lead us to conclude that CAPD with its effect on salt and water balance and the slower rate of ultrafiltration, controls blood pressure in dialysis patients better than does HD, making CAPD the preferred technique in diabetic patients with ESRD, particularly those with severe cardiovascular and cerebrovascular diseases.

6. RESIDUAL RENAL FUNCTION

As infections lessen in frequency and the number of long–term diabetic patients on CAPD increases, the problem of providing adequate dose of dialysis in patients on CAPD has become more important[74–76]. As is generally accepted, the preservation of residual renal function is important in the management of dialysis patients because of its contribution to the overall solute clearance and fluid removal. Furthermore it can permit liberal fluid and dietary intake and in some cases a reduction in the dose of dialysis.

Even with a complete urine collection the accuracy of the residual renal creatinine clearance in dialysis patients is limited because of the enchanced tubular creatinine secretion[30,77]. Alternative methods include measurement of the creatinine clearance during the administration of cimetidine and averaging the creatinine and urea clearances[75,77,78], although a more accurate determination requires measurement of the clearance of inulin or a radiolabeled compound such as iothalamate, diethylenetriamine pentaacetic acid (DTPA), or ethylenediamine tetracetic acid (EDTA)[30]. Recently the residual renal function in dialysis patients both on HD and CAPD has been measured with plasma clearance of iohexol, a nonionic and nonradiolabeled contrast agent, and produced reliable results[79,80]. The contribution of the residual renal function in achieving adequate dose of dialysis, as estimated by weekly creatinine clerarance and KT/V of urea, and consequently to outcome of these patients is now accepted[81–84]. It is now recommended that the aim should be a weekly KT/V urea of 2.1 and a weekly creatinine clearance of 60 to 70L. [81].

During the last 15 years, many studies have shown that CAPD preserves renal function better, sometimes for periods up to 5 years, than does HD[85–90]. This observation may be explained by the rapid changes in extracellural fluid volumes during HD that reduce blood pressure, renal blood flow, glomerular capillary pressure and thus produce ischemia of remaining nephrons[75]. Another more attractive and important explanation is that HD has a nephrotoxic effect because of the release of various cytokines, such as interleukin–1 and tumour necrosis factor, and reactive oxygen metabolites during the contact of the blood with HD membranes; these may direclty or indirectly damage residual renal function[91–94]. Also, recent studies have suggested that circulating "uremic toxins" stimulating the progression of glomerular sclerosis, may play a role in the progressive loss of nephrons and are eliminated by peritoneal dialysis, probably because of some of these substances are protein–bound[95–97]. On the other hand, at least theoretically, CAPD may be associated with steady glomerular capillary pressure in the remaining functioning glomeruli without any fluctuations to high or low levels which may protect residual renal function[32,75]. Thus, the recent demonstration that residual renal function declined more rapidly in intermittent automated peritoneal dialysis as compared to CAPD is relevant[98].

Every effort should be made to avoid hypotension and nephrotoxic drugs in order to maximally protect residual renal fucntion[11,75]. The protective effects of ACE inhibition in slowing the progression of diabetic nephropathy have recently reported, and strong consideration must be given for the use of ACE inhibitor therapy for hypertension control in diabetic CAPD patients[99]. Measures that contribute to maintenance of the residual renal function in CAPD patients have recently summarized[75]. These measures include avoidance of nonstreroidal anti–inflammatory drugs, excessive peritoneal ultrafiltration and ACE inhibitors when there is a possibility of renal atheromathosis, while controversial results with the prescription of loop diuretics have been described. The routine use of high doses of loop diuretics (furosemide, piretanide), eventually in combination with a thiazide[100] can without any doubt contribute to the maintenance of the residual diuresis. The careful use of loop diuretics could be beneficial to CAPD patients, in order to maintain a more normal extracellular volume, resulting in a reduced need for the use of hypertonic glucose solutions[75]. The better preservation of residual renal function has, also, other important clinical implications since endocrine function will also be better preserved, resulting in the maintenance of the erythropoietin synthesis[101], conversion of vitamin D to its active form[102], and a better elimination of ,2 mircroglobulin[75,103]. Finally, CAPD is a good first choice in patients with cardiac failure, severe liver disease, analgesic nephropathy, chronic urinary obstruction and cholesterol emboli[75], but without any doubt, the recent recommendation that dialysis should be started earlier than at the conventionally accepted time of commencement is the most provocative one[15,28,29,104].

7. VISUAL FUNCTION

Before they start on dialysis, during the end stage of renal failure, most diabetic patients already have irreversible retinal lesions usually accompanied with severe hypertension[28,35]. In diabetics on CAPD good blood glucose and hypertension control have been reported to improve visual function[105] whereas others have found that visual acuity deteriorates further [106]. The progression of retinal lesions is similar in CAPD and HD[107] whereas a study of 60 diabetics on CAPD showed improvement (22%), stabilisation (57%) and deterioration (21%)[35]. Blood pressure regulation may be of great importance in the stabilisation of visual acuity and preservation of vision[14,107]. Contrary to CAPD, HD often leads to rapid fluctuations in intravascular volume which combined with heparin administration and hypertension or hypotension during sessions may aggravate retinopathy in these patients[107].

8. PERIPHERAL VASCULAR DISEASE

Severe peripheral vascular disease is a common complication and a major problem in diabetics with ESRD which leads to ischemic gangrene of the extremities[15,22,35,108]. Diabetics are 15 times as likely as non–diabetics to require an amputation[11,109]. During the early years it was reported that CAPD might exacerbate peripheral vascular disease– an exacerbation that was associated with persistent hypotension[110]. In all diabetics the prevalence of gangrene of foot or leg ulcer is 10,2%. In a recent multicenter study of diabetic nephropathy with 6,487 patients assessed, foot ulcers were present in 2.2% of the patients and 2.5% had previously undergone lower limb amputation[111], while others recently reported 8.3% of patients with a current ulcer and a further 5.5% with a previous ulcer[112]. The results obtained in diabetics on CAPD are conflicting because some studies have reported a high rate of gangrene and amputations[15,35,113] whereas others had a low rate[34]. However, the prevalence of gangrene is similar in CAPD and HD[35,113].

The foot lesions seen in diabetes mellitus are due primarily to peripheral polyneuropathy and macrovascular diseases. The development of a foot ulcer often involves a complex interplay of a number of factors, but without either sensory loss or vascular disease foot ulceration does not occur[114]. Diabetic peripheral neuropathy creates an insensitive foot that is at risk for many types of trauma which damage the skin and set the stage for infection and ulceration[11,114]. The autonomic neuropathy that results form damage to sympathetic fibers further adds to the risk[114]. Typically, neuropathic ulcers occur at sites of high pressure, such as under the metatarsal heads, and are painless, whereas purely vascular lesions often arise at the ends of toes and are painful. About 80%–90% of diabetic foot lesions are accompanied by significant peripheral vascular insufficiency[115]. The gangrene and amputation rate can be reduced by correcting vascular risk factors, by aggressively treating hypertension and hyperlipidaemia and urging the patient to quit smoking. Also, by preventing hypotension, by avoiding intense ultrafiltration and high doses antihypertensive drugs, as well as a foot care program[25]. In case of ischemia with foot ulceration, revascularization to restore circulation may be required[115,116]. In the neuropathic ulcer, the key to healing is pressure relief. Identification by nephrologists of those patients at risk, an intensive patient education and a multidisciplinary approach to foot care can significantly decrease the amputation rate and lower the rate of hospitalizations for diabetic foot complications[35,116]. The pathogenesis of foot ulceration, the identification of the high–risk patient, a detailed clinical examination of the diabetic foot, the areas that need to be covered in an educational program and the management of foot ulcers, have been, recently, reviewed[114].

In a retrospective study, it has been reported that patients who are diabetic and receiving peritoneal dialysis (PD) have an increased rate of peripheral vascular disease complications if they are also receiving erythropoietin[117]. Erythropoietin may have the potential to increase clotting–related complications, but this observation, as well as the importance of factors that potentially affect the coagulation system need confirmation with prospective studies in the diabetic patient population.

9. PERIPHERAL AND AUTONOMIC NEUROPATHY

Peripheral neuropathy, which is an almost ubiquitous finding in diabetic patients with ESRD is induced by diabetes and uraemia, and tends to progress even after the initiation of both HD and CAPD. It is present in about two–thirds of patients and 25% have no peroneal nerve conduction[35]. Among patients with type I diabetes and nephropathy, about 70% have some degree of peripheral neuropathy[118]. Neuropathy has been associated with foot ulceration[119]. Clinical improvement and stabilisation have been reported on CAPD but deterioration has been also observed, and low nerve conduction velocity persists in most patients.[120]. Autonomic neuropathy, that results from damage to sympathetic fibers can lead to severe postural hypotension. Also, gastroparesis may contribute to malnutrition and micturition disorders after trasnplantation[35]. Autonomic neuropathy is extremely common in diabetic nephropathy, becoming almost universal when end–stage renal failure develops[114]. Gustatory sweating is a marker of this complication and is reported by 69% of patients with established diabetic nephropathy, and the two seem to be intimately linked[118]. Peripheral neuropathy, as reported above, creates an insensitive foot that is at risk for trauma and skin damage and, eventually, leads to favourable conditions for infection and ulceration[11]. Diabetic neuropathy is now the commonest cause of Charcot's neuroarthropathy of the foot and ankle[114]. During HD with its rapid fluctuations of intravascular volume, diabetic neuropathy may deteriorate.

10. PERITONEAL MEMBRANE FUNCTION

Biochemical data and peritoneal tests measuring the changes of the peritoneal function over time and clinical data supporting the ability of the peritoneum to assure a long–term survival for PD patients are the two different forms to find out how long PD can last. Peritoneal membrane function is assessed in terms of solute and water control. Diabetics maintain a steady biochemical state indicating good peritoneal membrane function[13,19,34,35]. In diabetics on CAPD peritoneal ultrafiltration capacity and peritoneal clearances are not different than in non–diabetics[19,28,34] and longitudinal studies of peritoneal permeability have shown stable solute transport characteristics for four or more years[13,19,121,122]. It allows the nephrologists to maintain adequate dialysis by increasing dialysate volume or exchange frequency as residual renal function decreases[123]. Ultrafiltration failure is not a frequent cause of technique failure in diabetics on CAPD and it is not different from those in non–diabetics[16,19,34,35]. Constant surveillance of dialysis and renal clearances with necessary adjustments to the dialysis prescription to maintain adequacy are required to optimise outcomes, since the correlation between several of the adequacy parameters and patient survival is widely accepted and it is now recommended that the target should be a weekly KT/V urea of 2.1. and a weekly creatinine clearance between 60 to 70L. [81].

11. PERITONITIS AND PERITONEAL CATHETER – RELATED INFECTIONS

For all CAPD patients, peritonitis is the most common complication and the major cause of hospitalization and "dropout", with recurrent peritonitis leading the list[13–16,124,125]. One–third of the patient transfers from PD to HD are due to peritonitis and catheter complications[125]. Whether diabetic patients are more susceptible to infection than non–diabetics and consequently are at greater risk of peritonitis is still debated. Many workers have reported no difference in the incidence of peritonitis between diabetics and non–diabetics [7,14,15,34,106] whereas others have found increased peritonitis rates in diabetics[28] and diabetes has been identified as a risk factor for the first episode of peritonitis[126]. In a recent multicenter study from the Italian Co–operative Peritoneal Dialysis Study Group, ten years (1980–1989) experience of CAPD, showed that the incidence of peritonitis was 0.95 and 0.65 per patient– year in diabetics and non– diabetics, but the probability and relative risk of first peritonitis episode were not significantly different between the two groups[16]. Moreover, during the last 3 years of the study, when Y–set widely used there was no difference in peritonitis incidence between diabetics and non– diabetics and between diabetics using or not using IP insulin administration. Isolated bacteria are not more different in diabetics than non-diabetics and most of these episodes are caused by skin bacteria[16,34,35,127]. During peritonitis, due to increased and rapid absorption of glucose, hyperglycaemia is frequent and insulin requirements increase[28,33,35]. However, rarely, inflammation may lead to increases in insulin absorption and insulin requirements may decrease[53]. In both diabetics and non– diabetics, peritonitis during CAPD requires the same antibiotic treatment; most episodes are mild and can be treated on an outpatient basis[28,34,35]. Although peritonitis may lead to fatal complications, usually treatment is successful and the reported mortality rate is generally low.[34,35]. In a recent study it was reported that peritonitis contributes to death in 5% of PD patients[124]. IP insulin administration does not seem to be a risk factor for peritonitis since diabetics not receiving insulin have higher peritonitis rate than those on either IP or SC insulin. Patients using a combination of IP and SC insuline have the lowest rate, according to the National CAPD Registry[128].

Peritoneal catheter–related infections (exit site, tunnel) are reported to be more common in diabetics than in non–diabetics[33,129,130]; others have found no difference in the incidence of exit site/ tunnel infection between diabetics (on any insulin administration schedule) and non–diabetics on CAPD[16,126,128]. Staphylococcus aureus nasal carriage, more common in diabetics than in non–diabetics, has been linked to exit site infections[129,131]. Also, repeated SC insulin infections are said to increase the risk of Staph. aureus nasal carriage in diabetics[132] and consequently IP insulin administration may reduce this risk[33]. However, this was not confirmed by others[34]. All above mentioned findings need confirmation by large studies.

Improvements in connectology (Y–set) have diminished peritonitis rates and will probably have a beneficial effect on the CAPD dropout rate in the future[16,35,127]. Further research is needed to understand the etiology of gram–negative peritonitis, prevention of peritonitis by modification of dialysate, catheter design, prophylactic antibiotic protocols, and management of chronic exit–site infections[133]. Staphylococcus aureus prophylaxis and ongoing assessment of patient technique with periodic refresher courses may also play a role in decreasing infections in both diabetic and non–diabetic patients[11].

12. MALNUTRITION

Mild to moderate malnutrition is reported in 30% to 40% of chronic peritoneal dialysis patients and severe malnutrition in another 5% to 7% of these patients[134]. Protein-calorie malnutrition remains a frequent complication of long–term CAPD, seems to be multifactorial (decreased intake, increased losses, altered metabolism, coexisting conditions, socioeconomic factors, age, and patient compliance) and worsen in diabetics[35,134–138]. It is a common cause of CAPD technique failure in diabetics on long–term dialysis and contributes to increased mortality[15,16,22,136, 137,139,140]. Gastroenteropathy leading to nausea, vomiting and diarrhoea, persistent urinary loss of protein and higher than non–diabetic protein losses in the dialysate[28,141] produce an increased incidence of mild to moderate malnutrition that is worse in diabetics than in non–diabetics[135–138,142,143]. Diabetic microangiopathy may produce an increased glomelural permeability with increased protein losses which during peritonitis are excessive. In association with inadequate food intake, possibly by insufficient dialysis, this loss may lead to malnutrition[28,34, 136–143]. As has been recognised, malnutrition has a negative effect on survival of both HD and CAPD patients[15,16,136,139,140,143]. Recently, the data from the CANUSA study showed an association between low residual renal function at the initiation of dialysis and a worse nutritional status at that time and also worse patients survival with worse initial nutritional status[144]. The inference from these findings is that starting dialysis earlier would prevent malnutrition and improve survival[145].

In order to assess the nutritional status of diabetic CAPD patients protein intake, based on both dietary recall and urea kinetics, must be determined in conjunction with evaluation of the dialysis dose[11]. In case of inadequate dialysis dose delivered, dialysate volume or exchange frequency should be increased. Increases in dialysis dose have been correlated with improved nutritional parameters[139]. If dialysis is adequate, dietary supplements and concentrated sources of protein, carbohydrate, or fat may be required[11]. Finally, malnourished diabetic patients on CAPD may benefit form IP administration of amino acids [27]. Peritoneal dialysis with amino acids containing solutions should be considered, although the improvement in nutritional parameters may be accompanied by a tendency towards acidosis and an increased blood urea nitrogen[27,139,146].

For patients with severe gastroparesis, a variety of gastric motility agents such as metoclopramide, domperidone, cisapride, and eryhtromycin can be used orally or itnraperitoneally. Frequent smaller feedings have also been recommended and eventually, it may be necessary to switch the patient from CAPD to nocturnal peritoneal dialysis (NPD), leaving the abdomen empty of dialysate during the day. This may be sufficient to allow increased oral intake during the day but the delivered dialysis dose must be adequate.

Studies evaluating the effect of dialysis dose on clinical outcomes should include an estimation of nutritional status[145]. Further research designed to define the role of recombinant human growth hormone and recombinant human insulin-like growth factor 1, especially in pediatric patients and in malnourished patients is required. Since these agents are essentially mitogens, detailed animal studies should precede large-scale human use of these agents[134].

13. HYPERLIPIDAEMIA

Lipid abnormalities complicate renal failure and the continuous absorption of dialysate glucose in CAPD patients produces an increase in circulating triglycerides, which tends to be proportional to the initial serum triglyceride level[21,147–150]. Peritoneal dialysis patients have more atherogenic lipid profiles than HD patients[61]. Hypertriglyceridaemia and, to a lesser extent, hypercholesterolaemia are frequent among CAPD patients whereas high-density lipoprotein (HDL) cholesterol varies[147–151]. Also, CAPD patients have higher apolipoprotein B levels, and a lower apoA/apoB ratio than HD patients [148–151]. It has been reported that CAPD patients appear to have smaller, denser, and more atherogenic low-density lipoprotein (LDL) cholesterol particles compared to HD patients[61]. Diabetics with lipid abnormalities on CAPD may be at higher risk of developing atherosclerotic disease[21,35,61,151]. The overall lipid profile of these patients will also include high beta very low–density lipoprotein (beta–VLDL) and lipoprotein(a) (Lp[a]) levels, that are not likely to be available for the practising clinician[61,152,153]. Thus, the effect of both diet and antihyperlipidaemic therapy are less clear on these atherogenic markers than on the more commonly measured ones[154]. It has been reported that renal failure interferes with the normal catabolism of Lp(a) and that both CAPD and HD patients have increased levels of Lp(a), an independent risk factor for cardiovascular disease[21,61,155–157], although these findings have not been confirmed by others[153,158]. Also, the possible mechanisms of the increased levels of Lp(a) such as, abnormal catabolism, absorption of glucose from the dialysate and protein loss in dialysis fluid[157] were not confirmed by others[153]. There were no significant differences in Lp(a) levels between men and women or between diabetic and non–diabetic patients[153].

The treatment of lipid abnormalities in dialysis patients has recently been reviewed and specific recommendations have been given[154, 159–161]. In cases where there are no identified risk factors and only mild to moderate increases in triglyceride levels, nonpharmacological measures such as regular exercise, smoking cessation, restriction of ethanol intake, avoidance of lipid–elevating medications, and dietary advice with weight and saturated fat reduction are the major goals. Reduction of CAPD glucose absorption is also important because of the elevated glucose levels require more insulin, increasing generation of free fatty acids and triglycerides. In cases where other risk factors are present, except the correction of these factors, a more aggressive approach with omega–3 fatty acids or fibric acid derivatives (fibrates) therapy has been recommended for the management of hypertriglyceridaemia. For patients with cholesterol abnormalities (increased total and LDL–cholesterol and decreased HDL–cholesterol) in addition to hypertriglyceridaemia, more thorough testing of lipids and lipoproteins may be indicated before the initiation of therapy with fibrates or HMG–CoA reductase inhibitors (statins). Fibrates and statins require careful monitoring of liver function tests and muscle enzymes. If persistent elevations of these parameters occur, drug must be discontinued and the use of the smallest effective dose is recommended[11]. Initial studies have shown these drugs to be well tolerated in dialysis patients but long–term studies will be needed to prove if amelioration of the risk factor of hyperlipidaemia translates into decreased cardiovascular mortality in the CAPD populations[159–161]. Our recent experience for patients with risk factors and hypertriglyceridaemia and/or hypercholesterolaemia showed that gemfibrozil (900mg, once daily, 30 minutes before eating), lipidil (100 mg twice or three times daily), pravastatin (10–20mg, once daily, with the evening meal), as well as omega–3 fatty acids (791mg EPA–527 mg DHA, twice daily with meal) are effective, safe and well–tolerated drugs even for long periods (up to 18 months)[162–165]. IP insulin administration has been reported to have a beneficial effect on lipoprotein profile[47,48], although this was not confirmed by others[36].

14. OTHER COMPLICATIONS – HOSPITALIZATION

Other complications such as the mechanical complications of peritoneal catheters, those resulting from increased intra–abdominal pressures (dialysate leaks, hernias, haemorrhoids), sclerosing peritonitis and others, are not influenced by diabetes and occur with the same frequency in diabetics and non–diabetics[28,35].

The frequency of hospitalization and success of rehabilitation depend on selection criteria and the age of the patients. In general, diabetes leads to a significant increase in hospital days among CAPD and HD patients[166]. In earlier studies, the overall hospitalization rate varied between 30 and 40 days/patient – year, about twice the number of days for non–diabetic patients of the same age, probably because of numerous complications and increased morbidity[7,120].

However, recent studies have reported lower hospitalization rates with an average of 20 to 23 days/patient – year [28,34] and a smaller difference than before (23 days vs. 17 days for diabetics and non–diabetics respectively)[28]. Diabetics on HD have similar rates of hospitalization[166,167]. Peritonitis is the main cause and accounts for 30–50% of the hospitalization days [34,120,167]. A more recent multicenter study reporting a ten years experience of CAPD in diabetics showed even lower hospitalization rates[16]. Days per patient–year of hospitalization were 18.4 and 14.3 respectively in diabetics and in non–diabetics. Peritonitis and, generally, CAPD–related problems were not the most important cause of hospitalization and this can be correlated to the low peritonitis incidence, mainly during the last years. The higher rate of hospitalization in diabetics was mainly related to clinical complications associated to diabetes rather than to CAPD – related problems[16]. It was reported that hospitalization rates for CAPD patients generally, have in recent years been steadily falling while those for HD patients have remained relatively stable[168]. Also, USRDS 1997 – Annual Data Report, shows that hospitalization rates among CAPD patients are slightly higher than for HD patients in each age–group, with the exception of those patients in the 65 and over age–group, where the two are equal[169], perhaps due to improvements in connection devices thereby reducing peritonitis risk or increased outpatient treatments of peritonitis in CAPD patients.

15. CAUSES OF CAPD FAILURE AND DEATH

The main cause of CAPD technique failure is peritonitis, with recurrent peritonitis leading the list, and to lesser extent, other severe abdominal complications such as loss of ultrafiltration, colonic perforation and sclerosing encapsulating peritonitis [14,15,22,170,171]. Other reasons for discontinuing dialysis are permanent access problems, malnutrition, and patient/partner choice. [35,170, 171]. A recent study from our center showed that the most frequent cause of CAPD failure was not peritonitis but inability to cope with treatment, probably because we use CAPD as the treatment of first choice but discontinue it if the patients cannot cope with it[34]. Technique failure leading to transfer to HD is common in diabetic population resulting in fewer diabetics on long–term CAPD[14,15,22,167]. It has been reported that the risk for changing modality treatment was 4.66 times greater for diabetics on CAPD than for those on HD, while the relative risk for non–diabetic CAPD patients was 3.74 times higher than non– diabetic HD patients[167]. However, a recent study on 301 diabetic and 1689 non–diabetic CAPD patients showed that the risk of technique failure did not differ between the two groups[16]. The USRDS 1997 Annual Data Report shows that the fraction of CAPD patients that switches to HD during the first few years of treatment is much larger than the fraction of HD patients that switches to CAPD[172]. Recurrent peritonitis, other medical complications but, also, a low delivered dose of CAPD could prompt some switching to HD once residual renal function is lost[170,172]. It has been reported that lack of compliance to the prescribed peritoneal dialysis program is a major reason for CAPD technique failure[173] and has also been proposed as a potential cause of excess mortality among CAPD patients[174]. Approximately 12% of CAPD patients reported that on average they miss one exchange per week, 6% miss 2 to 3 exchanges per week, 1% miss 4 to 6 per week[175]. Recent data (from USRDS)[59] showed that the rate of withdrawal from dialysis increased with age and was about three times higher in diabetics aged 20 to 44 years than non-diabetics of the same age group, and diabetes was associated with a higher rate of withdrawal in all age categories. The distribution of reasons for withdrawing from renal refplacement therapy is similar for diabetics and nondiabetics, with leading reasons chronic failure to thrive and acute medical complications.

The most frequent causes of death are of vascular origin, namely myocardial infarction, cardiac arrest and cerebrovascular accident, these account for more than 50% to 70% of the deaths[18,34,35,59]. Other causes include infections, malignancies and other infrequent causes[16,18,35,59]. The distribution of these causes is similar in patients on HD and CAPD[35,59,167]. Recent data from USRDS showed that myocardial infarction and other cardiac problems account for 50% of mortality in patients with ESRD, aged 45–64 years[18], and total cardiac causes account for 43.6% of mortality in all dialysis patients in 1993 to 1995 years in US[59]. Diabetic patients had threefold higher death rates than non–diabetics for myocardial infarction and other cardiac causes of death both on HD or CAPD[18]. In an other recent study, in the two groups (diabetics and non–diabetics on CAPD), cardiovascular diseases and cachexia were the two most frequent causes of death, with nearly twofold incidence in diabetics; infections other than peritonitis were the third cause of death in diabetics and occured over three times more often compared with non–diabetics[16]. According to USRDS data (1997 Annual Data Report)[59], the death rates due to cerebrovascular disease were more than two–fold higher in the older age group (65+vs 20–64) and almost twice as high among diabetics than nondiabetics. Death rates due to septicemia were much higher in CAPD than in HD patients, and in diabetics than in nondiabetics[59]. The higher infection deaths among PD patients may be related to several factors including: poor technique, peritoneal access, less overall clearance of small uremic toxins, possible deleterious effects of the dialysis fluid on macrophage function, malnutrition, or differences in baseline comorbidity between HD and CAPD patients[176]. Generally, among dialysis patients, diabetics have substantially higher adjusted death rates due to acute myocardial infarction, cardiac arrest, other cardiac causes, septicemia, cerebrovascular disease, and hyperkalemia than nondiabetics[59]. However, malignancy is almost two–fold higher for nondiabetics than diabetics, but this is probably related to the competing risk of cardiac, infections, and vascular causes of death in diabetics.

Recently, Bloembergen et al. reported a comparison of causes of death between patients treated with HD and PD[177]. Data were obtained from U.S. Renal Data System, for patients prevalent on January 1 of the years 1987, 1988, and 1989 (42,372 deaths occurring over 170,700 patient years at risk). There was a significantly increased mortality risk for PD compared to HD for all cause–of–death categories, except malignancy. The excess mortality observed in PD–treated patients can be accounted for, by infection (35%), acute myocardial infarction (24%), other cardiac causes (16%), cerebrovascular disease (8%), withdrawal (8%), and malignancy (6%). The increased risk of death due to other cardiac causes and withdrawal from dialysis in PD patients was found only among diabetics, and the increased risk due to acute myocardial infarction was accentuated among diabetics[177]. In a more recent study from the Lombardy Registry–Italia, the main causes of death of diabetic patients were cardiovascular diseases (56%), cachexia (18%), and infections(11%) [178]. Several factors may contribute to the observed higher risk of death, among PD patients, such as, selection of patients, lower amount of dialysis dose during the early years, poor patients compliance or medical care.

16. PATIENT AND TECHNIQUE SURVIVAL

According to USRDS–1997 Annual Data Report, there has been an overall improvement in survival from 1984 to 1994 and first–year mortality decreased dramatically and consistently for diabetic patients, from 44 per 100 patient years in 1984 to 27 per 100 patient years in 1994[179]. Survival rates of diabetic patients remain significantly lower than those of non–diabetics on CAPD[13–17,28,35,108,136,167,180,181], although one group has reported similar rates in the two groups[180]. The risk factors that reduce the survival of diabetics are age over 45 years, a previous or current cardiac disease, systolic blood pressure higher than 160mmHg and severe peripheral vascular disease[14,21,180]. The high mortality of diabetics on CAPD seems to be related to the comorbid conditions, especially the presence of cardiovascular disease at the start of dialysis; the course of heart disease does not seem to be affected by CAPD. The few diabetics, who have survived for long periods, were younger, free of or with minimal clinical cardiac disease, non–smokers, and with a higher predialysis serum creatinine and lower haematocrit[20]. In our center, seven diabetic patients have been on CAPD for more than five years (range: 65 to 109 months), they were older (5 over the age of 65) and at the beginning of dialysis had a variety of comorbid conditions (3 or more/patient)[13]; there was no difference in serum creatinine and haematocrit levels between these patients and those who did not survive for long periods.

After the second year patient survival decreases sharply, during the fourth year varies between 30%–57% and during the fifth year, between 17.4% to 40%[14,16,17,28,34,108,136,170, 171,178,180,181]. Some discrepancies may due to different numbers of patients in the various studies. It is interesting to note that blind diabetics live longer than the sighted ones[180].

The best method to compare survival rates between diabetics on CAPD and on HD is a randomised prospective study among large numbers of patients to avoid biases in selection common in the EDTA and USRDS registry[17,73,177,181,185] and in other surveys[182,183]. In some regions[184] selection criteria are based on race and sex and regional differences in survival of diabetics seem to exist. Since a prospective study of comparing diabetics on CAPD and HD will never be possible, the next best technique is a retrospective comparison of large numbers of patients dialysed with the two modalities, correcting for risk factors by the Cox proportional hazards model.

Analysis of the USRDS and EDTA data showed that mortality rates tended to be higher for HD than for CAPD in younger diabetic patients while the opposite was the case among older patients[17,73,177,181,185]. The relative risk of death was similar for patients younger than 60 years of age on HD and on CAPD during the 1984 and 1988 periods; for those older than 60 years, the relative risk of death was greater for CAPD patients in 1984 but had improved by 1988. Recent studies from the Michigan Kidney Registry using Cox proportional hazards analysis [186–188] in patients beginning dialysis in 1989 showed that diabetic patients aged 20 to 59 years old had a relative risk of death on CAPD 38% lower than on HD ($p<0.01$). Among diabetics older than 60 years, CAPD patiens had a 19% higher risk of death than those on HD, but this difference was not statistically significant ($p=0.08$). The higher mortality rate for older patients on CAPD probably reflects selection bias regarding treatment modality for diabetic patiens since older diabetic patients with severe cardiac and peripheral vascular diseases and other comorbid conditions are preferentially chosen for CAPD/CCPD treatment[8].

Survival of diabetic patients on CAPD has steadily improved since 1980, but the group as a whole still fares worse than non–diabetic patients[11,16,136]. In 1980, a diabetic had only a 45% chance of being alive after two years on dialysis compared with an approximately 60% chance of survival in non–diabetic patients with ESRD[11]. According to the 1994 USRDS report, two year survival on dialysis in 1990 has increased to 52.6% in diabetics versus an increase to about 65% in patients with other ESRD etiologies[17]. ESRD continues to be associated with a dismal long–term survival, with only 17.4% of the diabetic patients form 1987 surviving five years. Five–year survival for patients with ESRD due to glomerulonephritis, hypertension, and other causes were not much better, reported as 36.6%, 29.9% and 33.3%, respectively[17].

A recent, large comparative study of PD and HD (data from USRDS) [188] showed that, on average, prevalent patients treated with PD had a 19% higher adjusted mortality risk (relative risk (RR) = 1.19; $p<0.001$) than did those treated with HD. This risk was insignificant ($p>0.05$) and small for ages<55 years. It was accentuated in diabetics (RR=1.38; $p<0.001$). However, baseline differences in PD and HD treated patients are almost certain to exist. It is interesting that the Canadian experience is contrary to the U.S., with lower mortality among PD patients compared to HD patients for both diabetics and non diabetics of all ages. These discrepancies emphasise the need for large prospective studies with well matched patients and treatments and close monitoring on order to separate the effect of patient selection, differential dose of dialysis, nutrition, patients compliance, and medical quality of care from a possible adverse effect of PD.

Recent studies, have reported that after correcting for the influence of factors that significantly impair survival such as increased age, ischemic heart disease, cerebral and peripheral vasculopathy, malignant hypertension etc, the survival curves of the PD and HD patients did not differ[170,171,178]. Indeed, the evaluation of the outcomes of 155 HD and 139 PD patients who started dialysis in the same center throughout 1991–1996, showed survival curves similar with a probabiltiy of survival after 60 months of 36% for both modalities, strongly demonstrating that PD assures the same survival as HD when the two groups of patients are comparable[170]. Also, another recent study analyzing the survival of diabetic patients on PD (347pts) and on HD (545pts) admitted to dialysis between January 1983 and December 1993, showed that five–year survival of diabetic patients was 34% and no differences were found between PD and HD patients[178].

The lower technique survival rate for CAPD reflects the role of peritonitis as the main complication and the most frequent cause of CAPD failure. The more comorbid conditions of diabetics compared to non–diabetics account for a worse survival, higher relative risk of death, a higher need of partner, hospitatlization, and technique faillure[16,170,178]. The introduction of improved CAPD systems patricularly the Y–set system, and the institution of adequacy standards for CAPD may, as already shown in reccent studies[16,17], reduce the drop–out rates and lead to improved technique survival rates[8].

17. ADVANCED GLYCOSYLATION END–PRODUCTS

It has been established that persistent hyperglycaemia and the duration of diabetes are directly correlated with the complications of diabetes[189,190]. How hyperglycaemia causes irreversible tissue damage is still debated. A growing body of evidence has linked the formation and accumulation of irreversible glucose–derived "advanced glycosylation end–products" (AGEs) to a variety of chronic complications, including diabetic nephropahty[191,192]. The potential role of AGEs in diabetic renal and vascular disease has recently been reviewed[193–195]. AGE formation results from the spontaneous reaction of glucose and proteins, but also occurs on lipids and nucleic acids[196]. Specific receptors for AGEs have been identified on many cell types[191,197–199].

A receptor present on the macrophage, specifically recognizes proteins to which AGEs are bound (RAGE), enabling the cell to stimulate the removal and replacement of senescent macromolecules, cross–linked and denatured by long–term exposure to glucose. RAGE, a member of the immunoglobulin super family, is also expressed on endothelial and vascular smooth muscle cells. The binding of AGEs to RAGE results in the induction of cellular oxidant stress, with consequences for a range of cellular functions[199]. The excessive accumulation of AGEs in tissues is believed to exert its main pathological effect through abnormal permeability of blood vessels[191] resulting form an AGE–/RAGE–induced endothelial cell dysfunction [200] and also from the reduction in the negatively charged proteoglycan component of the basement membrane[191]. More recently, it has been reported from experimental studies in rats, using polyclonal antisera that there is co–localisation of AGEs and RAGE in sites of diabetic microvascular injury such as renal glomerulus, retina, aorta, and nerve bundles from mesenteric arteries[201]. This co–localisation suggests that this ligand–receptor interaction may represent an important mechanism in the genesis of diabetic complications[201].

Recent studies suggest that AGE damage could be compounded in chronic renal failure because of the renal retention of AGE–breakdown products which then recycle in the circulation at amplified levels[202–205]. Serum AGEs levels are inversely correlated with renal function[204]. Both, over–production and under–excretion, contribute to the highest concentrations of AGEs occuring in diabetics with ESRD. The accumulation of AGE–peptides in the circulation may act as an accelerating factor for the rapid evolution of diabetic complications. Also, it is a potential explanation for the rapid progression of diabetic nephropathy once this complication is initiated, as well as, a reason which might explain the excessively high morbidity and mortality of diabetic patients with ESRD[194].

AGEs are inefficiently cleared by conventional dialysis, so that circulating AGE–peptides accumulate dramatically in diabetic patients with ESRD on dialysis, with mean levels up to five–to –eight–fold compared to diabetics without clinical nephropathy[202,204]. Low molecular weight (<10Kd) AGE–peptides[196] are removed only one–third as well as creatinine by conventional HD[204,205]. High–flux dialysis was found to remove AGEs better than conventional HD, but AGE values return to predialysis concentrations within 3–5 hours[204]. AGE removal by CAPD was found to be between high–flux and conventional HD. Low–molecular weight AGE–peptides remain elevated about four–fold in diabetics on CAPD, in a range similar to patients on high–flux HD[204], and their clearance is inefficient compared to the clearance of creatinine and dialysate to plasma ratios are low[205]. Lamb et al reported in vitro formation of AGEs in peritoneal dialysis fluid[206] and, except haemoglobin–AGE, a circulating marker of advanced glycosylation[207], another specific AGE, pentosidine higher in peritoneal tissue in diabetics on PD compared to HD, presumably reflecting chronically high glucose levels in the peritoneal dialysate[208]. However, plasma levels were not affected by the presence or absence of diabetes itself.

The possible diabetiform effect of high dialysate glucose levels on the peritoneal membrane has been suggested from early on. [209]. As the peritoneum in CAPD is continually bathed in glucose concentrations at least one log greater than normal blood levels, it is not surprising that there should be some concern about the long–term effects of glucose–based dialysate[210]. The findings of peritoneal biopsies taken from patients after several years on CAPD, are indistinguishable from the microangiopathy encountered in diabetes mellitus[210]. *In vitro* and *ex vivo* studies have demonstrated that glycosylation and AGEs formation occur in conventional dextrose– containing dialysate[206,211]. The glycosylation rate is related to glucose concentration, is independent of other components of the fluid and an understanding of the chemistry and the factors involved in AGEs formation in dextrose dialysate has been established[212]. It is possible that icodextrin, a glucose polymer used in peritoneal dialysis, may *in vivo* cause less AGEs formation in peritoneal tissues, since *in vitro* studies have shown that the glycosylation rate with icodextrin (7.5%, 13.2 mmol/L) was more than tenfold lower than the weakest strength of dextrose used in peritoneal dialysis fluid (1.36%, 75 mmol/L) [213]. It has been reported that icodextrin – generating AGEs can be inhibited by aminoguanidine[213].

Dextrose degradation products, the inevitable consequence of heat sterilization of glucose–based dialysis solutions, are not only irritant to the peritoneum, but, as highly reactive chemicals, also responsible for long–term pathological effects on the peritoneal membrane itself[214]. Also, recently it was reported that dextrose degradation products promote a more rapid generation of AGEs in glucose– based peritoneal dialysate[213]. It is therefore highly likely that dextrose degradation products represent an underestimated pathogenetic agent in conjunction with AGEs formation in the long–term degeneration of the peritoneum[210].

In order to reduce the AGE burden, in addition to the control of hyperglycaemia, we need an alternative strategy which can interfere with the chemical pathway of glycosylation itself. Pimagedine (aminoguanidine) has been identified as the prototype of a new class of drugs which react with Amadori products in vivo and inhibit their formation of reaction AGEs [215,216]. In animal models of diabetic nephropathy, Pimagedine has been shown to ameliorate diabetic complications, preventing collagen cross–linking, reducing experimental retinopathy, and improving nerve action potential and conduction velocity[217,218]. It, also, reduces mesangial expansion and glomerular basement membrane thickness, and decreases albuminuria[219,220]. Also, it was recently reported that the use of aminoguanidine for 12 months in rats did not adversely affect renal function[221], and it prolonged significantly survival in a rat model of uremia due to diabetic nephropathy suggesting that aminoguanidine may prove beneficial in human diabetes[222]. Pimagedine is presently undergoing clinical trials in the United States, Canada and Europe,to assess progression of renal disease, effect on serum AGE profile, morbidity, mortality, and quality of life in diabetic patients with early renal disease. Unfortunately, recently , the early closure of European Pimagedine trial for no medical reasons was made known. [223,224].

18. CAPD IN IDDM (TYPE I) VS NIDDM (TYPE II) DIABETIC PATIENTS

There have been only a few studies of possible differences between insulin dependent (IDDM) and non–insulin dependent (NIDDM) diabetic patients on CAPD. Since the older diabetic patient is usually an insulin – resistant type II diabetic and a young diabetic patient is usually an insulin – deficient type I diabetic, it is very difficult to separate age from diabetes type when assessing reasons for differences in survival between older and younger diabetic patients receiving PD[61]. However, it is possible that the differences in survival between HD and PD noted in the elderly diabetic are not related to age as much as they are to the pathophysiological state underlying their diabetic state[61]. Four–and five–year patient and technique survival has been satisfactory and is almost equal between the two groups [225] whereas others have reported decreased 3–year patient and technique survival of NIDDM patients[226]. In our center [34], we found comparable patient and technique survival rates. In our Type I patients (most of whom were on IP insulin) we achieved a 50% lower rate of peritonitis than in our Type II patients whereas other workers found no difference in the peritonitis rate between patients using IP and those using SC isnulin[16,33,128]. Also median annual hospitalization was 7 days in Type I and 9 days in Type II, but the mean of 28 days/patient–year of hospitalization in Type II was about twice that in Type I (14 days/patient–year). A possible explanation of this difference is that the Type II diabetics have a higher average age and a higher incidence of peritonitis[34].

In a recent retrospective study, Zimmerman et al, found that diabetic patients younger than 55 years of age, mostly type I, had a survival on dialysis no significantly different than nondiabetics PD patients[227]. One–and five–year survival on PD of type I diabetics was 92% and 57%, respectively, while those of type II diabetics was 74% and 5% respectively. Also, of a total of 20 patients who survived on PD for more than 100 months, 7 were type I diabetics[228]. These results are consistent with the USRDS data suggesting a beter survival of younger PD diabetic patients and a worse survival for the older PD diabetic patients[73,177, 188].

It is possible that age is only a marker for diabetes type. Insulin–deficient type I diabetics may do well with the instillation of IP glucose and in many cases concomitant IP insulin delivery. Type II insulin–resistant diabetic patients may not fare with the addition of the absorbed IP glucose load, which may further elevate already elevated peripheral insulin levels. At present the response of the different types of diabetic patient to the glucose load is unclear[61]. It is not known if the continuous absorption of glucose and the lack of a fasting state in CAPD patients are related to the increased cardiovascular mortality, but the recent development of nonglucose–containing PD solutions may give us the answer[61]. Future prospective-controlled studies are needed to demonstrate all possible differences between Type I and Type II diabetic patients, and the possible reasons for these differences.

CONCLUSION

It is apparent that CAPD has certain unique beneficial features both medical and social that lead to better long–term outcomes in diabetic patients. Although the prevalence of many and severe comorbid conditions at the start of CAPD leads to increased mortality and morbidity, nephrologists must, in time, detect and treat cardiovascular disease, lipid abnormalities, neuropathy, and peripheral vascular disease in order to have an impact on patient and technique survival of CAPD diabetic patients. Also, the prevention of malnutrition is critical in lowering mortality, while as residual renal fucntion decreases, monitoring and adjustment of peritoneal dialysis regimen is needed to deliver an adequate dose of dialysis. CAPD with its potential medical benefits and its social advantages, has offered excellent treatment for diabetic patients with ESRD. Consequently there are signigificant reasons to recommend CAPD as first choice, renal replacement treatment for the majority of diabetic ESRD patients. Early renal transplantation and increased efforts at decreasing the rate of deterioration of renal function in diabetics remain the ideal approaches[229].

REFERENCES

1. United States Renal Data System 1994 Annual Data Report IV. Incidence and causes of treated ESRD. Am J Kidney Dis 1994; Suppl. 2: S48–S56.
2. Markell MS, Friedman EA. Diabetic nephropathy: Management of the end–stage patient. Diabetes Care 1992; 15: 1226–1238.
3. D' Amico G. Comparability of the different registries on renal replacement therapy. Am J Kindeny Dis 1995; 25: 113–118.
4. United States Renal Data System 1997 Annual Data Report II. Incidence and Prevalence of ESRD. Am J Kidney Dis 1997; 30(2): Suppl 1: S40–S53.
5. Mattem WD, Mc Gaghie WC, Rigby RJ, Nissenson AR, Dunhan CB, Khayrallah MA. Selection of ESRD treatment: An international study. Am J Kidney Dis 1989; 13: 457–464.
6. Passlick J, Grabensee B. CAPD and transplantation in diabetics. Clin Nephrol 1988; 30: Suppl. 1: S18–S23.
7. Amair P. Khanna R. Leibel B, Pierratos A, Vas S, Meema E, Blair G. Chisolm L, Vas M. Zingg W, Digenis G, Oreopoulos DG. Continuous ambulatory peritoneal dialysis in diabetics with end–stage renal disease. N Engl J Med 1982; 306: 625–630.
8. Khanna R. Dialysis considerations for diabetic patients. Kidney Int 1993; 43: Suppl. 40: S58–S64.
9. Markell MS, Friedman EA. Care of the diabetic patient with end–stage renal disease. Sem Nephrol 1990; 10: 274–286.
10. Cardella CJ. Peritoneal dialysis and renal transplantation. Perit Dial Bull 1985; 5: 149–151.
11. Johnston JR. Maintaining diabetic patients on long–term peritoneal dialysis. Sem Dial 1995; 8: 390–394.
12. Holley JL. PsycholÔgical factors causing technique failure in continuous peritoneal dialysis: The patient and the health care providers. Sem Dial 1995; 8: 395–396.
13. Balaskas EV, Yuan ZY, Gupta A, Meema HB, Blair G, Bargman J, Oreopoulos DG. Long–term continuous ambulatory peritoneal dialysis in diabetics. Clin Nephrol 1994; 42: 54–62.
14. Kemperman FAW, van Leusen R, van Liebergen FJHM, Oosting J, Boeschoten EW, Struijk DG, Krediet RT, Arisz L. Continuous ambulatory peritoneal dialysis (CAPD) in patients with diabetic nephropathy. Neth J Med 1991; 38: 236–245.
15. Rottembourg J, Issad B, Allouache M, Baumelou A, Deray G, Jacobs C. Clinical apsects of continuous ambulatory and continuous cyclic peritoneal dialysis in diabetic patients. Perit Dial Int 1989; 9: 289–294.
16. Viglino G, Cancarini GC, Catizone L, Cocchi R, De Vecchi A, Lupo A, Salomone M, Segoloni GP, Giangrande A. Ten years experience of CAPD in diabetics: comparison of results with non–diabetics. Nephrol Dial Transpalnt 1994; 9: 1443–1448.

17. United States Renal Data System 1994. Annual Data Report VI. Patient Survival. Am J Kidney Dis 1994; 24: Suppl. 2: S76–S87.
18. United States Renal Data System 1994. Annual Data Report VII. Causes of Death. Am J Kidney Dis 1994; 24: Suppl. 2: S88–S95.
19. Faller B, Lameire N. Evolution of clinical parameters and peritoneal function in a cohort of CAPD patients followed over 7 years. Nephrol Dial Transplant 1994; 9: 280–286.
20. Zimmerman SW, Johnson CA, O' Brien M. Long–term survivors on peritoneal dialysis. Am J Kidney Dis 1987; 10: 241–249.
21. Lameire N, Bernaert P, Lambert MC, Vijt D. Cardiovascular risk factors and their management in patients on continuous ambulatory peritoneal dialysis. Kidney Int 1994; 46: Suppl. 48: S31–S38.
22. Maiorca R, Vonesh E, Cancarini GC, Cantaluppi A, Manili L, Brunori G, Camerini C, Feller P, Strada A. A six–year comparison of patient and technique survivals in CAPD and HD. Kidney Int 1988; 34: 518–524.
23. Khanna R. Oreopoulos DG. Peritoneal access for chronic peritoneal dialysis. Int J Artif Organs 1985: 8: 1–6.
24. Khanna R, Nolph KD, Oreopoulos DG. "Peritoneal Access" In *The Essentials of Peritoneal Dialysis, Chapter 2.* Khanna R. Nolph KD, Oreopoulos DG, eds. Dordrecht: Kluwer Academic Publishers, 1993; pp. 19–34.
25. Balaskas EV. Oreopoulos DG. "Continuous ambulatory peritoneal dialysis in uremic diabetics". In *The Kidney and Hypertension in Diabetes Mellitus, 2nd ed.* Mogensen CE, ed. Boston. Dordrecht, London: kluwer Academic Publishers, 1994; pp. 469–485.
26. Hain H, Kessel M. Aspects of new solutions for peritoneal dialysis. Nephrol Dial Transplant 1987; 2: 67–72.
27. Gokal R. Peritoneal dialysis solutions: nutritional aspects. Perit Dial Int 1997; 17 (Suppl 3): S69–S72.
28. Scarpioni LL, Ballocchi S, Castelli A, Cecchettin M, Poisetti PG. Continuous ambulatory peritoneal dialysis in diabetic patients. Contrib Nephrol 1990; 84: 60–74.
29. Scarpioni L, Ballocchi S, Scarpioni R, Cristinelli L. Peritoneal dialysis in diabetics. Optimal insulin therapy on CAPD: intraperitoneal versus subcutaneous treatment. Perit Dial Int 1996; 16(Suppl 1): S275–S278.
30. Levey AS. Nephrology forum: measurement of renal function in chronic renal disease. Kideny Int 1990; 38: 167–184.
31. Viberti G, Wiseman MJ, Pinto JR, Messent J. "Diabetic Nephropathy". *In Joslin's Diabetes Mellitus, 13th ed,* Kahn CR, Weir GC, eds. Philadelphia: Lea and Febiger, 1994; pp 691–737.
32. Khanna R, Nolph KD, Oreopoulos DG. "Peritoneal Dialysis in Diabetics". *In The Essentials of Peritoneal Dialysis,* Khanna R, Nolph KD, Oreopoulos DG, eds. Dordrecht: Kluwer Academic Publishers, 1993; pp 99–108.
33. Tzamaloukas AH, Oreopoulos DG. Subcutaneous versus intraperitoneal insulin in the management of diabetes on CAPD: A review. Adv Perit Dial 1991; 7: 81–85.
34. Yuan ZY, Balaskas EV, Gupta A, Bargman JM, Oreopoulos DG. Is CAPD or Haemodialysis better? CAPD is more advantageous. Sem Dial 1992; 5: 181–188.
35. Khanna R. "Peritoneal dialysis in diabetic end–stage renal disease. "In *The Textbook of Peritoneal Dialysis,* Gokal R, Nolph KD, eds. Dordrecht: Kluwer Academic Publishers, 1994; pp 639–659.
36. Nevalainen PI, Lahtela JT, Mustonen J, Pasternack A. Subcutaneous and intraperitoneal insulin therapy in diabetic patients on CAPD. Perit Dial Int 1996; 16(Suppl 1): S288–S291.
37. Zingg W, Shirriff JM, Liebel B. Experimental routes of insulin administration. Perit Dial Bull 1982: 2: 24–27.
38. Duckworth WC. Insulin degradation: Mechanisms, products and significance. Endocrine Rev 1988; 9: 319–345.
39. Rubin J, Bell AH, Andrews M, Jones Q, Olanch A. Intraperitoneal insulin: a dose response curve. ASAIO Trans 1989; 35: 17–21.
40. Rubin J, Reed V, Adair C, Bower J, Klein E. Effect of intraperitoneal insulin on solute kinetics in CAPD. Am J Med Sci 1986; 291: 81–87.
41. Wideroe T, Smedy LC, Berg KJ, Jorstad S, Svartas IM. Intraperitoneal insulin absorption during intermittent and continuous peritoneal dialysis, Kidney Int 1983; 23: 22–28.
42. Madden MA, Zimmerman SW, Simpson DP. CAPD in diabetes mellitus: the risks and benefits of intraperitoneal insulin. Am J Nephrol 1982; 2: 133–139.

43. Twardowski ZJ, Nolph KD, Mc Gary TJ, Moore HL. Influence of temperature and time on insulin absorption to plastic bags. Am J Hosp Pharm 1983; 40: 583–586.
44. Saudek CD, Salem JL, Pitt HA, Waxman K, Rubio M, Jean Didier N, Turner D, Fischell RE, Charles MA. A preliminary trial of the programmable implantable medication system for insulin delivery. N Engl J Med 1989; 321: 574–579.
45. Schmitz O. Insulin–mediated glucose uptake in non–dialyzed and dialyzed uremic insulin dependent diabetic subjects. Diabetes 1985; 34: 1152–1159.
46. Grefberg N, Danielson BG, Nilson P, Berne C. Decreasing insulin requirements in CAPD patiens given intraperitoneally insulin. J Diabetic Compl 1987; 1: 16–19.
47. Selam JL. Kashyap M, Alberti KGMM, Lozano J, Hanna M, Turner D, Jean Didier N, Chan E, Charles MA. Comparison of intraperitoneal and subcutaneous insulin administration on lipids apolipoproteins, fuel metabolites, and hormones in Type I diabetes mellitus. Metabolism 1989; 38: 908–912.
48. Bagdade JD, Dunn FL. Effects of insulin treatment on lipoprotein composition and function in patients with IDDM. Diabetes 1992; 41(Suppl 2): 107–110.
49. Campbell PJ, Mandarino LJ, Gerich JE. Quantification of the relative impairment in actions of insulin on hepatic glucose production and peripheral glucose uptake in non insulin dependent diabetes mellitus. Metabolism 1988; 37: 15–21.
50. Duckworth WC, Saudek CD, Henry RR. Why intraperitoneal delivery of insulin with implantable pump in NIDDM? Diabetes 1992; 41: 657–661.
51. Fuller JH, Shipley MJ, Rose G, Jarrett RJ, Keen H. Coronary heart disease risk and impaired glucose tolerance: The White Hall Study. Lancet 1983; i: 1373–1376.
52. Schade DS, Duckworth WC. In search of the subcutaneous insulin degradation syndrome. N Engl J Med 1986; 315: 147–153.
53. Henderson IS, Patterson KR, Loung ACT. Decreased intraperitoneal insulin requirements during peritonitis on continuous ambulatory peritoneal dialysis BMJ 1985; 290: 1474.
54. Wanless IR, Bargman JM, Oreopoulos DG, Vas SL. Subcapsular steatonecrosis in response to peritoneal insulin delivery: A clue to the pathogenesis of steatonecrosis in obesity. Mod Pathol 1989; 2: 69–74.
55. Bargman JM. The impact of intraperitoneal glucose and insulin on the liver. Perit Dial Int 1996; 16(Suppl 1): S211–S214.
56. Harrison NA, Rainford DJ. Intraperitoneal insulin and the malignant omentum syndrome (Abstract). Nephrol Dial Transplant 1988; 3: 103.
57. Scalamogna A, Castelnova C, Crepaldi M, Guerra L, Graziani G, Cantaluppi A, Ponticelli C. Incidence of peritonitis in diabetic patients on CAPD: Intraperitoneal vs. subcutaneous insulin therapy. Adv Perit Dial 1987; 3: 166–170.
58. "A survey of diabetics in the CAPD/CCPD population". In *Continuous Ambulatory Peritoneal Dialysis in the USA*, Lindblad AS, Novak JW, Nolph KD, Stablein DM, Culter SJ, Steinberg SM, Vena DA, eds. Dordrecht: Kluwer Academic Publishers, 1989; pp 63–74.
59. United States Renal Data System – 1997 Annual Data Report. VI. Causes of Death. Am J Kidney Dis 1997; 30(2): Suppl 1: S107–S117.
60. Manske CL, Thomas W, Wang Y, Wilson RF. Screening diabetic transplant candidates for coronary artery disease: identification of a low risk subgroup. Kidney Int 1993; 44: 617–621.
61. Zimmerman S. The diabetic ESRD patient: specific needs. Perit Dial Int 1997; 17(Suppl 3): S9–S11.
62. Yu C–C, Wu M–S, Wu C–H, Yang C–W, Huang J–Y, Hong J–J, Fan Chiang C–Y, Leu M–L, Huang C–C. Predialysis glycemic control is an independent predictor of clinical outcome in type II diabetics on continuous ambulatory peritoneal dialysis. Perti Dial Int 1997; 17: 262–268.
63. Holler C, Auinger M, Ulberth F, Irsigler K, Eicosanoid precursors: potential factors for atherogenesis in diabetic CAPD patients? Perit Dial Int 1996; 16(Suppl 1): S250–S253.
64. Gundersen T, Kjekhus J. Timolol treatment after myocardial infarction in diabetic patients. Diabetes Carc 1983; 6: 285–290.
65. Kjekhus J, Gilpin E, Cali G, Blackey AR, Henning H, Ross J. Diabetic patients and beta–blockers after acute myocardial infarction. Eur Heart J 1989; 11: 43–50.
66. Nesto RW, Zarich SW, Jacoby RM, Kamalesh M. "Heart disease in diabetics" In *Joslin's Diabetes Mellitus, 13th ed*, Kahn CR, Weir GC, eds. Philadelphia: Lea and Febiger, 1994; pp 836–851.
67. Fuster V, Cohen M, Halperin J. Aspirin in the prevention of coronary disease (editorial) N Engl J Med 1989; 321: 183–185.

68. DAMAD Study Group. Effect of aspirin alone and aspirin plus dipyridamole in early diabetic retinopathy: A multi-center randomized controlled clinical trial. Diabetes 1989; 38: 491–498.
69. Young MA, Nolph KD, Dutton S, Prowant BF. Anti-hypertensive drug requirements in continuous ambulatory peritoneal dialysis. Perit Dial Bull 1984; 4: 85–88.
70. Di Paolo B, Di Liberato L, Fiederling B, Stuard S, Marini A, Bucciarelli S, Santoferrara A, Santarelli P, Albertazzi A. Incidence and pathophysiology of hypertension in continuous ambulatory peritoneal dialysis. Perit Dial Int 1993; 13: (Suppl. 2): S396–S398.
71. Stablein DM, Hamburger RJ, Lindbland AS, Nolph KD, Novak JW. The effect of CAPD on hypertension control: a report of the National CAPD registry. Perit Dial Int 1988; 8: 141–144.
72. Kraus MA, Hamburger RJ. Is peritoneal dialysis the preferred modality in the diabetic patient? Adv Perit Dial 1996; 12: 89–92.
73. Held PJ, Port FK, Turenne MN, Gaylin DS, Hamburger RJ, Wolfe RA. Continuous ambulatory peritoneal dialysis and hemodialysis: comparison of patient mortality with adjustment for comorbid conditions. Kidney Int 1994; 45: 1163–1169.
74. Churchill DN. Adequacy of peritoneal dialysis: How much dialysis do we need? Kidney Int 1994; 46: Suppl. 48: S2–S6.
75. Lameire N, Van Biesen W. The impact of residual renal function on the adequacy of peritoneal dialysis. Perit Dial Int 1997; 17(Suppl 2): S102–S110.
76. Gotch FA. The CANUSA Study. Perit Dial Int 1997; 17(Suppl 2): S111–S114.
77. van Acker BAC, Koomen GCM, Koopman MG, de Waart DR, Arisz L. Creatinine clearance during cimetidine administration for measurement of glomerular filtration rate. Lancet 1992; 340: 1326–1329.
78. Hilbrands LB, Artz MA, Wetzels JF, Koene RA. Cimetidine improves the reliability of creatinine as a marker of glomerular filtration. Kidney Int 1991; 40: 1171–1176.
79. Swan SK, Halstenson CE, Kasiske BL, Collins AJ. Determination of residual renal function with iohexol clearance in hemodialysis patients. Kidney Int 1996; 49: 232–235.
80. Marx MA, Shuler CL, Tattersall JE, Golper TA. Plasma iohexol clearance as an alternative to creatinine clearance for CAPD adequacy studies. Kidney Int 1995; 48: 1994–1997.
81. Churchill DN, Taylor DW, Keshaviah P. Adequacy of dialysis and nutrition in continuous peritoneal dialysis: association with clinical outcome. J Am Soc Nephrol 1996; 7: 198–207.
82. Faller B, Lameire N. Evolution of clinical parameters and peritoneal function in a cohort of CAPD patients followed over 7 years. Nephrol Dial Transplant 1994; 9: 280–286.
83. Lameire N, Vanholder R, Vijt D, Lambert MC, Ringoir S. A longitudinal five year survey of urea kinetic parameters in CAPD patients. Kidney Int 1992; 42: 426–432.
84. Blake PG. Targets in CAPD and APD prescription. Perit Dial Int 1996; 16(Suppl 1): S143–S146.
85. Rottembourg J, Issad B, Poignet JL, Stripoli P, Balducci A, Slama G, Gahl GM. "Residual renal function and control of blood glucose levels in insulin-dependent diabetic patients treated by CAPD". In *Prevention and Treatment of Diabetic nephropathy*, Keen H, Legrain M, eds. Boston, Lancaster: MTP Press Ltd, 1983; pp 339–359.
86. Rottembourg J, Issad B, Allouache M, Jacobs C. Recovery of renal function in patients treated by CAPD. Adv Perit Dial 1989; 5: 63–66.
87. Shekkarie MA, Port FK, Wolfe RA, Guire K, Humphrys R, van Amburg G, Ferguson CW. Recovery from end-stage renal disease. Am J Kidney Dis 1990; 15: 61–65.
88. Rottembourg J. Residual renal function and recovery of renal function in patients treated by CAPD. Kidney Int 1993; 43: Suppl. 40: S106–S110.
89. Nolph KD. Is residual renal function better preserved with CAPD than with hemodialysis? Am Kidney Fund Nephrol Lett 1990; 7: 1–7.
90. Iest CG, Vanholder RC, Ringoir SM. Loss of residual renal function in patients on regular hemodialysis. Int J Artif Organs 1989; 12: 154–159.
91. Herbelin A, Nguyen AT, Zingraft J, Urena P, Descamps-Latscha B. Influence of uremia and haemodialysis on circulating interleukin-1 and tumour necrosis factor alpha. Kidney Int 1990; 37: 116–125.
92. Shah AH. Role of reactive oxygen metabolites in experimental glomerular disease. Kidney Int 1989; 35: 1093–1106.
93. Schiffl H. Choice of dialysis membrane does not influence the outcome of residual renal function in *haemodialysis patients (Letter)*. Nephrol Dial Transplant 1995; 10: 611–612.
94. Van Stone JC. The effect of dialyzer membrane and etiology of Kidney disease on the preservation of residual renal function in chronic hemodialysis patients. ASAIO J 1995; 41: M 713–M716.

95. Motojima M, Nishijima F, Ikoma M, Kawamura T, Yoshioka T, Fogo AB, Sakai T, Ichikawa I. Role of "uremic toxin" in the progressive loss of intact nephrons in chronic renal failure. Kidney Int 1991; 40: 461–469.
96. Niwa T, Ise M. Indoxyl sulfate, a circulating uremic toxin, stimulates the progression of glomerular sclerosis. J Lab Clin Med. 1994; 124: 96–104.
97. Niwa T, Yazawa T, Kodama T, Vehara Y, Maeda K, Yamada K. Efficient removal of albumin – bound furancarbolic acid, an inhibitor of erythropoiesis, by continuous ambulatory peritoneal dialysis. Nephron 1990; 56: 241–245.
98. Hiroshige K, Yuu K, Soejima M, Takasugi M, Kuroiwa A. Rapid decline of residual renal function in patients on automated peritoneal dialysis. Perit Dial Int 1996; 16: 307–315.
99. Lewis FJ, Hunsicker LG, Bain RP, Rohde RD. The effect of angiotensin–converting enzyme inhibition on diabetic nephropathy. N Engl J Med 1993; 329: 1456–1462.
100. Fliser D, Schroder M, Neubeck M, Ritz E. Coadministration of thiazides increases the efficacy of loop diuretics even in patients with advanced renal failure. Kidney Int 1994; 46: 482–488.
101. Chandra M, Clemons GK, McVicar M, Wilkes B, Mossey RT. Serum erythropoietin levels and hematocrit in end–stage renal disease: influence of the mode of therapy. Am J Kidney Dis 1988; 12: 208–213.
102. Jongen MJM, Van der Vijgh WSF, Lip P, Netelenbos JC. Measurements of vitamin D metabolites in anephric subjects. Nephron 1984; 36: 230–236.
103. Montenegro J, Martinez I, Saracho R, Gonzalez R. ,2 microglobulin in CAPD. Adv. Perit Dial 1992; 8: 369–372.
104. Schulman G, Hakim RM. Improving outcomes in chronic hemodialysis patients: should dialysis be initiated earlier? Sem Dial 1996; 9: 225–229.
105. Rottembourg J. Remaoun M. Maiga K, Bellio P, Issad R, Boudjemma A, Cossette PY. Continuous ambulatory peritoneal dialysis in diabetic patients. The relationship of hypertension to retinopathy and cardiovascular complications. Hypertension 1985; 7: Suppl. 2: 125–130.
106. Tzamaloukas AH, Rogers K, Ferguson BJ, Leymon PC, Sena P, Merlin TL, Avasthi PS. Management of diabetics on CAPD with subcutaneous insulin. Adv Perit Dial 1988; 4: 126–132.
107. Diaz–Buxo JA, Burgess WP, Greenman M, Chandler JT, Farmer CD, Walker PJ. Visual function in diabetic patients undergoing dialysis: comparison of peritoneal and haemodialysis. Int J Artif Organs 1984; 7: 257–262.
108. Catalano C, Goodship THJ, Tapson TS, Venning MK, Taylor RMR. Proud G, Tunbridge WM, Elliot RW, Ward MK, Alberti KGMM, Wilkinson R, Renal replacement therapy for diabetic patients in Newcastle–upon–Tyne and northern region, 1964–1988. BMJ 1990; 301: 535–540.
109. Bild DE, Selby IV, Sinnock P, Brower WAS, Braveman P, Shostack JA. Lower extremity amputation in people with diabetes. Diabetes Care 1989; 12: 24–31.
110. Brown PM, Johnston KW, Fenton SA, Cattran DC. Symptomatic exacerbation of peripheral vascular disease with chronic ambulatory peritoneal dialysis. Clin Nephrol 1981; 16: 258–261.
111. Young MJ, Boulton AJM, Macleod AF, Williams DRR, Sonksen PH. A multicentre study of the prevalence of diabetic peripheral neuropathy in the United Kingdom hospital clinic population. Diabetologia 1993; 36: 150–154.
112. Apelqvist J, Bitzen P, Larsson J, Nyberg P, Schersten P. Foot lesions common in a diabetic population older than 25 years. Diabetic Med. in press.
113. Tzamaloukas AH, Murata GH, Harford AM, Sena P, Zager PG. Eisenberg B, Wood B, Simon D, Goldman RS, Kanig SP, Avasthi PS, Saddler MC. Hand gangrene in diabetic patients on chronic dialysis. ASAIO Trans 1991; 37: 638–643.
114. Shaw JE, Boulton AJM, Gokal R, Management of foot problems in diabetes. Perit Dial Int 1996; 16(Suppl 1): S279–S282.
115. Lo Gerfo FW, Gibbons GW. "Vascular disease of the lower extremities in diabetes mellitus: Etiology and management". In *Joslin's Diabetes Mellitus, 13th ed,* Kahn CR, Weir GC, eds. Philadelphia. Lea and Febiger, 1994; pp 970–975.
116. Levin ME. The diabetic foot: A primer for nephrologists. Sem Dial 1991; 4: 258–264.
117. Wakeen M, Zimmerman SW, Bidwell D. Peripheral vascular disease in diabetic patients on PD receiving rhu–erythropoietin. J Am Soc Nephrol 1993; 4: 420.
118. Shaw JE, Parker R, Bulton AJM. Risk factors for foot disease in diabetic nephropathy. Eur J Clin Invest 1995; 25(Suppl 2): A59.
119. Young MJ, Breddy JL, Veves A, Boulton AJM. The prediction of neuropathic foot ulceration using vibration perception thresholds. Diabetes Care 1994; 17: 557–561.

120. Khanna R, Wu G, Prowant B, Jastrzebska J, Nolph KD, Oreopoulos DG. "Continuous ambulatory peritoneal dialysis in diabetics with end–stage renal disease: A combined experience of two North American centers". *In Diabetic Renal–Retinal Syndrome 3*, Friedman E, L' Esperance F, eds. New York: Grune and Stratton, 1986: pp 363–381.
121. Coronel F, Tornero F, Macia M, Sanche A, De Oleo P, Naranjo P, Barrientos A. Peritoneal clearances, protein losses and ultrafiltration in diabetic patients after four years on CAPD. Adv Perit Dial 1991: 7: 35–38.
122. Lee HB, Park MS, Chung SH, Lee YB, Kim KS, Hwang SD, Moon C. Peritoneal solute clearances in diabetics. Perit Dial Int 1990; 10: 85–88.
123. Johnston JR, Bernardini J, Holley J, Piraino B. Effect of increasing exchange volume or frequency on CAPD efficiency. Adv Perit Dial 1995; 11: 97–100.
124. Fried L, Bernardini J, Johnston JR, Piraino B. Peritonitis influences mortality in PD patients. J Am Soc Nephrol 1995; 6: 530.
125. Burkart J, Schreiber M, Tabor T, Korbet S, Stallard R, and PD Collaborative Group. Prospective, multicenter evaluation of patient transfer from PD to HD in 1995. Perit Dial Int 1996; 16(Suppl 2): S66.
126. Lindblad AS, Novak JW, Nolph KD. *Continuous Ambulatory Peritoneal Dialysis in the USA. Final report of the National CAPD registry 1981–1988.* Dordrecht; Kluwer Academic Publishers, 1989; pp 30, 37, 258.
127. Holley JL, Bernardini J, Piraino B. Infecting organisms in continuous ambulatory peritoneal dialysis patients on the Y set. Am J Kidney Dis 1994; 23: 569–573.
128. Lindblad AS, Nolph KD, Novak JW, Friedman EA. A survey of the NIH CAPD Registry population with end–stage renal disease attributed to diabetic nephropathy. J Diabetic Compl 1988; 2: 227–232.
129. Luzar MA, Coles GA, Faller B, Slingeneyer A, Dah GD, Briat C, Wone C, Knefati Y, Kessler M, Peluso F. Staphylococcus aureus carriage and infection in patients on continuous ambulatory peritoneal dialysis. N Engl J Med 1990; 322: 505–509.
130. Holley JL, Bernardini J, Piraino B. Risk factors for tunnel infections in continuous peritoneal dialysis. Am J Kidney Dis 1991: 18: 344–348.
131. Lye WC, Leong SO, van der Stratten J, Lee EJC. Staphylococcus aureus CAPD–related infections are associated with nasal carriage. Adv Perit Dial 1994; 10: 163–165.
132. Tuazon CU. Staphylococcus aureus among insulin–injecting diabetic patients: An increased carried rate. JAMA 1975; 231: 1272.
133. Piraino B. Infectious complications of peritoneal dialysis. Perit Dial Int 1997; 17(Suppl 3): S15–S18.
134. Teehan BP, Churchill DN, Kopple JD, Kohaut EC. NIH peritoneal dialysis workshop nutrition subcommittee: research recommen–dations. Perit Dial Int 1997; 17(Suppl 3): S58–S59.
135. Harty J, Gokal R. Nutritional status in peritoneal dialysis. J Renal Nutr 1995; 5: 2–10.
136. Avram MM, Fein PA, Bonomini L, Mittman N, Loutoby R, Avram DK, Chattopadhyay J. Predictors of survival in continuous ambulatory peritoneal dialysis patients: A five–year prospective study. Perit Dial Int 1996; 16(Suppl 1): S 190–S194.
137. Scanziani R, Dozio B, Bonforte G, Surian M. Nutritional parameters in diabetic patients on CAPD. Adv Perit Dial 1996; 12: 280–283.
138. Espinosa A, Gueto – Manzano AM, Velazquez – Alva C, Hernandez A, Cruz N, Zamora B, Chaparro A, Irigoyen E, Correa – Rotter R. Prevalence of malnutrition in Mexican CAPD diabetic and nondiabetic patients. Adv Perit Dial 1996; 12: 302–306.
139. Heimburger O, Bergstrom J, Lindholm B. Maintenance of optimal nutrition in CAPD. Kidney Int 1994; 46: Suppl. 48: S39–S46.
140. Churchill DN, Taylor DW, Keshaviah PR, and the Canada–USA (CANUSA) Peritoneal Dialysis Study Group. Adequacy of dialysis and nutrition in continuous peritoneal dialysis patients; association with clinical outcomes. J Am Soc Nephrol 1996; 7: 198–207.
141. Krediet RT, Zuyderhoudt FMJ, Boeschoten EW, Arisz L. Peritoneal permeability to proteins in diabetic and non–diabetic continuous ambulatory peritoneal dialysis patients. Nephron 1986; 42: 133–140.
142. Young CA, Kopple JD, Lindholm B, De Vecchi A, Scalamogna A, Castelnova C, Oreopoulos DG, Anderson GH, Bergstrom J, et al. Nutritional assessment of continuous ambulatory peritoneal dialysis patients: an international study. Am J Kidney Dis 1991; 17: 462–471.

143. Marckmann P. Nutritional status of patients on haemodialysis and peritoneal dialysis. Clin Nephrol 1988; 29: 75–78.
144. McKusker FX, Teehan BP, Thorpe KE, Keshaviah PR, Churchill DN, for the CANUSA Study Group. How much peritoneal dialysis is required for the maintenance of a good nutritional state? Kidney Int 1996; 50(Suppl 56): S56–S61.
145. Churchill DN. Nutrition and adequacy of dialysis. Perit Dial Int 1997; 17(Suppl 3): S60–S62.
146. Jones M, Hamburger R, Charytan C, Sandroni S, Bernard D, Piraino B, Schreiber M, Gehr T, Fein P, Friedlander M, et al. Treatment of malnutrition in peritoneal dialysis (PD) patients with a 1.1% amino– acid (AA) dialysis solution. Perit Dial Int 1995; 15: Suppl 1: S 42.
147. Appel G. Nephrology forum: Lipid abnormalities in renal disease. Kidney Int 1991; 39: 169–183.
148. Avram MM, Goldwasser P, Burrell DE, Antignani A, Fein PA, Mittman N. The uremic dislipidemia: A cross–sectional and longitudinal study. Am J Kidney Dis 1992: 20: 324–335.
149. Attman PO, Samuelsson O, Alaupovic P. Lipoprotein metabolism and renal failure. Am J Kidney Dis 1993; 21: 573–592.
150. Keane WF. Lipids and the Kidney. Kidney Int 1994; 46: 910–920.
151. Babazono T, Miyamae M, Tomonaga O, Omori Y. Cardiovascular risk factors in diabetic patients undergoing continuous ambulatory peritoneal dialysis. Adv Perit Dial 1996; 12: 120–125.
152. Cheung AK, Wu LL, Kablitz C, Leypoldt JK. Atherogenic lipids and lipoproteins in hemodialysis patients. Am J Kidney Dis 1993; 22: 271–276.
153. Guindeo C, Vega N, Fernandez AM, Palop L, Aguilar JA, Moreda A, Cia P. Lipoprotein (a) levels in patients undergoing continuous ambulatory peritoneal dialysis. Perit Dial Int 1996; 16(Suppl 1): S236–S240.
154. Appel GB. How should the lipid abnormalities of dialysis patients be treated? Sem Dial 1995; 8: 15–16.
155. Bartens W, Wanner C. Lipoprotein (a): new insights into an atherogenic lipoprotein. J Clin Invest Med 1994; 72(8): 558–567.
156. Webb AT, Reaveley DA, O' Donell M, O' Connor B, Seed M, Brown EA. Lipoprotein (a) in patients on maintenance hemodialysis and continuous ambulatory peritoneal dialysis. Nephrol Dial Transplant 1993; 8: 609–613.
157. Anwar N, Bhatnagar D, Short CD, Mackness MI, Durrington PN, Prais H. Serum lipoprotein (a) concentrations in patients undegoing continuous ambulatory peritoneal dialysis. Nephrol Dial. Transplant 1993; 8: 71–74.
158. kandoussi A, Cachera C, Pagniez D, Dracon M, Fruchart JC, Tacquet A. Plasma level of lipoproteins Lp(a) is high in predialysis or hemodialysis, but not in CAPD. Kidney Int 1992; 42: 424–425.
159. Jacobs C. How should the lipid abnormalities of dialysis patients be treated? Sem Dial 1995; 8: 17–19.
160. Markell MS. How should the lipid abnormalities of dialysis patients be treated? Sem Dial 1995; 8: 19–21.
161. Iaina A, Weintraub M. How should the lipid abnormalities of dialysis patients be treated? Sem Dial 1995; 8: 21–22.
162. Balaskas EV, Bamihas GI, Karamouzis M, Sioulis A, Tourkantonis A. Gemfibrozil treatment of hypertriglyceridemia in CAPD patients. Perit Dial Int 1996; 16: Suppl. 2: S57.
163. Balaskas EV, Bamihas GI, Pidonia I, Gutsaridis N, Tourkantonis A. The effect of Pravastatin on hyperlipaemia in CAPD patients. Perit Dial Int 1996; 16: Suppl. 2: S58.
164. Balaskas EV, Bamihas GI, Pidonia I, Giousef H, Tourkantonis A. Omega –3 fatty acids in the management of dyslipaemia in CAPD patients. Perit Dial Int 1996; 16: Suppl. 2: S58.
165. Balaskas EV, Bamichas G.I, Tourkantonis A. Management of lipid abnormalities in patients on CAPD. Perit Dial Int 1997; 17: 308–309.
166. Burton PR, Walls J. A selection adjusted comparison of hopsitalization on continuous ambulatory peritoneal dialysis and haemodialysis. J Clin Epidemiol 1989; 42: 531–539.
167. Serkes KD, Blagg CR, Nolph KD, Vonesh EF, Shapiro F. Comparison of patient and technique survival in continuous ambulatory peritoneal dialysis (CAPD) and hemodialysis: A multicenter study. Perit Dial Int 1990; 10: 15–19.
168. Habach G, Port FK, Mauger E, Wolfe RA, Bloembergen WE. Hospitalization among US dialysis patients: Hemodialysis versus peritoneal dialysis. J Am Soc Nephrol 1995; 5: 1940–1948.
169. United States Renal Data System–1977 Annual Data Report IX. Hospitalization. Am J Kidney Dis 1997; 30(2): Suppl 1: S145–S159.

170. Cancarini GC, Brunori G, Zani R, Zubani R, Pola A, Sandrini M, Zein H, Maiorca R. Long–term outcomes of peritoneal dialysis. Perit Dial Int 1997; 17(Suppl 2): S115–S118.
171. Maiorca R, Cancarini GC, Zubani R, Camerini C, Manili L, Brunori G, Movilli E. CAPD viability: a long–term comparison with hemodialysis. Perit Dial Int 1996; 16: 276–287.
172. United States Renal Data System – 1997 Annual Data Report III. Treatment modalities for ESRD patients. Am J Kidney Dis 1997; 30(2): Suppl 1: S54–S66.
173. Banks JE, Langenohl KM, Brandes JC. Inadequate dialysis is a major reason for transfer from CAPD to hemodialysis. Perit Dial Int 1992; 12(Suppl 1): 97.
174. Port FK, Wolfe RA, Bloembergen WE, Held PJ, Young EW. The Study of outcomes for CAPD versus Hemodialysis patients. Perit Dial Int 1996; 16: 628–633.
175. United States Renal Data System–1997 Annual Data Report IV. The USRDS Dialysis Morbidity and Mortality Study: Wave 2. Am J Kidney Dis 1997; 30(2): Suppl 1: S67–S85.
176. Bloembergen WE, Port FK. Epidemiological perspective on infections in chronic dialysis patients. Adv Renal Replacement Therapy 1996; 3: 201–207.
177. Bloembergen WE, Port FK, Mauger EA, Wolf R.A. A comparison of cause of death between patients treated with hemodialysis and peritoneal dialysis. J Am Soc Nephrol 1995; 6: 184–191.
178. Marcelli D, Spotti D, Conte F, Tagliaferro A, Limido A, Lonati F, Malberti F, Locatelli F. Survival of diabetic patients on peritoneal dialysis or hemodialysis. Perit Dial Int 1996; 169(Suppl 1): S283–S287.
179. United States Renal Data System – 1997 Annual Data Report V. Patient mortality and survival. Am J Kidney Dis 1997; 30(2): Suppl 1: S86–S106.
180. Chandran PKG, Lane T, Flynn CT. Patient and technique survival for blind and sighted diabetics on continuous ambulatory peritoneal dialysis: a ten years analysis. Int J Artif Organs 1991; 14: 262–268.
181. Brunner EP. End–stage renal failure due to diabetic nephropathy: data from the EDTA registry. J Diabetic Compl. 1989; 3: 127–135.
182. Hamburger RJ, Mattern WD, Schreiber MJ, Doerblom R, Sorkin M, Zimmerman SW. A dialysis modality decision guide based on their experience of six dialysis centers. Dial Transplant 1990; 19: 66–69.
183. Gokal R, Friedman EA, Rottembourg J, Tzamaloukas AH, Beeker GJ. Peritoneal dialysis in diabetic ESRD patients. Dial Transplant 1991; 20: 59–66.
184. Wolfe RA, Port FK, Hawthorne VM, Guire KE. A comparison of survival among dialytic therapies of choice: in–center haemodialysis versus continuous ambulatory peritoneal dialysis at home. Am J Kidney Dis 1990; 15: 433–440.
185. U.S. Renal Data System. USRDS 1991 Annual Data Report. Bethesda. NIH; August 1991; D.38, D.40, E.56, E.57.
186. Nelson CB, Port FK, Wolf RA, Guire KE. Comparison of continuous ambulatory peritoneal dialysis and hemodialysis patients survival with evaluation of trends during the 1980s. J Am Soc Nephrol 1992; 3: 1147–1155.
187. Nelson CB, Port FK, Wolfe RA, Guire KE. Dialysis patient survival: Evaluation of CAPD vs HD using 3 techniques. Perit Dial Int 1992; 12: Suppl.1: 144.
188. Bloembergen WE, Port FK, Mauger EA, Wolfe RA. A comparison of mortality between patients treated with hemodialysis and peritoneal dialysis. J Am Soc. Nephrol 1995; 6: 177–183.
189. Lasker RD. The diabetes control and complications trial. Implications for policy and practice. N Engl J Med 1993; 329: 1035–1036.
190. Diabetes Control and Complications Trial Research Group. The effect of intensive treatment of diabetes on the development and progression of long–term complications in insulin–dependent diabetes mellitus. N Engl J Med 1993; 329: 977–986.
191. Brownlee M, Cerami A, Vlassara H. Advanced glycosylation end products in tissue and the biochemical basis of diabetic complications. N Engl J Med 1988; 318: 1315–1321.
192. Bucala R, Cerami A. Advanced glycosylation: chemistry, biology, and implications for diabetes and aging. Adv Pharmacol 1992; 33: 1–34.
193. Vlassara H. Advanced glycation in diabetic renal and vascular disease. kidney Int 1995; 48: Suppl. 51: S43–S44.
194. Makita Z. Toxicity of glucose: is AGE the answer? Nephrol Dial Transplant 1995; 10: Suppl. 7: 33–37.
195. Williams ME. Dam (AGE) in diabetic ESRD: Role of advanced glycosylation. Sem Dial 1996; 9: 1–4.

196. Vlassara H. Recent progress on the biological and clinical significance of advanced glycosylation end–products. J Lab Clinic Med 1994; 124: 19–30.
197. Vlassara H, Brownlee M, Cerami A. High–affinity receptor–mediated uptake and degradation of glucose–modified proteins: A potential mechanism for the removal of senescent macromolecules. Proc Natl Acad Sci USA 1985; 82: 5588–5592.
198. Vlassara H, Brownlee M, Cerami A. Novel macrophage receptor for glucose–modified proteins is distinct form previously described scavenger receptors. J Exp. Med 1986; 164: 1301–1309.
199. Schmidt AM, Hori O, Cao R, Yan SD, Brett J, Wautier JL, Ogawa S, Kuwabara K, Matsumoto M, Stern D. RAGE: A novel cellular receptor for advanced glycation end products. Diabetes 1996; 45: S77–S80.
200. Wautier JL, Zoukourian C, Chappey O, Wautier MP, Guillausseau PJ, Cao R, Hori O, Stern D, Schmidt AM. Receptor – mediated endothelial cell dysfunction in diabetic vasculopathy. Soluble receptor for advanced glycation end products, blocks hyperpermeability in diabetic rats. J Clin Invest 1996; 97: 238–243.
201. Soulis T, Thallas V, Youssef S, Gilbert RE, Mc William BG, Murray–Mc Intosh RP, Cooper ME. Advanced glycation end products and their receptors co–localise in rat organs susceptible to diabetic microvascular injury. Diabetologia 1997; 40: 619–628.
202. Makita Z, Radoff S, Rayfield J, Yang Z, Skolnik E. Friedman EA, Cerami A, Vlassara H. Advanced glycosylation end products in patients with diabetic nephropathy. N Engl J Med 1991; 325: 836–842.
203. Makita Z, Vlassara H, Cerami A, Bucala R. Immunochemical detection of advanced glycosylation end products in vivo. J Biol Chem 1992; 267: 5133–5138.
204. Makita Z, Bucala R, Rayfield EJ, Friedman EA, Kaufman AM, Korbet SM, Barth RH, Winston JA, Fuh H, Manogue KR, Cerami A, Vlassara H. Reactive glycosylation end–products in diabetic uremia and treatment of renal failure. Lancet 1994; 343: 1519–1522.
205. Korbet SM, Makita Z, Friedman EA, Vlassara H. Advanced glycosylation end products in continuous ambulatory peritoneal dialysis patients. Am J Kidney Dis 1993; 22: 588–591.
206. Lamb EJ, Cattell WR, Dawnay AB St. J. In vitro formation of advanced glycasion end products in peritoneal dialysis fluid. Kidney Int 1995; 47: 1768–1774.
207. Makita Z, Vlassara H, Rayfield EJ, Cartweight K, Friedman E, Rodby R, Cerami A, Bucala R. Hemoglobin–AGE: a circulating marker of advanced glycosylation Science 1992; 258: 651–653.
208. Friedman MA, Wu YC, James MS, Schulak A, Monnier VM, Hrielk DE. Influence of pentosidine in patients with end–stage renal disease. Am J Kidney Dis 1995; 25: 445–451.
209. Dobbie JW, Zaki MA, Wilson LS. Ultrastructural studies on the peritoneum with special reference to chronic ambulatory peritoneal dialysis. Scott Med J 1981; 26: 213–223.
210. Dobbie JW. Advanced glycosylation end products in peritoneal tissue with different solutions. Perit Dial Int 1997; 17(Suppl 2): S27–S30.
211. Friedlander MA, Wu YC, Elgawish A, Monnier V, Early and advanced glycosolation end–products. Kinetics of formation and clearance in peritoneal dialysis. J Clin Invest 1996; 97: 728–735.
212. Dawnay AB. Advanced glycation end–products in peritoneal dialysis. Perit Dial Int 1996; 16(Suppl 1): S50–S53.
213. Dawnay AB, Millar DJ. Glycation and advanced glycation end–product formation with icodextrin and dextrose. Perit Dial Int 1997; 17: 21–28.
214. Dobbie JW. Serositis: Comparative analysis of histological findings and pathogenetic mechanisms in non–bacterial serosal inflammation. Perit Dial Int 1993; 13: 256–259.
215. Edelstein D, Brownlee M. Mechanistic studies of advanced glycosylation end product inhibition by aminoguanidines. Diabetes 1992; 41: 26–29.
216. Yagihashi S, Kamijo M, Baba M, Yagihashi N, Najai K. Effect of aminoguanidine on functional and structural abnormalities in peripheral nerve of stz–induced diabetic rats. Diabetes 1992; 41: 47–52.
217. Chibber R, Molinatti PA, Wong JSK, Mirlees D, Kohner EM. The effect of aminoguanidine and tolrestat on glucose toxicity in bovine retinal capilary pericytes. Diabetes 1994; 43: 758–763.
218. Brownlee M, Vlassara H, Kooney P, Ulrich A, Cerami A. Aminoguanidine prevents diabetes – induced arterial wall protein cross–linking. Science 1986; 232: 1629 – 1632.
219. Brownlee M. Glycation and diabetic complications. Diabetes 1994; 43: 837–841.
220. Soulis–Liparota T, Cooper M, Papazoglou D, Clarke B, Jerums G. Retardation by aminoguanidine of development of albuminuria, mesangial expansion, and tissue fluorescence in streptozocin–induced diabetic rat. Diabetes 1991; 40: 1328–1334.

221. Waz WR, Van Liew JB, Feld LG. Nitric oxide – inhibitory effect of aminoguanidine on renal function in rats. Kidney Blood Press Res 1997; 20: 211–217.
222. Friedman EA, Distant DA, Fleishhacker JF, Boyd TA, Cartwright K. Aminoguanidine prolongs survival in azotemic–induced diabetic rats. Am J Kidney Dis 1997; 30(2): 253–259.
223. A curious stopping rule from Hoechst Marion Roussel. Lancet (Editorial) 1997; 350(9072): p. 155.
224. Viberti G. Early closure of European Pimagedine trial. Steering Committee. Safety Committee. Lancet 1997; 350(9072): 214–215.
225. Abraham G, Zlotnik N, Ayiomamitis A, Oreopoulos DG. Drop– out of diabetic patients form CAPD. Adv Perit Dial 1987; 3: 199–204.
226. Rubin J, Hsu H. Continuous ambulatory peritoneal dialysis: ten years at one facility. Am J Kideny Dis 1991; 17: 165–169.
227. Zimmerman SW, Oxton LL, Bidwell D, Wakeen M. Long–term outcome of diabetic patients receiving peritoneal dialysis. Perit Dial Int 1996; 16: 63–68.
228. Abdel –Rahman E, Wakeen M, Zimmerman SW. Characteristics of long–term peritoneal dialysis survivors J Am Soc Nephrol 1995; 6: 516.
229. Schmitz O, Mogensen CE. How can the care of diabetic ESRD patients be improved? Sem Dial 1991; 4: 24–25.

50. RENAL TRANSPLANTATION FOR DIABETIC NEPHROPATHY

Eli A. Friedman, M.D.
Department of Medicine, State University of New York, Health Science Center at Brooklyn, Brooklyn, N.Y., USA

BACKGROUND

Registries listing the demographics of end-stage renal disease (ESRD) in the United States (US), Japan, and most nations in industrialized Europe show that diabetes mellitus, in 1998, is the leading cause of renal failure world-wide. More than a decade ago, Mauer and Chavers presciently predicted that "Diabetes is the most important cause of ESRD in the Western World [1]". Furthermore, in every European and North American registry of renal failure patients, both the incidence and prevalence of diabetic patients has risen continuously over the past ten years. According to the most recent (1997) report of the United States Renal Data System (USRDS), of 257,266 US patients undergoing either dialytic therapy or a kidney transplant in 1995, 80,667 had diabetes [2], a prevalence rate of 31.4%. Moreover, of 71,875 new (incident) cases of ESRD in 1995, 28,740 (40%) had diabetes (figure 50-1).

The incidence to prevalence ratio of 1.27 in 1995 reflects a disproportionately high mortality during the course of treatment in diabetic ESRD patients. Because early trials of maintenance hemodialysis in diabetic ESRD patients approached disaster, neither prolonging useful life nor gaining rehabilitation [3], a near unanimity among nephrologists concluded that individuals with diabetic nephropathy should be excluded from ESRD therapy. Indeed, this excess morbidity and mortality, in uremic diabetics previously discouraged their acceptance for renal transplantation in the belief that their rehabilitation was unobtainable. A decidedly negative view of the value of proffering renal transplants to diabetic ESRD patients persists through the 1990s in many locations as evidenced by a 1993 report from Groote Schuur Hospital which concludes: "Despite very strict selection criteria, the results of renal transplantation in diabetic patients remains poor. Better treatment strategies are needed to justify acceptance of these patients for transplantation[4]."

Elsewhere in the world, a more favourable assessment of the utility of renal

Mogensen, C.E. (ed.), THE KIDNEY AND HYPERTENSION IN DIABETES MELLITUS.

transplantation in the diabetic ESRD patient is the opinion of groups with large experience. As summarized by the center with the largest contribution to pioneering treatment kidney failure in diabetes: "Kidney transplants results in diabetic recipients have exceeded the expectations of 20 years ago, both at our institution and others.

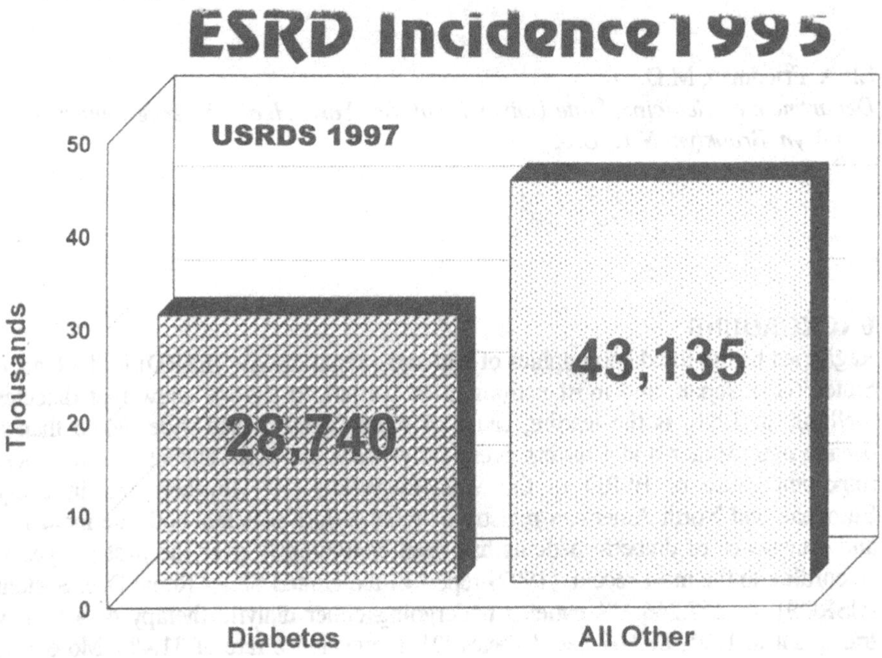

Figure 50-1 Demographic data presented in the 1997 report of the United States Renal Data System (USRDS) shows that the proportion of incident ESRD patients whose diagnoses was listed as diabetes was 40% in 1995. The USRDS does not distinguish between type 1 and type 2 diabetes in their reporting forms. Registries in Europe and Japan also list diabetes as the disease accounting for the greatest number of incident and prevalent ESRD cases.

We currently advocate a kidney transplant for all uremic diabetic patients [5]". Central to the improved prognosis for diabetic kidney transplant recipients is recognition that careful regulation of hypertension and hyperglycaemia reduces stress in the peri- and post-transplant period. Caution is appropriate when extrapolating results in treating the uremic diabetic from one institution to another. Variables which affect outcome and are not always identified are listed in table 50-1. Comparing treatment of diabetic ESRD patients in Norway and the US illustrates this caveat.

Firstly, about 10% of Americans with diabetes are thought to have insulin-dependent diabetes mellitus (Type 1) while as many as 50% of Norwegians with diabetes have Type 1. As detailed elsewhere in this text, distinguishing type 1 from the predominant form of diabetes mellitus (Type 2) separates two disorders with markedly different inheritance and clinical courses. to illustrate, we surveyed the race and gender of 232 of 1450 (16%) diabetic patients undergoing maintenance hemodialysis at 14 centres in Brooklyn and found the largest patient subset consisted of 87 black women, who comprised 37.5% of the total study population [6]. Type 2 was clearly diagnosed in 139 or 59.9% of surveyed diabetic patients on hemodialysis, but diabetes type could not be determined in 24 (10.3%) of patients.

Table 50-1 Variables in comparing diabetic kidney transplant recipients

Diabetes type
Mean age
Race
Socioeconomic status
Co-morbid conditions
Skill of surgeon and group
Immunosuppressive regimen
Available support services
(podiatry, ophthalmology, cardiology, nephrology, psychiatry)

Secondly, what is applicable for younger type 1 patients may be inappropriate for older persons with Type 2 diabetes. However, an extensive overlap in signs and symptoms often blurs distinction between diabetes type. Nagai found that of 551 patients diagnosed as having diabetes with onset before the age of 30 years, 337 (61.2%) had type 2. In Japanese diabetic individuals, diabetic retinopathy and nephropathy are as frequent in those who are young at onset of type 2 as in type 1 diabetes. Defining the faulty limits of present diabetes classification systems, Abourizk and Dunn remarked that: "Clinicians treating diabetic patients encounter numerous insulin-taking diabetic subjects who clinically are neither type 1 nor type 2". Further to the point, these workers reviewed 348 consecutive diabetic patients of mean age 53 years, evaluated in the north-eastern US, and concluded that diabetes type could not be established in 35% of whites, 57% of blacks, and 59% of Hispanics. Even with the recently revised Report of the Expert Commitee on the Diagnosis and Classification of Diabetes Mellitus [8] in hand, recommendations pertaining to kidney transplantation in diabetics *by diabetes type* must be interpreted with awareness of the above difficulty. For example, a combined pancreas-kidney transplant generally thought of as applicable only in type 1 diabetes may have a role in therapy of individuals with type 2 diabetes who no longer evince insulin synthesis (C-peptide negative).

TYPE 1 VERSUS TYPE 2 DIABETES

As a generalization, the majority (70 to 95% depending upon race) of those with diabetes in Europe and the US have type 2 diabetes: Some population subsets such as 100% full blooded Native American have absolutely no persons afflicted with type 1 despite a high endemicity (exceeding 50% of the population) of type 2 diabetes. In both type 1 and type 2 diabetes, ESRD is the end-point of a well-described progression following, in sequence, microalbuminuria, fixed proteinuria and azotemia [9,10,11], associated with the pathologic changes of nodular and diffuse intercapillary glomerular sclerosis and afferent and efferent arteriolonephrosclerosis.

After 20-30 years of type 1 diabetes, about 30-40% of patients manifest irreversibly failed kidneys [12]. Over the past forty years, a decreasing proportion of diabetic individuals with type 1 develop ESRD, reflecting the impact of enhanced blood pressure and blood glucose control. While previously, renal failure was thought relatively rare in type 2 [13], recent reports of a single population followed longitudinally indicate an approximately equal risk of nephropathy in both major diabetes types. For example, in Rochester, Minnesota, Humphrey et al. found equivalent rate of renal failure over 30 years in cohorts of 1,832 type 2 and 136 type 1 diabetic patients [14]. Complementing this study, a report from Heidelberg, Germany reached the same conclusion, noting that after 20 years of diabetes, a serum creatinine level >1.4 mg/dl was present in 59% of type 1 and 63% of type 2 diabetic subjects [15]. The message to be extracted from these and other studies is that ESRD is not an unusual conclusion of diabetic nephropathy in type 2 diabetes, in the U.S., Europe and Japan, the large majority of new diabetic ESRD cases occur in patients with type 2 diabetes. Indeed, among 550 diabetic individuals (91% were Black or Hispanic) undergoing maintenance hemodialysis in seven ambulatory dialysis units in Brooklyn in October 1997, 97% had type 2 diabetes. While the ratio of type 2 to type 1 diabetes in the general population is lower in Caucasians than in Blacks, Hispanics, or Native Americans, the much greater prevalence of type 2 compared to type 1 diabetes is present in all ESRD programs reported thus far.

UREMIA THERAPY

Planning long-term management for the uremic diabetic patient requires matching life style, availability of desired regimen, and social support systems. Understandably, a small proportion of uremic diabetic patients (usually those with extensive extrarenal complications) opt for passive suicide by declining further dialysis or a kidney transplant [16]. After exclusion of a reversible, profound depression, those individuals wishing to terminate ESRD care – a blind, double lower limb amputee with intractable heart failure, for example – should be guided to a hospice or provided with emotional support at home to minimize agonal discomfort.

Table 50-2 Choices for ESRD management in Diabetic Nephropathy

HEMODIALYSIS	
	Home hemodialysis
	Facility hemodialysis
PERITONEAL DIALYSIS	
	Intermittent (IPD)
	Continuous Ambulatory (CAPD)
	Continuous Cyclic (machine) (CCPD)
KIDNEY TRANSPLANTION	
	Living donor kidney
	Cadaver donor kidney
KIDNEY and PANCREAS TRANSPLANTATION	
HEMOFILTRATION (Europe)	

Interventional options in therapy must be presented in clearly understood terms in order to enlist the patient as an active member of the renal team. Listed in table 50-2 are those options in ESRD therapy available to diabetic patients including kidney transplantation and peritoneal or hemodialysis, performed at a facility or in the patient's home. The decision to perform self-dialysis at home demands unusually strong patient motivation, appropriate space, and an empathetic partner. As reported by the USRDS in 1997, for patients under treatment in 1995, survival and rehabilitation of those few (0.5%) diabetic persons who elect home hemodialysis is markedly superior to facility hemodialysis. Approximately 68% of diabetic individuals with ESRD in the US in 1995 were treated with facility hemodialysis. Peritoneal dialysis in 1995, was utilized to treat about 12% of diabetic ESRD patients attaining survival equivalent to that of maintenance hemodialysis. Kidney transplantation, the best ESRD option in diabetes (vide infra) in 1995 in the US was applied to fewer than one in five ESRD patients with diabetes (18%).

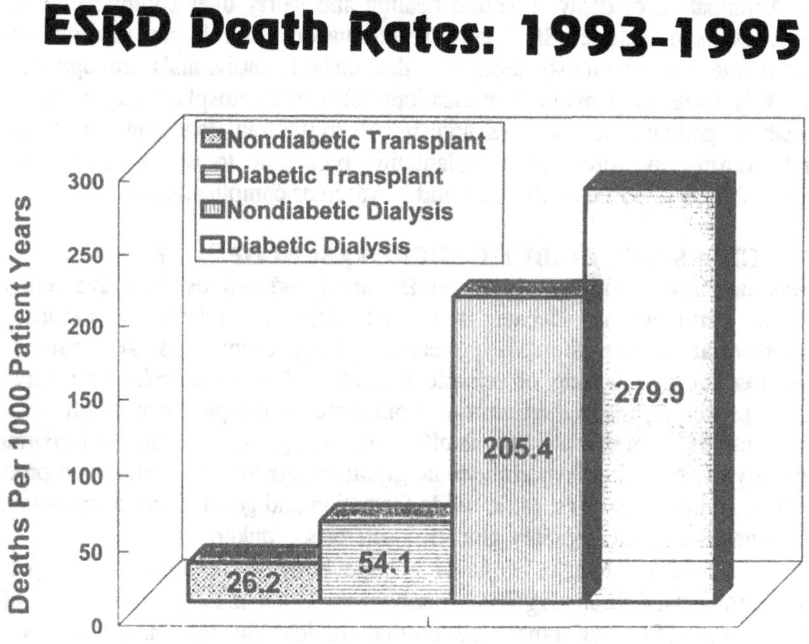

Figure 50-2 Extracted from the 1997 report of the United States Renal Data System (USRDS), the fate of diabetic and non-diabetic ESRD patients treated between 1993 and 1995 is shown by treatment modality. For this analysis, survival of peritoneal and hemodialysis patients was grouped. Note that within both transplant and dialysis subsets, diabetic patients had much greater mortality than did non-diabetic patients.

KIDNEY TRANSPLANTATION

The combination of diabetes and uremia presents a major challenge in surgical management [17]. Nevertheless, multiple reports document the consensus belief that long-term survival of the uremic diabetic patient with a well functioning renal transplant is greater than that afforded by other renal replacement therapy [18]. By 1985, at centres performing a large number of kidney transplants, patient and graft survival in renal transplantation in diabetic patients improved to be about equal to non-diabetic patients. Analysis of national statistics in the US notes than in 1991, diabetic persons comprised 23% of first renal transplant recipients. In the diabetic recipient cohort, renal allograft survival was not different from other causes of ESRD, excepting the superior functional survival in IgA nephropathy. At its best, one year post-renal transplant, of 995 diabetic recipients in a study of combined pancreas and kidney transplants was a remarkable 84% [19]. The most optimistic current assessments of short- and long-term outcome in diabetic renal allograft recipients indicate success rates equivalent to that obtained in nondiabetic recipients as exemplified in reports by Ekberg and Christenssen [20] and Aswad, Shidban, Bogaard et al [21]. Although approximately 10% of diabetic renal allograft recipients die during the first post-transplant year, a remarkable 100% survival was achieved in Malmö, Sweden, in the diabetic subset transplanted between 1988 and 1993. Anticipation of delayed wound healing and worry over complicating sepsis are not reasons to exclude ESRD patients with diabetes from kidney transplantation. Nor is it true – as previously thought – that diabetic individuals are significantly more likely to develop major complications following transplant surgery than are non-diabetic patients. Nevertheless, adjustments to the treatment plan must be made prior to, during and after the transplantation procedure to accommodate for the unique problems imposed by diabetes and its vascular complications [22].

PATHOGENESIS OF DIABETIC MICROVASCULOPATHY

Kidneys in diabetic individuals are under stress induced by hemodynamic and metabolic perturbations. Debate is intense over the relative importance of intraglomerular hypertension [23] versus hyperglycaemia as key causes of glomerulosclerosis. Lacking of reliable indicator of renal morphologic damage, however, precise timing of the transition from diabetes as a purely metabolic disease to that of multisystem vasculopathy is often a clinical guess. The relative importance of capillary hypertension, hyperlipidemia, glycation, advanced glycated end-product formation, sorbitol synthesis, nitric oxide formation and genetic predetermination to the pathogenesis of intercapillary glomerulosclerosis is unknown.

No single mechanism explains a large body of seemingly incompatible experimental data. The *hyperglycemia school* to which the author belongs, infers from the results of kidney transplantation that ambient glucose concentration is the main risk factor for glomerular damage. Support for this thesis is drawn from several observations:

1. Recurrent intercapillary glomerulosclerosis and renal failure can develop in kidneys obtained from non-diabetic donors that are transplanted into diabetic recipients [24].

2. Kidney graft recipients who become diabetic only after administration of corticosteroid drugs (steroid diabetics) may develop typical diabetic glomerulopathy – nodular and diffuse intercapillary glomerulosclerosis.

3. In isolated case reports, early diabetic glomerulopathy may be reversed by establishment of a euglycemic environment, as shown by disappearance of

glomerulosclerosis in two cadavic donor kidneys obtained from a diabetic donor after transplantation into nondiabetic recipients [25]. Further to the point, if nephromegaly is accepted as an early morphologic change in diabetic nephropathy, then the reduction in renal size induced by sustained euglycemia in type 1 diabetes is evidence that correction of euglycemia reverses morphologic injury [26].

COMBINED PANCREAS PLUS KIDNEY TRANSPLANTION

For many uremic individuals with type 1 diabetes, a combined kidney plus pancreas transplant has evolved as an important option because of its ability to offer superior glycemic control and improved quality of life. As both kidney graft survival and overall mortality are approximately equivalent following kidney alone versus dual organ transplantation alone at many centres, neither the survival of the patient nor the success of the kidney transplant need by jeopardized by the addition of a pancreas graft. Further on the positive side of the ledger, anecdotal reports indicate that recipients of combined pancreas and kidney transplants have greater stabilization of diabetic eye disease than do kidney recipients. On the other hand, a sombre review of the surgical risk of 445 consecutive pancreas transplants from the pioneer University of Minnesota program noted that relaparotomy was required in 32% of recipients while perioperative mortality was 9% [27]. Based on "serious surgical complication" rate of 35%, these workers advise that donors over 45 years old not be used while recipients over 45 years old be given a kidney graft alone.

It is true that recipients of combined pancreas plus kidney grafts experience greater morbidity, a reality that can be justified by the evidence that a pancreas graft will both prevent recurrent morbidity, a reality that can be justified by the evidence that a pancreas graft will both prevent recurrent diabetic nephropathy, and may result in improvements in sensory/motor neuropathy. Newer immunosuppressive drug regimens may improve the outlook for pancreas transplantation. For example, matched-pair analysis of pancreas and kidney graft recipients immunosuppressed with tacrolimus plus prednisone had an 88% first year survival compared with 73% immunosuppressed cylclosporine plus prednisone [28]. Switching from cyclosporine to tacrolimus with or without mycopheolate mofetil appeared to increase enhanced graft survival rates with a low rate of rejection episode.

Consequent to a dual organ transplant, but not after a solitary kidney transplant, lipid perturbations revert to normal perhaps foreshadowing better cardiovascular outcomes as well. In those with normal or "mild" renal disease, the decision to proffer an isolated pancreas transplant is more complex. In several reports, success rates for solitary pancreas transplants are lower than after combined organ replacement. Suitable candidates for an isolated pancreas graft are those younger than 45 years suffering repeated bouts of disabling hypoglycemia or ketoacidosis unresponsive to other measures. More difficult to judge is whether or when individuals who have advancing diabetic complications with relatively intact renal function (creatinine clearance > 70 mL/min) should be considered for an isolated pancreas transplant. Presently, such operations must be classed as investigational. An encouraging report from the Minnesota Transplant Team observed that a successful pancreas transplant after five or more years of euglycemia will reverse established pathologic changes of diabetic nephropathy including disappearance of nodular glomerular lesions [29]. Pancreas transplantation will remain an important option in the treatment of type 1 diabetes until alternative strategies are developed that can provide equal glycemic control with less or no immunosuppression or less overall morbidity.

ADVANCED GLYCOSYLATION END-PRODUCTS (AGEs)

As a constantly occurring process, reducing sugars such as glocuse react non-enzymatically and reversibly with free amino groups in proteins to form small amounts of stable Amadori products through Schiff base adducts. With progressive ageing, spontaneous further irreversible modification of proteins by glucose results in the formation of a series of compounds termed advanced glycosylated end-products (AGE's), a heterogeneous family of biologically and chemically reactive compounds with crosslinking properties. In diabetes, this continuos process of protein modification is magnified by high ambient glucose concentrations [30].

Hyperglycemia is the prime determinant of protein binding by Amadori products [31]. After dehydration and rearrangements Amadori products become highly reactive carbonyl compounds including 3-deoxyglucosane (3-deoxy-D-erythro-hexos-2-ulose, 3-DG) [32] which in turn reacts with free amino groups, leading to crosslinking and so called "browning" of proteins as AGEs accumulate in the Maillard reaction. Determining which AGE compounds are the active mediators of protein injury has produced inferential evidence indicting N^{ε}-(carboxymethyl) L-lysine (CML) [33], pyrraline, pentosidine [34], and crosslinks [35]. Recent reports by Niwa and co-workers indicate that several imidazolones, the reaction products of the guanindino group of arginine with 3-DG, are common etitopes of AGE-modified proteins produced in vitro and are significantly increased in erythrocytes of diabetic patients. Employing immunologic histopathologic techniques, imidazolone has been demonstrated in nodular lesions and expanded mesangial matrix of glomeruli and renal arteries in diabetic nephropathy [36]. CML, an oxidative product of glycated proteins, accumulates in arteries, atherosclerotic plaques, and in foam cells and serum proteins in diabetic patients suggesting that it may be an endogenous marker of oxidative tissue damage and glomerulopathy in diabetic individuals [37].

Binding to specific receptors on endothelial cells [38], AGEs increase vascular permeability, procoagulant activity, adhesion molecule expression, and monocyte influx, actions that may contribute to vascular injury [39]. Normally excreted by the kidney, the plasma concentration of AGEs is inversely proportional to the glomerular filtration rate. As diabetic patients develop renal insufficiency, there is a progressive and marked increase in plasma and tissue levels of AGEs. Compounding the complexity of AGE action is the demonstration by Vlassara's group that renal excretion of AGEs in digested foods is suppressed in individuals with diabetic nephropathy, a perturbation that may contribute to progressive elevation of plasma AGE levels as residual renal function declines [40].

Following administration of AGEs to non-diabetic rabbits and rats, vascular dysfunction resembling that seen in diabetes is observed [41]. Furthermore, treatment of non-diabetic rats for four weeks with AGE-modified albumin causes glomerular hypertrophy and increased extracellular matrix production in association with activation of the genes for collagen, laminin, and transforming growth factor-β [42].

Treatment with AGEs alone in concentrations that achieve plasma concentrations equivalent to those seen in diabetic animals [43]. AGE-treated rats had a 50 percent expansion in glomerular volume, basement membrane widening, and increased mesangial matrix, indicating significant glomerulosclerosis compared to untreated controls.

AGEs in the rat impair a variety of important nitric oxide-mediated processes including neurotransmission, wound healing [44], blood flow in small vessels, and decreased cell proliferation [45]. It follows that, the toxicity of AGEs may be mediated in part by their interference with the actions of nitric oxide [46]. Brownlee reviewed the importance of glycosylation of proteins to the progression of diabetic microangiopathy through the mechanism of formation of advanced glycosylation end-products (AGEs) [47].

Renal failure is associated with both a high serum level of AGEs and accelerated vasculopathy in diabetes. Vlassara et al injected AGEs to non-diabetic rats and rabbits and showed that physiologic and morphologic changes typical of diabetes resulted [48].

Diabetic uremic patients accumulate advanced glycosylated end-products in "toxic" amounts that are not decreased to normal by hemodialysis or peritoneal dialysis, but fall sharply, to within the normal range, within days of restoration of renal function by renal transplantation [49]. *It is this persistent high level of AGEs in dialysis patients which we postulate is responsible to the greater mortality in diabetics of dialytiĉ therapy as compared with a functioning renal transplant.*

AMINOGUANIDINE

Aminoguanidine (empirical formular of CH6N4) is a nucleophilic hydrazine derivative. It has an HC1, a molecular weight of 110.5 and a chemical structure as depicted:

$H_2N - C - NHNH_2$

||

NH

Given to aminoguanidine streptozotocin-induced diabetic rats aminoguanidine pharmacologically inhibits formation of AGEs. In a 9 months trial from the onset of experimental diabetes, aminoguanidine prevented the widening of the glomerular basement membrane that is typical of diabetes [50]. Induced diabetic retinopathy is also prevented in rats by treatment with aminoguanidine which blocks retinal capillary closure, the principal pathohysiologic abnormality, underlying diabetic retinopathy [51]. Similarly, experimental diabetic neuropathy in the rats also is minimized by treatment with aminoguanidine as judged by motor nerve conduction velocity and the accumulation of AGEs in nerves [52]. Recently, in streptozotocin-induced diabetic rats made azotemic by surgical reduction of renal mass, aminoguanidine treated rats were found to have significantly ($p<0.04$) superior survival to that of untreated azotemic diabetic rats [53].

The rationale for preventing AGE formation as a means of impeding development of diabetic complications has been reviewed [54,55]. An especially appealing aspect of this approach to preventing diabetic complications is the elimination of the necessity for the patient to attain euglycemia [56]. Aminoguanidine treatment significantly prevents NO activation and limits tissue accumulation of AGEs. Corbett et al speculate that aminoguanidine inhibits interleukin-1 beta-induced nitrite formation (an oxidation product of NO) [57].

In a derivative study [58], aminoguanidine but not methylguanidine, inhibited AGE formation from L-lysine and G6P while both guanidine compounds were equally effective in normalizing albumin permeation in induced-diabetic rats. A role for a relative or absolute increase in NO production in the pathogenesis of early diabetic vascular dysfunction was also inferred as was the possibility that inhibition of diabetic vascular functional changes by aminoguanidine may reflect inhibition of NO synthase activity rather than, or in addition to, prevention of AGE formation. Aminoguanidine is also a glucose competitor for the same protein-to-protein bond [59] that becomes the link for the formation and accumulation of irreversible and highly reactive advanced glycation end-products (AGE) over long-lived fundamental molecules such as the constituents of arterial wall collagen, GBM, nerve myelin, DNA and others. How aminoguanidine prevents renal, eye, nerve and other microvascular complications in animals models of diabetes is under active investigation by Brownlee and associates [60], and others in diverse specialities [61].

Concurrent multicenter clinical trials are in progress to evaluate the effect of aminoguanidine (Pimagidine) on the course of diabetic nephropathy after onset of clinical proteinuria in type 1 and type 2 diabetes. Adults with documented diabetes, fixed proteinuria ≥ 500 mg/day, and a plasma creatinine concentration ≥ 1.0 mg/dL (88 μmol/L) in men have been randomly assigned to treatment with aminoguanidine or placebo for four years. The effect of treatment on the amount of proteinuria, progression of renal insufficiency, and the course of retinopathy will be monitored. An additional multicenter clinical trial of aminoguanidine in diabetics undergoing maintenance hemodialysis was initiated in mid-1996. The hypothesis under evaluation is that the higher mortality of diabetic persons on dialysis (both peritoneal and hemodialysis) as contrasted with survival of diabetic patients after a kidney transplant, reflects, in part, toxicity of AGEs the level of which falls to near normal after a successful allograft is in situ.

CO-MORBIDITY

Co-morbidity, extrarenal coincident disease, distinguishes diabetic ESRD from non-diabetic ESRD patients (table 50-3).

By means of a scoring system (table 50-4) the severity of co-morbid illness in two patients or groups of patients can be expressed quantitatively and compared. We have found the co-morbid index to be a useful tool in the pre-transplant assessment of diabetic ESRD patients whether receiving dialytic therapy or renal allografts as therapy.

Table 50-3 Progressive diabetic complications post renal transplantation

1. Retinopathy, glaucoma, cataracts.
2. Coronary artery disease. Cardiomyopathy.
3. Cerebrovascular disease.
4. Peripheral vascular disease: limb amputation.
5. Motor neuropathy. Sensory neuropathy.
6. Autonomic dysfunction: diarrhea, dysfunction, hypotension.
7. Myopathy.
8. Depression

Table 50-4 Variables in morbidity in diabetic kidney transplant recipients. The co-morbidity index.

1. Persistent angina or myocardial infaction.
2. Other cardiovascular problems, hypertension, congestive heart failure, cardiomyopathy.
3. Respiratory disease.
4. Autonomic neuropathy (gastroparesis, obstipation, diarrhea, cystopathy, orthostatic hypo-sion.
5. Neurologic problems, cerebrovascular accident or stroke residual.
6. Musculoskeletal disorders, including all varieties of renal bone disease.
7. Infections including AIDS but excluding vascular access-site or peritonitis.
8. Hepatitis, hepatic insufficiency, enzymatic pancreatic insufficiency.
9. Hematologic problems other than anemia.
10. Spinal abnormalities, lower back problems or arthritis.
11. Vision impairment (minor to severe – decreased acuity to blindness) loss.
12. Limb amputation (minor to severe – finger to lower extremity).
13. Mental or emotional illness (neurosis, depression, psychosis).

To obtain a numerical Co-Morbidity Index for an individual patient, rate each variable from 0 to 3 (0=absent, 1=mild – of minor import to patient's life, 2=moderate, 3=severe). By proportional hazard analysis, the relative significance of each variable can be isolated from the other 12.

CARDIOVASCULAR DISEASE

Stress on the cardiovascular system may follow the intentional volume expansion during surgery. Pre-transplant cardiovascular evaluation in the diabetic patient is a vital facilitating step prior to kidney transplantation. Should severe coronary artery disease be discovered, revascularization of the myocardium by coronary artery bypass or angioplasty becomes a stipulated requirement to reconsideration of kidney transplantation [62]. Khauli et al first reported the use of coronary angiography for detecting the presence and severity of coronary artery disease and left ventricular dysfunction in 48 diabetic patients scheduled for a kidney transplant [63]. The benefit of pre-transplant myocardial revascularization was inferred by the uniform successful outcome in 23 diabetic patients, none of whom died. The remarkably good two-year patient and graft survival for living donor and cadaver donorrecipients given "standard" immunosuppresion with azathioprine and prednisone was 81% and 68% and 61% and 32% respectively.

We concur with Khauli et al who "discourage transplantation" in patients who have "the simultaneous presence of >70 percent arterial stenosis and left ventricular dysfunction." A reasonable policy was proffered by Philipson et al who studied 60 diabetic patients being considered for a kidney transplant and advised that "patients with diabetes and end-stage renal disease who are at highest risk for cardiovascular events can be identified, and these patients probably should not undergo renal transplantation "[64]. The basis for this position was an analysis of treatment outcome in which only seven patients had a negative thallium stress test, four of whom received a kidney transplant, without subsequent "cardiovascular events". By contrast, of 53 diabetic patients with either a positive or non-diagnostic stress thallium tests, cardiac catheterization was employed to identify 26 patients with mild or no coronary disease or left ventricular dysfunction; 16 patients in this group received kidney transplants without cardiovascular incident. In a subset of ten patients with moderate heart disease, of whom 8 received renal transplant, two died of heart disease, while of thirteen patients with severe coronary artery disease or left ventricular malfunction, eight died before receiving a transplant, three from cardiovascular disease. What may be the most important finding by Khauli et al is that 38% of diabetic ESRD patients had coronary artery disease. Risk of cardiac death in the uremic diabetic is so great [65] that pre-kidney transplant evaluation – including a thorough history and physical examination – should include an electrocardiogram, echocardiogram, thallium stress test, and, if needed coronary artery catheterization and Holter monitoring [66]. More recently, a simplified cardiac evaluation employing echocardiography after administration of dobutamine has been advocated for pre-transplant screening in diabetic ESRD patients [67], but the specificity and sensitivity of this technique have been questioned [68].

Kidney transplantation should not be performed in diabetics who evince arrhythmias on minimal exercise, EKG changes on stress, and/or an ischemic myocardium with occluded coronary vessels. An additional benefit of thorough pre-transplant cardiac evaluation is the guidance gained to assist in regulation of volume expansion during the operative procedure.

SCREEENING FOR CARDIOVASCULAR DISEASE

All diabetics with ESRD who have experienced symptomatic peripheral vascular disease require evaluation pre-operatively with non-invasive Doppler flow studies, and in some instances, angiography to avoid placement of the renal allograft in an area of compromised arterial flow. Specifically, arteries supplying a lower extremity with marginal peripheral flow must not be used to revascularize an organ allograft, because the extremity may be placed in jeopardy of amputation [69]. diabetic ESRD patients frequently have nearly occlusive arthrosclerotic narrowing of the internal iliac artery forcing use of the external iliac artery for the arterial anastomosis to the allograft. In this circumstance, a local proximal endarterectomy of the external iliac artery can be performed.

MORTALITY

Death in diabetic renal transplant recipients, as in diabetics on dialytic therapy is most often attributed to cardiac disease or a myocardial infarction (MI) (figure 50-4). Despite careful evaluation of the coronary and peripheral vascular systems prior to renal transplantation, there is a high incidence of extremity amputation and cardiovascular death in diabetic renal allograft recipients followed for three or more years [70], due to progression of diabetic macro and microvasculopathy [71].

Age is a correlate of survival in all ESRD patients. Consistent with this generalization, diabetic renal transplant recipients over 40 years of age have a higher mortality than that of younger diabetic renal transplant recipients, mainly due to a higher rate of cardiovascular death [72]. When comparing different modalities applied to ESRD in diabetes, it should be kept in mind that the increased risk of cardiovascular death post-transplant in older patients is also present should the same patient be managed by dialytic therapy. Restated, arteriosclerotic heart disease is the leading cause of death in diabetics treated by dialytic therapy or kidney transplantation. The latest USRDS long-term survival results for ESRD due to diabetes (1997 Report of 1995 data) are shown in figure 50-3, which underscores the clear advantage of renal transplantation both from cadaver donor and living related donor kidneys over dialytic therapy.

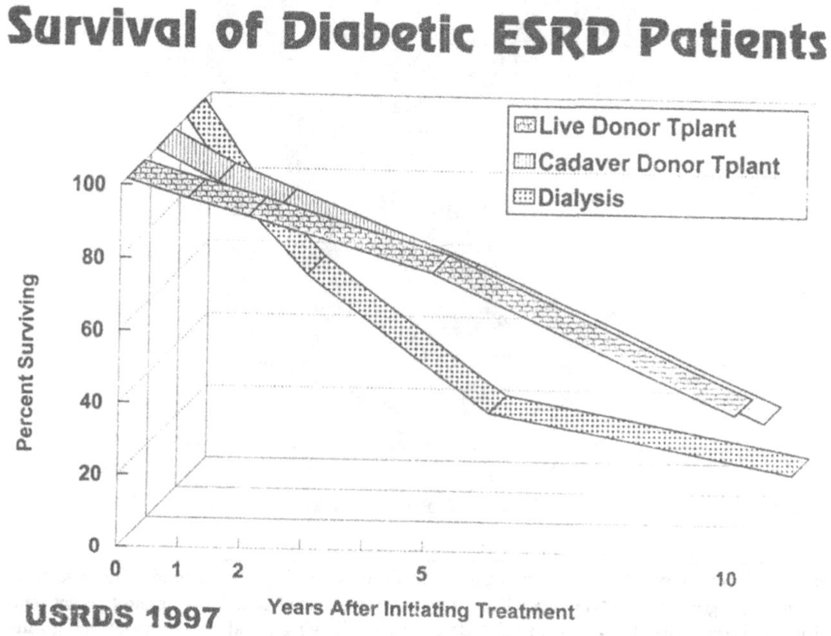

Figure 50-3 Long-term observation of diabetic ESRD patients shown in selected data from the most recent report of the United States Renal Data System (USRDS) depicts two key points; 1. Dialysis patients are nearly all dead within a decade. Renal transplant recipients have superior survival though more than one-half die within a decade whether treated with a living donor or cadaver donor kidney. The burden of advanced glycosylated end-product (AGE) toxicity in dialysis patients may explain the difference in outcome between modalities.

POST-TRANSPLANT MANAGEMENT

Diabetic recipients of renal transplants spend more days during frequent hospitalization than do non-diabetic patients [73]. Post-transplant hospitalization are prompted mainly by suspicion of allograft failure, infections, or cardiac disease. Perturbations in plasma glucose levels due to changing doses of corticosteroids usually can be managed at home. When wide swings in glucose concentration, including alternating hypo and extreme hyperglycemia (hyperosmolar non-ketonic coma) become life threatening, hospital admission is wise.

Restoration of normal renal function is a diabetic who developed ESRD because of diabetic nephropathy does not reverse concomitant advanced extrarenal micro- and macrovasculopathy.

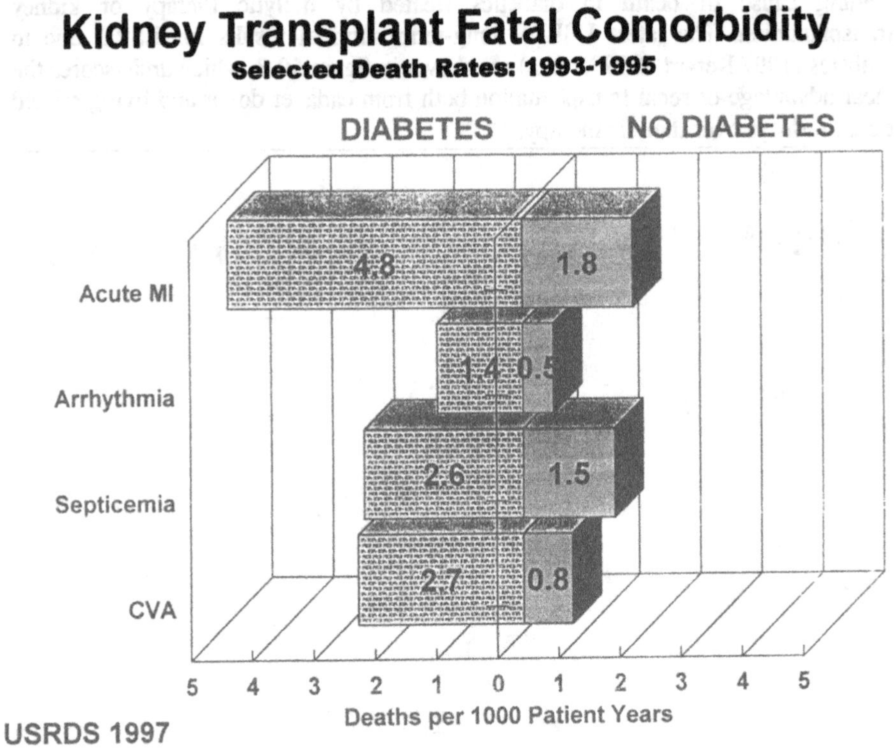

Figure 50-4 Management of renal transplant recipients with diabetes demands the inventory and treatment of progressive comorbid conditions. As shown in selected data from the most recent report of the United States Renal Data System (USRDS), deaths following a kidney transplant are greater for myocardial infaction, septicemia, and cerebrovascular disease in diabetic than in non-diabetic patients.

What distinguishes the diabetic from the non-diabetic renal transplant recipient are the multiple organ system perturbations associated with long-standing diabetes. Starting with the immediate post-transplant period, management of the diabetic renal transplant recipient is often complex demanding attention from diverse subspecialists. For example, distinguishing between acute allograft rejection, acute tubular necrosis, and cyclosporine drug nephrotoxicity in an oliguric newly transplanted patient may be impossible. In many instances, determining a single pathogenetic mechanism after interpretation of renal scans, sonograms, biopsies, and tests of glomerular and tubular function is still largely an art based on experience.

AUTONOMIC NEUROPATHY

Thoughout transplant surgery, and the day or two before oral feeding is resumed, metabolic control of plasma glucose concentration is best effected by frequent – hourly when needed – measurements of glucose and an intravenous infusion of 1-4 units per hour of regular insulin. Bethanechol, which may be given in combination with metoclopramide or cisapride, also improves gastric motility. Constipation, sometimes evolving into obstipation, is a frequent problem following transplantation; Effective stimulants to resume spontaneous defecation are early ambulation, stool softening agents, and suspension of cascara. Autonomic neuropathy may, at the other extreme, induce explosive and continuous liquid diarrhea enervating and dehydrating the post-operative diabetic patient. In our experience, loperamide given hourly in doses as high as 4 mg/hr almost always halts diarrhea. Another troublesome manifestation of diabetic autonomic neuropathy is diabetic cystopathy, a functional urinary bladder outflow obstruction. Encouragement to the patient adapting to a regimen of frequent voiding and self-application of manual external pressure above the pubic symphysis (Credé Manuever) plus administration of oral bethanechol usually permits resumption of spontaneous voiding. Repeated self-catheterization of the bladder may be the only means to avoid an indwelling catheter when an atonic bladder is unresponsive to the above protocol.

IMPOTENCE

Caused by arterial insufficiency and diabetic neuropathy, erectile impotence is common in diabetic dialysis patients and, in a minority of patients, may improve after a successful kidney transplant. Unless due to psychiatric cause, impotence in diabetes has a poor prognosis. Resort to a penile prostheses, or pre-coital intrapenile injections and more recently intraurethral instillation or oral administration of prostaglandins may be appropriate for rehabilitation when impotence persists.

LIFE QUALITY

Diabetic renal transplant recipients enthusiastically rate their quality of life as equivalent to that of the general population in the US. Rehabilitation of the diabetic transplant recipient often hinges on a team approach to management which minimizes the time devoted to multiple visits to different specialists. Typically, the diabetic transplant recipient is expected to make repeated visits to ophthalmologists, podiatrist, endocrinologist, nephrologist and internist (figure 50-5). Success of the renal transplant team depends upon collaboration with an ophthalmologist skilled in laser surgery and a podiatrist experienced in preventive management of diabetic feet. Progressive vasculopathy even in those given a renal transplant before initiation of a dialysis regimen, does not prevent worsening many diabetic patients become increasingly disabled due to progressive extrarenal disease processes [74].

RECURRENT NEPHROPATHY

Recurrent diabetic glomerulopathy, along with allograft rejection, cyclosporine toxicity and single kidney hyperfiltration pose threats to renal allograft integrity. First detectable as GBM thickening with mesangial expansion after two years [75] and later as characteristic glomerulosclerosis in recipients with type 1 [76], after five or more years [77] recurrent diabetic nephropathy may present as a nephrotic syndrome followed by progressive azotemia and finally and sadly as recurrent ESRD. Approximately half of those given a living related kidney survive their first post-transplant decade. After kidney transplantation, survival of diabetic recipients may be longer than a decade [78]. Of 265 ESRD patients with type 1 at the University of Minnesota, who were given a renal transplant between December 1966

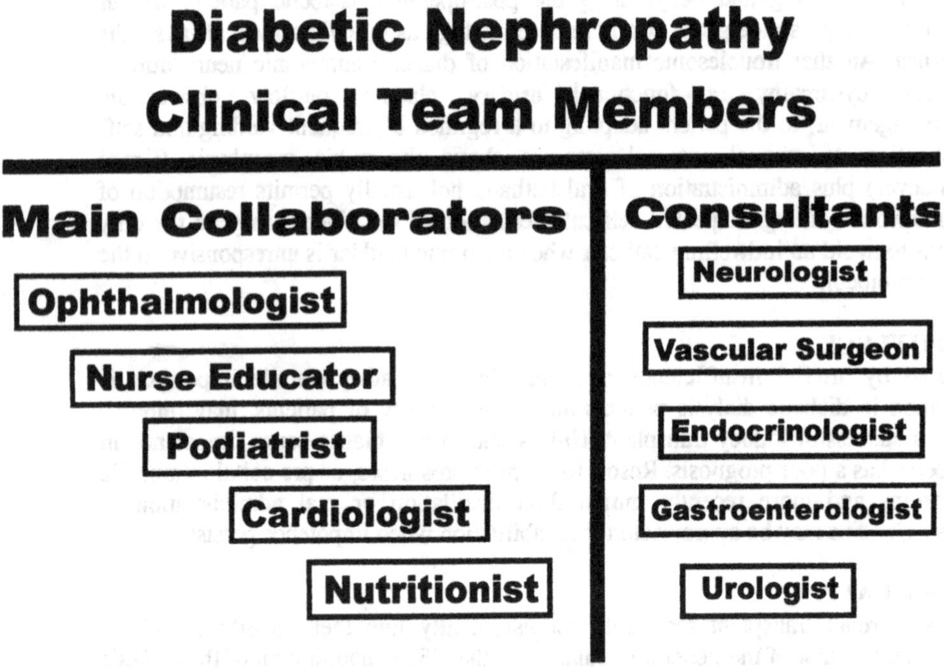

Figure 50-5 Defining a Life Plan for each ESRD patient reduces stress imparted by indecision and confusion. Key collaborators are listed on the left while frequent consultants are listed on the right. Not included though perhaps equally important is "The Patient" who should be an active participant in all decision making.

and April 1978, 100 were alive with a functioning graft 10 years later, an actual patient and primary graft survival of 40% and 32% respectively. HLA-identical recipients of living related kidneys attained a remarkable actual 10-year functional graft survival of 62%. 23 recipients died in the second decade after kidney transplantation; death from cardiovascular disease occurred in 10, continuing the pattern observed during the first decade.

CONCLUSIONS

Diabetes is the disorder most often linked with development of end-stage renal disease (ESRD) in the USA, Europe, South America, Japan, India, and Africa. Kidney disease is as likely to develop in long-duration type 2 as in type 1 diabetes mellitus. Nephropathy in diabetes follows a predictable course starting with microalbuminuria through proteinuria, azotemia and culminating in ESRD. When compared with other causes of ESRD, the diabetic patient sustains greater mortality and morbidity due to concomitant (co-morbid) systemic disorders especially coronary artery and cerebrovascular disease. A functioning kidney transplant provides the uremic diabetic patient better survival with superior rehabilitation than does either peritoneal or maintenance hemodialysis. For the minority (<8%) of diabetic ESRD patients who have type 1 diabetes, performance of a combined pancreas and kidney transplant may cure diabetes and permit full rehabilitation. No matter which ESRD therapy has been elected, optimal rehabilitation in diabetic ESRD patients requires that effort be devoted to recognition and management of co-morbid conditions.

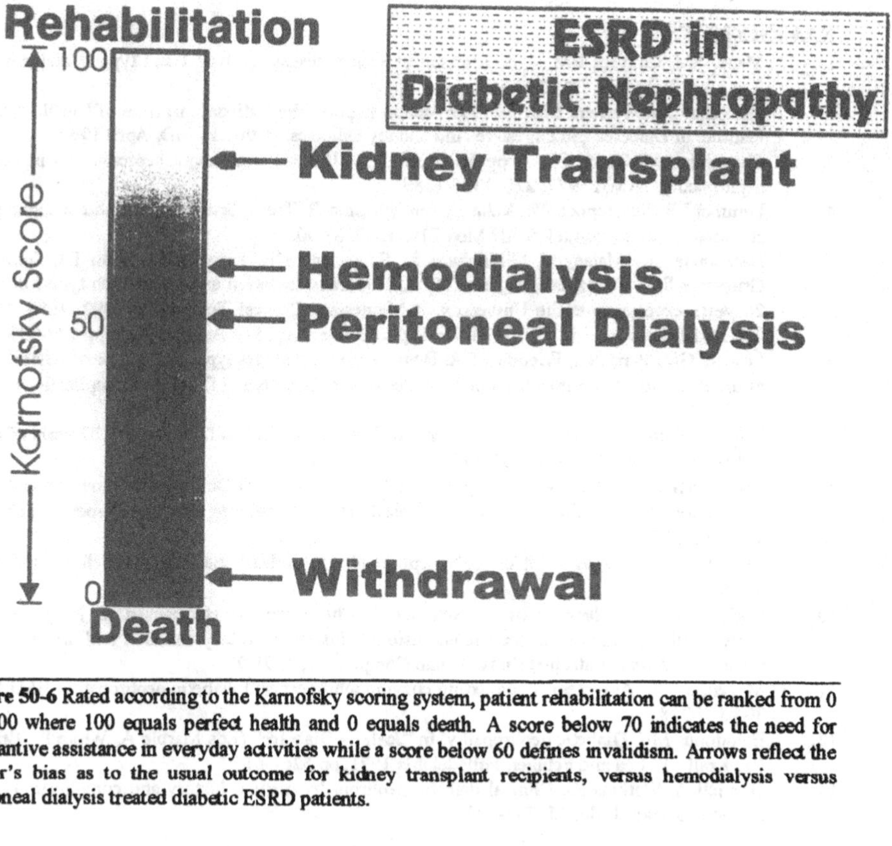

Figure 50-6 Rated according to the Karnofsky scoring system, patient rehabilitation can be ranked from 0 to 100 where 100 equals perfect health and 0 equals death. A score below 70 indicates the need for substantive assistance in everyday activities while a score below 60 defines invalidism. Arrows reflect the author's bias as to the usual outcome for kidney transplant recipients, versus hemodialysis versus peritoneal dialysis treated diabetic ESRD patients.

Survival in treating ESRD in diabetes by dialytic therapy and renal transplantation is continuously improving. This inexorable progress in therapy reflects multiple small advances in understanding of the pathogenesis of extrarenal micro- and macrovasculopathy in an inexorable disease, coupled with safer immunosuppresion. Pertubed biochemical reactions underlying the pathogenesis of diabetic vasculopathy – especially the adverse impact of accumulated advanced glycosylated end-products (AGEs) – raises the possibility of blocking end-organ damage without necessarily correcting hyperglycemia. In this context, trials of aminoguanidine are now being conducted. A functioning kidney transplant provides the uremic diabetic patient a greater probability for survival with better rehabilitation than does either CAPD or maintenance hemodialysis (figure 50-6). For the minority (<10%) of diabetic ESRD patients who have type 1 diabetes, serious consideration should be devoted to performance of a combined pancreas and kidney transplant to effect a cure of the diabetes so long as the pancreas functions [79]. No matter which ESRD therapy has been elected, optimal rehabilitation in diabetic ESRD patients requires that effort be devoted to recognition and management of co-morbid conditions. Uremia therapy, whether CAPD, hemodialysis or a kidney transplant should be individualized to the patient's specific medical and family circumstances.

REFERENCES

1. Mauer SM, Chavers BM. A comparison of kidney disease in type I and type II diabetes. Adv Exp Med Biol 1985; 189: 299-303.
2. US Renal Data System, USRDS 1997 Annual Report. The National Institutes of Health, National Institute of Diabetes and Digestive And Kidney Diseases. Bethesda, MD, April 1997.
3. Chavamian M, Gutch CF, Kopp KF Kolff WJ.. The sad truth about hemodialysis in diabetic nephropathy. JAMA 1972; 222: 1386-1389.
4. Lemmer ER, Swanepoel CR, Kahn D, van-Zyl-Smit R. Transplantation for diabetic nephropathy at Groote Schuur Hospital. S Afr Med J 1993; 83: 88-90.
5. Basadonna G, Matas AJ, Gillingham K, Sutherland DE, Payne WD, Dunn DI, Gores PF, Gruessner RW, Arrazola I, Najarian JS. Kidney transplantation in patients with type I diabetes: 26 years experience at the University of Minnesota. Clinical Transplants 1992, 1993. Paul I, Terasaki JM, Cecka Eds. UCLA Tissue Typing Laboratory, Los Angeles, Cal., pp 227-235.
6. Lowder GM, Perri NA, Friedman EA. Demographics, diabetes type, and degree of rehabilitation in diabetic patients on maintenance hemodialysis in Brooklyn. J Diabetec Complications, 1988; 2: 218-226.
7. Nagai N. Clinical statistics of 551 patients with diabetes mellitus found before 30 years of age. J Tokyo Wom Med Coll. 1982; 52:904-915.
8. The Expert Committee on the Diagnosis and Classification of Diabetes Mellitus. Report of the Expert Committee on the Diagnosis and Classification of Diabetes Mellitus. Diabetes Care 1997; 20: 1183-1197.
9. Mogensen CE. Management of early nephropathy in diabetic patients. Annu Rev Med 1995; 46:79-93.
10. Christensen CK, Christiansen JS, Schmitz A, Christensen T, Hermansen K, Mogensen CE. Effect of the continuous subcutaneous insulin infusion on kidney function and size in type 1 patients. A 2 year controlled study. J Diab Compl 1987; 1: 91-95.
11. Mogensen CE. Angiotensin converting enzyme inhibitors and diabetic nephropathy. BMJ 1992; 304:327-328.
12. Balodimus MC. Diabetic nephropathy. In "Joslin's Diabetes" (Eds Marble A, White P, Bradley RF, Krall LP) Lea and Febiger, Philadelphia 1971; pp 526-561.
13. Grenfell A, Watkins PJ. Clinical diabetic nephropathy: natural history and complications. Clin Endocrin Metab, 1986; 15: 783-805.

14. Humphrey LL, Ballard DJ, Frohnert PP, Chu CP, ,O'Fallon WM, Palumbo PJ. Chronic renal failure in non-insulin-dependent diabetes mellitus. Ann Intern Med 1989; 10: 788-796.
15. Hasslacher CH, Ritz E, Wahl P, Michael C. Similar risks of nephropathy in patients with type I or type II diabetes mellitus. Nephrol Dial Transplant, 1989; 4: 859-863.
16. Neu S, Kjellstrand CM. Stopping long-term dialysis. An empirical study of withdrawal of life-supporting treatment. N Engl J Med 1986; 314: 14-20
17. Khauli RB, Steinmuller DR, Novick AC et al. A critical look at survival of diabetics with end-stage renal disease: Transplantation versus dialysis therapy. Transplantation, 1986; 41: 598-602.
18. Rettig and Levinsky (ed.) Institute for Medicine (US) Kidney failure and the federal government access to kidney transplantation. Nat Academy of Sciences, 1991; p167-186.
19. Cecka JM, Terasaki PI. The UNOS Scientific Renal Transplant Registry – 1991. Clinical Transplants 1991 (Terasaki PI. ed.) UCLA Tissue Typing Lab., Los Angeles, CA, 1992; p. 1-11.
20. Ekberg H, Christensson A. Similar treatment success rate after renal transplantation in diabetic and non-diabetic patients due to improved short- and long-term diabetic patient survival. Transpl Int 1996; 9: 557-564.
21. Aswad S, Shidman H, Bogaard T, Asai P, Khetan U, McEvoy K, Satterthwaite, Mendez RG, Mendez R. Renal transplantation in diabetic patients in the 1990s (Abst) J Am Soc Nephrol 1997; 7: 1902.
22. Patterson AD, Dornan TL, Peacock I, et al. Cause of death in diabetic patients with impaired renal function. An audit of a hospital diabetic clinic population. Lancet 1987; 1: 313-316.
23. Lewis EJ, Hunsicker LG, Bain RP, Rhode RD. The effect of angiotensin-converting –enzyme inhibition on diabetic nephropathy. N Engl J Med 1993; 329: 1456-1462.
24. Maryniak RK, Mendoza N, Clyne D, Balakrishnan K, Weiss MA. Recurrence of diabetic nodular glomerulosclerosis in a renal transplant. Transplantation 1985; 39: 35-38.
25. Abouna G, Adnani MS; Kumar MS, Samhan SA. Fate of transplanted kidneys with diabetic nephropathy. Lancet 1986; 1: 622-624.
26. Tuttle KR, Bruton L, Perusek MC, Lancaster JL, Kopp DT, DeFronzo R. Effect of strict glycemic control on renal hemodynamic response to amino acids and renal enlargement in insulin-dependent diabetes mellitus. N Engl J Med 1991; 324: 1626-1632.
27. Gruessner RW, Sutherland DE, Troppmann C, Benedetti E, Hakim N, Dunn DL, Gruesnner AC. The surgical risk of pancreas transplantation in the cyclosporine era. An oveview. J Am Coll Surg 1997; 185: 128-144.
28. Gruessner RW. Tacrolimus in pancreas transplantation: a multicenter analysis. Tacrolimus Pancreas Transplant Study Group. Clin Transpl 1997; 11: 299-312.
29. Fioretto P, Steffes MW, Sutherland DER, Goetz FC, Mauer M. Successful pancreas transplantion alone reverses established lesions of diabetic nephropathy in man. J Am Soc Nephrol (Abst) 1997; 8: 111A.
30. Brownlee M. Glycation and diabetic complications. Diabetes 1994; 43: 837-841.
31. Vlassara H. Protein glycation in the kidney. Role in diabetes and aging. Kidney Int 1996; 49: 1795-1804.
32. Kato H, Hayase F, Shin DB, Oimomi M, Baba S 3-Deoxyglucosone, an intermediate product of the Maillard reaction.,Prog Clin Biol Res 1989; 304: 69-84.
33. Reddy S, Bichler J, Wells-Knecht KJ, Thorpe SR, Baynes JW. N^{ε}-(Carboxymethyl)lysine is a dominant advanced glycation end product (AGE) antigen in tissue proteins. Biochemistry 1995; 34: 10872-10878
34. Freilander MA, Witko-Sarsat V, Nguyen AT, Wu YC, Labrunte M, Verger C, Jungers P, Descamps-Latscha B. The advanced glycation endproduct pentosidine and monocyte activation in uremia. Clin Nephrol 1996; 45: 379-382.
35. Sell DR, Monnier VM. Structure elucidation of a senescence cross-link from human extracellur matrix. J Biol Chem 1989; 264: 21597-21602.
36. Niwa T, Kaatsuzaki T, Miayzaki S, et al. Immunohistochemical detection of imidazolone, a novel advanced glycation end product, in kidneys and aortas of diabetic patients. J Clin Invest 1997; 99.1272-1280.
37. Schleicher ED, Wagner E, Nerlich AG. Increased accumulation of the glycoxidation product N(epsilon)-(carboxymethyl)lysine in human tissues in diabetes and aging. J Clin Invest 1997; 99: 3:457-468.

38. Schmidt AM, Hori O, Chen JX, et al. Advanced glycation end-product interacting with their endothelial receptor induce expression of vascular cell adhesion molecule-1 (VCAM-1) in cultured human endothelial cells and in mice. J Clin Invest 1995; 96: 1395-1403.
39. Renard C, Chappey O, Wautier MP, Nagashima M, Lundh E, Morser J, Zhao L, Schmidt AM, Scherrmann JM, Wautier JL. Recombinant advanced glycation end product receptor pharmacokinetics in normal and diabetic rats. Mol Pharmacol 1997; 52: 54-62.
40. Koschinsky T, He CJ, Mitsuhashi T, Cucala R, Liu C, Buenting C, Heitmann K, Vlassara H. Orally absorbed reactive glycation products (glycotoxins): an enviromental risk factor in diabetic nephropathy. Proc Natl Avcad Sci USA, 1997; 94: 6474-6479.
41. Vlassara H, Fuh H, Makita Z, Krungkrai S, Cerami A, Bucala R. Exogenous advanced glycosylation end products induce complex vascular dysfunction in normal animals: A model for diabetic and aging complications. Proc Natl Acad Sci USA 1992; 89: 12043-12047.
42. Yang CW, Vlassara H, Peten EP, He CJ, Striker GE, Striker JL. Advanced glycation end-products up-regulate gene expression found in diabetic glomerular disease. Proc Natl Acad Sci USA, 1994; 91: 9436-9440.
43. Vlassara H. Serum advanced glycosylation end products: A new class of uremic toxins? Blood Purif 1994; 12: 54-59.
44. Knowx LK, Stewart AG, Hayward PG, Morrison WA. Nitric oxide synthase inhibitors improve skin flap survival in the rat. Microsurgery 1994; 15:708-711.
45. Tilton RG, Chang K, Corbett JA, Misko TP, Currie MG, Cora NS, Kaplan HJ, Williamson JR. Endotoxin-induced uveitis in the rat is attenuated by inhibition of nitric oxide production. Invest Ophthalmol Vis Sci 1994; 35: 3278-3288.
46. Hogan M, Cerami A, Bucala R. Advanced glycosylation end-products block the antiproliferative effect of nitric oxide. Role in the vascular and renal complications of diabetes mellitus. J Clin Invest 1992; 90: 1110-1105.
47. Brownlee M. Glycosylation of proteins and microangiopathy. Hosp Pract (Off ed) 27, 1992; (suppl 1): 46-50
48. Vlassara H, Fuh H, Makita Z, Krungkrai S, Cerami A, Cucala R. Exogenous advanced glycosylation end products induce complex vascular dysfunction in normal animals: a model for diabetic and aging complications. Proc Natl Acad Sci USA, 1992; 89: 12043-12047.
49. Makita Z, Radoff S, Rayfield EJ, Yang Z, Skolnik E, Delaney V, Friedman EA, Cerami A, Vlassara H. Advanced glycosylation end products in patients with diabetic nephropathy. New Engl J Med 1991; 325: 836-842.
50. Ellis EN, Good BH. Prevention of glomerular basement membrane thickening by aminoguanidine in experimental diabetes mellitus. Metabolism 1991; 40: 1016-1019.
51. Hammes HP, Martin S, Federlin K, Geisen K, Brownlee M. Aminoguanidine treatment inhibits the development of experimental diabetic retinopathy. Proc Natl Acad Sci USA, 1991; 88: 11555-11558.
52. Yagihashi S, Kamijo M, Baba M, Yagihashi M, Nagai K. Effect of aminoguanidine on functional and structural abnormalities in peripheral nerve of STZ-induced diabetic rats. Diabetes 1992; 41: 47-52.
53. Friedman EA, Distant DA, Fleishhacker JP, Boyd TA, Cartwright K. Aminoguanidine prolongs survival in azotemic induced diabetic rats. Amer J Kidney Dis 1997; 30:253-259.
54. Brownlee M. Pharmacological modulation of the advanced glycosylation reaction. Prog Clin Biol Res 1989; 304:235-248.11.
55. Nicholls K, Mandel TE. Advanced glycosylation end-products in experimental murine diabetic nephropathy: effect of islet isografting and of aminoguanidine. Lab Invest, 1989; 60: 486-491.
56. Lyons TJ, Dailie KE, Dyer DG, Dunn JA, Baynes JW. Decrease in skin collagen glycation with improved glycemic control in patients with insulin-dependent diabetes mellitus. J Clin Invest, 1991; 87: 1910-1915.
57. Corbett JA, Tilton RG, Chang K, Hasan KS, Ido Y, Wang JL, Sweetland MA, Lancaster Jr., Williamson JR, McDaniel ML. Aminoguanidine, a novel inhibitor of nitric oxide formation, prevents diabetic vascular dysfunction. Diabetes, 1992; 4:552-556.
58. Tilton RG, Chang K, Hasan KS, Smith SR, Petrash JM, Misko TP, Moore WM, Currie MG, Corbett JA, McDaniel ML, et al. Prevention of diabetic vascular dysfunction by guanidines. Inhibition of nitric oxide synthase versus advanced glycation end-product formation. Diabetes, 1991; 42; 221-232.

59. Sensi M, Pricci F, Andreani D, DiMario U. Advanced non-enzymatic glycation (AGE) their relevance to aging and the pathogenesis of late diabetic complications. Diabetes Res 1991; 16:1-9.
60. Edelstein D, Brownlee M. Mechanistic studies of advanced glycosylation end-product inhibition by aminoguanidine. Diabetes, 1992; 41: 26-29.
61. Eika B, Levin RM, Longhurst PA. Collagen and bladder function in streptozotocin-diabetic rats: effects of insulin and aminoguanidine. J Urol 1992; 148:167-172.
62. Braun WE, Phillips D, Vidt DG, et al. The course of coronary artery disease in diabetics with and without renal allografts. Transplant Proc, 1983; 15: 1114-1119.
63. Khauli RB, Steinmuller DR, Novick AC, et al. A critical look at survival of diabetics with end-stage renal disease: Transplantation versus dialysis therapy. Transplantation, 1986; 41: 598-602.
64. Philipson JD, Carpenter BJ, Itzkoff J, Hakala TR, Rosenthal JT, Taylor RJ, Puschett JB. Evaluation of cardiovascular risk for renal transplantation in diabetic patients. Am J Med, 1986; 81: 630-634.
65. Corry RJ, Nghiem DD, Shanbacher B, et al. Critical analysis of mortality and graft loss following simultaneous renal – pancreatic duodenal transplantation. Transplant Proc, 1987; 19: 2305-2306.
66. Gill JB, Ruddy TD, Newell JB, et al. Prognostic importance of thallium uptake by the lungs during exercise in coronary artery disease. N Engl J Med, 1987; 317: 1485-1489.
67. Bates JR, Sawada SG, Segar DS, Spaedy AJ, Petrovic O, Fineberg NS, Feigenbaum H, Ryan T. Evaluation using dobutamine stress echocardiography in patients with insulin-dependent diabetes mellitus before kidney and/or pancreas transplantation. Am J Cardiol 1996; 77:175-179.
68. Hennesy TG, Codd MB, Kane G, McCarthy C, McCann HA, Sugrue DD. Evaluation of patients with diabetes mellitus for coronary artery disease using dobutamine stress echocardiography. Coron Artery Dis 1997; 8: 171-174.
69. Fanning WJ, Henry ML, Sommer BG, et al. Extremity and renal ischemia following renal transplantation. Vascular Surg. 1986; 23: 231-234.
70. Abendroth D, Landgraft R, Illner WD, et al. 1990. Beneficial effects of pancreatic transplantation in insulin-dependent diabetes mellitus patients. Transplant Proc, 1990; 22: 696-697.
71. Gonzales-Carrillo M, Moloney A, Bewick M, et al. Renal transplantation in diabetic nephropathy. Br Med J, 1982; 285: 1713-1716.
72. Yuge J and Cecka JM. Sex and age effects in renal transplantation. Clinical transplants 1991, (Terasaki PI ed) UCLA Tissue and Typing Lab, 1992; p. 261.
73. Najarian JS, Sutherland DER, Simmons RL, et al. Ten year experience with renal transplantation in juvenile onset diabetics. Ann Surgery, 1979; 190:487-500.
74. Milde FK, Hart LK, Zehr PS. Pancreatic transplantation. Impact on the quality of life of diabetic renal transplant recipients. Diabetes Care, 1995; 18:93-95.
75. Østerby R, Nyberg G, Hedman L, Karlberg I, Persson H, Svalander C. Kidney transplantation in type 1(insulin-dependent) diabetic patients. Diabetologia, 1991; 9:668-674.
76. Bohman SO, Wilczek H, Jaremko G, et al. Recurrence of diabetic nephropathy in human renal allografts: Preliminary report of a Biopsy Study. Transplant Proc, 1984; 16: 649-653.
77. Mauer SM, Goetz FC, McHugh LE, et al. Long-term study of Normal Kidneys transplanted into patients with type 1 diabtes. Diabetes, 1989; 38:516-523.
78. Najarian JS, Kaufman DB, Fryd DS, McHugh L, Mauer SM, Ramsey RC, Kennedy WR, Navarro X, Goetz FC, Sutherland DE. Long-term survival following kidney transplantation in 100 type 1 diabetic patients. Transplantation, 1989; 1: 106-113.
79. Remuzzi G; Ruggenenti P, Mauer SM. Pancreas and kidney/pancreas transplants: experimental medicine or real improvement? Lancet 1994; 343:27-31.

51. PREVENTION OF DIABETIC RENAL DISEASE WITH SPECIAL REFERENCE TO MICROALBUMINURIA

Carl Erik Mogensen, William F. Kerne, Peter H. Bennett, George Jerums, Hans-Henrik Parving, Philippe Passa, Michael W. Steffes, Gary E. Striker and Gian Carlo Viberti

Reprinted from The LANCET 1995; 346: 1080-1084 with permission from the journal.

In the past year six sets of recommendations on the prevention of diabetic nephropathy, with special reference to microalbuminuria, have been published [1-6]. The background to this activity was the large and increasing number of diabetic patients in whom end-stage renal failure (ESRD) develops and who therefore require dialysis or renal transplantation. Throughout the world about half a million patients are registered as being on renal replacement therapy, and diabetic nephropathy is the cause in nearly one-fifth of them [7]. These data are extrapolated from countries which have registries but in many areas, especially in the densely populated countries of the Far East, accurate information on numbers of patients with ESRD is not yet available. Moreover, the half-million figure probably underestimates the number of diabetic patients with ESRD because selection criteria for renal replacement therapies vary from country to country. Both insulin dependent (IDDM) and non-insulin-dependent (NIDDM) diabetic patients contribute to the increase in ESRD. Prevention of diabetic renal disease, or at least the postponement or slowing down of the disease process, has emerged as a key issue. Our strategy is to develop programmes for all patients with diabetes, focused on early detection of renal disease followed by intervention.

Increased urinary albumin excretion also predicts early mortality in NIDDM [8,9], and the same relation is observed in the general population too [10-13], possibly associated with the metabolic syndrome, of which raised blood pressure (BP) is an important component. The association with vascular disease is important [10,12,13]. Microalbuminuria is common in poorly treated individuals with essential hypertension [14]. It is not yet known if screening for microalbuminuria and subsequent treatment will improve outcome in hypertensive non-diabetic patients or in the general population. In diabetes, however, the evidence is strong.

Since the six programmes proposed do differ an agreed unifying, global strategy for screening and treatment would be welcome. In this report we aim at a consensus on the detection, prevention, and treatment of diabetic nephropathy. We focus on microalbuminuria because this is the first clinically easy identifiable sign of risk of diabetic nephropathy and other vascular complications and because we believe that prevention is best achieved at this early stage.

Table 51-1. SCREENING AND CONFIRMATORY PROCEDURES

Document	Proposed yearly screening and confirmatory procedure	BP screening; demarcation for interview	Confounding factors of microalbuminuria	Comments on associated abnormalities
St. Vincent [1]	First morning urine A/C ratio or AC, confirmed by 3 overnight UAE (or by continued monitoring of A/C ratio).	Yearly measurements; ≥140/90 below 60 yr, ≥160/90 above 60 yr	Heavy exercise, urinary tract infection, acute illness, cardiac failure	Cardiovascular disease, dyslipidaemia
WHO [2]	UAE (not specified) at least once a year for all with IDDM >5 yrs and aged 12, and all with NIDDM until age 70. Confirm by repeat testing and measure 6-monthly	BP at least annually; ≥140/90 below 60 yrs or increases in BP by 5 mmHg	Heavy exercise, urinary tract infection, acute illness, high protein intake, metabolic decompensation, cardiac failure	Other long-term complications
Australia [3]	Spot urine A/C ratio or AC for screening. Timed urine more accurate. Confirm microalbuminuria by UAE (2 out of 3). Micral test or other bedside test useful.	140/90 in young individuals. Measured in supine position after 5 min at rest at every visit	..	Retinopathy, dyslipidemia, foot complications, discourage smoking
ADA consensus [4]	UAE in a timed urine or A/C ratio in random urine. Sensitive strips may be used. Quantitative sensitive albumin determination for confirmation	Frequent BP monitoring, >130/85 (short comments on »elderly«)	See table in document	Retinopathy often present
National Kidney Foundation [5]	At least once a year of A/C ratio in first morning urine (or random urine). Should be confirmed. Different dipstick available for measurements of low albumin concentrations	Monitoring advisable; 140/90	Heavy exercise, urinary tract infection, acute febrile illness, heart failure, non-steroidal anti-inflammatory agents	Dyslipidaemia, discourage smoking
National Institutes of Health [6]	Yearly screening, not specified	>130/85	..	Microalbuminuria designates patients at risk for other complications

A/C ratio = albumin/creatinine ratio; AC = albumin concentration. UAE = urinary albumin excretion rate.

SCREENING

The screening and confirmatory procedures [1-6] for microalbuminuria (figure 51-1) are summarised in table 51-1. Several procedures for urine sampling have been proposed 24h urine collection, overnight collection, short-term collection in the clinic, and albumin-creatinine ratios in random or early morning (first voided) urine. There are no formal studies with long-term follow-up to demonstrate which procedure is best but there is consensus that screening can easily be done by measuring a urinary albumin-creatinine ratio. We propose to use of the first voided morning urine for this procedure [15,16]. Patients can easily provide this sample and there is little water intake during the night or physical activity while asleep so the urine sample is concentrated, allowing for easier detection of albumin. It is unlikely that dilution due to high urine volume will result in underestimation of albumin excretion (slight overestimation cannot be excluded) [17-20]. Even so, because of the potential variability in urine volume, we recommended measuring creatinine concentration too and using the ratio. Urinary albumin excretion is 30-50% lower during the night, possibly due to lower night-time BP and glomerular filtration rate (GFR) [15]. An alternative to the early morning albumin-creatinine ratio could be overnight or 24 h urine collection but these are difficult in practice. Albumin excretion can vary by as much as 40% due to natural fluctuations so several tests should be done [16].

Panel : **Definition of microalbuminuria.**

Excretion rate 20-200 µg/min or 30-300 mg/24 (hours)
Albumin/creatinine ratio 2.5-25 mg/mmol* Europe (+elsewhere)
Albumin/creatinine ratio 30-300 mg/g USA (+elsewhere)
Albumin concentration (early morning urine) 30-300 mg/L
Confounders: mainly variability (about 40%), posture or diurnal variation, exercise, urinary tract infection, other diseases.
*3.5 as lower limit has been proposed in females because of lower creatinine excretion.

Figure 51-1

Irrespective of the procedure used, two or all of three samples over a 3-6 month period should test positive before microalbuminuria is confirmed [16]. It is generally recommended that diabetic patients be screened at least once a year [1] but some prefer more frequent testing [21,22]. Inexpensive immunoturbidimetric assays are now routine in many clinical laboratories [22]. Screening can also be done satisfactory by »dip stix« [23] but an abnormal result should be confirmed.

Once microalbuminuria has been confirmed two strategies for future testing may be used. There is nothing to choose, medically, between an early morning albumin-creatinine ratio at every clinic visit or further monitoring by overnight collections on several occasions [1] so the convenience of the patient and his or her compliance should be considered.

There are several confounding factors for microalbuminuria, such as exercise, urinary tract infection, acute illness and cardiac failure, besides blood glucose decompensation, but usually these can easily be recognised, being detectable at routine clinical and laboratory examinations [15]. Patients with microalbuminuria should be screened more frequently and carefully for neuropathy, retinopathy, cardiovascular disease, as well as dyslipidemia, because they are at high risk of such complications [1-6].

All recommendations propose careful BP screening [1-6], because BP is often raised in microalbuminuric patients. BP should be monitored under standard conditions, after at least 5 min at rest, with the patient sitting. However, recommendations on the level of BP that is to be identified as increased varies with age (table 51-2). 24 h ambulatory BP may be used when »white coat« hypertension (especially with normoalbuminuria) is suspected [21].

We propose that BP consistently equal to or higher than 140/90 mmHg below age of 60 and higher than 160/90 mmHg above age 60 serves as a minimum indication for intervention. This accords with proposals from several hypertension-related organisations, although age is not always taken into consideration [24-26]. However, this approach may still lead to pharmacological undertreatment of young diabetic microalbuminuric patients. In the Systolic Hypertension in the Elderly Program (SHEP) study, also containing diabetic patients, one inclusion crition was a systolic BP of 160 mmHg or more.

Systolic BP was reduced from 170 to 144 mmHg during active treatment, which reduced the incidence of stroke significantly [27].

We propose that treatment aimed at renal disease should begin when microalbuminuria is detected, irrespective of BP, especially in young diabetic individuals [5]. Early antihypertensive treatment, especially with angiotensin-converting enzyme (ACE) inhibitors will reduce and/or stabilise microalbuminuria and preserve GFR [28] (see below).

It would be useful to monitor GFR (e.g., by single-shot isotopic decay methods) but this is usually too demanding for routine practice [1]. It is also questionable whether this procedure is required, because GFR is usually still normal or supranormal at least in IDDM patients with microalbuminuria [29,30]. Creatinine clearance is not a satisfactory marker of true GFR, and collection difficulties, especially in diabetic patients, frequently confound interpretation, although not all clinicians would agree with the issues [31,32].

Yearly or half-yearly serum creatinine measurements would be reasonable requirements.

PREVENTION AND INTERVENTION IN IDDM (table 51-2)

Good blood glucose control will postpone or prevent microalbuminuria and overt renal disease [33] and should be aimed at all patients with IDDM. For example, the Diabetes Control and Complications Trial Research Group (DCCT) [33] showed that intensive blood glucose control care can reduce the incidence of microalbuminuria. Usually microalbuminuric patients have poorer control than patients with normal albumin excretion. However, life style issues and hypoglycaemic events need to be taken into account. Some groups propose glycosylated haemoglobin (HbA_{1c}) level of 7.0-7.5% as the range to aim at (normal HbA_{1c} is 5.5%) [34] but this is not easy to achieve and interventions other than tight glucose control must be tried.

Table 51-2. PREVENTION AND INTERVENTION RELATED TO IDDM

Document	Glycemic intervention or IIT	»Normotensive« micro- albuminuria	»Hypertensive« micro- albuminuria	What to monitor
St. Vincent [1]	Best possible metabolic control, especially for primary prevention of MA	ACE-I delays progression to overt nephropathy; AHT must be tailored	ACE-I delays progression to overt nephropathy; AHT must be tailored	BP, MA
WHO [2]	DCCT used as reference; meticulous glycaemic control	AHT if DBP rises by 5 mmHg in a year below 60 yrs of age	Meticulous control of hypertension, with particular attention to AHA that prevents increases in intracapillary pressure	Albumin excre tion rate, HbA_{1C}, BP, creatinine, lipids
Australia [3]	Rate of increase in MA related to glycaemic control; best glycaemic control advisable	Some AHA, especially ACE-I, reduce MA and delay progression to CON	Drug treatment should be considered if BP ≥140/90; ACE-I generally preferred; target BP 120-130/80 in young patients	BP, MA, creatinine, potassium, lipids
ADA Consensus [4]	DCCT used as reference; reduce glucose levels to near-normal as possible	Increasing evidence to support the use of ACE-I to reduce MA; insufficient duration for determining long-term effect (pregnancy contraindication)	Any AHA can reduce BP, but certain AHA may have advantages in diabetic patients	MA, BP, creatinine, potassium
National Kidney Foundation [5]	DCCT used as reference; best possible glycaemic control is goal	ACE-I appropriate	ACE-I appropriate; if 130/85 or lower not achieved addition of loop diuretic recommended	MA, BP
National Institutes of Health [6]	Intensified control of blood glucose.	ACE-I should be initiated	ACE-I as part of hypertensive regimen	BP, MA

A/C ratio=albumin/creatinine ratio; AC=albumin concentration; UAE=urinary albumin excretion rate; MA=microalbuminuria; AHA=antihypertensive agents; BP=blood pressure; ACE-I=ACE-inhibitor; IIT=intensified insulin treatment; CON=clinical overt nephropathy.

There is general agreement that so-called normotensive IDDM patients (BP <140/190 mmHg at age below 60 and <160/90 mmHg above age 60) should receive antihypertensive treatment with an ACE inhibitor as soon as microalbuminuria has been clearly confirmed by several tests and provided that the best possible blood glucose control has been obtained for several months. Older age should still be considered as a relative modulating factor in the indication [5]. The longest follow-up trial in young IDDM patients with microalbuminuria has been 8 years [36] and long-term data on mortality and ESRD (final end-points) are not yet available. ACE inhibitors are beneficial in diabetic patients with overt renal disease [37], but other agents may also be effective [38].

For patients with hypertensive microalbuminuric all recommendations stress tight control of BP. ACE inhibitors are generally preferred because their effect on albuminuria may to some extent be independent of their influence on systemic BP. ACE inhibitors can be used in combination with other drugs [39]. In general, the target BP is 120-130/80-85 mmHg, especially in young patients. However, no clear-cut long-term data are currently available to define the exact target. A J-shaped curve (more complications with low BP) has not been documented in diabetic patients. Microalbuminuria should at least be stabilised, and ideally it should be reduced by 20-30% per year. It is also suggested that the antihypertensive regimens should be tailored individually. Although some reduction in dietary protein intake has also been proposed [1], there are inadequate data to evaluate the long-term consequences of and compliance with this approach in microalbuminuric patients.

During treatment BP and microalbuminuria must be monitored, every 1-3 months at first. Monitoring of serum creatinine and serum potassium is also crucial, especially during treatment with an ACE inhibitor. However, serum potassium rarely increases worryingly in microalbuminuric patients; if it does, a low-dose diuretic may be added [38].

PREVENTION AND INTERVENTION IN NIDDM (table 51-3)

There are no formal trials of tight blood glucose control in NIDDM but most experts extrapolate from the DCCT [33], especially in young patients, and we propose that the best possible control should be achieved in patients with NIDDM.

Antihypertensive treatment in »normotensive« microalbuminuric NIDDM patients has not been studied prospective in trials on large numbers patients. One 5-year intervention study using ACE-inhibition [40] in young and lean NIDDM patients, many of whom were normotensive, noted that microalbuminuria was reduced, and renal function (serum creatinine) was preserved. Early ACE inhibition may slow the progression of renal disease in such patients with microalbuminuria, even when BP is »normal«.

In hypertensive microalbuminuric NIDDM patients all agree on the need for careful control of BP [1-6,24-26]. Therapy must be tailored individually but ACE inhibition is usually appropriate, though patients with concomitant diseases may benefit from , say, a calcium antagonist or cardioselective beta blocker. Usually, these patients also show sodium retention [41] and even oedema, so low doses of diuretic agents may be prescribed. Again, microalbuminuria and BP need regular monitoring, together with serum creatinine and serum potassium. In elderly people with cardiovascular disease, initiation of treatment with an ACE inhibitor in moderate doses may result in some deterioration of renal function and an increase in serum potassium. We recommend starting an ACE inhibitor at a low dose, gradually titrating the dose to achieve the desired reduction in BP and urine albumin excretion without adversely affecting serum potassium or serum creatinine. The recommendations on GFR monitoring for discussed IDDM are also relevant to NIDDM.

COMMENTS

The proposed screening and confirmatory procedures and the recommended interventions in diabetic patients with microalbuminuria are straightforward (figure 51-2). Renal biopsy is not indicated routinely in microalbuminuric individuals [42], unless a rapid or unexplained clinical progression of renal involvement is evident.

Table 51-3. PREVENTION AND INTERVENTION RELATED TO NIDDM

Document	Glycaemic intervention or IIT	»Normotensive« microalbuminuria patients, ACE-inhibition?	»Hypertensive« microalbuminuria patients.	What to monitor
St. Vincent [1]	Best possible metabolic control in particular primary prevention of MA	ACE-I delays progression to overt nephropathy; AHT must be tailored individually	ACE-I delays progression to overt nephropathy; AHT must be tailored individually	BP, MA
WHO [4]	DCCT used as reference. Meticulous glycaemic control.	Antihypertensive treatment if DBP increases by 5 mmHg in a year in those aged ≥60 years	Meticulous control of hypertension, with particular attention to AHA that prevents increases in intracapillary pressure within the kidney.	Albumin excretion rate HbA_{1C} BP Creatinine Lipids
Australia [3]	Intensified glycaemic control not proven beneficial in NIDDM, but advisable	Some AHA, especially ACE-I have been shown to reduce MA, delay progression to CON and to preserve renal functions in normotensive patients	As in IDDM, but higher target BP (140/90) in elderly	As in IDDM, with more emphasis on cardiovas-cular status
ADA 0consensus [4]	Optimised metabolic control (however, no results from clinical trials available in NIDDM)	Studies show that ACE-I can reduce MA and may slow progression of »ne-phropathy«	Any AHA that reduce BP may be used, but some AHA may have certain advantages	MA+BP, creatinine, potassium
National Kidney Foundation [5]	No clear data. However, best glycaemic control possible should be the goal	ACE-I appropriate	ACE-I appropriate	MA, BP
National Institutes of Health [6]	..	Insufficient data	(Not discussed)	..

A/C ratio=albumin/creatinine ratio; AC=albumin concentration; UAE=urinary albumin excretion rate. MA=microalbuminuria; AHA=antihypertensive agents; BP=blood pressure; ACE-I=ACE-inhibitor; *IIT=intensified insulin treatment; CON=clinical overt nephropathy.*

Several studies suggest that good blood glucose control (HbA_{1c} below 7.5-8.0%) in the diabetic patients will preserve renal function and prevent development of microalbuminuria [34,43,44]. Attained BP and rate of progression are correlated in microalbuminuric patients as well as in patients with overt renal disease [7,38]. Intervention studies confirm this [38] so careful antihypertensive treatment is recommended. No studies have demonstrated a harmful effect of reducing BP below 140/90 mmHg. Most investigations show that BP should be reduced in young individuals to 125/80 mmHg or so along with stabilisation of or reduction in microalbuminuria. A new concept is »antihypertensive« or renoprotective treatment, even when the BP is not at conventional hypertensive levels [5]. Treatment should begin with small doses, especially in the normotensive and in elderly diabetic patients. Titration of antihypertensive therapy can then occur with monitoring of urinary albumin and serum creatinine and potassium. Other potential risk factors such as plasma lipids and smoking should be evaluated and consideration given to intervention. When clinically suspected, investigations for renal artery stenosis should be done.

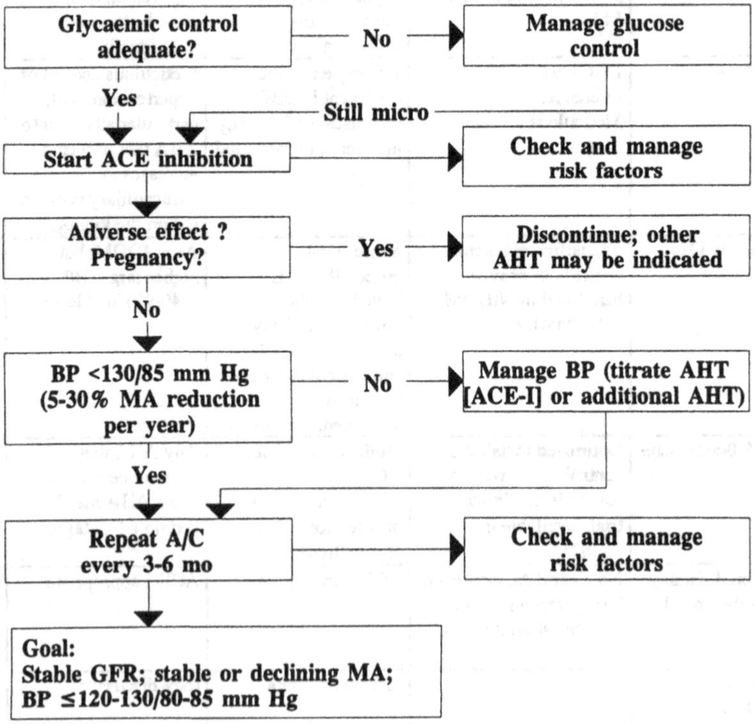

Figure 51-2. Microalbuminuria in diabetes. (Slightly modified from Bennett et al. [5]).

We propose to early morning urine for screening with measurement of albumin-creatinine ratio.The programme outlined here is very highly cost effective [45]; mainly because ESRD treatment is so expensive. However, a considerable increase in the lifespan of Early morning urinary albumin concentration seems also to be predictor of poor outcome [15,16].diabetic patients with hypertension and microalbuminuria is likely, This having been seen in diabetic patients with overt renal disease treated with an ACE inhibitor and other antihypertensive treatments [37,46-48]. The history of the development is recently given elsewhere [49].

In IDDM patients with microalbuminuria end-points such as mortality or and ESRD are far off and a favourable effect in respect of these has yet to be convincingly demonstrated in an intervention trial. In elderly NIDDM microalbuminuric patients, in whom the incidence of cardiovascular mortality is very high, different studies are in progress aimed at demonstrating a beneficial effect of various antihypertensive regimens.

REFERENCES

1. Viberti GC, Mogensen CE, Passa P, Bilous R, Mangili R. »St Vincent declaration, 1994: Guidelines for the prevention of diabetic renal failure.« In *The Kidney and Hypertension in Diabetes Mellitus, 2nd ed*, Mogensen CE, ed. Boston, Dordrecht, London: Kluwer Academic Publishers, 1994; pp 515-527.
2. Anon. Prevention of Diabetes Mellitus: report of a WHO study group. WHO Tech Rep Ser 844. Geneva: WHO, 1994: 55-59.
3. Jerums G, Cooper M, Gilbert R, O'Brien R, Taft J. Microalbuminuria in diabetes. Med J Aust 1994; 161: 265-268.
4. Consensus development conference on the diagnosis and management of nephropathy in patients with diabetes mellitus. Diabetes Care 1994; 17: 1357-1361.
5. Bennett PH, Haffner S, Kasiske BL, Keane WF, Mogensen CE, Parving H-H, Steffes MW, Striker GE. Screening and management of microalbuminuria in patients with diabetes mellitus - recommendations to the scientific advisory board of the National Kidney Foundation from an ad hoc committee of the council on diabetes mellitus of the National Kidney Foundation. Am J Kidney Dis 1995; 25: 107-112.
6. Striker GE. Report on a workshop to develop management recommendations for the prevention of progression in chronic renal disease Bethesda (MA) April 1994. Nephrol Dial Transplant 1995; 10: 290-292.
7. Mogensen CE. Systemic blood pressure and glomerular leakage with particular reference to diabetes and hypertension. J Intern Med 1994; 235: 297-316.
8. Jarrett RJ, Viberti GC, Argyropoulos A, Hill RD, Mahmud U, Murrells TJ. Microalbuminuria predicts mortality in non-insulin-dependent diabetes. Diabetic Med 1984; 1: 17-19.
9. Mogensen CE. Microalbuminuria predicts clinical proteinuria and early mortality in maturity-onset diabetes. N Engl J Med 1984; 310: 356-360.
10. Yudkin JS, Forrest RD, Jackson CA. Microalbuminuria as a predictor of vascular disease in non-diabetic subjects. Islington diabetes Survey. Lancet 1988; ii: 530-533.
11. Damsgaard EM, Frøland A, Jørgensen OD, Mogensen CE. Microalbuminuria as a predictor of increased mortality in elderly people. BMJ 1990; 300: 297-300.
12. Mogensen CE. Microalbuminuria: An important warning sign from the laboratory. J Diabetic Compl 1994; 8: 135-136.
13. Feldt-Rasmussen B, Borch-Johnsen K, Deckert T, Jensen G, Jensen JS. Microalbuminuria: An important diagnostic tool. J Diabetic Compl 1994; 8: 137-145.
14. Parving H-H, Jensen HÆ, Mogensen CE, Evrin PE. Increased urinary albumin excretion rate in benign essential hypertension. Lancet 1974; i: 1190-1192.

15. Mogensen CE, Vestbo E, Poulsen PL, Christiansen C, Damsgaard EM, Eiskjær H, Frøland A, Hansen KW, Nielsen S, Mau Pedersen M. Microalbuminuria and potential confounders. A review and some observations on variability of urinary albumin excretion. Diabetes Care 1995; 18: 572-581.
16. Mogensen CE. Microalbuminuria as a predictor of clinical diabetic nephropathy. Kidney Int 1987; 31: 673-689.
17. Gatling W, Knight C, Hill RD. Screening for early diabetic nephropathy: Which sample to detect microalbuminuria? Diabetic Med 1985; 2: 451-455.
18. Marshall SM, Alberti KGMM. Screening for early diabetic nephropathy. Ann Clin Biochem 1986; 23: 195-197.
19. Cowell CT, Rogers S, Silink M. First morning urinary albumin concentration is a good predictor of 24-hour urinary albumin excretion in children with type 1 (insulin-dependent) diabetes. Diabetologia 1986; 29: 97-99.
20. Hutchinson AS, O'Reilly DSTJ, MacCuish AC. Albumin excretion rate, albumin concentration, and albumin/creatinine ratio compared for screening diabetics for slight albuminuria. Clin Chem 1988; 34: 2019-2021.
21. Mogensen CE: Management of early nephropathy in diabetic patients. With emphasis on microalbuminuria. Ann Rev Med 1995; 46: 79-94.
22. Mogensen CE, Poulsen PL, Heinsvig EM. »Abnormal albuminuria in the monitoring of early renal changes in diabetes.« In *Concepts for the Ideal Diabetes Clinic. Diabetes Forum Series, Volume IV*. Mogensen CE, Standl E, eds. Berlin, New York: Walter de Gruyter, 1993; pp 289-313.
23. Poulsen PL, Mogensen CE. Evaluation of a new semiquantitative stix for microalbuminuria. Diabetes Care 1995; 18: 732-733.
24. Anon. Fifth report of the joint national committee on detection, evaluation, and treatment of high blood pressure (JNC V). Arch Intern Med 1993; 153: 154-183.
25. Anon. Guidelines for management of mild hypertension: memorandum from a WHO/ISH meeting. Clin Exp Hypertens 1993; 15: 1363-1395.
26. The National High Blood Pressure Education Program Working Group. National high blood pressure education program working group report on hypertension. Hypertension 1994; 23: 145-148.
27. SHEP Cooperative Research Group. Prevention of stroke by antihypertensive drug treatment in older persons with isolated systolic hypertension. Final results of the systolic hypertension in the elderly program (SHEP). JAMA 1991; 265: 3255-3264.
28. Mogensen CE. Renoprotective role of ACE inhibitors in diabetic nephropathy. Br Heart J 1994; 72: Suppl.: 38-45.
29. Hansen KW, Mau Pedersen M, Christensen CK, Schmitz A, Christiansen JS, Mogensen CE. Normoalbuminuria ensures no reduction of renal function in type 1 (insulin dependent) diabetic patients. J Intern Med 1992; 232: 161-167.
30. Schmitz A. Renal function changes in middle-aged and elderly Caucasian Type 2 (non-insulin-dependent) diabetic patients - a review. Diabetologia 1993; 36: 985-992.
31. Tsalamandris C, Allen TJ, Gilbert RE, Sinha A, Panagiotopoulos S, Cooper ME, Jerums G. Progressive decline in renal function in diabetic patients with and without albuminuria. Diabetes 1994; 43: 649-655.
32. Lane PH, Steffes MW, Mauer SM. Glomerular structure in IDDM women with low glomerular filtration rate and normal urinary albumin excretion. Diabetes 1992; 41: 581-586.
33. The Diabetes Control and Complications Trial Research Group. The effect of intensive treatment of diabetes on the development and progression of long-term complications in insulin-dependent diabetes mellitus. N Engl J Med 1993; 329: 977-986.
34. Dahl-Jørgensen K, Brinchmann-Hansen O, Bangstad H-J, Hanssen KF. Blood glucose control and microvascular complications - what do we do now? Diabetologia 1994; 37: 1172-1177.
35. Viberti GC, Mogensen CE, Groop L, Pauls JF for the European Microalbuminuria Captopril Study Group. Effect of captopril on progression to clinical proteinuria in patients with insulin-dependent diabetes mellitus and microalbuminuria. JAMA 1994; 271: 275-279.
36. Mathiesen ER, Hommel E, Hansen HP, Parving H-H. Preservation of normal GFR with long term captopril treatment in normotensive IDDM patients with microalbuminuria. Am Soc. of Nephrology, Vol. 8, Sep. 1997; 115A.

37. Lewis EJ, Hunsicker LG, Bain RP, Rohde RD, for the Collaborative Study Group. The effect of angiotensin-converting-enzyme inhibition on diabetic nephropathy. N Engl J Med 1993; 329: 1456-1462.
38. Parving H-H, Rossing P. The use of antihypertensive agents in prevention and treatment of diabetic nephropathy. Current Opinion in Nephrology and Hypertension 1994; 3: 292-300.
39. Mogensen CE, Hansen KW, Nielsen S, Mau Pedersen M, Rehling M, Schmitz A. Monitoring diabetic nephropathy: Glomerular filtration rate and abnormal albuminuria in diabetic renal disease: Reproducibility, progression studies and efficacy of antihypertensive intervention. Am J Kidney Dis 1993; 22: 174-187.
40. Ravid, M, Savin H, Jutrin I, Bental T, Katz b, Lishner M. Long-term stabilizing effect of angiotensin-converting enzyme inhibition on plasma creatinine and on proteinuria in normotensive type II diabetic patients. Ann Intern Med 1993; 118: 577-581.
41. Weidmann P, Ferrari P. Central role of sodium in hypertension in diabetic subjects. Diabetes Care 1991; 14: 220-232
42. Østerby R. Microalbuminuria in diabetes mellitus - is there a structural basis? Nephrol Dial Transplant 1995: Editorial Comments: 10: 12-14.
43. Krolewski AS, Laffel LMB, Krolewski M, Quinn M, Warram JH. Glycosylated hemoglobin and the risk of microalbuminuria in patients with insulin-dependent diabetes mellitus. N Engl J Med 1995; 332: 1251-1255.
44. Viberti GC. A glycemic threshold for diabetic complications? N Engl J Med 1995; 332: 1293-1294.
45. Borch-Johnsen K, Wenzel H, Viberti GC, Mogensen CE. Is screening and intervention for microalbuminuria worthwhile in patients with insulin dependent diabetes? BMJ 1993; 306: 1722-1725.
46. Mathiesen ER, Borch-Johnsen K, Jensen DV, Deckert T. Improved survival in patients with diabetic nephropathy. Diabetologia 1989; 32: 884-886
47. Parving H-H, Hommel E. Prognosis in diabetic nephropathy. BMJ 1989; 299: 230-233.
48. Hasslacher C, Borgholte G, Ritz E, Wahl P. Impact of hypertension on prognosis of IDDM. Diabete Metab (Paris) 1989; 15: 338-342.
49. Mogensen CE. Diabetic renal disease: the quest for normotension - and beyond. Diabetic Med 1995; 12: 756-769.

ADDENDUM

A recent position statement from American Diabetes Association is in agrement with above chapter proposing ACE-1 in normotensive microalbuminuric IDDM-patients "*Subsequently, many studies have shown that in hypertensive patients with type 1 diabetes, ACE inhibitors can reduce the level of albuminuria and can reduce the rate of progression of renal disease to a greater degree than other antihypertensive agents that lower blood pressure by an equal amount. Other studies have shown that there is benefit in reducing the progression of microalbuminuria in normotensive patients with type 1 diabetes and normotensive and hypertensive patients with type 2 diabetes*".[50].

50. American Diabetes Association. Diabetes Care, vol. 21, suppl. 1, Jan. 1998; S50-53.

52. COMBINATION THERAPY FOR HYPERTENSION AND RENAL DISEASE IN DIABETES

Imelda P. Villarosa, MD and George L. Bakris, MD, F.A.C.P
The Rush Hypertension Center, Rush Presbyterian/St Luke's Medical Center, Chicago IL, USA

INTRODUCTION

More than 75% of individuals with diabetes, microalbuminuria and hypertension require two or more antihypertensive medications to attain the currently recommended level of arterial pressure control i.e., substantially less than 130/85 mmHg [1-3]. To achieve this blood pressure goal, it is common to add a medication whose antihypertensive action potentiates the initially selected drug [4,5]. To further improve compliance and reduce drug side effect profiles, fixed-dose combinations of antihypertensive drugs with complementary modes of action have been recently developed [5]. These medications combine a lower dose of two different antihypertensive drugs that, in a fixed dose combination, reduce arterial pressure to a greater extent compared to either alone. The history of various fixed-dose antihypertensive drug combinations is shown in Table 52-1. The evolution of fixed-dose combination antihypertensive therapy is beyond the scope of this chapter. The reader, however, is referred to a recent review on the topic [5]. This chapter will focus on the available evidence from both animal models of hypertension and renal disease as well as clinical studies that examine the efficacy of different classes of antihypertensive medications, either alone or combined, to either halt or prevent development of renal disease. The discussion will primarily, but not exclusively, focus on angiotensin converting enzyme (ACE) inhibitors and calcium channel blockers (CCBs).

RENAL MORPHOLOGY AND HEMODYNAMICS

Brief overviews of the renal hemodynamic and morphologic changes that occur in the diabetic kidney are presented. This is done in an effort to improve the understanding of how and why, at a comparable blood pressure level, combinations of various antihypertensive medications slow progression of diabetic nephropathy to a greater extent than either of the individual components.

Early changes observed in the diabetic kidney include an increase in efferent arteriolar tone and a loss of autoregulation [6-7]. These changes lead to an increase in intraglomerular capillary pressure, which results in cell stretch and activation of various autocrine and paracrine factors associated with tissue injury [7-8]. In addition, glomerular membrane permeability is increased and microalbuminuria ensues, a surrogate marker for the presence and progression of diabetic nephropathy [9-12]. The *earliest* morphologic change is mesangial matrix expansion and in some cases interstitial inflammation, the latter portends a poor renal prognosis [12,13].

Table 52-1. Historical Evolution of Fixed Dose Combination

1960's
Ser-Ap-Es (reserpine-hydralazine-hydrochlorothiazide)
Methyldopa/thiazide diuretic
1970's
Thiazide/ Various[K^+] Sparing Diuretic
Thiazide/Spironolactone
β Blocker/thiazide diuretic
Clonidine/thiazide diuretic
1980's
ACE inhibitor/thiazide diuretic
1990's
(Low dose) β Blocker /thiazide diuretic
Calcium Channel Blocker/ACE inhibitor
β Blocker/Dihydropyridine Calcium Channel Blocker
Angiotensin II Receptor Blocker/Diuretic

INDIVIDUAL ANTIHYPERTENSIVE AGENTS

Experimental evidence demonstrates that reductions in intraglomerular capillary pressure, through either profound reductions in arterial pressure or dilation of the efferent arteriole, slow progression of diabetic renal disease [7,12,14]. Drugs that reduce efferent arteriolar tone and intraglomerular pressure include the ACE inhibitors and potassium channel openers (hydralazine, minoxidil). In clinical studies, however, only the ACE inhibitors demonstrate a consistent and persistent reduction in both albuminuria and proteinuria as well as an attenuated progression in nephropathy associated with type I diabetes and possibly from type II diabetes [15-24]. Moreover, while blood pressure reduction itself slows progression of both diabetic and non-diabetic renal disease, the ACE inhibitors appear to preserve renal function to even greater extent than other agents do [15,18,22-25].

Antihypertensive agents that do not reduce intraglomerular pressure may still slow progression of diabetic nephropathy. This may relate to their specific effects on synthesis or degradation of mesangial matrix proteins. Notably, nondihydropyridine CCBs, verapamil and diltiazem preserve renal morphology in a manner similar to ACE inhibitors [20,26-31]. This subclass of CCBs affects the synthesis of various matrix proteins such as heparan sulfate and glucoaminoglycan as well as fibroblast turnover

[31-32]. Prevention of mesangial expansion or glomerulosclerosis has never been shown for either α blockers or dihydropyridine CCBs in animal models of diabetes [12,14,33].

To further bolster the argument that dihydropyridine CCBs do not protect against morphologic progression of renal disease, studies using 24 hour blood pressure monitoring in a rat model of renal insufficiency were performed. Animals were randomized to four different CCBs, two long acting dihydropyridines, amlodipine or felodipine, as well as the nondihydropyridine agents, verapamil and diltiazem. Given similar levels of blood pressure reduction, only verapamil prevented development of glomerulosclerosis and proteinuria [29-30]. Conversely, the long acting CCBs amlodipine and felodipine did not protect against development of renal injury or proteinuria at comparable blood pressure levels, figure 52-1. A lack of morphologic protection and increase in proteinuria was also noted in a salt-sensitive, DOCA-salt, rat model as well as the SHR model [34].

This lack of effect on albuminuria by dihydropyridine CCBs is also seen clinically [9,10,35]. Results from a recent clinical trial of patients with type II diabetes and microalbuminuria
randomized to either lisinopril or nifedipine retard were found to have a significantly greater reduction in albumin excretion when compared to the CCB [24]. Moreover, this occurred in spite of similar reductions in blood pressure. In a separate study, an increase in protein excretion of as much as 50 % has also been shown in Type II diabetic African-Americans with albuminuria randomized to isradipine [23].

The reason for this absence of effect on albuminuria by dihydropyridine CCBs relates to a lack of effect on glomerular membrane permeability, in spite of blood pressure reduction [9,10]. Results from a recently completed two year randomized, prospective trial in 28 type II diabetic patients with nephropathy, demonstrates *no alteration* of glomerular membrane permeability or albuminuria with once-daily nifedipine whereas there was a clear *reduction* in membrane permeability and albuminuria with once-daily diltiazem [9].

There are four long term (≥ 3 year follow-up) clinical studies that examine the effects of long acting dihydropyridine CCBs on both changes in albuminuria as well as progression of renal
disease [25,36-38]. The longest-term study with dihydropyridine CCBs comes from the Melbourne Diabetes Study Group. This group has now followed patients with both incipient and established diabetic nephropathy for a period of more than three years. They note that the initial reductions in albuminuria seen with nifedipine retard did not persist beyond the first year [36]. Moreover, the rate of decline in renal function in the group randomized to nifedipine was significantly faster than the group randomized to the ACE inhibitor [37].

In a separate study, Zucchelli et.al. followed patients with chronic renal disease, randomized to either nifedipine or an ACE inhibitor, for three years [38]. At study end, no significant differences in proteinuria or the slopes of glomerular filtration rate (GFR) declines were noted. However, in the third year, people randomized to nifedipine were more than five times more likely to start dialysis. A third study of patients with early diabetic nephropathy, randomized to either an ACE inhibitor or amlodipine and followed for three years, noted no difference between groups in reduction of microalbuminuria [39]. Interestingly, however, this is the only study, to date, that demonstrates an acute reduction in GFR with amlodipine. Thus, the results of this small study may be the result of a reduction in GFR. Lastly, a subanalysis of a recent international trial among patients with non-diabetic renal disease demonstrates that those who received nifedipine retard to control blood pressure in the placebo group had a significantly faster rate of decline in GFR as well as a much shorter time to dialysis [40]. Additional data that may bolster these observations may come from the ongoing Appropriate Blood Pressure Control in Diabetes (ABCD) trial.

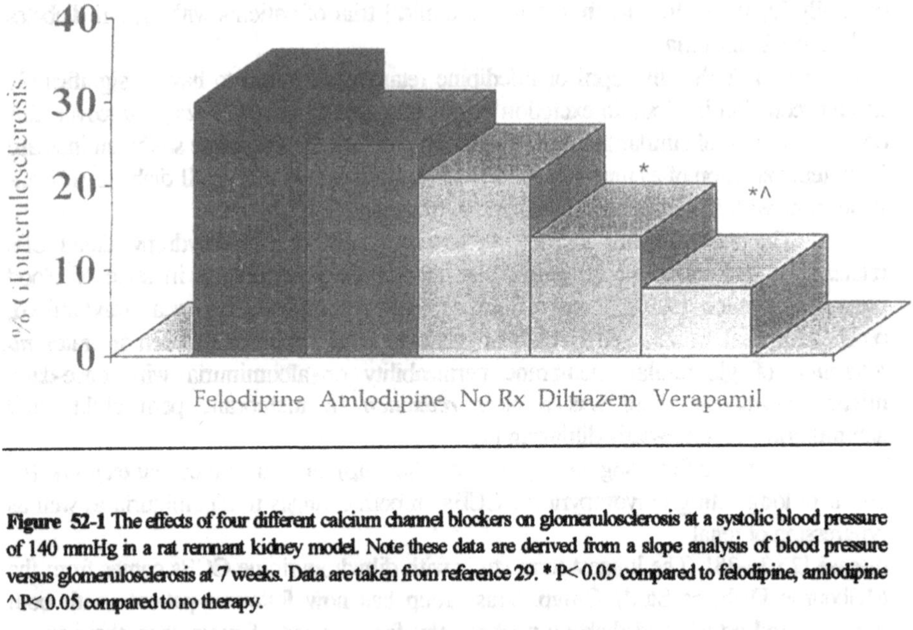

Figure 52-1 The effects of four different calcium channel blockers on glomerulosclerosis at a systolic blood pressure of 140 mmHg in a rat remnant kidney model. Note these data are derived from a slope analysis of blood pressure versus glomerulosclerosis at 7 weeks. Data are taken from reference 29. * P< 0.05 compared to felodipine, amlodipine ^ P< 0.05 compared to no therapy.

This ongoing randomized, double-blind trial of 900 type II diabetic patients is designed to assess whether, at a given blood pressure level, a dihydropyridine CCB will slow progression of nephropathy to a comparable degree as an ACE inhibitor [41].

In contrast to the dihydropyridine CCBs, three different meta-analyses noted that nondihydropyridine CCBs reduce albuminuria and slow the decline in GFR among patients with established diabetic nephropathy [42-44]. This observation is further supported by two recent long term (≥ 5 years) studies in patients with established nephropathy from type II diabetes. These investigations revealed that long acting verapamil or diltiazem slowed progression of established diabetic renal disease to a degree similar to an ACE inhibitor [20,45].

Many factors may contribute to the disparate effects of the different subclasses of CCBs on both surrogate end-points as well as progression of renal disease. These differences are reviewed, in detail, elsewhere [46]. It is clear, however, that arterial pressure reduction is the ultimate goal that uniformly leads to preservation of renal function. Thus, since the majority of patients with diabetic nephropathy require more than one medication to reduce arterial pressure, a combination of antihypertensive agents, individually shown to reduce arterial pressure and albuminuria as well as preserve renal morphology and function, is preferred, figure 52-2. Since preliminary evidence supports the notion that both ACE inhibitors and nondihydropyridine CCBs slow progression of diabetic renal disease to a greater extent than conventional blood pressure lowering agents, it is predicted that a combination of these two classes of agents will provide better renal protection than either alone. Unfortunately, few animal or human studies have examined this hypothesis. The remainder of the chapter will review the data that examine this and associated hypotheses.

COMBINATION ANTIHYPERTENSIVE THERAPY

Few animal studies have evaluated the effects of an ACE inhibitor/CCB combination on various aspects of renal disease [26-28,47-48]. Unfortunately, only one of these studies actually controlled for blood pressure differences, so that a meaningful comparison could be made between the combination and its individual components [48]. This study showed that combination therapy with a fixed-dose of an ACE inhibitor, benazepril, and dihydropyiridine CCB, amlodipine, prevented progression to glomerulosclerosis observed with amlodipine alone. This combination also blunted the rise in albuminuria in contrast to amlodipine alone, which had no effect on this variable. These findings were also observed in a recent clinical study that examined changes in proteinuria and GFR with this combination [49]. Lastly, a series of case reports demonstrate a reduction in proteinuria after cessation of once daily nifedipine among patients with diabetic nephropathy who were also receiving other antihypertensive therapy [50]. Interestingly, while proteinuria dropped in these patients, mean arterial pressure increased by an average of 7 mmHg.

In contrast to dihydropyridine CCB/ ACE inhibitor combinations, animal studies that combine a nondihydropyridine CCB with an ACE inhibitor have demonstrated a potentiation of ACE inhibitor associated reductions in proteinuria[26-28]. Two of these studies also showed relatively greater preservation of renal morphology [26,27]. Moreover, the fixed-dose combination of verapamil with trandolapril showed protection of glomerular morphology, in the absence of blood pressure control [27]. The potentiating antiproteinuric effects of the fixed-dose combination, verapamil plus trandolapril, has also been observed in a recent randomized, multicenter, clinical trial of patients with nephropathy secondary to type II diabetes with comparable blood pressure control [51]. Thus, while ACE inhibitors appear to protect the kidney from the neutral effects of dihydropyridine CCBs, they potentiate the positive effects of nondihydropyridine CCBs.

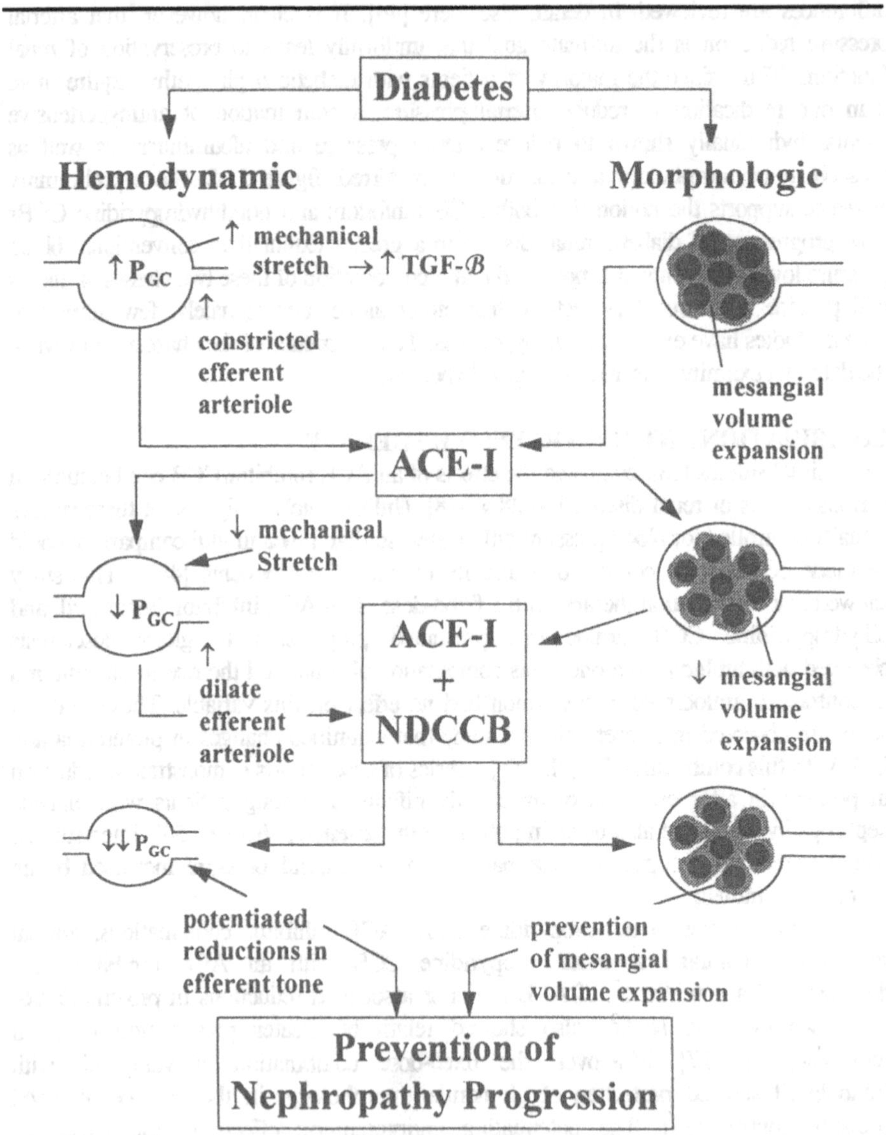

Figure 52-2- A representation of the renal hemodynamic and morphologic effects of ACE inhibitors (ACE-I) and nondihydropyridine calcium channel blockers (NDCCB), P_{GC}- Intraglomerular capillary pressure

***Adapted from Kilaru PK and Bakris GL. Calcium channel blockade and/or ACE inhibition in diabetic hypertensive nephropathy. IN Combination Drug Therapy for Hypertension . Opie LH and Messerli F, (eds). Lippincott-Raven Publ., Philadelphia, 1997, pp.123-138.

Aside from the additive antiproteinuric effects of fixed-dose nondihydropyridine CCB/ACE inhibitor combinations, clinical studies have also shown that fixed-dose combinations have a side effect profile generally less than that the individual components used separately [52]. Schneider, et al has shown that in patients with type II diabetes and hypertension, this combination did not aggravate insulin resistance nor elevate lipid levels unlike patients who were treated with ?-blockers and chlorthalidone [53]. Additionally, a four year follow-up study of patients with nephropathy secondary to type II diabetes demonstrated that the combination of verapamil plus lisinopril resulted in a slower decline in GFR, a lower amount of albuminuria and the lowest side effect profile [54]. No other long term clinical studies have formally evaluated either fixed-dose or reduced dose combination therapy on progression of diabetic renal disease. Lastly, in anesthesized dogs, the verapamil-trandolapril combination prevented hypoxemia-induced vasoconstriction of the coronary arteries [55]. This would be clearly beneficial, since cardiovascular disease is the most common cause of death among patients with diabetic nephropathy [56].

CONCLUSIONS

It is critically important that effective arterial pressure reduction be achieved in diabetic patients to not only preserve renal function but to also reduce cardiovascular mortality. Since most patients with diabetic nephropathy require a minimum of two medications to control their blood pressure to the newly recommended goal, combination therapy is highly recommended. Given the difficulties with medication compliance in this patient group along with the socioeconomic cost of diabetic nephropathy and its impact on the quality of life, the advantages of fixed dose combinations are obvious [57]. Of the many possible combinations, a nondihydropyridine CCB/ACE inhibitor combination may be preferred not only because of a low side effect profile but also because each agent has been individually shown to reduce cardiovascular mortality following myocardial infarctions [58]. This has not been shown for dihydropyridine CCBs [59,60].

In light of these few studies, however, there are insufficient data to assess whether fixed-dose antihypertensive therapy offers a distinct advantage to reduce renal and cardiovascular mortality over its individual components used together. The evidence does suggest, however, that low dose combinations of a nondihydropyridine CCB with an ACE inhibitor yields additive effects on glomerular membrane permeability and may, in longer term studies, slow progression of diabetic nephropathy to a greater extent than an ACE inhibitor alone. This hypothesis is further supported by a recent meta-analysis of experimental and clinical studies that examined changes in glomerular permeability in the context of renal disease progression [61].

REFERENCES:

1. National High Blood Pressure Education Program Working Group on Hypertension and Renal Disease. 1995 Update of the working group reports on chronic renal failure and renovascular hypertension. Arch Intern Med. 1996;156 :1938-1947.
2. Bakris GL. Pathogenesis of hypertension in diabetes. Diabetes Reviews 1995;3(3):460-476

3. The Sixth Report of the Joint National Committee on Prevention, Detection, Evaluation, and Treatment of High Blood Pressure (JNC VI). Arch Intern Med, 1997; 157:2413-2446.
4.. Waeber B, Brunner HR. Main objectives and new aspects of combination treatment of hypertension. J Hypertens 1995; 13 (Suppl):S15-S19.
5. Epstein M and Bakris GL. Newer approaches to antihypertensive therapy using fixed dose combination therapy: Future perspectives. Arch Intern Med. 1996;156:1969-1978.
6. Griffin KA, Picken MM and Bidani AK. Deleterious effects of calcium channel blockade on pressure transmission and glomerular injury in rat remnant kidneys. J Clin. Invest 1995; 96: 793-800.
7. Kilaru P and Bakris GL: ACE inhibition or calcium-channel blockade: Renal implications of combination therapy versus a single agent. J Cardiovasc Pharmacol.1996;28(Suppl 4):S34-S44.
8. Bakris GL, Walsh MF, Sowers JR. Endothelium,mesangium interactions:Role of insulin-like growth factors . IN: Endocrinology of the Vasculature (Sowers JR, ed). Humana Press Inc. New Jersey, 1996, pp.341-356.
9. Smith AC, Toto R, Bakris GL. Differential effects of calcium channel blockers on size selectivity of proteinuria in diabetic glomerulopathy. Kidney Int. In press.
10. Bakris GL. Microalbuminuria: Prognostic Implications. Curr Opin in Nephrol and Hypertens 1996;5(3):219-233.
11. Drumond MC , Kristal B , Myers BD , Deen WM Structural basis for reduced glomerular filtration capacity in nephrotic humans. J Clin Invest 1994 ;94(3):1187-1195
12. Bakris GL, Mehler P, and Schrier R. Hypertension and Diabetes. IN Schrier RW and Gottschalk CW (eds.) Diseases of the Kidney 6th ed., Little Brown and Company, 1996, Chapter 54, pp.1281-1328
13. Steffes MW, Osterby R, Chavers B, and Mauer SM. Mesangial expansion as a central mechanism for loss of kidney function in diabetic patients. Diabetes 1989;38:1077-1081.
14. Anderson S, Rennke HG, Brenner BM. Nifedipine versus fosinopril in uninephrectomized diabetic rats. Kidney Int 1992;41:891-897.
15. Ravid M, Lang R, Rachmani R, Lishner M. Long-term renoprotective effect of angiotensin-converting enzyme inhibition in non-insulin-dependent diabetes mellitus. Arch Intern Med 1996;156:286-289
16. Parving H, Hommel E, Nielsen M, Giese J: Effect of captopril on blood pressure and kidney function in normotensive insulin dependent diabetics with nephropathy. Br Med J 1989;299:533-536.
17. Bakris GL, Slataper R, Vicknair N, Sadler R: ACE inhibitor mediated reductions in renal size and microalbuminuria in normotensive, diabetic subjects. J Diab Compl 1994;8:2-6.
18. Viberti G; Mogensen CE; Groop LC; Pauls JF. Effect of captopril on progression to clinical proteinuria in patients with insulin-dependent diabetes mellitus and microalbuminuria. European Microalbuminuria Captopril Study Group JAMA 1994;271(4):275-9.,
19. Sakamoto N: Effects of long-term enalapril treatment on persistent microalbuminuria in well-controlled hypertensive and normotensive NIDDM patients. Diabetes Care 1994;17:420-424
20. Bakris GL, Copley JB, Vicknair N, Sadler R, Leurgans S. Calcium channel blockers versus other antihypertensive therapies on progression of NIDDM associated nephropathy: Results of a six year study. Kidney Int. 1996;50:1641-1650.
21. Lebovitz HE, Wiegmann TB, Cnaan A: Renal protective effects of enalapril in hypertensive NIDDM: role of baseline albuminuria. Kidney Int Suppl 1994;45:S150-S155.
22. Lewis EJ, Hunsicker LG, Bain RP, Rohde RD for the Collaborative Study Group. The effect of angiotensin converting enzyme inhibition on diabetic nephropathy. N Engl J Med 1993;329:1456-1462.
23. Guasch A, Parham M, Zayas CF, Campbell O, Nzerue C, Macon E. Contrasting effects of calcium channel blockade versus converting enzyme inhibition on proteinuria in African Americans with non-insulin dependent diabetes mellitus and nephropathy. J Am Soc Nephrol 1997;8: 793-798.

24. Agardh CD, Garcia-Puig J, Charbonnel B, Angelkort B, Barnett AH. Greater reduction of urinary albumin excretion in hypertensive Type II diabetic patients with incipient nephropathy by lisinopril than by nifedipine. J Human Hypertens 1996;10:185-192.
25. Maschio G, Alberti D, Janin G, Locatelli F, Mann JEF, Motolese M, Ponticelli C, Ritz E, Zucchelli P, and the Angiotensin-Converting-Enzyme Inhibition in Progressive Renal Insufficiency Study Group. Effect of the angiotensin-converting-enzyme inhibitor benazepril on the progression of chronic renal insufficiency. N Engl J Med 1996;334:939-945
26. Gaber L, Walton C, Brown S, Bakris, GL: Effects of different antihypertensive treatments on morphologic progression of diabetic nephropathy in uninephrectomized dogs. Kidney Int 1994;46:161-169
27. Munter K, Hergenroder S, Jochims K, Kirchengast M. Individual and combined effects of verapamil or trandolapril on glomerular morphology and function in the stroke prone rat. J Am Soc Nephrol 1996;7:681-686
28. Brown SA, Walton CL, Crawford P & Bakris GL. Long-term effects of different anti-hypertensive regimens on renal hemodynamics and proteinuria. Kidney Int 1993, 43:1210-1218.
29. Picken M, Griffin K, Bakris GL and Bidani A. Comparative effects of four different calcium antagonists on progression of renal disease in a remnant kidney model. J Am Soc Nephrol. 1996;7:1586[abstract]
30. Griffin K, Picken M, Bakris GL and Bidani A. Calcium antagonists and the remnant kidney model:relative antihypertensive and glomeruloprotective efficacies. Am J Hypertens 1996; 9:38 (abstract)
31. Jyothirmayi GN, Reddi AS: Effect of diltiazem on glomerular heparan sulfate and albuminuria in diabetic rats. Hypertension 1993; 21:765-802.
32. Andrawis NS and Abernathy DR. Effect of calcium antagonists on RNA synthesis of NIH 3T3 cells. Am J Med Sci 1993;306:137-140.
33. Jyothirmayi GN, Alluru I, Reddi AS. Doxazosin prevents proteinuria and glomerular loss of heparan sulfate in diabetic rats. Hypertension 1996;27:1108-1114
34. Dworkin LD, Tolbert E, Recht PA, Hersch JC, Feiner H, Levin RI. Effects of amlodipine on glomerular filtration, growth and injury in experimental hypertension. Hyperten. 1996; 27:245-250
35. Abbott K, Smith AC, Bakris GL. Effects of dihydropyridine calcium antagonists on albuminuria in diabetic subjects. J. Clin Pharmacol. 1996;36:274-279.
36. Gilbert RE, Jerum G, Allen T, Hammond J, Cooper ME on behalf on Diabetic Nephropathy Study Group. Effect of different antihypertensive agents on normotensive microalbuminuria patients with IDDM and NIDDM. J Am Soc Nephrol 1994;5:377 (abstract).
37. Campbell D on behalf of the Melbourne Nephropathy Study Group. ACE inhibitors versus calcium channel blockade. Fifth International Symposium on Hypertension associated with Diabetes Mellitus. International Society of Nephrology 1997, pp.32.
38. Zucchelli P, Zuccala A, Borghi M, et. al., Long term comparison between captopril and nifedipine in the progression of renal insufficiency Kidney Int 1992 42:452-458.
39. Velussi M, Brocco E, Frigato F, Zolli M, Muollo B, Maioli M, Carraro A, Tonolo G, Fresu P, Cernigoi A, Fioretto P, Nosadini R. Effects of cilazapril and amlodipine on kidney function in hypertensive NIDDM patients. Diabetes 1996;45:216-222
40. Locatelli F. AIPRI Trial: Secondary Analysis. Progression of Renal Disease Symposium. International Society of Nephrology Meeting, 1997
41. Estacio RO, Savage S, Nagel NJ, Schrier RW. Baseline characteristics of participants in the Appropriate Blood Pressure Control in Diabetes Trials. Controlled Clin Trials 1996; 17:242-257.
42. Gansevoort RT, Sluiter WJ, Hemmelder MH, de Zeeuw D, de Jong PE Antiproteinuric effect of blood pressure lowering agents: a meta-analysis of comparative trials. Nephrol Dial Transplant 1995;10:1963-1974
43. Weidmann P, Scneider M, Bohlen L et. al. Therpeutic efficacy of differentantihypertensive drugs in human diabetic nephropa: An updated meta-analysis. Nephrol Dial Transpl 1995;10(Suppl 9):39-45

44. Maki DD, Ma JZ, Louis TA, Kasiske BL: Effect of antihypertensive agents on the kidney. Arch Intern Med 1995 ;155:1073-1082.
45. Bakris GL, Mangrum A, Copley JB, Vicknair N, Sadler R. Calcium channel or beta blockade on progression of diabetic renal disease in African-Americans. Hypertension 1997;29:744-750
46. Tarif N and Bakris GL Preservation of renal function: the spectrum of effects by calcium channel blockers. Nephrol Dial Transpl, 1997;12: 2244-2250.
47. Wenzel RO, Helmchen U, Schoeppe W, Schwietzer G. Combination treatment of enalapril with nitrendipine in rats with renovascular hypertension. Hypertension 1994;23: 114-122.
48. Bakris GL, Griffin KA, Picken MM, and Bidani AK. Combined effects of an angiotensin converting enzyme inhibitor and a calcium antagonist on renal injury. J Hypertension 1997;15: 1181-1185.
49. Fogari R, Zoppi A, Mugellini A, Lusardi P, Destro M, Corradi L. Effect of benazepril plus amlodipine vs. benazepril alone on urinary albumin excretion in hypertensive patients with type II diabetes and microalbuminuria. Clin Drug Invest 1996:11:50-55.
50. Hess B. Reduced proteinuria after cessation of long acting osmotic release nifedipine GITS in diabetic nephropathy. Nephrol Dial Transplant. 1997;12:1772 (letter).
51. Bakris GL, Weir M, DeQuattro V, Rosendorff C, McMahon G. Renal effects of a long acting ACE inhibitor, trandolapril or nondihydropyridine calcium blocker, verapamil alone or in a fixed dose combination in diabetic nephropathy: a randomized double blind placebo controlled multicenter study. Nephrology; 1997; 3: 271 [abstract]
52. Holzgreve H. Safety profile of the combination of verapamil and trandolapril. J Hypertens. 1997;15(suppl 2): S51-S53.
53. Schneider M, Lerch M, Papiri M, Buechel P, Boehlen L, Shaw S, Risen W, Weidmann P. Metabolic neutrality of combined verapamil-trandolapril treatment in contrast to beta-blocker-low-dose chlorthalidone treatment in hypertensive type II diabetes. J Hypertens. 1996;14:669-677.
54. Lash JP and Bakris GL. Effects of ACE inhibitors and calcium antagonists alone or combined on progression of diabetic nephropathy. Nephrol. Dial and Transpl.1995;10 (Suppl.9):56-62
55. Lee JJ, Boulanger CM, Kirchengast M, Vanhoutte PM. Trandolapril plus verapamil inhibits the coronary vasospasm induced by hypoxia following ischemia-reperfusion injury in dogs. Gen Pharm. 1996;27(6):1057-1059.
56. Nelson RG, Knowler WC, Pettitt DJ, Bennett PH. Kidney diseases in diabetes. In Diabetes In America National Institutes of Health Pub. No.95-1468, 2nd edition, 1995, pp. 349-400
57. Simeon G, Bakris G. Socioeconomic impact of diabetic nephropathy: can we improve the outcome? J Hypertens 1997;15 (Suppl 2):S77-S82.
58. Yusuf S, Lessem J, Jha P, Lonn E. Primary and secondary prevention of myocardial infarction and strokes: an update of randomly allocated, controlled trials. J Hypertens 1993; 11 (Suppl 4):S61-S73.
59. Furberg CD, Psaty BM and Meyer JV. Dose-related increase in mortality in patients with coronary heart disease. Circulation 1995;92:1326-1331.
60. Estacio RO, Jeffers BW, Hiatt WR, Biggerstaff SL, Gifford N, Schrier RW. The effect of nisoldipine as compared with enalapril on cardiovascular outcomes in patients with non-insulin-dependent diabetes and hypertension. N Engl J Med. 1998; 338: 645-652.
61. Perna A and Remuzzi G. Abnormal permeability to proteins and glomerular lesions: a meta-analysis of experimental and human studies. Am J Kidney Dis 1996;27:34-41.

53. MICROALBUMINURIA IN PATIENTS WITH ESSENTIAL HYPERTENSION. CARDIOVASCULAR AND RENAL IMPLICATIONS

Stefano Bianchi, Roberto Bigazzi and Vito M. Campese
U.O. di Nefrologia, Spedali Riuniti, Livorno, Italy, and Division of Nephrology, University of Southern California, Los Angeles, USA.

Supported in part by NIH Grants 1 RO1 HL 47881

INTRODUCTION

The availability of methods to quantitate small amounts of urinary albumin excretion non detectable by the albustix, has allowed early recognition of renal disease in several pathological conditions, such as diabetes mellitus and essential hypertension. The term microalbuminuria indicates amounts of urinary albumin excretion above the 95% confidence interval of the normal population, but below amounts detectable by semiquantitative methods (30-300 mg/24 hours or 20-200 μg/min) [1,2,3]. Several studies have indicated that microalbuminuria is a marker of glomerular damage, and predicts the development of overt proteinuria and progressive renal failure in patients with insulin-dependent diabetes mellitus (IDDM) [4,5,6,7,8] and non-insulin-dependent diabetes mellitus (NIDDM) [9,10]. In both IDDM and NIDDM patients, microalbuminuria also predicts cardiovascular morbidity and mortality [11,12,13,14]. Treatment of hypertension and administration of angiotensin-converting enzyme inhibitors, even in normotensive patients are of benefit in arresting the progression of diabetic renal disease both in IDDM [15,16,17,18,19] and NIDDM patients [20,21,22]. Some evidence also indicates that microalbuminuria may predict cardiovascular events and perhaps early renal damage in patients with essential hypertension.

The purpose of this manuscript is to review the incidence of microalbuminuria and its relationship with blood pressure levels and cardiovascular risk factors in patients with essential hypertension. Moreover, we will discuss the evidence supporting the role of microalbuminuria in predicting

Mogensen, C.E. (ed.), THE KIDNEY AND HYPERTENSION IN DIABETES MELLITUS.

cardiovascular as well as renal complications and the effects of antihypertensive treatment on microalbuminuria in patients with essential hypertension.

MICROALBUMINURIA IN ESSENTIAL HYPERTENSION: INCIDENCE AND RELATIONSHIP WITH LEVELS OF BLOOD PRESSURE.

The prevalence of microalbuminuria in patients with essential hypertension varies enormously among different studies with rates ranging between 5 and 37 percent [23,24,25,26]. A wide variability of UAE has also been shown among normotensive healthy subjects [27,28,29]. Several studies have failed to find a correlation between office blood pressure and urinary albumin excretion in patients with essential hypertension [24,30]. Other studies, however, have observed a significant correlation between those two variables [31,32,33,34]. Similarly, in normotensive healthy subjects, a correlation between office blood pressure and UAE has been shown in some [35,36] but not in other studies [27]. Usually, better correlations between levels of blood pressure and UAE are observed when continuous ambulatory measurements are used instead of occasional blood pressure readings in the office. Opsahl et al [30] observed a better correlation between 24 h ambulatory blood pressure and UAE than between office blood pressure and UAE. Giaconi et al [37] found a significant correlation between day-time average diastolic blood pressure and UAE, whereas Cerasola et al observed a significant correlation between 24 hr systolic and diastolic blood pressure and UAE [38].

We have recently shown that patients with essential hypertension and microalbuminuria manifest a blunted or absent nocturnal dipping of blood pressure (Fig 53-1). Hypertensive patients with no nocturnal dipping of blood pressure (non-dippers) displayed greater UAE than "dippers" [39]. An association between reduced nocturnal dipping of blood pressure and increased UAE has been shown by others in patients with essential hypertension [40] and patients with type 1 [41,42,43] or type 2 [44,45] diabetes mellitus. Patients with increased 24 hour systolic and diastolic blood pressure also are more likely to evolve from the phase of normal UAE to the phase of microalbuminuria [46,47]. In all, these studies suggest that in patients with essential hypertension as well as in those with both IDDM and NIDDM, levels of blood pressure measured throughout the 24 hour correlate with UAE better than casual measurements of blood pressure taken in the office.

MICROALBUMINURIA AND SERUM LIPIDS

In patients with essential hypertension, the combined presence of microalbuminuria and hyperlipidemia is frequent. In these patients, higher levels of UAE correlate significantly with higher serum levels of triglycerides and apolipoprotein B, and lower serum levels of HDL cholesterol [27,48,49] We have also shown higher serum levels of lipoprotein (a), low-density lipoprotein (LDL) cholesterol and a greater LDL/HDL ratio in hypertensive patients with microalbuminuria than in those without microalbuminuria. Using multiple regression analysis we observed that lipoprotein (a) and nocturnal blood pressure values were among several variables that best correlate with microalbuminuria

[50]. In a non selected population, Metcalf et al [51] observed a close correlation between microalbuminuria and cholesterol intake. In normotensive nondiabetic obese subjects, Basdevant et al [52] observed a significant association among microalbuminuria, serum cholesterol and apolipoprotein B.

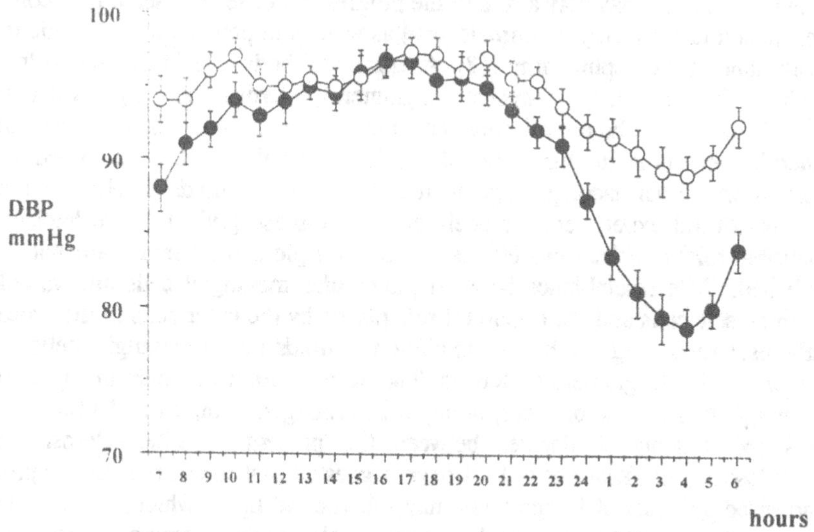

Figure 53-1 Mean hourly diastolic blood pressure (DBP) values in essential hypertensive patients with (open circles) and without (closed circles) microalbuminuria. [Adapted from ref. 39 with permission]

Microalbuminuria and hyperlipidemia are frequently linked independently of diet and/or body weight. Jensen et al [36] described low levels of apoprotein A-1 and HDL cholesterol in healthy subjects with microalbuminuria. Haffner et al [53] observed higher serum levels of triglycerides and lower HDL cholesterol in non diabetic subjectswith microalbuminuria than in subjects without microalbuminuria. Normotensive nondiabetic subjects with microalbuminuria also showed a significant reduction in serum HDL cholesterol levels and the HDL/LDL cholesterol ratio in comparison to subjects without microalbuminuria [35].

One possible explanation for the association between microalbuminuria and hyperlipidemia is that the urinary loss of protein may cause the increase in serum levels of lipoproteins. This is supported by the evidence that urinary losses of large amounts of proteins may lead to increased serum levels of total and LDL cholesterol [54,55] as well as lipoprotein (a) [56,57,58]. Moreover, recent studies in diabetic patients have indicated that even losses of small amounts of albumin in the urine may cause substantial alterations of serum lipoproteins [59,60].

An alternative explanation for the association between microalbuminuria and hyperlipidemia is that hyperlipidemia causes renal damage and the increase in urinary excretion of albumin. Hyperlipidemia is a well-known independent risk factor for atherosclerosis and cardiovascular disease [61,62,63,64]. Many authors believe that lipid abnormalities may contribute to renal damage by a mechanism analogous to atherogenesis. According to this hypothesis increased levels of lipoproteins accelerate generalized atherosclerosis as well as intrarenal micro and macrovascular disease, resulting in microalbuminuria. Recent studies have shown that hyperlipidemia may play a role in the progression of renal disease [65] both in experimental nephropathy in animals [66] as well as in patients with diabetic [67] or with nondiabetic nephropathy [68]. A substantial body of evidence supports the hypothesis that lipids may be involved in glomerulosclerosis and the progression of renal disease. Cholesterol-enriched diets may cause albuminuria and glomerulosclerosis in different animal species, particularly when combined with hypertension. Pharmacologic agents that lower serum lipids ameliorate renal injury in several experimental models of renal disease [69]. The mechanism(s) responsible for the deleterious effects of lipids on glomerular injury are not well established. The resemblance between glomerular mesangial cells and vascular smooth muscle cells and the important role played by the latter cells in the process of atherosclerosis suggests that accumulation of lipids in the mesangial cells may cause or accelerate glomerulosclerosis. The accumulation of lipids in mesangial cells or glomerular macrophages, along with collagen, laminin and fibronectin, also supports some similarities between the process of atherosclerosis and glomerulosclerosis. Klahr et al [70] have suggested that mesangial cells exposed to increased amounts of lipoproteins may incorporate lipids which, in turn, may stimulate their proliferation and excessive glomerular basement membrane deposition leading to progressive glomerulosclerosis. LDL can also promote adherence of monocytes to endothelial cells, a potentially important factor in the progression of inflammatory glomerular diseases [71].

MICROALBUMINURIA, INSULIN RESISTANCE AND HYPERINSULINEMIA IN ESSENTIAL HYPERTENSION

Several investigators have described the presence of insulin resistance and hyperinsulinemia in a substantial number of patients with essential hypertension [72,73], and suggested hyperinsulinemia as a risk factor for atherosclerotic cardiovascular diseases [74,75,76].

The mechanisms by which insulin resistance, hyperinsulinemia, or both may increase the risk of cardiovascular disease are not well-defined. Whether hyperinsulinemia and microalbuminuria are directly related has not been determined. To test this possibility we measured the plasma insulin response to an oral glucose load in hypertensive patients with or without microalbuminuria and normotensive healthy subjects. In the hypertensive patients, the plasma insulin response to a glucose load (evaluated as the insulin area under the curve, AUC) was significantly enhanced compared with the control subjects. When the hypertensive patients were subdivided according to their urinary albumin excretion rate, the microalbuminuric patients had significantly higher insulin AUC values. In addition, a significant direct correlation was found to exist between insulin AUC and the urinary albumin excretion rate [77]. Using the euglycemic clamp technique, we have also observed a 35% reduction of the peripheral glucose uptake stimulated by insulin in patients with essential hypertension and microalbuminuria [78]. This appeared to be secondary to a reduction of glycogen synthesis since the glucose oxidation was not altered. Because during an euglycemic clamp approximately two-thirds of glycogen synthesis occur in skeletal muscles [79], the abnormality in glycogen synthesis in hypertensive patients with microalbuminuria has to occur primarily in skeletal muscle cells. Like in other forms of insulin resistance, it is possible that the activation of glycogen synthase by insulin may be impaired [80]. Haffner et al (53) observed a greater plasma insulin response to glucose in nondiabetic subjects with microalbuminuria compared with those without microalbuminuria and similar results were reported by Woo et al in nondiabetic chinese subjects [81]. Nosadini et al showed a significant correlation between UAE and insulin resistance in patients with essential hypertension as well as in patients with type II diabetes mellitus [82,83]. An association between insulin resistance and microalbuminuria has also been described by Falkner et al [84] in young African-Americans. It seems therefore possible to conclude that microalbuminuria is a consistent correlate of iperinsulinemia and insulin resistence in normotensive or hypertensive individuals. It is also noteworthy that patients with type 1 and 2 diabetes and microalbuminuria manifest greater insulin resistance than diabetics without microalbuminuria [85,86,87].

The significance of the association between hyperinsulinemia, insulin resistance and microalbuminuria in essential hypertension is uncertain. Because microalbuminuria [51,52] and insulin resistance [88,89] occur in nondiabetic normotensive subjects with genetic predisposition for hypertension, microalbuminuria and enhanced plasma insulin response to glucose could be both genetically determined and cosegregate with the hypertensive status. Alternatively, insulin resistance and hyperinsulinemia, or both, are causally related to microalbuminuria. Finally, enhanced plasma insulin response to glucose, insulin resistance and microalbuminuria could be a consequence of hypertension.

Insulin could directly or indirectly increase UAE through a variety of mechanisms. Insulin could lead to arteriosclerosis, renal damage and microalbuminuria through its effects on blood pressure and lipid metabolism, or through its throphic actions. The structure of an atherosclerotic plaque is characterized by excessive amounts of lipid and collagen, foam macrophages and proliferation of smooth muscle cells [90]. Insulin could be responsible for all these abnormalities. Insulin infusion into femoral arteries of animals induced intimal and medial proliferation and accumulation of cholesterol and fatty acids [91]. In vitro, insulin can stimulate the proliferation of smooth muscle cells and collagen deposition. This action could be directly or indirectly mediated by growth-promoting factors [92]. Insulin can increase cholesterol and triglycerides synthesis and enhance LDL-receptor activity in arterial smooth muscle cells, fibroblasts and mononuclear cells [93,94].

An alternative hypothesis is that insulin may alter glomerular hemodynamics and/or glomerular permeability directly or in association with other factors such as catecholamines, angiotensin II, glucagone and sodium [95]. It is worth mentioning that insulin may contribute to the salt-sensitivity of blood pressure by causing sodium retention [96,97] or via activation of the sympathetic nervous system [98,99], and that salt-sensitive individuals manifest an abnormal renal hemodynamic response to high salt intake characterized by increased filtration fraction and intraglomerular pressure. Salt-sensitive individuals manifest greater UAE than salt resistant patients, and high salt intake causes a further rise in UAE in the former than in the latter group [100]. Thus, it is conceivable that directly or indirectly insulin may contribute to alterations of renal hemodynamics leading to greater urinary albumin excretion rate.

Insulin could increase UAE by altering glomerular membrane permeability. Infusions of insulin increase UAE both in normal subjects [101] and in patients with type I diabetes mellitus [102]. This suggests that insulin may increase the permselectivity of the glomerular basement membranes. This can be studied by measuring albumin transcapillary escape rate (TER). It is of note that patients with type I [103] as well as type II diabetes mellitus [104,105] and microalbuminuria manifest greater TER than patients without microalbuminuria. An increase in TER has also been shown in patients with severe atherosclerosis [106] and in patients with moderate to severe hypertension [107]. An increase in TER has been described even in normotensive healthy subjects with microalbuminuria [108], and an acute administration of insulin increases TER in these subjects [109].

Hyperinsulinemia could contribute to microalbuminuria by altering endothelial function. Alterations of endothelial function have been described in IDDM and NIDDM patients [110,111]. In patients with type 1 and 2 diabetes mellitus serum concentrations of von Willebrand factor are increased to suggest an alterations of endothelial function [112,113]. Stehouwer et al have shown an increase in von Willebrand factor years prior to the appearance of microalbuminuria in patients with type 1 diabetes [114]. Pedrinelli et al [115] have observed higher serum levels of von Willebrand factor in hypertensive patients with microalbuminuria than in those with normal UAE. In all, this evidence suggests that alterations of the permeability of endothelial cells can contribute to microalbuminuria in diabetic patients and in individuals with essential hypertension.

Finally, both insulin resistance and microalbuminuria could be the result of alterations of the microcirculation caused by long standing hypertension. This explanation seems less likely, because hyperinsulinemia, insulin resistance and microalbuminuria may precede the appearance of high blood pressure and are not found in all patients with established hypertension.

MICROALBUMINURIA AND CARDIOVASCULAR DISEASE

The increasing interest in the significance of microalbuminuria in essential hypertension derives, in large part, from the recognition that an increase in UAE is associated with an increased incidence of cardiovascular morbid events, such as left ventricular hypertrophy [38,116,117], myocardial ischemia [118,119], and hypertensive retinopathy [120]. In a large group of patients with essential hypertension we observed [50] that those patients who displayed an increase in urinary albumin excretion, also manifested an increased thickness of the carotid artery, (Fig 53-2) a recognized marker of atherosclerosis and coronary heart disease [121]. In a population of hypertensive patients older than 40 years of age, Yudkin et al [122] observed a greater incidence of coronary heart disease and peripheral vascular disease in patients with microalbuminuria than in those without microalbuminuria. After a follow-up of 3.6 years, the mortality rate was 33% in patients with increased UAE, and only 2% in patients with normal UAE. In a mixed group of normotensive and hypertensive individuals, Haffner et al [53] observed a greater prevalence of myocardial infarction in patients with than in those without microalbuminuria. The difference in cardiovascular events in patients with microalbuminuria persisted even when patients with hypertension were excluded. Similar results have been obtained by Winocour et al [35].

In a population of elderly patients without diabetes mellitus after a follow-up of 62-83 months, Damsgaard et al [28] observed a greater incidence of strokes and other cardiovascular events in subjects with increased UAE than in those with normal UAE. Kuusisto et al [123] studied the impact of hyperinsulinemia and microalbuminuria, alone or in combination, on the incidence of cardiovascular events in 1069 elderly subjects followed for an average of 3.5 years. Forty-eight percent of males and 60.8% of females had hypertension. The incidence of fatal and non-fatal cardiovascular events was significantly greater in patients with than in those without microalbuminuria. However, the incidence of cardiovascular events was only slightly, but not significantly increased in patients with increased serum insulin levels. In subjects with increased UAE and serum insulin the incidence of fatal and non-fatal cardiovascular events was greater than in patients with normal UAE and serum insulin levels. The presence of both microalbuminuria and hyperinsulinemia increased the probability of fatal and non-fatal cardiovascular events, even after adjusting for other risk factors, such as male sex, cigarette smoking, hypertension and serum cholesterol levels. In a major health screening at the State University Hospital in Copenaghen, among 1254 hypertensive patients with essential hypertension there was a positive independent relationship between UAE as a continuos variable and cardiovacular disease [26].

To evaluate whether the presence of microalbuminuria is associated with an increased risk of cardiovascular events we performed a retrospective cohort analysis of 141 hypertensive individuals followed-up for approximately 7 years. Fifty-four patients had microalbuminuria and 87 had normal UAE. At baseline, the two groups had similar age, weight and blood pressure, but serum cholesterol, triglycerides, and uric acid were higher and HDL cholesterol lower in patients with microalbuminuria than those with normal UAE. During follow-up, 12 cardiovascular events occurred in the 54 patients with microalbuminuria and only 2 events in the 87 patients with normal UAE. Multiple regression analysis showed that UAE cholesterol and diastolic blood pressure were independent predictors for the cardiovascular outcome [124].

In conclusion, the presence of microalbuminuria in patients with essential hypertension carries an increased risk of cardiovascular events. Although the mechanisms underscoring this association are not clear, it is plausible that the increased incidence of cardiovascular events in these patients may be due to the presence of hormonal and metabolic disturbances with atherogenic potential.

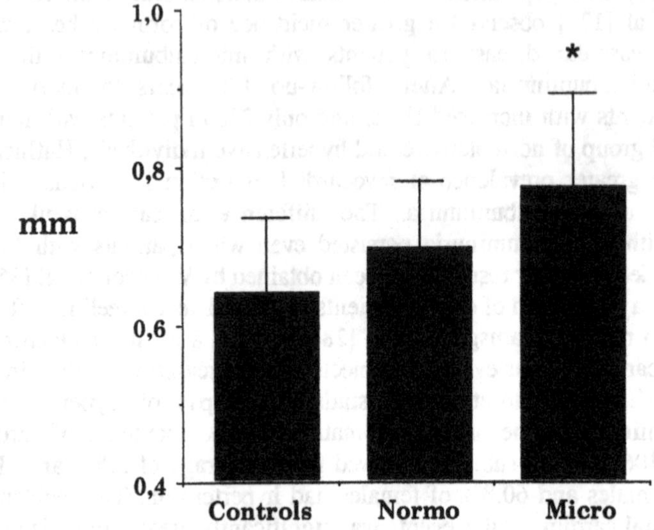

Figure 53-2 Thickness of the media-intima carotid artery in hypertensive patients with normal urinary albumin excretion (normo), patients with microalbuminuria (micro) and normotensive healthy subjects (controls). The difference between patients with microalbuminuria and patients with normal urinary albumin excretion was significant (p<0.01) [From ref. 50 with permission].

MICROALBUMINURIA AND NEPHROANGIOSCLEROSIS.

Data from the United States Renal Data System (USRDS) show that over the past decade, the incidence of renal failure as a consequence of essential hypertension has steadily increased [23]. This phenomenon is particularly striking when one considers that definite progress has been made in the treatment of established hypertension and in the prevention of other cardiovascular complications. Can we predict the patients at risk for developing renal failure due to hypertension, and more specifically is microalbuminuria such a predictor ?

Schmieder et al followed-up for 6 years a group of hypertensive subjects with normal renal function and observed no correlation between baseline urinary protein excretion and worsening of renal function [125]. Ruilope et al studied hypertensive subjects with and without microalbuminuria mantained on antihypertensive therapy consisting of diuretics and β-blockers alone or in combination for 5 years. They observed that patients who at baseline evaluation manifested microalbuminuria, showed a greater reduction of renal function than patients without microalbuminuria [126].

To evaluate whether the presence of microalbuminuria is associated with an increased risk of renal progression, we performed a retrospective cohort analysis of 141 hypertensive individuals followed for approximately 7 years [124]. Creatinine clearance decreased more in patients with microalbuminuria than in those with normal UAE (-12.1±2.77 vs. -7.1±0.88 ml/min; P<0.05).

In all, the available data suggests that hypertensive individuals with microalbuminuria may experience greater deterioration of renal function than patients with normal UAE.

ANTIHYPERTENSIVE THERAPY AND MICROALBUMINURIA

The notion that the presence of microalbuminuria predicts cardiovascular complications, has induced investigators to determine the effect of antihypertensive drugs on UAE, on the assumption and hope that this may result in greater cardiovascular and renal protection.

In patients with severe hypertension, reduction of blood pressure appears to uniformly result in decreased UAE [33,127]. Studies in patients with stage 1-2 hypertension have given conflicting results. Some studies have shown that antihypertensive drugs of different classes have equal effect on UAE, whereas other studies have shown that ACE-inhibitors reduce UAE more effectively than other commonly used antihypertensive drugs, despite similar effects on blood pressure.

In a cross-over study of patients with stage 1-2 hypertension Erley et al observed that a calcium antagonist, an ACE-inhibitor, a ß-blocker and an alpha-blocker had similar effects on blood pressure and UAE when administered each for 12 weeks [128]. Other studies using ß-blockers [129,130] or calcium channel antagonists [131] as single agents, have shown that reduction of blood pressure is associated with a decrease in UAE. This would suggest that the rise in blood pressure is the single most important factor determining the rise in UAE. Other investigators, however, have observed no effect of calcium channel antagonists [132,133] or activators of the K-channel [134] on UAE. De Venuto et al [135] observed that captopril and not a calcium channel blockler decreased UAE in patients with essential hypertension despite similar antihypertensive action. In patients with essential hypertension and normal renal function, we have also shown that despite similar antihypertensive efficacy, enalapril decreased UAE whereas no effects could be detected with a calcium channel antagonists, a ß-blocker or a diuretic [136,137]. The effect of ACE-inhibitors on UAE appears to persist even after therapy for 2 years [138], similar to what observed in hypertensive patients with type I diabetes mellitus [139]. Several other investigators have confirmed that ACE-inhibitors reduce UAE in patients with essential hypertension [140,141,142]. The greater antiproteinuric action of ACE-inhibitors compared with other antihypertensive agents has been attributed to selective vasodilation of the glomerular efferent arterioles with consequent decrease of intraglomerular hydrostatic pressure [143]. The antiproteinuric action of ACE-inhibitors is potentiated by dietary salt-restriction and reduced by high salt intake [146]. On the other hand, a direct effect of these drugs on glomerular basement membrane permselectivity cannot be ruled out. Whether a greater reduction of UAE translates into lesser incidence of cardiovascular and renal events remains to be determined with large prospective studies.

REFERENCES

1. Keen H, Chlouverakis C. An immunoassay method for urinary albumin at low concentrations. Lancet 1963; ii: 913-914.
2. Krans HMJ, Porta M, Keen H. Diabetes Care and research in Europe: The St Vincent Declaration Action Programme. World Health Organization, Copenhagen, 1992; pp 29-32.
3. Viberti GC, Hill RD, Jarret RD, Argyropoulos A, Mahmud U, Keen H. Microalbuminuria as a predictor of clinical nephropathy in insulin-dependent diabetes mellitus. Lancet 1982; i: 1430-1432.
4. Parving H-H, Oxenboll B, Svendsen PA, Christensen JS, Andersen AR. Early detection of patients at risk of developing diabetic nephropathy: a longitudinal study of urinary albumin excretion. Acta Endocrinol 1982; 100: 550-555.
5. Mogensen CE, Christensen CK. Predicting diabetic nephropathy in insulin-dependent patients. New Engl J Med 1984; 31: 89-93.
6. Nathan DM. Long-term complications of diabetes mellitus. N Engl J Med 1993; 328: 1676-1685.
7. Jones SL, Viberti GC. Hypertension and microalbuminuria as predictors of diabetic nephropathy. Diabetes Metab 1989; 15 (5 pt 2): 327-332.
8. Mathiessen ER, Saurbrey N, Hommel E, Parving HH. Prevalence of microalbuminuria in children with type 1 (insulin-dependent) diabetes mellitus. Diabetologia 1986; 29: 640-643.
9. Wirta O, Pasternack A, Mustonen J, Oksa H, Koivula T, Helin H. Albumin excretion rate and its relation to kidney disease in non-insulin-dependent diabetes mellitus. J Intern Med 1995; 237:367-373.
10. Mogensen CE. Microalbuminuria predicts clinical proteinuria and early mortality in maturity-onset diabetes. N Engl J Med 1984; 310: 356-360.
11. Messent JW, Elliot TG, Hill RG, Jarret RJ, Keen H, Viberti GC. Prognostic significance of microalbuminuria in insulin-dependent diabetes mellitus: a twenty-three year follow-up study. Kidney Int 1992; 41: 836-839.
12. Mau Pedersen M, Christensen CK, Mogensen CE. Long-term (18 years) prognosis for normo- and microalbuminuria type 1 (insulin-dependent) diabetic patients. Diabetologia 1992; 35:A60.
13. Jarret RJ, Viberti GC, Argyropoulos A, Hill RD, Mahmud U, Murrels TJ. Microalbuminuria predicts mortality in non-insulin-dependent diabetics. Diabet Med 1984; 1(1):17-19.
14. Schmitz A, Vaeth M. Microalbuminuria: a major risk factor in non-insulin-dependent diabetes. A ten-year follow-up study of 503 patients. Diabet Med 1988; 5: 126-134.
15. Mogensen CE. Antihypertensive treatment inhibiting the progression of diabetic nephropathy. Acta Endocrinol. 1980; 238: 103-108.
16. Johnson CI, Cooper ME, Nicolls GM. Meeting report of the International Society of Hypertension Conference on Hypertension and Diabetes. J Hypertens 1992; 10 (4): 393-397.
17. Mogensen CE, Hansen KW, Pedersen NN, Christensen CK. Renal factors influencing blood pressure threshold and choice of treatment for hypertension in IDDM. Diabetes Care 1991; 4 (suppl 4): 13-26.
18. Viberti GC, Mogensen CE, Groop LC, Pauls JF for the European Microalbuminuria Captopril Study Group. Effect of captopril on progression to clinical proteinuria in patients with insulin-dependent diabetes mellitus and microalbuminuria. JAMA 1994; 271: 245-326.
19. Wiegmann TBB, Herron KG, Chonko AM, MacDougall ML, Moore WV. Effect of angiotensin-converting enzyme inhibition on renal function and albuminuria in normotensive type 1 diabetic patients. Diabetes 1992, 41: 62-67.
20. Baba T, Murabayashi S, Takebe K. Comparison of the renal effects of angiotensin converting enzyme inhibitor and calcium antagonist in hypertensive type 2 (non-insulin-dependent) diabetic patients with microalbuminuria: a randomized controlled trial. Diabetologia 1989; 32(1): 40-44.
21. Ravid M, Savin H, Jutrin I, Bental T, Katz B, Lishner M. Long-term stabilizing effect of angiotensin –converting-enzyme inhibition on plasma creatinine and on proteinuria in normotensive type II diabetic patients. Ann Intern Med 1993; 118: 577-581.
22. Marre M, Hallab M, Billiard A, Le Jeune JJ, Bled F, Girault A, Fressinaud P. Small doses of ramipril to reduce microalbuminuria in diabetic patients with incipient nephropathy independent of blood pressure changes. J Cardiovasc Pharmacol 1991; 18 (suppl 2): S165-S168.
23. Gerber LM, Shmukler C, Alderman MH. Differences in urinary albumin excretion rate between normotensive and hypertensive white and non-white subjects. Arch Intern Med 1992; 152: 373-377.
24. Bigazzi R, Bianchi S, Campese VM, Baldari G. Prevalence of microalbuminuria in a large population of patients with mild to moderate essential hypertension. Nephron 1992; 61: 94-97.

25. Redon J, Liao Y, Lozano JV, Miralles A, Baldo E. Factors related to the presence of microalbuminuria in essential hypertension. Am J Hypertens 1994; 7(9 Pt1): 801-807.
26. Jensen JS, Feldt-Rasmussen B, Borch-Johnson K, Clausen P, Appleyard M, Jensen G. Microalbuminuria and its relation to cardiovascular disease and risk factors. A population-based study of 1254 hypertensive individuals. J Human Hypertens 1997; 11: 727-732.
27. Gosling P, Beevers DG. Urinary albumin excretion and blood pressure in the general population. Clinical Sc. 1989; 76: 39-42.
28. Damsgaard EM, Froland A, Jorgensen OD, Mogensen CE. Microalbuminuria as predictor of increased mortality in elderly people. BMJ 1990; 300: 297-300.
29. Watts GF, Morris RW, Khan K, Polak A. Urinary albumin excretion in healthy adult subjects: reference values and some factors affecting their interpretiaton. Clin Chim Acta 1988; 172: 191-198.
30. Opsahl JA, Abraham PA, Halstenson CE, Keane WF. Correlation of office and ambulatory blood pressure measurements with urinary albumin and N-acetyl-beta-D-glucosaminidase excretions in essential hypertension. Am J Hypertens 1988; 1: S117-S120.
31. Pedersen EB, Mogensen CE. Effect of antihypertensive treatment on urinary albumin excretion, glomerular filtration rate and renal plasma flow in patients with essential hypertension. Scand J Clin Lab Invest 1976; 36: 231-237.
32. Parving H-H, Jensen HE, Mogensen CE, Evrin PE. Increased urinary albumin excretion in benign essential hypertension. Lancet 1974; i: 1190-1192.
33. James A, Fotherby MB, Potter JF. Screening tests for microalbuminuria in non-diabetic elderly subjects and their relation to blood pressure. Clin Sci 1995; 88: 185-190.
34. West JNW, Gosling P, Dimmitt SB, Littler WA. Non-diabetic microalbuminuria in clinical practice and its relationship to posture, exercise and blood pressure. Cli Sci 1991; 81: 373-377.
35. Winocour PH, Harland J, Miller JP, Laker MF, Alberti KGM. Microalbuminuria and associated risk factors in the community. Atherosclerosis 1992; 93: 71-81.
36. Jensen JS, Borch Johnsen K, Jensen G, Feldt-Rasmussen B. Atherosclerotic risk factors are increased in clinically healthy subjects with microalbuminuria. Atherosclerosis 1995; 112: 245-252.
37. Giaconi S, Levanti C, Fommei E, Innocenti F, Seghieri G, Palla L, Palombo C, Ghione S. Microalbuminuria and casual and ambulatory blood pressure monitoring in normotensive and in patients with borderline and mild essential hypertension. Am J Hypertens 1989; 2: 259-26.
38. Cerasola G, Cottone S, Mule G, Nardi E, Mangano MT, Andronico G, Contorno A, Li Vecchi M, Gaglione P, Renda F, Piazza G, Volpe V, Lisi A, Ferrara L, Panepinto N, Riccobene R. Microalbuminuria, renal dysfunction and cardiovascular complication in essential hypertension. J Hypertens 1996; 26: 915-92.
39. Bianchi S, Bigazzi R, Baldari G, Sgherri GP, Campese VM. Diurnal variation of blood pressure and microalbuminuria in essential hypertension. Am J Hypertens 1994; 7: 23-29.
40. Redon J, Liao Y, Lozano JV, Miralles A, Pasqual JM, Cooper RS. Ambulatory blood pressure and microalbuminuria in essential hypertension: role of circadian variability. J Hypertens 1994; 12 (8): 947-953.
41. Berrut G, Hallab M, Bouhanick B, Chameau AM, Marre M, Fressinaud P. Value of ambulatory blood pressure monitoring in type I (insulin-dependent) diabetic patients with incipient diabetic nephropathy. Am J Hypertens 1994; 7: 222-227.
42. Weigmann TB, Herron KG, Chonko AM, MacDougall MI, Moore WV. Recognition of hypertension and abnormal blood pressure burden with ambulatory blood pressure recordings in type 1 diabetes mellitus. Diabetes 1990; 39: 1556-1560.
43. Almdal T, Norgaard K, Feldt-Rasmussen B, Deckert T. The predictive value of microalbuminuria in IDDM: a five year follow-up study. Diabetes Care 1994; 17: 120-125.
44. Fogari R, Zoppi A, Malamani GD, Lazzeri P, Albonico B, Corradi L. Urinary albumin excretion and nocturnal blood pressure in hypertensive patients with type II diabetes mellitus. Am J Hypertens 1994; 7(9 pt1): 803-813.
45. Equiluz-Bruck S, Schnack C, Kopp HP, Schernthaner G. Non dipping of nocturnal blood pressure is related to urinary albumin excretion rate in patients with type 2 diabetes mellitus. Am J Hypertens 1996; 9: 1139-1143.
46. Poulsen PL, Hansen KW, Mogensen CE. Ambulatory blood pressure and abnormal albuminuria in type 1 diabetic patients. Kidney Int 1994; 45: S34-S40.

47. Nosadini R, Cipollina MR, Solini A, Sambataro M, Morocutti A, Doria A, Fioretto P, Brocco E, Muollo B, Frigato F. Close relationship between microalbuminuria and insulin resistance in essential hypertension and non-insulin-dependent diabetes mellitus. J Am Soc Nephrol 1992; 3: S56-S63.
48. Pontremoli R, Sofia A, Ravera M, Nicoletta C, Viazzi F, Tirotta A, Ruello N, Tomolillo C, Castello C, Grillo G, Sacchi G, DeFerrari G. Prevalence and clinical correlates of microalbuminuria in essential hypertension: The MAGIC Study. Microalbuminuria: A Genoa Investigation on complications. Hypertension 1997; 30: 1135-1143.
49. Mimran A, Ribstein J, DuCailar G. Is microalbuminuria a marker of early intrarenal vascular dysfunction in essential hyperfunction? Hypertension 1994; 23 (part 2): 1018-1021.
50. Bigazzi R, Bianchi S, Nenci R, Baldari D, Baldari G, Campese VM. Increased thickness of the carotid artery in patients with essential hypertension and microalbuminuria. J Hum Hypertens 1995; 9: 827-833.
51. Metcalf PA, Baker JR, Scragg RK, Dryson E, Scott AJ, Wild CJ. Dietary nutrients intake and microalbuminuria in people at least 40 years old. Clin Chem 1993; 39:2191-2198.
52. Basdevant A, Cassuto D, Gibault T, Raison J, Guy-Grand B. Microalbuminuria and body fat distribution in obese subjects. Int J Obes Relat Metab Disord 1994; 18: 806-811.
53. Haffner SM, Stem MP, Gruber KK, Hazuda HP, Mitchell BD, Patterson JK. Microalbuminuria. A marker for increased cardiovascular risk factors in non-diabetic subjects? Arteriosclerosis 1990; 10: 727-31.
54. Kaysen GA, Hyperlipidemia of the nephrotic syndrome. Kidney Int 1991; 3 (suppl 31): S8-S15.
55. Keane WF, Peter JV, Kasiske BL. Is the aggressive management of hyperlipidemia in nephrotic syndrome mandatory? Kidney Int 1992; 42 (suppl 38): S134-S141.
56. Newmark SR, Anderson CF, Donadio JV, Ellefson RD. Lipoprotein profiles in adult nephrotics. Mayo Clin Proc 1975; 50: 359-366.
57. Thomas ME, Freestone AL, Persaud JW, Varghese Z, Moorhead JF. Raised lipoprotein(a) [Lp(a)] levels in proteinuric patients. J Am Soc Nephrol 1990; 1: 344A.
58. Karådi I, Romics L, Pålos G, Domån J, Kaszås I, Hesz A, Kostner GM. Lp(a) lipoprotein concentration in serum of patients with heavy proteinuria of different origin. Clin Chem 1989, 10: 2121-2123.
59. Jenkins AJ, Steel JS, Janus ED, Best JD. Increased plasma apoprotein(a) levels in IDDM patients with microalbuminuria. Diabetes 1991; 40: 787-790.
60. Kapelrud H, Bangstad HJ, Dahl-Jorgensen K, Berg K, Hanssen KF. Serum Lp(a) lipoprotein concentrations in insulin-dependent diabetic patients with microalbuminuria. Brit Med J 1991; 303: 675-678.
61. Kannel WB, Castelli WP, Gordon T. Cholesterol in the prediction of atherosclerosis disease. New perspectives based on the Framingham Study. Ann Intern Med 1979; 90: 85-91.
62. Gordon T, Kannel WB, Castelli WP, Dawber TR. Lipoproteins, cardiovascular disease and death. The Framingham Study. Arch Intern Med 1981; 141: 1128-1131.
63. Scanu AM. lipoprotein(a): a genetic risk factor for premature coronary heart disease. JAMA 1992; 267: 3326-3329.
64. Willeit J, Kiechl S, Santer P, Oberhollenzer F, Egger G, Jarosch E, Mair A. Lipoprotein (a) and asymtomatic carotid artery disease. Evidence of a prominent role in the evolution of advanced carotid plaques: the Bruneck Study. Stroke 1995; 26: 1582-1587.
65. Keane WF. Lipids and the kidney. Kidney Int 1994; 46: 910-920.
66. Keane WF, Kasiske BL, O'Donnel MP, Kim Y. Hypertension, hyperlipidemia and renal damage. Am J Kidney Dis 1993; 21 (suppl 2): 43-50.
67. Mulec H, Johnson SA, Bjorck S. Relationship between serum cholesterol and diabetic nephropathy. Lancet 1990; i: 1537-1538.
68. Tolins JP, Stone BG, Raij L. Interactions of hypercholesterolemia and hypertension in initiation of glomerular injury. Kidney Int 1992; 41: 1254-1261.
69. Keane WF, Mulcahy WS, Kasiske BL, Kim Y, O'Donnell MP. Hyperlipidemia and progressive renal disease. Kidney Int 1991; 39 (suppl 31): S41-S48.
70. Klahr S, Schreiner G, Ichikawa I. The progression of renal disease. New Engl J Med 1988; 318: 1657-1666.
71. Alderson LM, Endemann G, Lindsey S, Pronczuk A, Hoover RL, Hayes KC. LDL enhances monocyte adhesion to endothelial cells in vitro. Am J Pathol 1986; 123: 334-342.

72. Ferrannini E, Buzzigoli g, Bonadonna R, Giorico MA, Oleggini M, Graziadei L, Pedrinelli R, Brandi L, Bevilacqua S. Insulin resistance in essential hypertension. N Engl J Med 1987; 317: 350-357.
73. Swislocki AL, Hoffman BB, Reaven GM. Insulin resistance, glucose intolerance and hyperinsulinemia in patients with hypertension. Am J Hypertens 1989; 2: 419-423.
74. Fuller JH, Shipley MJ, Rose G, Jarret RJ, Keen H. Coronary heart disease risk and impaired glucose tolerance. The Whitehall Study. Lancet 1880; i: 1373-1376,
75. Stern MP, Haffner SM. Body fat distribution and hyperinsulinemia as risk factors for diabetes and cardiovascular disease. Arteriosclerosis 1986; 6: 123-130.
76. Zavaroni I, Bonora E, Pagliara M, Dall'Aglio E, Luchetti L, Buonanno G, Bonati PA, Bergonzani M, Gnudi L, Passeri M, Reaven G. Risk factors for coronary artery disease in healthy persons with hyperinsulinemia and normal glucose tolerance. N Engl J Med 1989; 320: 702-706.
77. Bianchi S, Bigazzi R, Valtriani C, Chiapponi I, Sgherri G, Baldari G, Natali A, Ferrannini E Campese VM. Elevated serum insulin levels in patients with essential hypertension and microalbuminuria. Hypertension 1994; 23: 681-687.
78. Bianchi S, Bigazzi R, Quinones Galvan A, Muscelli E, Baldari G, Pecori N, Ciociaro D, Ferranini E, Natali A. Insulin resistance in microalbuminuric hypertension: sites and mechanism. Hypertension 1995; 26: 789-795.
79. Shulman GI, Landerson PW, Wolfe MH, Ridway EC, Wolfe RR. Quantitation of muscle glycogen synthesis in normal subjects and subjects with non-insulin-dependent diabetes by 13C nuclear magnetic resonance spectroscopy. N Eng J Med 1990; 322: 223-228.
80. Felber JP, Ferranini E, Golay A, Meyer HU, Theibaud D, Churcod B, Maeder E, Jequier E, DeFronzo A. Role of lipid oxidation in pathogenesis of insulin resistance of obesity and type II diabetes. Diabetes 1987; 36: 1341-1350.
81. Woo J, Cockram CS, Swaminathan R, Lau E, Chan A, Cheung R. Microalbuminuria and other cardiovascular risk factors in nondiabetic subjects. Int J Cardiol 1992; 37: 345-350.
82. Doria A, Fioretto P, Avogaro A, Carraro A, Morocutti A, Trevisan R, Frigato F, Crepaldi G, Viberti GC, Nosadini R. Insulin resistance is associated with high sodium-lithium countertransport in essential hypertension. Am J Physiol 1991; 261: 684-691.
83. Nosadini R, Semplicini A, Fioretto P, Lusiani L, Trevisan R, Donadon V, Zanette G, Nicolosi GL, dall'Aglio V, Zanuttini D, Viberti GC. Sodium-lithium countertransport and cardiorenal abnormalities in essential hypertension. Hypertension 1991; 18: 191-198.
84. Falkner B, Kushner H, Levison S, Canessa M. Albuminuria in association with insulin and sodium-lithium countertransport in young African americans with borderline hypertension. Hypertension 1995; 25: 1315-1321.
85. Yip J, Mattock MB, Morocutti A, Sethi M, Trevisan R, Viberti G. Insulin resistance in insulin-dependent diabetic patients with microalbuminuria. Lancet 1993; 342: 883-887.
86. Groop L, Ekstrand A, Forsblom C, Widen E, Groop P-H, Teppo A-M, Eriksson J. Insulin resistance, hypertension and microalbuminuria in patients with type 2 (non-insulin-dependent) diabetes mellitus. Diabetologia 1993; 36: 642-647.
87. Niskanen L, Laakso M. Insulin resistance is related to albuminuria in patients with type II (non-insulin-dependent) diabetes mellitus. Metabolism 1993; 42: 1541-1545.
88. Ferrari P, Weidmann P, Shaw S, Giachino D, Riesen W, Alleman Y, Heynen G. Altered insulin sensitivity hyperinsulinemia and dyslipidemia in individuals with a hypertensive parent. Am J Med 1991; 91: 589-596.
89. Grunfeld B, Balzareti M, Romo M, Gimenez M, Gutman R. hyperinsulinemia in normotensive offspring of hypertensive parents. Hypertension 1994; 231 (suppl 1): I12-I15.
90. Ross R. The pathology of artherosclerosis: an update. N Engl J Med 1986; 314: 488-500.
91. Cruz AB, Amaturzio DS, Grande F, Hay LJ. Effect of intraarterial insulin on tissue cholesterol and fatty acids in alloxan diabetic dogs. Circ. Res 1961; 9: 39-43.
92. Capron L, Jamet J, Kazandjian S, Housset E. Growth promoting effects of diabetes and insulin on arteries. Diabetes 1988; 35: 973-978.
93. Oppenheumer MJ, Sundquist K, Bierman EL. Down-regulation of high-density lipoprotein receptor in human fibroblats by insulin and IGF-I. Diabetes 1989; 38: 117-122.
94. Krone W, Greten H. Evidence for post-transcriptional regulation by insulin of 3 Hydroxy-3-methylglutaryl coenzyme. A reductase and sterol synthesis in human mononuclear leucocytes. Diabetologia 1984; 26: 366-369.
95. Sholey JW, Meyer TW. Control of glomerular hypertension by insulin administration in diabetic rats. J Clin Invest 1989; 83: 1384-89.

96. DeFronzo RA, Cooke CR, Andres R, Faloona GR, David PJ. The effect of insulin on renal handling of sodium, potassium, calcium and phosphate in man. J Clin Invest 1975; 55: 845-855.
97. Baum M. Insulin stimulates volume absorption in the proximal convoluted tubule. J Clin Invest 1987; 56: 335-340.
98. Christensen NJ, Gundersen HJG, Hegedus L, Jacobsen F, Mogensen CE, Osterby R, Vittinghus E. Acute effects of insulin on plasma noradrenaline and the cardiovascular system. Metabolism 1980; 29: 1138-1145.
99. Rowe JW, Young JB, Minaker KL, Stevens AL, Pallotta J, Landsberg L. Effect of insulin and glucose infusions on sympathetic nervous system activity in normal man. Diabetes 1981; 30: 219-225.
100. Bigazzi R, Bianchi S, Baldari D, Sgherri G, Baldari G, Campese VM. Microalbuminuria in salt-sensitive patients: a marker for renal and cardiovascular risk factors. Hypertension 1994; 23: 195-199.
101. Hilsted J, Christensen NJ. Dual effect of insulin on plasma volume and trancapillary albumin transport. Diabetologia 1992; 35: 99-103.
102. Mogensen CE, Christensen NJ, Gundersen HJG. The acute effects of insulin on hearth rate, blood pressure, plasma noradrenaline and urinary albumin excretion. Diabetologia 1980; 18: 453-457.
103. Norgaard K, Jensen T, Feldt-Rasmussen B. Transcapillary escape rate of albumin in hypertensive patients with type 1 (insulin-dependent) diabetes mellitus. Diabetologia 1993; 36: 57-61.
104. Feldt-Rasmussen B. Increased transcapillary escape of albumin in type 1 (insulin-dependent) diabetic patients with microalbuminuria. Diabetologia 1986; 29: 282-286.
105. Nannipieri M, Rizzo L, Rapuano A, Pilo A, Penno G, Navalesi R. Increased transcapillary escape of albumin in microalbuminuric type II diabetic patients. Diabetes Care 1995; 18:1-9.
106. Jensen JS. Renal and systemic transvascular albumin leakage in severe atherosclerosis. Arterioscler Thromb Vasc Biol 1995; 15: 1324-1329.
107. Parving H-H, Jensen HE, Westrup M. Increased transcapillary escape rate of albumin and IgG in essential hypertension. Scand J Lab Invest 1977; 37: 223-227.
108. Jensen JS, Borck-Johnsen K, Jensen J, Feldt-Rasmussen B. microalbuminuria reflects a generalized transvascular albumin leakness in clinically healthy subjects. Clin Sci 1995; 88: 629-633.
109. Nestler JE, Barlascini GO, Tetrault GA, Fratkin MJ, Clore JN, Blackard. Increased transcapillary escape of albumin in nondiabetic men in response to hyperinsulinemia. Diabetes 1990; 39: 1212-1217.
110. Elliot TG, Cockroft JR, Groop PH, Viberti GC, Ritter JM. Inhibition of nitric oxide synthesis in forearm vasculature of insulin-dependent diabetic patients; blunted vasocontriction in patients with microalbuminuria. Clin Sci 1993; 83: 687-693.
111. Stehouwer CDA, Nauta JJP, Zeldenrust GC, Hackeng WHL, Donker AJM, den Ottolander GJH. Urinary albumin excretion, cardiovascular disease, and endothelial dysfunction in non-insulin-dependent diabetes mellitus. Lancet 1992; 340: 319-323.
112. Stehouwer CDA, Zellenrath P, Polak BCP, Baarsma GS, Nauta JJP, Donker AJM, den Ottolander GJH. von Willebrand factor and development of diabetic nephropathy in insulin-dependent diabetes mellitus. Diabetes 1991; 40: 971-976.
113. Chen JW, Gall MA, Deckert M, Jensen JS, Parving H-H. Increased serum concentration of von Willebrand factor in non-insulin-dependent diabetics with and without diabetic nephropathy. J Am Soc Nephrol 1995; 3: 447.
114. Stehouwer CDA, Fisher HR, van Kuijk AW, Polak BC, Donker AJ. Endothelial dysfunction precedes development of microalbuminuria in IDDM. Diabetes 1995; 44:561-564.
115. Pedrinelli R, Giampietro O, Carmassi F, Melillo E, Dell'Omo G, Catapano G, Matteucci E, Talarico R, Morale M, De Negri F, Di Bello V. Microalbuminuria and endothelial dysfunction in essential hypertension. Lancet 1994; 344: 14-18.
116. Redon J, Gomez-Sanchez MA, Baldo E, Casal MC, Fernandez ML, Miralles A, Gomez-Pajuelo C, Rodicio JL, Ruilope LM. microalbuminuria is correlated with left ventricular hypertrophy in male hypertensive patients. J Hypertens 1991; 9 (suppl 6): S148-S149.
117. Pedrinelli R, Bello VD, Catapano G, Talarico L, Materazzi F, Santoro G, Giusti C, Mosca F, Melillo E, Ferrari M. Microalbuminuria is a marker of left ventricular hypertrophy but not hyperinsulinemia in non diabetic atherosclerotic patients. Arteriosclerosis and Thrombosis 1993; 13: 900-906.
118. Agewall S, Persson B, Samuelsson O, Ljunman S, Herlitz H, Fageberg B. Microalbuminuria in treated hypertensive men at high risk of coronary disease. The Risk Factor Intervention Study Group. J Hypertens 1993; 11: 461-469.

119. Horton RC, Gosling P, Reeves CN, Payne M, Nagle RE. Microalbumin excretion in patients with positive exercise electrocardiogram tests. Eur Heart J 1994; 15: 1353-1355.
120. Cerasola D, Cottone S, D'Ignoto G, Grasso L, Mangano MT, Carapelle E, Nardi E, Andronico G, Fulantelli MA, Marcellino T, Seddio G. Microalbuminuria as a predictor of cardiovascular damage in essential hypertension. J Hypertens 1989; 7(suppl 6): S332-333.
121. Salonen JT, Salonen R. Ultrasonographically assessed carotid morphology and the risk of coronary heart disease. Aterioscleerosis and Thrombosis 1991; 11: 1245-1249.
122. Yudkin JS, Forrest RD, Jackson CA. Microalbuminuria as predictor of vascular disease in non-diabetic subjects. Islington Diabetes Survey. Lancet 1988 ii: 530-83.
123. Kuusisto J, Mykkanen L, Pyorealea K, Laakso M. Hyperinsulinemic microalbuminuria. A new risk indicator for coronary heart disease. Circulation 1995; 9: 831-837.
124. Bigazzi R, Bianchi S, Baldari G, Vito M Campese. Microalbuminuria in patients with hypertension predicts cardiovascular and renal events. Am J Hypertens 1997; 10 (part 2): 78A.
125. Schmieder RE, Veelken R, Gatzka CD, Ruddel H, Schachinger H. Predictors for hypertensive nephropathy: results of a 6-year follow-up study in essential hypertension. J Hypertens 1994; 13: 357-365.
126. Ruilope LM, Campo C, Rodriguez-Artalejo F, Lahera V, Garcia Robles R, Rodicio JL. Blood pressure and renal function: therapeutic implications. J Hypertens 1996; 14: 1259-1263.
127. Chrisensen CK. Rapidly reversible albumin and B_2-microglobulin hyperexcretion in recent severe essential hypertension. J Hypertens 1983; 1: 45-51.
128. Erley CM, Haefele U, Heyne N, Braun N, Risler T. Microalbuminuria in essential hypertension. Reduction by different antihypertensive drugs. Hypertension 1993; 21: 810-815.
129. Laville M, Doche C, Fauvel JP, Pozet N, Hadj-Aissa A, Zech P. Effect of beta-blockade on albumin excretion rate in essential hypertension. Nephron 1990; 54: 183-184.
130. Hartford M, Wendelhag I, Berglund G, Wallentin I, Ljungman S, Wikstrand J. Cardiovascular and renal effects of long-term antihypertensive treatment. JAMA 1988; 259: 2553-2557.
131. Schmieder RE, Ruddel H, Schlebusch H, Rockstroh J, Schachinger H, Schulte W. Impact of antihypertensive therapy with isradipine and metoprolol on early markers of hypertensive nephropathy. Am J Hypertens 1992; 5: 318-321.
132. Persson B, Andersson OK, Wysocki M, Hedner T, Karlberg B. Calcium antagonism in essential hypertension: effect on renal hemodynamics and microalbuminuria. J Intern Med 1992; 213: 247-252.
133. Ruilope LM, Lahera V, Alcazar JM, Praga M, Campo C, Rodicio JL. Randomly allocated study of the effects of standard therapy versus ACE inhibition on microalbuminuria in essential hypertension. J Hypertens 1994; 12: S59-S63.
134. Krusell LR, Chrisensen CK, Lederballe-Pedersen O. Renal effects of pinacidil in hypertensive patients on chronic beta-blocker therapy. Eur J Clin pharmacol 1986; 30: 641-647.
135. De Venuto G, Andreotti C, Mattarei M, Pegoretti G. Long-term captopril therapy at low doses reduces albumin excretion in patients with essential hypertension and no sign of renal impairment. J Hypertens 1985; 3: S143-S145.
136. Bianchi S, Bigazzi R, Baldari G, Campese VM. Microalbuminuria in patients with essential hypertension. Effects of an angiotensin converting enzyme inhibitor and of a calcium channel blocker. Am J Hypertens 1991; 4: 291-296.
137. Bianchi S, Bigazzi R, Baldari G, Campese VM. Microalbuminuria in patients with essential hypertension. Effects of several antihypertensive drugs. Am J Med; 93;525-528.
138. Bigazzi R, Bianchi S, Baldari D, Sgherri G, Baldari G, Campese VM. Long-term effects of a converting enzyme inhibitor and a calcium channel blocker on urinary albumin excretion in patients with essential hypertension. Am J Hypertens 1993; 6: 108-113.
139. Hermans MP, Brichard SM, Colin I, Borgies P, Ketelslegers JM, Lambert AE. Long-term reduction of microalbuminuria after 3 years of angiotensin-converting-enzyme inhibition by perindopril in hypertensive insulin-treated diabetic patients. Am J Med 1992: 92: S102-S107.
140. Reams GP, Lau A, Knaus V, Bauer JH. Short and long term effects of spirapril on renal hemodynamics in patients with essential hypertension. J Clin Pharmacol 1993; 33: 348-353.
141. Puig JG, Mateos FA, Ramos TH, Lavilla MP, Capitan MC, Gil A. Albumin excretion rate and metabolic modifications in patients with essential hypertension. Effects of two angiotensin converting enzyme inhibitors. Am J Hypertens 1994; 7: 46-51.
142. Domingues LJ, Barbagallo M, Kattah W, Garcia D, Sowers J. Quinapril reduces microalbuminuria in essential hypertension and in diabetic hypertensive subjects. Am J Hypertens 1995; 8: 808-814.

143. Heeg JE, DeJong PE, van der Hem GK, de Zeeuw D. Reduction of proteinuria by converting enzyme inhibition. Kidney Int 1989; 36: 272-279.

54. A COMPARISON OF PROGRESSION IN DIABETIC AND NON-DIABETIC RENAL DISEASE: SIMILARITY OF PROGRESSION PROMOTERS

Gerjan Navis, Paul E. De Jong, Dick De Zeeuw.
Department of Internal Medicine, Division of Nephrology and Department of Clinical Pharmacology, State University, Groningen, The Netherlands.

The prevention of progressive renal function loss remains the major challenge for nephrologists today. Traditionally the progressive nature of renal function loss was attributed to the underlying disease, with a major role for hypertension [1]. The hypothesis, however, that common mechanisms account for the progressive renal function loss in many different renal conditions regardless the nature of initial renal damage[2] was fueled by several observations. These include the linear renal function deterioration that occurs in many patients regardless their initial renal disease [3], as well as the similarity in histopathological abnormalities in end-stage kidneys with different underlying diseases. Systemic [4] and glomerular [5] hypertension, proteinuria [6] and lipid abnormalities [7] are assumed to be common mediators in the pathogenesis of focal segmental glomerulosclerosis, the alleged final common pathway of progressive renal disease [8]. Here we will briefly review current knowledge on progressive renal function loss in human diabetic and non-diabetic renal disease and on the response to intervention treatment. As to diabetic patients we will, for the sake of brevity, mainly focus on patients with type I (insulin-dependent) diabetes. We will specifically address the question whether current clinical evidence supports the hypothesis that common mechanisms underlie progressive renal function loss in diabetic and non-diabetic renal disease; this will help to devise future prevention strategies.

NATURAL HISTORY

The assessment of progression rate

As progression to end stage renal failure usually takes many years, it is not surprising that few studies provide data in terms of hard end points such as end stage renal failure or death. In view of the constant rate of renal function loss in many patients, the rate of decline of GFR is usually considered a useful surrogate end point [9], provided it is measured with accuracy, taking into account the methods of measurement, and the frequency and duration of follow-up in relation to the rate of decline [10,11].

The use of progression rate as a surrogate end point, however, entails several pitfalls. The unreliability of creatinine-derived indices has recently extensively been reviewed [12]. When progression rate is used as a surrogate end point, moreover, it should be kept in mind that the assumption of linear deterioration of renal function may not always be true. Whereas in patients with nephropathy due to IDDM, linear progression appears to be the rule [13], among patients with non-diabetic renal disease [6, 14] or with NIDDM [15] considerable subpopulations (up to one-fifth or a quarter of the patients) may have stable renal function, or non-linear progression. Such a heterogeneity in patient populations might partly explain the difficulties in reproducing clear-cut renoprotective effects obtained by specific treatment modalities in experimental animals, in particular for nondiabetic renal disease [10,16].

THE INITIATION OF RENAL DAMAGE

In diabetic nephropathy the natural history is relatively well-characterized, as, contrary to non-diabetic renal disease, most patients come to medical attention years before renal abnormalities develop. It is still not understood why some 30 to 40 per cent of diabetic patients develop nephropathy whereas others don't; familial clustering, however, suggests genetically determined susceptibility [17]. In patients in whom nephropathy occurs, a typical, biphasic clinical course of renal function has been demonstrated, with elevated glomerular filtration rate in the early stages, followed by micro-albuminuria [9]. The elevated GFR presumably reflects glomerular hypertension, due to afferent arteriolar dysfunction with increased transmission of systemic blood pressure to glomerular capillaries. Glomerular hypertension, leading to glomerular capillary damage and protein leakage is thought to play an important role in the initiation and perpetuation of renal damage in these patients [18,19]. The transition from normoalbuminuria to microalbuminuria is associated with a slight increase in systemic blood pressure [20]. When micro-albuminuria progresses to overt proteinuria, usually in association with a further rise in arterial blood pressure, glomerular filtration rate decreases, and gradual progression to end-stage renal failure occurs, albeit with large interindividual differences in progression rate [9,13].

In non-diabetic renal disease the factors that initiate renal damage are of a heterogeneous nature, and can include primarily glomerular or vascular, or tubulo-interstitial damage. Little is known about possible factors preceding the development of non-diabetic renal disease, as by the time patients come to medical attention overt renal damage is usually present. Patients with hypertension may form an exception to this rule. Remarkably, microalbuminuria [21] as well as glomerular hyperfiltration [22], the two hallmarks of incipient diabetic nephropathy, can be found in subsets of patients with essential hypertension. Although for this category of patients the prognostic value of microalbuminuria and glomerular hyperfiltration for long term renal function is poorly defined, these findings nevertheless suggest that similar pathways of early renal damage may be involved in hypertension and in diabetes. For primary glomerular or tubulo-interstitial disorders, such data are lacking altogether.

If long-term renal function loss is determined by common perpetuating factors one would expect progression of renal function loss to be more or less similar in different renal disorders. Whether or not the underlying disease determines progression rate, however, remains controversial. Some studies found no effect of underlying disease on progression rate [3,23] but in many other studies progression was related to the diagnostic category. In those studies, glomerulonephritis and diabetic nephropathy invariably had a faster progression rate than chronic pyelonephritis, analgesic nephropathy or hypertensive nephrosclerosis [6,24,25,26,27,28,29]. In most studies, polycystic kidney disease is associated with a faster progression rate as well [14,26,29,30,31] although this is not a uniform finding [6, 24]. Current evidence, therefore, seems to indicate that the nature of the underlying disease is not indifferent to the long-term course of renal function. Of note, in conditions where the primary cause of damage can be reliably eliminated (such as obstructive uropathy, analgesic abuse, or primary hypertension) the course of renal function is more favorable than in conditions where the initiating factors cannot (or not reliably) be annihilated (such as diabetic nephropathy, glomerulonephritis, or polycystic kidney disease). This suggests that either primary causes still exert effect, or that they trigger the alleged common perpetuating factors to a greater extent than other conditions.

COMMON PROGRESSION PROMOTERS

In diabetic as well as non-diabetic populations [3] considerable interindividual variability is apparent in the rate of renal function loss for any given disease. Many studies investigated the determinants of this variability (see also Table 54-1), thus attempting to assess the clinical relevance of common progression promoters identified in experimental renal disease, such as systemic and glomerular hypertension, proteinuria and lipid abnormalities. In the interpretation of these studies, however, the close interaction of these factors as to their effects on long-term renal function [2] should be kept in mind. As a consequence, their respective contributions are often hard to dissect.

In both diabetic and non-diabetic renal disease [6,26,30,31,32] the severity of proteinuria is a predictive factor for progression rate. Interestingly, Wight [30] showed that differences in progression rate between most renal conditions were no longer apparent after correction for proteinuria (with the sole exception of polycystic kidney disease). Moreover, the association between proteinuria and progression not only occurs in conditions where proteinuria might reflect activity of the primary glomerular disorder, such as diabetic nephropathy and glomerulonephritis, but also in chronic pyelonephritis [6]. Taken together, this evidence strongly suggests that, once a certain renal disorder is present, the severity of proteinuria rather than the underlying disorder per se predicts renal outcome. The case of polycystic kidney disease [33,34] however, illustrates that disease-specific mechanisms may predominate over common mechanisms in some conditions.

As to hypertension, in IDDM the development of hypertension is closely associated with transition from normoalbuminuria to microalbuminuria [20] and subsequently with further progression to overt proteinuria and progressive renal function loss [35,36,37] .

Table 54-1. Clinical characteristics of progressive renal function loss in diabetic and non-diabetic renal disease

	diabetic nephropathy	*non-diabetic nephropathy*
	natural history	
renal function loss	invariably progressive	progressive in many patients
predictors of progression	diabetes control proteinuria blood pressure cholesterol DD genotype ACE gene	underlying disease proteinuria blood pressure cholesterol DD genotype ACE gene
	prevention of progressive renal function loss	
protein restriction	probably effective	effective
antihypertensive therapy	effective	effective; benefit proportional to severity of proteinuria.
predictors renoprotection	initial antiproteinuric effect initial renal hemodynamic effect	initial antiproteinuric effect initial renal hemodynamic effect
	response to specific renoprotective drugs	
ACE inhibitors	reduce proteinuria reduce progression rate independent from blood pressure effect??	reduce proteinuria reduce progression rate independent from blood pressure effect??
non-ACE inhibitor antihypertensives	reduce proteinuria in a strongly pressure-dependent fashion	slight, pressure-dependent effect on proteinuria

In non-diabetic renal disease as well, high blood pressure is usually associated with a poor renal outcome [23,26,30,31], and moreover, the antihypertensive response to treatment is associated with reduction of the rate of renal function loss, as discussed below [4]. Moreover, blood pressure was a strong predictor for end stage renal failure in the large MRFIT cohort [38]. Yet, somewhat surprisingly, several studies in renal patients failed to demonstrate that blood pressure was an independent determinant of progression rate [6,25,26]. In these studies, however, proteinuria and blood pressure were closely related and a predominant effect of proteinuria might obscure the role of a co-linear factor such as blood pressure.

In both diabetic and non-diabetic renal disease lipid profile affects progression rate; an elevated serum cholesterol is associated with a faster progression rate in several studies [39,40].

Interestingly, recent studies identified a genetic factor, that is, an insertion/deletion polymorphism for the ACE-gene, to be an important determinant of the rate of renal function loss in patients with nondiabetic renal disease [41] as well as diabetic nephropathy [42] with an increased rate of renal function loss in patients homozygous for the D-allele. The mechanism of the increased renal risk in DD homozygotes is still unknown; in particular it is still unsure whether the ACE genotype is a mere marker of increased renal risk or whether it may play a causal role. Higher serum and tissue ACE-levels are present in DD-homozygotes, and there is some evidence suggesting that the D allele can be associated with a blunted response to ACE-inhibition in diabetic nephropathy [43,44] as well as non-diabetic proteinuric patients [45]. As other reports, however, yielded conflicting results [46], this issue awaits further clarification by prospective studies.

RESPONSE TO RENOPROTECTIVE TREATMENT

As a matter of clinical common sense, renoprotective treatment should, first, aim at eliminating primary damaging factors. This may halt progression in some patients with specific disorders, such as obstructive uropathy [6] and analgesic nephropathy [47] . In diabetes, strict metabolic control can reverse early hyperfiltration, and retard the progression of renal function loss [48]. Progressive renal function loss in the large proportion of patients in whom the initial cause of renal damage is no longer present [3] however, prompted the development of additional treatment strategies aimed at intervention with factors thought to be involved in the alleged final common pathway for progressive renal function loss; i.e, systemic and glomerular pressure, proteinuria and lipid abnormalities.

Research has mainly focussed on two intervention strategies: antihypertensive treatment and reduction of protein intake. Reduction of blood pressure is considered the cornerstone of therapy for renal patients: it effectively slows renal function loss in diabetic [49] and in non-diabetic renal disease [4,23] (Table 54-1). Restriction of dietary protein intake has elicited extensive discussion over the last decades as to its efficacy and feasibility, but recent analyses have shown that a low protein intake indeed is associated with a reduction in the rate of renal function loss in both diabetic and non-diabetic renal patients [50,51].

Short-term responses to renoprotective therapy are of interest to see whether they are prognostic for long-term protection. If so, this may not only help to titrate therapy but also to unravel the mechanisms of renoprotection. Indeed, such predictive responses have been identified. The magnitude of the early renal hemodynamic response (i.e a slight drop in GFR that may reflect a fall in glomerular hydostatic pressure) to renoprotective intervention be it antihypertensive treatment [52] or a low protein diet appears to predict the long term course of renal function [53]. Likewise, the efficacy of the initial antiproteinuric effect predicts the course of long term renal function in both diabetic [54] and non-diabetic nephropathy [55,56,57]. With the notable exception of the MDRD study [58], the reduction in blood pressure did not predict the subsequent course of renal function. This supports the hypothesis that specific renal effects, such as a reduction in proteinuria, are causally involved in long-term renoprotection [8].

The question whether ACE-inhibitors, by virtue of specific renal effects, offer better renoprotection than other antihypertensives has been subject of many studies. These were motivated by findings in experimental animals that ACE-inhibition protects against progressive renal damage not only by reducing systemic blood pressure, but also by a fall in glomerular capillary pressure [18] and in proteinuria. In man, renoprotective properties of ACE inhibitors beyond reduction of blood pressure are for instance suggested by studies in normotensive diabetic patients where treatment with ACE inhibition was able to reverse microalbuminuria [59] and to prevent progression to overt proteinuria [60], in the absence of a blood pressure effect. In overt diabetic nephropathy as well as non-diabetic renal disease ACE inhibitors can reduce proteinuria [61,62,63], progression rate [64] and the risk to reach end stage renal failure or death [65,66,67]. Moreover, ACEi provided more effective long-term renoprotection than control antihypertensives in several studies in diabetic and non-diabetic patients [68,69]. Blood pressure effects, however, may explain the differences in long term renoprotection, as in these studies ACE inhibition generally induced more effective blood pressure reduction than the control regimens [69]. Some studies in non-diabetic patients, however, failed to demonstrate an advantage of ACE inhibitors over control antihypertensives [69,70]. Patient selection may be involved in the discrepancies between different comparative trials, as the advantage of ACE inhibitors over other antihypertensives appeared to be most readily apparent in patients with a rapid progression rate associated with proteinuria, that is, in patients with diabetic nephropathy and in non-diabetic patients with overt proteinuria [71]. In fact, the advantage of the ACE-inhibitor has been found to be proportional to the severity of pre-treatment proteinuria [56]. Taken together with the predictive value of the antiproteinuric response for long term renoprotection, this suggests that the antiproteinuric effect may be pivotal in providing renoprotection.

The antiproteinuric efficacy of ACE inhibitors versus other antihypertensives in diabetic and non-diabetic renal patients has been subject of several reviews [72,73,74]. From these analyses some interesting inferences emerge. First, the meta-analyses confirmed the notion that the antiproteinuric effect of ACE inhibitors cannot solely be accounted for by their effect on blood pressure. Second, it was shown that non-ACE inhibitor antihypertensives, with the exception of nifedipine, also lower proteinuria (albeit to a lesser extent than ACE-inhibitors) provided a pronounced fall in blood pressure is achieved. Finally, it was shown that this blood pressure-related fall in proteinuria with non-ACE inhibitor therapy was more pronounced in diabetic patients than in non-diabetic patients. This is consistent with the hypothesis that in diabetic nephropathy, due to afferent arteriolar dysfunction, increased transmission of systemic blood pressure to the glomerular capillary bed plays an important role in abnormal glomerular hemodynamics and protein leakage.

Interestingly, in large scale trials in non-diabetic patients the long- term benefit of lower blood pressure (whether or not achieved with ACE inhibitors) on renal function was more pronounced in proteinuric patients [58,65,75]. Thus, like diabetic patients (in whom proteinuria is the hallmark of renal involvement), proteinuric patients with non-diabetic renal disease display greater renal sensitivity to the effect of elevated systemic blood pressure than their non-proteinuric counterparts. Whether this similarity simply reflects the long-term benefits of reduction of proteinuria secondary to the lower blood pressure, or whether proteinuria is a marker (or even a mediator) of the susceptibility of the glomerular vascular bed to hypertensive damage is as yet unknown.

CONCLUSIONS AND IMPLICATIONS FOR RENOPROTECTIVE TREATMENT

From the studies summarized here it appears that promoters for progression in patients with diabetic and non-diabetic nephropathy are more or less similar. Moreover, predictors for efficacy of long-term renoprotective therapy are similar as well. This supports the hypothesis that common mechanisms underlie progressive renal function loss in diabetic and many non-diabetic renal patients, with the possible exception of specific diagnostic categories, such as polycystic kidneys [34], where disease-specific mechanisms may be the main determinants of progression. The similarities are readily apparent for patients with proteinuria, supporting the assumption that proteinuria is pivotal in the alleged common mechanisms [8].

Several implications for renoprotective treatment can be derived from the studies reviewed here. First, these data suggest that to provide renoprotection in proteinuric patients (with or without diabetes) target blood pressure should be lower than in non-proteinuric patients. For diabetic patients the need for a low target blood pressure has already gained acceptance, as emphasized recently [76]. For non-diabetic proteinuric patients, data from the MDRD study demonstrated that the lowest mean arterial pressure attained ($\leq$92 mmHg, corresponding to 125/75 mmHg) provided improved renoprotection, without signs of a J-shape pattern [77]. From a renal perspective, therefore, target mean arterial blood pressure in proteinuric patients may have to be even lower than 90 mmHg. For such an aggressive approach to be feasible, short-term titration criteria predictive for long-term renoprotection are virtually indispensable.

Second, the predictive value of the antiproteinuric response to antihypertensive treatment for long-term renoprotection implicates that proteinuria is presumably a useful parameter to monitor and titrate blood pressure to a long-term renoprotective level. This may even implicate that, in proteinuric patients, reduction of proteinuria is a major, and perhaps the main target of renoprotective therapy. In fact, for diabetic patients, such an approach has been advocated in the recent recommendations to start ACE-inhibitor therapy in normotensive patients with microalbuminuria, with the purpose of preventing progression to overt nephropathy [76]. Based on current evidence, therefore, it would be of interest to evaluate the

long-term renoprotective potential of treatment strategies that target at elimination of proteinuria for non-diabetic patients as well.

REFERENCES

1. Ellis A. Natural history of Bright's disease; clinical, histological and experimental observations. The vicious circle in Bright's disease. Lancet 1942; i:72-76.
2. Klahr Sm Schreiner G, Ichikawa I. The progression of renal disease. N Engl Med 1988; 318:1657-1666.
3. Mich WE, Buffington G, Lemaan J, Walser M. Progression of renal failure: a simple method of estimation. Lancet 1976; ii:1326-1331.
4. Alvestrand A, Gutierrez A, Bucht H, Bergström J. Reduction of blood pressure retards the progression of chronic renal failure in man. Nephrol Dial Transplant 1988; 3: 624-631.
5. Brenner BM, Meyer TW, Hostetter TW. Dietary protein and the progressive nature of kidney disease: role of hemodynamically mediated glomerular injury in the pathogenesis of progressive glomerular sclerosis of aging, renal ablation and intrinsic renal disease. N Engl J Med 1982; 307: 652-659.
6. Williams PS, Fass G, Bone JM. Renal pathology and proteinuria determine progression in untreated mild/moderate chronic renal failure. Quart J Med 1988; 67: 343-354.
7. Keane WF, Kasiske B, O'Donnell MP, Kin Y. The role of altered lipid metabolism in the progression of renal disease. Am J Kidney Dis 1991; 17:S38-S42.
8. Remuzzi G, Bertani T. Is glomerulosclerosis a consequence of altered glomerular permeability to macromolecules? [editorial]. Kidney Int 1990; 38:384-94.
9. Mogensen CE. Natural history and potential prevention of diabetic nephropathy in insulin-dependent and non-insulin-dependent diabetic patients. In: Prevention of progressive chronic renal failure. El Nahas A, Mallick NP, Anderson S, (eds). Oxford 1993; pp 278-279.
10. Levey AS. Measurement of renal function in chronic renal disease. Kidney Int 1990; 38:167-184.
11. Apperloo AJ, de Zeeuw D, de Jong PE. Precision of GFR determinants for long term slope calculations is improved by simultaneous infusion of ^{125}I-iothalamate and ^{131}I-Hippuran. JASN 1996; 7: 567-572.
12. Walser M, Drew HH, LaFrance LD. Creatinine measurements often yield false estimates in chronic renal failure. Kidney Int 1988; 34: 412-418.
13. Jones RH, Mackay JD, Hayakawa H, Parsons V, Watkins PJ. Progression of diabetic nephropathy. Lancet 1979; i:1105-1106.
14. Bergström J, Alvestrand A, Bucht H, Gutierrez A, Stenvinkel P. Is renal failure always progressive? Contrib Neprol 1989, 75:60-67.
15. Gall M-A, Nielsen FS, Smidt UM, Parving H-H. The course of kidney function in type 2 (non-insulin-dependent) diabetic patients with diabetic nephropathy. Diabetologia 1993; 36: 1071-1078.
16. Williams PS, Mallick NP. The natural history of chronic renal failure. In: Prevention of progressive chronic renal failure. El Nahas AM, Mallick NP, Anderson S (eds). Oxford 1993, p210-259.
17. Tarnow L. Genetic pattern in diabetic nephropathy. Nephrol Dial Transplant 1996; 11:410-412.
18. Zatz R, Meyer TW, Rennke HG, Brenner BM. Predominance of hemodynamic rather than metabolic factors in the pathogenesis of diabetic glomerulopathy. Proc Natl Acad Sci 1985; 82: 5963-5967.
19. Parving H-H, Kastrup H, Smidt UM, Andersen AR, Feldt-Rasmussen B, Sandahl Christiansen J. Impaired autoregulation of glomerular filtration rate in type 1 (insulin-dependent) diabetic patients with nephropathy. Diabetologia 1984; 27: 547- 552.
20. Poulsen PL, Hansen KW, Mogensen CE. Ambulatory blood pressure in the transition from normo- to microalbuminuria: a longitudinal study in IDDM. Diabetes 1994; 43: 1248-53.
21. Parving H-H, Jensen HE, Mogensen CE. Increased urinary albumin excretion in benign essential hypertension. Lancet 1974; 231-237.
22. du Cailar G, Ribstein J, Mimran A. Glomerular hyperfiltration and left ventricular mass in mild never-treated essential hypertension. J Hypertens 1990; 9 suppl. 6: S158-S159.

23. Brazy PC, Fitzwilliam JF. Progressive renal disease: role of race and antihypertensive medications. Kidney Int 1990; 37:1113-1119.
24. Ahlem J. Incidence of human chronic renal insufficiency. A study of the incidence and pattern of renal insufficiency in adults during 166-71 in Gothenburg. Acta Med Scand 1975; suppl 582:1-50.
25. Stenvinkel P, Alvestrand A, Bergström J. Factors influencing progression in patients with chronic renal failure. J Int Med 1989; 226: 183-188.
26. Locatelli F, Marcelli D, Comelli M, Alberti D, Graziani G, Buccianti G, Redaelli B, Giangrande A et al. Proteinuria and blood pressure as causal components of progression to end-stage renal failure. Nephrol Dial Transplant 1996; 11;461-67.
27. Rutherford WE, Blondin J, Miller JP,Greenwalt AS, Vavra JD. Chronic progressive renal disease: rate of change of serum creatinine concentration. Kidney Int 1977; 11: 62-70.
28. Hannedouche T, Chaveau P, Fehrat A, Albouze G, Jungers. Effect of moderate protein restriction on the rate of progression of renal failure. Kidney Int 1989; 36 (suppl 27) S91-95.
29. Rosman JB, Langer K, Brandl M, Piers-Becht TPM, van der Hem GK, ter Wee PM, Donker AJM. Protein-restricted diets in chronic renal failure: a four-year follow-up shows limited indications. Kidney Int. 1989; 36 (suppl 27): S96-102.
30. Wight JP, Salzano S, Brown CB, El Nahas AM. Natural history of chronic renal failure: a reappraisal. Nephrol Dial Transplant 1992; 7: 379-383.
31. Oldrizzi L, Rugiu C, Valvo E, Lupo A, Loschiavo C, Gammaro L, Tessitore N, Fabris A, Panzetta G, Maschio G. Progression of renal failure in patients with renal disease of diverse etiology on protein-restricted diet. Kidney Int 1985; 27: 553-557.
32. Mallick NP, Short CD, Hunt LP. How far since Ellis? Nephron 1987; 46:113-24.
33. Woo DJ. Apoptosis and loss of renal tissue in polycystic kidney diseases. N Engl J Med 1995; 333: 18-25.
34 Grantham JJ. Polycystic kidney disease: there goes the neighbourhood. N Engl J Med 1995; 333:56-57.
35. Hasslacher C, Ritz E, Terpstra J, Gallasch G, Kunowski G, Rall C. Natural history of nephropathy in type 1 diabetes. Hypertension 1985; 7 (suppl II): II74-II78.
36. Mogensen CE, Christensen CK. Blood pressure changes and renal function in incipient and overt diabetic nephropathy. Hypertension 1985; 7 (suppl II): II64-II73.
37. Rossing P, Hommel E, Smidt U, Parving H-H. Impact of blood pressure and albuminuria on the progression of diabetic nephropathy in IDDM patients. Diabetes 1993; 42: 715-719.
38. Klag MJ, Whelton PK, Randall BL, Neaton JD, Brancati FL, Ford CE, Shulman NB, Stamler J. Blood pressure and end-stage renal disease in men. N Engl J Med 1996; 334:13-18.
39. Apperloo AJ, de Zeeuw D, de Jong PE. Short-term antiproteinuric response to antihypertensive therapy predicts long-term GFR decline in patients with non-diabetic renal disease. Kidney Int 1994; 45 (suppl 45): S174-178.
40. Mulec H, Johnson S-A, Björck S. Relation between serum cholesterol and diabetic nephropathy. Lancet 1990; 335:1536-1538.
41. van Essen GG, Rensma PL, de Zeeuw D, de Jong PE. Association between angiotensin-converting enzyme gene polymorphism and failure of renoprotective therapy. Lancet 1996; 347:94-95.
42. Parving H-H, Jacobsen P, Tarnow L, Rossing PP, Lecrof L, Poirier O, Cambien F. Effect of deletion polymorphism of the angiotensin converting enzyme gene on progression of diabetic nephropathy during inhibition of angiotensin converting enzyme: observational follow-up study. BMJ 1996; 313: 591-594..
43. Rossing K, Rossing P, Jacobsen P, Tarnow L, Cambien F, Parving H-H. (1996) Role of angiotensin-converting enzyme (ACE) gene polymorphism and antiproteinuric effects of ACE inhibition in diabetic nephropathy. J Am Soc Nephrol 7:1364(A).
44. The Euclid Study Group. Differences in albumin excretion rate response to lisinopril by ACE-genotype in insulin-dependent diabetes (IDDM) Diabetologia 1996; 39: suppl1: A60.
45. van der Kleij FGH, Schmidt A, Navis GJ, Haas M, Yilmaz N, de Jong PE, Mayer G, de Zeeuw D. ACE I/D polymorphism and short term response to ACE inhibition; role of sodium status. Kidney Int 1997; 52; suppl. 63; S23-S26.

46. Yoshida H, Mitarai T, Kawamura T, Kitajima T, Miyazaki Y, Nagasawa R, Kawaguchi Y, Kubo H, Ichikawa I, Sakai O. Role of the deletion polymorphism of the angiotensin-converting enzyme gene in the progression and therapeutic responsiveness of IgA nephropathy. J Clin Invest 1995; 96: 2162-2169.
47. Hauser AC, Derfler K, Balcke P. Progression of renal insuffiency in analgesic nephropathy: impact of drug abuse. J Clin Epidemiol 1991; 44: 53-56.
48. Diabetes Control and Complications Trial Research Group. The effect of intensive treatment of diabetes on the development and progression of long-term complications in insulin-dependent diabetes mellitus. N Engl J Med 1993; 329: 977-86.
49. Parving H-H, Andersen AR, Smidt UM, Svendsen PA. Early aggressive antihypertensive treatment reduces rate of decline in kidney function in diabetic nephropathy. Lancet 1983; 1175-1179.
50. Pedrini MT, Levey AS, Lau J, Chalmers TC, Wang PH. The effect of dietary protein restriction on the progression of diabetic and non-diabetic renal disease: a meta-analysis. Ann Int Med 1996; 124:627-632.
51. Levey AS, Adler S, Caggiula AW, England BK, Greene T, Hunsicker LG. Effects of dietary protein restriction on the progression of advanced renal disease in the Modification of Diet in Renal Disease. (MDRD) Study. Am J Kidney Dis 1996; 27: 652-663.
52. Apperloo AJ, de Zeeuw D, de Jong PE. A short term antihypertensive treatment induced fall in glomerular filtration rate predicts long term stability of renal function. Kidney Int 1997; 51:793-797.
53. El Nahas AM, Masters-Thomas A, Brady AS, Farrington K, Wilkinson V, Hilson AJW, Varghese Z, Moorhead JFI. Selective effect of low protein diets in chronic renal diseases BMJ 1984; 289: 1337-1341.
54. Rossing P, Hommel E, Smidt UM, Parving H-H. Reduction in albuminuria predicts diminished progression in diabetic nephropathy. Kidney Int. 1994; 45 (suppl 45): S145-149.
55. Gansevoort RT, de Zeeuw D, de Jong PE. Long-term benefits of the antiproteinuric effect of ACE-inhibition in non-diabetic renal disease. Am J Kidney Dis 1993; 2: 202-206.
56. The GISEN Group: Randomised placebo-controlled trial of effect of ramipril on decline in glomerular filtration rate and risk of terminal renal failure in proteinuric, non-diabetic nephropathy. Lancet 1997; 349:1857-1863.
57. Praga M, Hernández E, Montoyo C, Andrés A, Ruilope L, Rodicio JL. Long-term beneficial effects of angiotensin-converting enzyme inhibition with nephrotic proteinuria. Am J Kidney Dis 1992; 20: 240-248.
58. Klahr S, Levey AS, Beck GJ, Caggiula AW, Hunsicker L, Kusek JW, Striker G, et al. The effects of dietary protein restriction and blood pressure control on the progression of chronic renal disease. N Engl Med 1994; 330: 877-884.
59. Rudberg S, Aperia A, Freyschuss U, Persson B. Enalapril reduces microalbuminuria in young normotensive Type 1 (insulin-dependent) diabetic patients irrespective of its hypotensive effect. Diabetologia 1990; 33: 470-476.
60. Mathiesen ER, Hommel E, Giese J, Parving H-H. Efficacy of captopril in postponing nephropathy in normotensive insulin dependent diabetic patients with microalbuminuria. Br Med J 1991; 303:81-87.
61. Heeg JE, de Jong PE, van der Hem GK, de Zeeuw D. Efficacy and variability of the antiproteinuric effect of lisinopril. Kidney Int 1989; 36: 272-279.
62. Bjõrck S, Nyberg G, Mulec H, Granerus G, Herlitz H, Aurell M. Beneficial effects of angiotensin converting enzyme inhibition on renal function in patients with diabetic nephropathy Br Med J 1986; 293: 471-474.
63. Heeg JE, de Jong PE, van der Hem GK, de Zeeuw D. Reduction of proteinuria by angiotensin converting enzyme inhibition. Kidney Int 1987; 32: 78-83.
64. Björck S, Mulec H, Johnson SA, Nordén G, Aurell M. Renal protective effect of enalapril in diabetic nephropathy. Br Med J 1992; 304: 339-343.
65. Lewis EJ, Hunsicker LG, Bain RP, Rohde RD et al. The effect of angiotensin-converting enzyme inhibition on diabetic nephropathy. N Engl J Med 1993; 329: 1456-1462.
66. Maschio G, Alberti D, Janin G, Locatelli F, Mann JFE, Motolese M, Ponticelli C, Ritz E, Zuchelli P et al. Effect of the angiotensin converting enzyme inhibitor benazepril on the progression of chronic renal insufficiency. N Engl J Med 1996; 334-945.

67. Kamper A-L, Strandgaard S, Leyssac PP. Late outcome of a controlled trial of enalapril treatment in progressive chronic renal failure. Hard end-points and influence of proteinuria. Nephrol Dial Transplant 1995; 10:1182-1188.
68. Hannedouche T, Landais P, Goldfarb B, El Esper N, Fournier A, Godin M, Durand D, Chanard J, Mognon F, Suc J-M, Grünfeld J-P. Randomized controlled trial of enalapril and beta-blockers in non-diabetic chronic renal failure. Br J Med 1994; 309-833-837.
69. Giatras I, Lau J, Levey A. for the angiotension converting enzyme inhibition and progressive renal disease study group. Effect of angiotensin converting enzyme inhibitors on the progression of non-diabetic renal disease: a meta-analysis of randomized trials. Ann Int Med 1997; 127: 337-345.
70. van Essen GG, Apperloo AJ, Rensma PL, Stegeman CA, Sluiter WJ, de Zeeuw D, de Jong PE. Are ACE-inhibitors superior to beta-blockers in retarding progressive renal function decline? Kidney Int 1997; 52; suppl 63; S58-S62.
71. Navis GJ, de Zeeuw D, de Jong PE. ACE-inhibitors: panacea for progressive renal disease? Lancet 1997; 349: 1852-1853.
72. Gansevoort RT, Sluiter WJ, Hemmelder MH, de Zeeuw D, de Jong PE. Antiproteinuric effect of blood-pressure lowering agents; a meta-analysis of comparative trials. Nephrol Dial Transplant 1995; 10:1963-1974.
73. Maki DD, Ma JZ, Louis TA, Kasiske BL. Long-term effects of antihypertensive agents on proteinuria and renal function. Arch Int Med 1995; 155: 1073-1080.
74. Weidmann P, Schneider M, Böhlen L. Therapeutic efficacy of different antihypertensive drugs in human diabetic nephropathy.: An updated meta-analysis. Nephrol Dial Transplant 1995; 10 (suppl 9): 39-45.
75. Petersson JC, Adler S, Burkart JM, Greene T, Herbert LA, Hunsicker LG, King AJ, Klahr S, Massry S, Seifter JL, for the MDRD study group. Blood pressure control, proteinuria and the progression of renal disease. Ann Int Med 1995; 123: 754-762.
76. Mogensen CE, Keane WF, Bennett PH, Jerums G, Parving H-H, Passa P, Steffes MW, Striker GE, Viberti GC. Prevention of diabetic renal disease with special reference to microalbuminuria. Lancet 1995; 346: 1080-1084.
77. Lazarus JM, Bourgoignie JJ, Buckalew VM, Greene T, Levey AS, Milas NC, Parandi L, Peterson JC, Porush JG, Rauch S, Soucie JM, Stollar C for the Modification of Diet in Renal Disease Study Group. Achievement and safety of a low blood pressure goal in chronic renal disease. Hypertension 1997; 29: 641-650.

INDEX

F

G

H

I

K

L

M

N

O

P

R

U

V

W